W9-AXY-511

PEDIATRIC Physical Therapy

THIRD EDITION

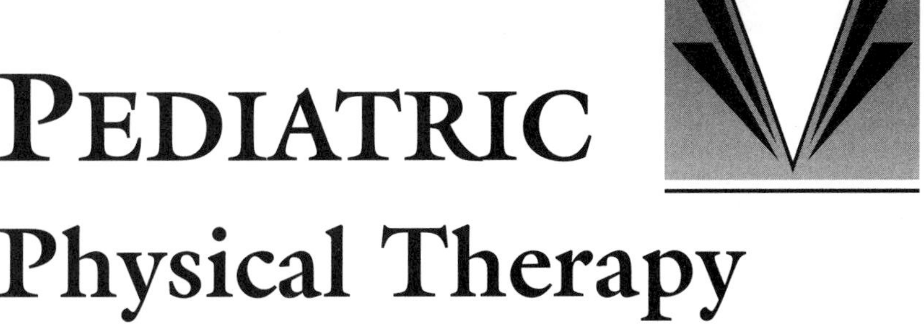

PEDIATRIC Physical Therapy

THIRD EDITION

Jan Stephen Tecklin, M.S., P.T.
Professor
Department of Physical Therapy
Beaver College
Glenside, Pennsylvania

WITH 13 CONTRIBUTORS

Lippincott Williams & Wilkins
Philadelphia • New York • Baltimore

Acquisitions Editor: Margaret N. Biblis
Sponsoring Editor: Amy Amico
Production Editor: Jahmae Harris
Production Manager: Helen Ewan
Production Coordinator: Patricia McCloskey
Design Coordinator: Nicholas Rook

Third Edition

Printed in the United States of America. For information write Lippincott Williams & Wilkins, 227 East Washington Square, Philadelphia, PA 19106.

Library of Congress Cataloging-in-Publication Data

Pediatric physical therapy / Jan Stephen Tecklin ; with 13 contributors.
p. cm.
Includes bibliographical references and index.
ISBN 0-7817-1010-3
1. Physical therapy for children. I. Tecklin, Jan Stephen.
[DNLM: 1. Physical Therapy—in infancy & childhood. WB 460 P371 1998]
RJ53.P5P43 1998
615.8'2'083—dc21
DNLM/DLC
for Library of Congress 98–18730
CIP

Care has been taken to confirm the accuracy of the information presented and to describe generally accepted practices. However, the authors, editors, and publisher are not responsible for errors or omissions or for any consequences from application of the information in this book and make no warranty, express or implied, with respect to the contents of the publication.

The authors, editors, and publisher have exerted every effort to ensure that drug selection and dosage set forth in this text are in accordance with current recommendations and practice at the time of publication. However, in view of ongoing research, changes in government regulations, and the constant flow of information relating to drug therapy and drug reactions, the reader is urged to check the package insert for each drug for any change in indications and dosage and for added warnings and precautions. This is particularly important when the recommended agent is a new or infrequently employed drug.

Some drugs and medical devices presented in this publication have Food and Drug Administration (FDA) clearance for limited use in restricted research settings. It is the responsibility of the health care provider to ascertain the FDA status of each drug or device planned for use in their clinical practice.

9 8 7 6 5 4 3 2 1

In loving memory of my mother, Natalie Rosen Tecklin

August 20, 1925–February 28, 1992

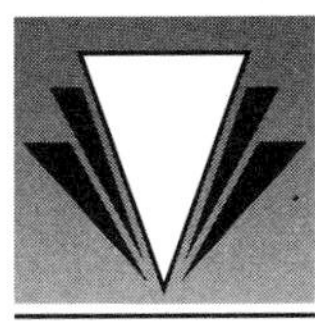

Contributors

Dolores B. Bertoti, MS, PT, PCS
Assistant Professor
Alvernia College
Reading, Pennsylvania
Instructor in Pediatrics
Beaver College
Glenside, Pennsylvania

Amy Both, MHS, PT
Assistant Professor of Physical Therapy
Medical College of Ohio
Toledo, Ohio

Susan K. Brenneman, PT, MS
Education/Development Coordinator
Occupational & Physical Therapy Department
University of Pennsylvania Health System
Philadelphia, Pennsylvania

Julaine M. Florence, MHS, PT
Director, Clinical Studies
Neuromuscular Division
Department of Neurology
Washington University School of Medicine
St. Louis, Missouri

Lauri Grigsby de Linde, OTR/L
Senior Staff Occupational Therapist
Burn Center and Plastic Surgery
St. Christopher's Hospital for Children
Philadelphia, Pennsylvania

Emilie Kallenbach Aubert, MA, PT
Associate Professor, Physical Therapy
Marquette University
Milwaukee, Wisconsin

Susan E. Klepper, PhD, PT
Owner, Pediatric Physical Therapy Services
Ewing, New Jersey
Adjunct Clinical Instructor in Physical Therapy
Columbia University
New York, New York

Karen Yundt Lunnen, MS, PT
Assistant Professor
Western Carolina University
Cullowhee, North Carolina

Christine R. Morgan, PT
Staff Physical Therapist
Wake County Public School System
Raleigh, North Carolina

Shirley Albinson Scull, MS, PT
Service Line Director, Pediatric Rehabilitation
Director, Department of Physical Therapy
Children's Seashore House
Philadelphia, Pennsylvania

Meg Stanger, MS, PT, PCS
Director of Occupational and Physical Therapy
Children's Hospital of Pittsburgh
The Children's Institute
Pittsburgh, Pennsylvania

Jane L. Styer-Acevedo, PT
Pediatric Coordinator
General Healthcare Resources, Inc.
Plymouth Meeting, Pennsylvania

Elena Tappit-Emas, MHS, PT
School District of Philadelphia
Philadelphia, Pennsylvania
Former, Senior Physical Therapist
Myelomeningocele Clinic
Children's Memorial Hospital of Chicago
Chicago, Illinois

Jan Stephen Tecklin, MS, PT
Professor
Department of Physical Therapy
Beaver College
Glenside, Pennsylvania

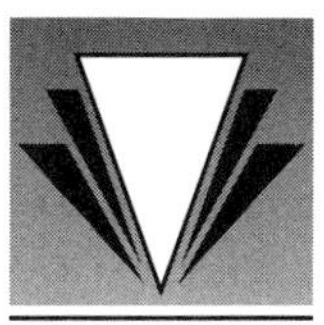

Preface

The acceptance within our profession of the first edition of *Pediatric Physical Therapy* was very gratifying, and I reiterate my thanks to the authors of that edition. Of course, the responsibility in preparing the second edition also was great. Yet, the publication of the third edition of Pediatric Physical Therapy is as exciting for me as the previous two. The excitement springs from the coming to fruition of the project, the inclusion of new material and several new authors, and from the on-going acceptance and widespread use of the text throughout the physical therapy community.

The various chapters have all been revised and updated with the following chapters deserving particular note. Chapter Two by Susan Brennemannn has several tests of development added to the earlier group. Chapter Four on Cerebral Palsy by Jane Styer-Acevedo has had major revisions and additions as has Chapter Five on Spina Bi-fida written by Elena Emas. Amy Both has written an entirely new chapter on Traumatic Brain Injury that offers a very practical approach to assessment and treatment planning for this group of children. Dolores Bertoti has completely re-written Chapter Eight about mental retardation using Down Syndrome as a model. Emilie Aubert, also a new author for the third edition, has provided a major revision to the chapter on Adaptive Equipment. I am very pleased to have had Meg Stanger develop a completely new chapter regarding Orthopedics and Limb Deficiency in Children. This chapter offers a very contemporary and thorough approach. Susan Klepper joined Shirley Scull and was the primary author for the revised chapter on Juvenile Rheumatoid Arthritis. Laurie de Linde updated her comprehensive chapter regarding burns in children. I offered added material to the pulmonary disorder chapter that reflects many of the new approaches to airway clearance, particularly for children with cystic fibrosis. And, finally Karen Yundt Lunnen completely rewrote the chapter on physical therapy in the schools to incorporate many of the more contemporary issues from the IDEA legislation.

I would like to offer my most sincere thanks to each of the authors who battled deadlines, requests for more information, various injuries and illnesses, and the usual crises of life to ultimately help me compile this third edition.

I would also like to recognize several individuals from the Lippincott-Raven family without whose insight and expertise my job as editor would have been much more onerous. Those individuals include Allied Health Editor Margaret Biblis, and editorial assistants Patty Moore, early in the course, and Amy Amico, who was so helpful in bringing all the materials together towards the end. Each is a true professional.

Jan Stephen Tecklin, M.S., P.T.

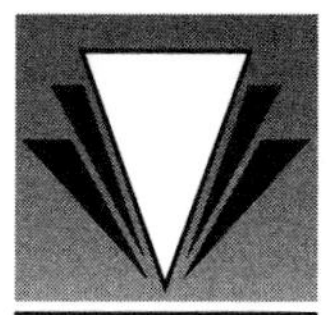

Contents

Normal Motor Development

(Chapter 1 for the 3rd edition was compiled from the first 2 editions of Pediatric Physical Therapy, authored by Cindy Goldberg and Ann Van Sant, respectively)

What is motor development? Why is the study of motor development important to physical therapists? Why should I study motor development if I don't expect to work with children? Does any of this information relate to clinical practice outside the realm of pediatrics?

These questions are frequently asked by professional students in physical therapy as they begin to study motor development. They are very important questions, and each is answered in the following.

What is motor development? *Motor development is the process of change in motor behavior that is related to the age of the individual.* The focus on the relationship between age and motor behavior makes the study of motor development unique from other viewpoints. Motor development includes age-related changes in both posture and movement, the two basic ingredients of motor behavior. Although this chapter concentrates on the motor development of infants and children, developmental processes occur throughout the human life span. Adolescents, young adults, and those in their thirties, forties, and beyond are also undergoing developmental changes in motor behavior.

What causes these changes? For many years, physical therapists attributed much of the change we see in motor behavior to changes occurring within the central nervous system (CNS). Developmental change in motor abilities was thought to reflect maturation of the CNS. Recently, however, we have started to realize that the nervous system is not the only structure that determines developmental change. Changes in other body systems, such as the musculoskeletal and cardiorespiratory system, also influence motor development. Of course, the environment in which we live also exerts a very strong and systematic influence on motor development. So the causes of motor development are many. Each system—whether a body system or a specific environmental system—interacts in complex and fascinating ways to effect change in motor behavior as one grows older.

Why is it important for a physical therapist to understand motor development? The changes that occur in the motor behavior of an infant are truly remarkable. At birth, the infant is almost helpless, but by the first birthday, the child has acquired an impressive degree of physical independence. The child has moved from helplessness to competence in gross motor activities such as sitting, creeping, and standing and in fine motor skills that include manipulating many types of objects. Many children are walking by their first birthdays. The natural pattern of progression toward physical independence can be a very useful guide when designing a treatment plan to help individuals overcome their limitations and gain independence. *The planning of treatment is facilitated by an understanding of the natural process by which physical independence is acquired.*

Why should I study motor development if I don't expect to work with children? Does any of this information relate to clinical practice outside the realm of pediatrics? Physical impairments arising from disease or trauma may affect functional independence at any age. When independence is altered, the natural pattern by which individuals first gain self-sufficiency is a very useful guide as you help an individual regain physical independence. Knowing about motor development is just as important for those working with young adults or the elderly as it is for those who work with children or adolescents. To understand how one attains control over their posture and movements through acquisition of skills that are a part of our daily lives is useful information for therapists in every type of practice setting. What we know about developmental change in one period of the life span can be used to assist individuals of all ages.

This chapter reviews the motor behaviors characteristic of the prenatal period, infancy, and childhood. Beginning with the prenatal period, the discussion of the variety and clearly well-adapted movements of the fetus sets the stage for understanding the great change the individual undergoes as the force of gravity is experienced immediately on birth. The remarkable progress of the infant in attaining a great degree of physical independence during the first postnatal year is outlined. The discussion will explore the range of factors known to influence motor behavior during the early periods of development. The motor accomplishments of childhood are reviewed, and the important achievements are outlined. Finally, at the end of the chapter, a brief discussion of contemporary issues in motor development is included that will be helpful for all therapists trying to understand the factors that underlie motor behavior, regardless of the age of the individuals with whom they might work.

Prenatal Development of Motor Behavior

A distinct language has been developed to describe periods and characteristics of motor development before birth. The prenatal period of development is also known as the *gestational period*. The gestational period typically lasts between 38 and 40 weeks, which translates to approximately 9 months of pregnancy. The prenatal period is a time of rapid developmental change.

The age of the developing individual before birth is measured using a variety of conventions. *Menstrual age* (MA) is the term used when the age of the individual is calculated from the first day of the mother's last menstrual period. Menstrual age is typically measured in weeks. The term *gestational age* (GA) is in more common use in recent years and is roughly equivalent to menstrual age. The prenatal stage of development can be divided into three distinct periods: the germinal period, the embryonic period, and the fetal period.

The *germinal period* begins at the time of fertilization and lasts 2 weeks. It is during this period that the fertilized egg, called the zygote, undergoes rapid cell division. The zygote travels through the fallopian tube to the uterus and, by the end of the germinal period, becomes attached to the uterine wall. The *embryonic period* begins 2 weeks after conception and lasts about 6 weeks. During this time, the developing individual is known as an embryo. The embryonic period is characterized by rapid *morphologic changes.* This is the time when the cells are rapidly dividing, growing, and differentiating to take on specialized functions. At the end of the embryonic period, the developing individual is about 2 inches long and is recognizable as a human being. The *fetal period* begins at 7 weeks MA and ends at birth. It is during the fetal period that motor behavior first appears. During the fetal period, the developing individual is referred to as a fetus. Table 1-1 offers an overview of developmental characteristics.

Two Views of Motor Development During the Fetal Period

Before the 1970s, our knowledge of motor behavior during the fetal period was limited because we could not visualize the fetus. The methods used to record fetal activity included maternal reports of fetal movements, listening through the uterine wall with a stethoscope, or in some instances, echocardiography or electromyography to detect movement through the mother's abdomen.

Without the ability to visualize the fetus in utero, physicians and researchers proposed that the motor behavior of aborted infants could be studied to understand fetal movement. Hooker (1944), an anatomist and researcher, studied aborted fetuses who were not able to sustain vital functions necessary for extrauterine life. His research served as a classic foundation for understanding how human motor behavior evolves before birth. Early theorists in physical therapy, such as Margaret Rood and Dorothy Voss, studied Hooker's findings in order to understand more fully the earliest forms of human movement. They applied what they learned from Hooker to their assessments of motor behavior, as well as to sequence the motor skills they included in their treatment programs.

DEVELOPMENT OF MOTOR RESPONSES TO STIMULATION

According to Hooker (1944), motor behavior can be evoked at the age of approximately 8 weeks MA. In his studies, the fetus was kept in an isotonic bath at body temperature. He used the tip of a hair to apply tactile stimulation to the skin of the fetus. He carefully filmed and recorded any motor response to the tactile stimulation. The earliest responses were obtained only when touch was applied around the mouth, the *perioral area.* The motor responses were characterized as withdrawal movements. The fetus laterally flexed and rotated the head so that the mouth was moved away from the site of the stimulus. Hooker termed these reflexes "avoiding" reactions. Applying stimuli to older fetuses, he found the area sensitive to tactile stimulation had spread from the mouth in all directions: up toward the nose, out to the sides of the face, down the chin, and in even older individuals, to the neck and upper chest. The expanding area of cutaneous sensitivity was accompanied by an increasingly wider ranging withdrawal response. In older fetuses, not only were neck flexion and rotation seen, but the trunk and pelvis would also laterally flex and

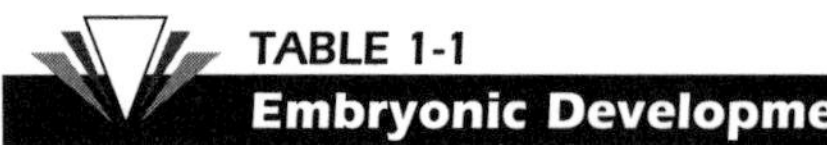

TABLE 1-1
Embryonic Development*

Gestational Age	Developmental Characteristics
First Month	
2 1/2 wks	Shape and length are determined. Neural plate begins for brain. Heart begins as a single tube; may beat; no blood is circulating yet.
3 wks	Cells differentiate into three layers: 1. Ectoderm—outer layer: becomes the skin, hair, nails, sensory and skin glands and all nervous tissue. 2. Mesoderm—middle layer: becomes muscles, bones circulatory organs, and some of the endocrine glands. 3. Endoderm—inner layer: becomes digestive organs, liver, alimentary tract, linings, and more of the endocrine glands.
28 days Length 1/5 in.	Head region is differentiated, taking up one third of the length of the body. Brain and primitive spinal cord are developed. Rudimentary eyes, ears, and nose appear. Initial limb buds appear.
Second Month 6 wks	Embryo becomes more human looking with the features becoming more identifiable. Deciduous teeth form.
8 wks Length 1 in. Weight 2/3 oz	Embryo now becomes a fetus. Organs become functional.
End of Third Month Length 3 in. Weight 3/4 oz	More activity begins: Turns head, bends elbow, makes fist, fans toes, and moves hips. Movement not detected by mother, however, hiccups will be felt.
Fourth Month Length 6 in. Weight 4 oz	Fingerprints appear. Mother begins to feel movements.
Fifth Month Length 12 in. Weight 1 lb	Fetus turns and moves about easily. Regular sleep and wake patterns develop. Sucking reflex is present. Heartbeat becomes regular.
Sixth Month Length 14 in. Weight 2 lb.	Hair grows thicker. Eyes open and close.
Seventh Month Length 16 in. Weight 2 1/2 lbs	
Eighth and Ninth Months	Strong growth phase starts. Fetal movements begin to slow down.

*Adapted from Kaluger G, Kaluger MF: *Human Development: The Span of Life*. St. Louis: CV Mosby, 1974.

rotate away from the side of stimulation. These wide-ranging responses were termed "total body responses." In 11-week-old fetuses, when the palms of the hands were touched, partial finger closure resulted. In fetuses of the same age or just slightly older, touch on the sole of the foot would bring about plantar flexion of the toes. As with the first responses seen in the perioral area, upper and lower limb responses were wider ranging in older fetuses, involving flexion and withdrawal from stimuli applied to the palm or sole. In older fetuses, areas of cutaneous sensitivity were found in more proximal areas of the limbs, eventually including the whole upper and lower limbs.

Responses of older fetuses encompassed an increasing number of body regions, and the character of the responses also changed. Rather than withdrawing from the site of stimulation, there was an increase in the frequency of responses that moved the face toward the source of stimulation. This gradual change in direction—from movements away from the stimulus at about 8 weeks to moving toward the stimulus by 12 weeks—has important consequences. The fetus that moves away from stimuli is demonstrating what might be interpreted as a very primitive survival function by protecting the area from harm. Yet after birth, the individual must not withdraw from all touch received in the perioral area or feeding would be impossible. In a relatively short period of time, by the age of 14 to 15 weeks MA, all the preliminary feeding movements, including mouth opening and closing, sustained lip closure, and tongue movements, were found to be present. In fetuses of 29 weeks MA, audible sucking was observed. The character of trunk and limb responses was also different in older fetuses. Rather than continuing as widespread, total body responses, some actions were confined to local areas, and the responses were more variable in their form. In fetuses of 13 or 14 weeks MA, Hooker described the character of movement as being graceful and flowing. At this age, responses that involved action of the whole body could include complete sequences of action. For example, movements such as head and trunk extension were followed by rotation and flexion. The action sequences were described as "anticipatory" of postnatal life, as they seemed to include patterns of action typically seen after birth, such as rolling or reaching out.

Hooker's studies were long regarded by physical therapists as an important source of information regarding motor development during the prenatal period. Yet the assumption that the aborted fetus demonstrates behavior typical of intrauterine fetal behavior has been questioned. Some argue that the environment of the aborted fetus is drastically different from the intrauterine environment and that motor behavior observed outside the uterus is not representative of the normal motor development that occurs in the intrauterine environment. A second criticism of these studies is that the fetuses studied were in the process of dying during the study. Fetuses born as young as Hooker reported could not breathe to sustain life. Many of the reactions observed may have been a result of decreased oxygen in the blood. Further, the aborted fetus may have had serious abnormalities that triggered the early birth. If that was the case, the movements observed and described by Hooker may not be typical of the normal population of infants born at term or 37 to 42 weeks GA.

DEVELOPMENT OF SPONTANEOUS MOVEMENTS

Spontaneous movements represent a different class of movements than do reflexive responses. Rather than being evoked, spontaneous movements arise without an apparent stimulus. Reflexes are evoked responses, and their initiation depends on a stimulus. Spontaneous movements arise without external stimuli and can be considered to be self-initiated. Spontaneous movements are not necessarily "voluntary." In fact, the term "voluntary movement" can be problematic when discussing early development. Volition implies intent and purpose, and we have no reliable way of determining the intent of the very young individual.

Until recently, researchers and physicians concentrated on describing reflexes or evoked responses of the fetus and young infants and ignored spontaneous actions. This tendency to focus on reflexes is likely a rsult of our scientific culture that values well-controlled experiments. The preference for the controlled experimental approach to documenting human behavior may have led to the general belief that infants were capable only of "reflexive movement." In an experimental approach to the study of movement, spontaneous movements were considered to be random events, nonpurposeful, and interfering with the study.

In the 1970s, the technologic advance of ultrasonographic monitoring of the fetus brought about a revolution in our understanding of the development of movement during the fetal period. Milani-Comparetti, an Italian pediatric neuropsychiatrist, observed and interpreted the ultrasonographic records of more than 1000 pregnant women. These women went on to deliver normal healthy babies. Milani-Comparetti had, until the time of his ultrasound study, been a firm believer in reflexes as the fundamental unit of human motor behavior. However, his observations of the ultrasonographic records of normally developing fetuses changed his most basic concepts of motor development. Milani-Comparetti was impressed with the spontaneous and frequent nature of early fetal movement. He could find no stimuli evoking the natural movements of the developing individual.

He described the sequential appearance of spontaneous action across the fetal period and contributed to a great understanding of human movement by describing *primary movement patterns* (PMPs). According to Milani-Comparetti, PMPs are the fundamental units of action from which all human movements develop. These action patterns arise spontaneously and later become linked to sensory stimuli to form *primary automatisms.* A primary automatism is similar to a reflex. His concept that spontaneous movements arise *before* primary automatisms was revolutionary, particularly for those who felt the reflex was the basic unit of motor behavior from which all other movements originated.

Milani-Comparetti's colorful and rich descriptions of the well-adapted movements of the fetus while in utero is an excellent example of how modern technology can be applied to aid our understanding of human movement. He described earliest fetal movements as "jumping." Jumping appeared spontaneously in fetuses of about 10 weeks GA. A series of jumps continued in succession until the fetus had attained a new resting posture on the uterine floor. The earliest form of jumping involved extension of the lower limbs and flexion of the upper limbs. Later, apparently owing to fetal growth within confined intrauterine space, the upper limbs were brought forward and extended down in front of the body during jumping.

Locomotor movements, which enabled the fetus to climb up and over the placenta, were described as a part of the motor behavior at 17 weeks GA. Milani-Comparetti described a wide range of very well-adapted fetal movements, including exploring the face and body with the hands, reaching out to grasp and move the umbilical cord, and so forth. Spontaneous thumb-sucking and swallowing movements were documented. Responses to auditory and visual stimuli appeared before birth. Sound or light were applied to the abdominal wall of the mother to examine responsiveness to stimuli. Initially, responses of alarm were observed, with both hands being raised to shield the face in a seemingly protective pattern.

Milani-Comparetti discussed how the earliest responses were used ultimately "to be born."

Locomotion was used to move into position for birth with the head down, engaged in the pelvic outlet. The jumping movements were used to thrust against the uterine wall to initiate or cooperate in the birthing process. Breathing movements, sucking, and swallowing were preparatory for feeding following birth, and auditory and visual responsiveness prepared the infant for receiving information about the new postnatal environment. One cannot read Milani-Comparetti's work without a general sense that the fetus is behaving in a manner that reflects progressive adaptation to the uterine environment, as well as anticipation of the birthing process that is to come at the end of the gestational period.

SUMMARY

There are two distinctly different views of the fetal period and thus of the origins of human movement. One point of view is based on research conducted on fetuses outside the uterine environment, and one is based on research conducted on fetuses as they function within the uterus. The latter, more natural study of prenatal movements reveals a very active and spontaneously moving fetus. The research conducted in an extrauterine environment portrayed fetal movements as reflexes. These viewpoints were influenced by the technology available to the researchers at the time they conducted their studies, but they were also influenced by the prevailing scientific perspectives of the times in which they were developed. Physical therapists have become interested recently in self-generated movement, after a long period of concentration on reflexes and reactions of our patients. We now realize how very important it is to foster self-initiated actions, for they are an integral part of human movement from the very beginning. As a result, the work of Milani-Comparetti in describing the very earliest of self-initiated movements is of great interest to therapists and is revolutionary in nature. Milani-Comparetti's unique perspective stands in direct contrast to the traditional view of the fetus as a passive, reflexive being.

Planes of Movement and Postural Alignment

Prior to discussing the specific patterns and skills associated with normal motor development, it seems useful to present the scheme by which movement is often described. The human body has a wide variety of combinations of movement available. As a result of these combinations, a person can negotiate movement safely over various types of terrain, on surfaces with poor friction, and when balance is lost, the person can either regain an upright position or use the hands for protection during a fall. The development of equivalent or balanced strength in opposing groups of muscles is considered by many as important for achieving good posture. Failure of this development of equivalent strength can distort proper alignment, which can ultimately lead to inefficient movement and reduced endurance. The body's structures must endure greater strain and increased mechanical load when muscles are not balanced and when bones and joints are improperly aligned.

In terms of movement, the body is divided into three planes—frontal, sagittal, and transverse. The frontal plane divides the body into anterior and posterior portions, the sagittal plane divides the body into right and left portions, and the transverse plane divides the body into upper and lower portions. Movement *within* the sagittal plane occurs with flexion and extension against gravity. Antigravity movement also occurs during lateral flexion *within* the frontal plane. In the transverse plane, movement occurs with rotation about the axis of the body. The reference points change when movement occurs *across* the plane of motion. Movement *across* the frontal plane becomes anterior and posterior; movement *across* the sagittal plane becomes side-to-side or lateral. Because normal movement is rarely unidimensional, in order to achieve proper postural alignment, one must be able to combine and control movement within and across all planes.

Normal postural muscle tone is also important for smooth movement through the planes of motion. Muscle tone has been described by many as the condition of muscle that, although not an active contraction, determines the posture of the body, the range of motion at the joints, and the feel of the muscle. Normal muscle tone is high enough to permit movement against gravity, yet low enough to allow complete freedom of movement *within* and *across* the various planes and in response to various stimuli.

Motor Development During Infancy

Infancy is considered to be the period from birth until the child is able to stand and walk. Typically, infancy lasts approximately 1 year. This period is very instructive for physical therapists. The neonate, essentially helpless in the face of gravity, gradually develops the ability to align body segments with respect to each other and with respect to the environment, achieving what is called the "normal posture" of upright stance. The gravity-filled environment in which the infant must function is almost completely conquered during that first year. The newborn infant, able to life the head only momentarily, gains the ability to hold the head in an increasingly vertical posture. The flexed posture of the newborn gives way to the extended posture of upright stance. Along the way, infants acquire locomotor skills: first rolling, then crawling and creeping, then walking with support, until they finally achieve that important milestone of independent locomotion, as shown in Table 1-2.

In the following discussion, the motor accomplishments of the first year of life are discussed for each of the four quarters during the first postnatal year. A quarter comprises a 3-month period. This division of the first year into four periods is a useful way of understanding the rapid motor accomplishments of the infant. In each quarter, the behavior of the infant will be discussed for each of four body positions: the supine position, the prone position, sitting, and standing. Rather than focusing on a monthly sequence of motor milestones, the accomplishments of the infant in each quarter are outlined.

The First Quarter: Head Alignment

The newborn infant is termed a neonate—a period that lasts 2 weeks. The posture of the neonate is characterized by flexion, thought to derive, to some degree, from the flexed posture imposed in utero during the prenatal period. After the seventh month of gestation there is limited space for movement of the fetus. The flexed posture has also been attributed to the degree of nervous system development. Specifically, the regions of the brain responsible for the motor abilities involved in extending the body against the force of gravity are thought not to be fully developed at this time. As a result of the flexed posture, when the baby is placed in a prone position the arms and legs curl under the trunk, thus forcing the baby's weight forward onto the shoulder girdle. Although this early flexor posture places the child in a difficult position from which to move, the baby can develop one of the most basic and important skills—lifting and rotating the head from side to side. This motion of the head is the child's first active movement against gravity and is accomplished using a combination of muscles that extend and rotate the neck. This is a major accomplishment of the first quarter.

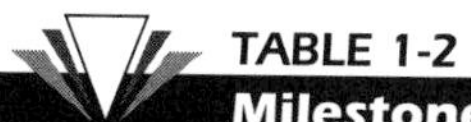

TABLE 1-2
Milestones of Motor Development for the First Year of Life*

Functional Accomplishment	Average Age of Accomplishment (in Months)	Normal Age Range (in Months)
Holds head erect and steady	0.8	0.7–4
Turns from side to back	1.8	0.7–5
Sits with support	2.3	1–5
Turns from back to side	4.4	2–7
Sits alone (momentarily)	5.3	4–8
Rolls from back to stomach	6.4	4–10
Sits alone (steadily)	6.6	5–9
Early stepping movements (with support)	7.4	5–11
Pulls to standing position	8.1	5–12
Walks with help	9.6	7–12
Stands alone	11.0	9–16
Walks alone	11.7	9–17

*From Bayley N *Bayley Scales of Infant Development,* New York: Psychological Corp.: 1969.

THE SUPINE POSITION

When the infant is supine, the head and upper trunk rest on the support surface with the head turned to one side (Fig. 1-1). The lower trunk is often flexed so that the buttocks do not fully contact the bed. Both upper and lower limbs are held in a relatively symmetric posture of acute flexion during the first few days following birth. The feet may be positioned close to the buttocks, and the hands are often contacting the trunk. Typically the hips are held in flexion and kept up off the support surface by the action of the hip adductor muscles. The knees are flexed, and the ankles are held in an acute degree of dorsiflexion. The arms are held in forward flexion close to the body. The elbows and hands are flexed.

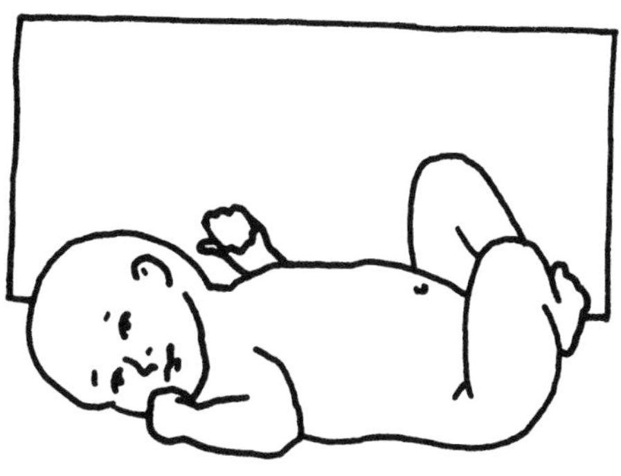

Figure 1-1 ▪ First quarter, supine position.

Because of the predominance of flexion, some resistance is encountered when the infant's limbs are passively moved into extension. Elbows, knees, and hips rebound into flexion after being passively straightened. This tendency to hold a flexed posture and to rebound into flexion when released from an extended position is termed "flexor tone." The physiologic mechanisms responsible for this phenomenon are not clearly understood. The posture is thought to reflect both the elasticity of soft tissue that had been confined in a flexed posture during the late fetal period and CNS activity at this early point in postnatal development.

The acutely flexed posture of the newborn infant is normal but gradually wanes. By the end of the first quarter, the degree of flexion in the limbs has lessened. The feet and arms are no longer held off the support surface. This change is thought to result from active extension movements on the part of the infant as well as the pull of gravity.

The posture of the infant's upper limbs changes during the first quarter. After a month or so, *when the head is in a relatively central or midline position,* flexion of the upper limbs begins to give way to an abducted and extended arm posture. Initially, this posture is seen when the infant is sleeping or when the whole body moves in an expression of delight or happiness. When the infant cries, an acute flexion posture will reappear. *When the head is turned fully to the right or left,* an asymmetric posture of the upper and lower limbs may be seen. The upper limb toward which the face is turned is frequently abducted to the side with the elbow extended. The lower limb on the face side is extended. The other upper limb is abducted and laterally rotated so that it rests on the bed with the elbow flexed. This posture of the upper limbs is commonly called an asymmetric tonic neck reflex posture.

Movements in the first quarter involve bouts of stretching, kicking and thrusting of the extremities, and turning and twisting of the head and trunk. The frequency and degree of movement is related to the "state of the infant." Prior to feeding, infants tend to be most active. They are more quiet and sleepy after feedings. Infants are capable of focusing on objects held a short distance from their face and will turn to track the object, bringing the head to a midline position but not beyond. The infant cannot track objects beyond the midline until the end of the first quarter.

It is not uncommon for an infant to roll from a supine to a side-lying position during the first quarter. This rolling usually results from a combination of head turning with head and trunk extension. A roll from supine to prone is usually an accidental event early in the second quarter. Consistent rolling will not appear until late in the second quarter or during the third quarter.

While in a supine position, the baby engages in a great deal of hand and foot play and begins to explore its body. The baby's body schema improves as the baby plays with its hands, gives sensory input to the feet, and explores its body in preparation for later activities. The baby engages in these activities with the head most commonly in midline more than moving from side to side. This midline orientation allows convergence of the eyes and hands, which come together for exploration.

THE PRONE POSITION

In the prone position, the newborn infant lies in flexion with the head turned to one side. The neonate has the capacity to lift and turn the head from one side to the other. A newborn infant placed prone will be able to keep the nose and mouth unobstructed and free for breathing. At the beginning of the first quarter, the upper limbs are held relatively close to the body in a flexed position. The lower limbs are flexed up under the infant, keeping the lower abdomen up off the bed. The hips and knees are acutely flexed and the feet are in dorsiflexion.

When awake and in the prone position, the infant spends much time actively extending the head and trunk against the force of gravity. The infant repeatedly lifts the head. It appears as if the infant is actively seeking a midline orientation, but the head is often off center and bobs up and down. Occasionally, the efforts are so great that the upper trunk is lifted as well so that the infant is supporting weight on the forearms, which are medially rotated and tucked under the trunk (Fig. 1-2). The ability of the baby to lift is upper chest off the supporting

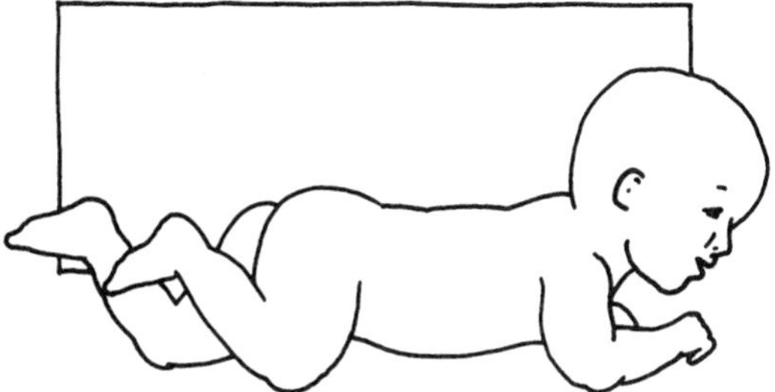

Figure 1-2 ▪ First quarter, on-elbows position.

surface depends on the balanced action of flexors and extensors working together. This so-called *"on-elbows" posture* becomes increasingly frequent throughout the first quarter. With the increased frequency of active extension of the head and trunk come attempts to straighten the elbows under the body and support the weight of the upper trunk on the hands. The infant frequently pushes up and then falls, rocking forward on the trunk with the arms flexed and pulled back in retraction. This sequence of pushing up and then falling into prone becomes increasingly common toward the end of the first quarter.

SITTING AND STANDING

During the first quarter, the infant cannot sit or stand alone. This is not a problem of strength, as the infant is able to develop sufficient tension in the muscles to support body weight fully in the standing position. Assistance is needed because the baby has no ability to balance. The sophisticated control and coordination of muscles that sustains the ability to balance has not yet developed.

When held in a sitting position, the baby has a rounded back (Fig. 1-3). The head is typically held in a flexed position forward of vertical. However, unless the infant is very sleepy, the chin does not droop; rather, it is held up off the chest by active contraction of the neck extensors. The head bobs, with intermittent loss of head position. Head bobbing seen during sitting is similar to the intermittent head lifting observed in the prone position.

During the course of the first quarter, the steadiness of the head increases. By the end of the first quarter, most infants hold their head steady and in alignment with the trunk. The ability to keep the head aligned is termed "head control." Babies first straighten the head with respect to the trunk, but later, they develop the ability to keep the head aligned with respect to gravity. That is, the baby can keep the head in what is called a *normal position.*

Although unable to stand alone, when provided support for balance, the newborn infant is able to maintain the standing position. This ability is referred to as primary standing (Fig. 1-4). Typically, this standing pattern is characterized by crossed feet and asymmetry in the lower limbs. The baby may stand on its toes. Toward the end of the first quarter, this primary standing pattern begins to wane and is increasingly difficult to demonstrate. At that time, the baby is moving into a period of *astasia.* Quite literally, astasia means "without stance." When someone tries to stand the baby up, the legs

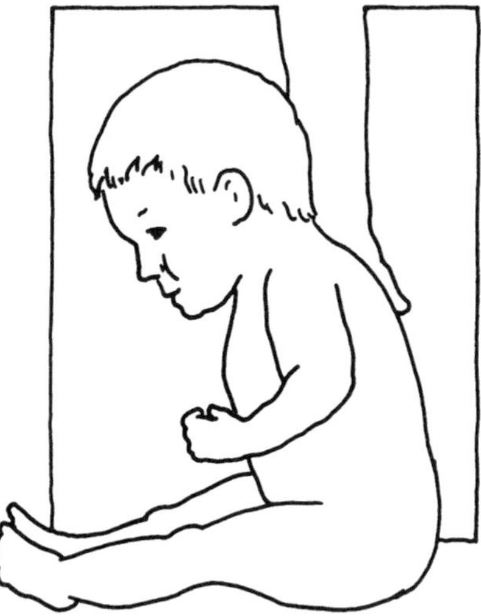

Figure 1-3 ▪ First quarter, supported in sitting.

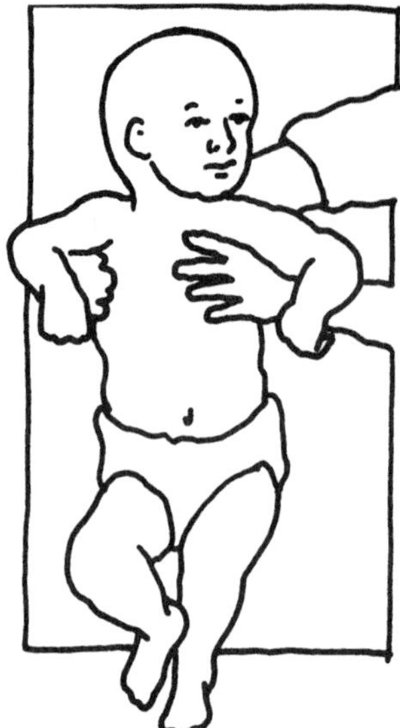

Figure 1-4 ▪ First quarter, supported, primary standing.

give way and the infant sinks into flexion, not accepting or supporting weight through the lower limbs. Astasia may appear toward the end of the first quarter and can last into the second quarter.

In summary, sitting and standing are not independent postures in the first quarter. But the infant shows promise of what is to come. By struggling against the force of gravity, the infant gains control of the head and has taken a large stride toward conquering the force of gravity that rendered the baby helpless at the time of birth.

The Second Quarter: Pushing Up and Sitting Up

The second quarter is marked by great strides in combating the force of gravity. The infant begins this quarter with the competence to keep the head aligned with respect to the body and progresses within the quarter to the ability to sit alone for brief periods and to push up onto the hands and knees. These postures provide the foundation for later accomplishments, but by themselves, they permit a wider range of interaction with the surrounding world. Sitting and getting up on hands and knees are important milestones on the way to physical independence. Accomplishments in supine, prone, sitting, and standing positions are outlined in the following sections.

THE SUPINE POSITION

When the infant is supine, a great deal of activity can be observed. The baby frequently lifts the legs off the support surface, bringing them toward the hands and face. The infant reaches out for the feet with the hands and struggles to bring the feet to the mouth for exploration (Fig. 1-5).

Although the infant does not consistently roll from the supine position, the extreme postures involving lifting of the lower limbs and extension with rotation of the head of the head and neck are precursors to the ability to roll.

This struggle can lead to a loss of the supine position. The weight of the legs, when carried to the right or left, may turn the baby to a side-lying position. This apparent loss of control of the lower limbs during lifting may be one of the

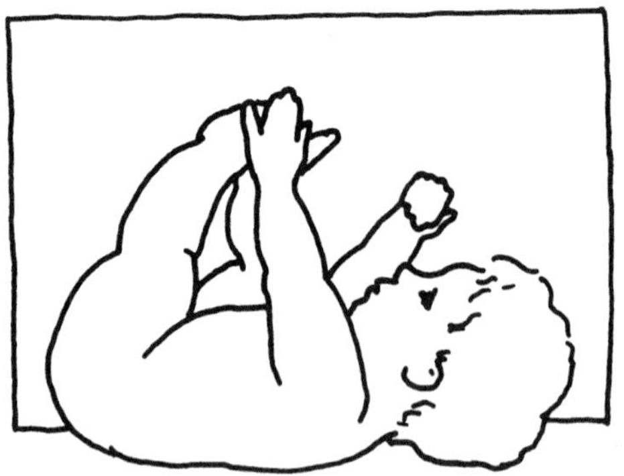

Figure 1-5 ▪ Second quarter, supine position, reaching for feet.

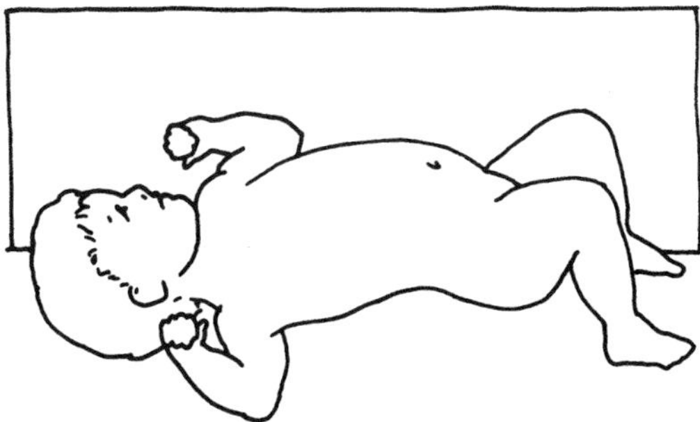

Figure 1-6 ■ Second quarter, bridging position.

factors that lead to the ability to roll out of the supine position. Most infants attempt to actively roll over during this period and some actually accomplish this skill during the second quarter, but it is more often an achievement of the third quarter.

The infant also places the feet on the supporting surface with the hips and knees flexed. This posture serves as a starting position for strong bursts of extension that lift the buttocks and spine off the surface. This is termed "bridging" (Fig. 1-6). Some babies push themselves to the far reaches of their cribs by a series of bridging movements. At other times, the infant will demonstrate strong rotation of the head and neck to one side, coupled with extension, as if to look up and over one shoulder. The action of turning and looking can also lead to rolling out of the supine position to a side-lying posture during the second quarter. Although the infant does not consistently roll from the supine position, the extreme postures involving lifting of the lower limbs and extension with rotation of the head of the head and neck are precursors to the ability to roll.

THE PRONE POSITION

The intermittent lifting and bobbing of the head associated with the effort to gain an erect posture in the prone position during the first quarter gradually begins to involve the trunk musculature. Early in this quarter, the baby struggles in the prone position to elevate the trunk off the supporting surface, first getting up on elbows and then pushing up on hands. The baby spends a great deal of time pushing up (Fig. 1-7) and then dropping back into the prone position, pivoting on the stomach with arms and legs elevated off the support surface. This pivoting posture is termed "pivot prone" or the airplane position (Fig. 1-8).

The baby learns to play on extended arms, attempts to reach for toys, and tries to shift weight through a greater range in the lateral direction. This shifting of weight is more mature in quality and is characterized by elongation on the weight-bearing side. Later in this period, when the baby plays on extended arms, there is less loss of control in the forward (cephalad) direction as the baby's center of gravity moves caudally giving the child greater control in this position. The baby may shift weight laterally while on extended arms; however, because this task is difficult, the baby may revert to a position with the forearm propped up in order to reach for a toy. When the center of gravity shifts laterally, it is not uncommon for the child to fall out of the hands-and-knees posture. A tendency

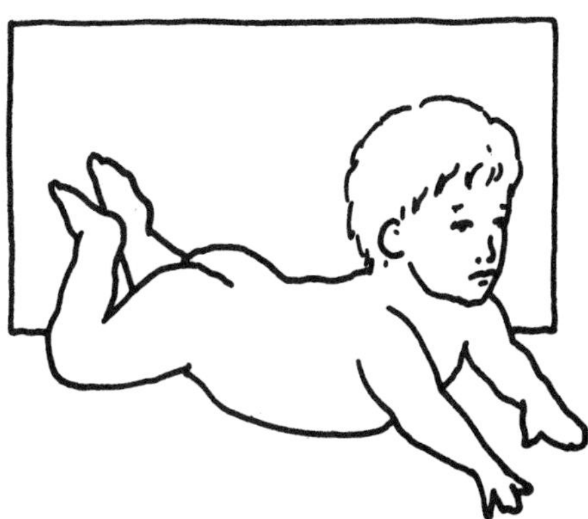

Figure 1-7 ■ Second quarter, pushing up on hands.

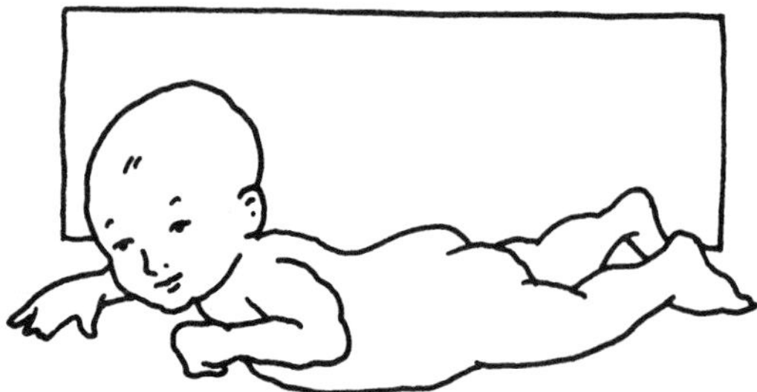

Figure 1-8 ■ Second quarter, pivot prone position.

to rock seems to be a self-initiated balancing exercise and eventually leads to a very steady and stable hands-and-knees posture.

It is not uncommon for the baby to push back while up on hands and thus to push across the support surface while in prone. This is termed *crawling,* defined as the locomotor pattern of moving forward or backward by pushing and pulling with the extremities while the abdomen is in contact with the support surface. Crawling begins during the second quarter. *Creeping* is a locomotor pattern characterized by elevation of the abdomen up off the support surface. Typically, babies crawl before creeping. Crawling is a second quarter accomplishment, whereas creeping usually appears in the third or fourth quarter.

When crawling, babies tend to push backward first, later developing the capacity to move forward. Initial attempts at crawling are characterized by a lack of coordination of the movements of the extremities. Soon, a consistent pattern evolves that is very effective for moving about the floor.

Babies in the United States tend to spend much time in the prone position, particularly when compared to British children, who are more often placed in the supine position to play. Experience in a common or preferred position is an important determinant of the sequence of motor skill accomplishments. Often, children who spend a great deal of time in a preferred posture will demonstrate advances in the achievement of motor milestones accomplished from that posture, whereas skills in other postures might lag slightly. It is important to remember that some babies prefer the supine position, whereas others like sitting. In these instances, skills in the preferred posture often outdistance skills of the other postures. Differences in accomplishments among postures often reflect the child's preferences. These differences are to be expected as an expression of the infant's individuality and are a part of normal development.

The infant will also begin to push up on hands and knees during the second quarter. Usually, this is accomplished by first pushing up on hands and then flexing the lumbar spine and hips, pulling the knees up under the chest. Initially, the hands-and-knees position is an unstable posture, but with time, the child becomes quite competent at pushing back into the hands-and-knees posture and will engage in bouts of rocking: repetitively shifting weight back and forth from the hands to the knees. Because the child does not have good control of the hips, if weight is shifted to one side or the other, it is not uncommon for the child to fall out of the hands-and-knees posture. The rocking action seems to be a self-initiated balancing exercise and eventually leads to a very steady and stable hands-and-knees posture.

THE SITTING POSITION

The second quarter is the time when the infant develops a steady and erect sitting posture. The infant's increasing ability to control the upper trunk is often illustrated by the placement of the mother's hands while she supports the child in sitting. It is as though the mother knows intuitively how much freedom to allow the child to work against the force of gravity. The experience of struggling in a protected but challenging sitting posture helps the infant develop competence in sitting.

The baby first sits alone while propped forward on the hands (Fig. 1-9). The posture of the trunk and upper limbs is very similar to the posture attained when pushing up on hands in

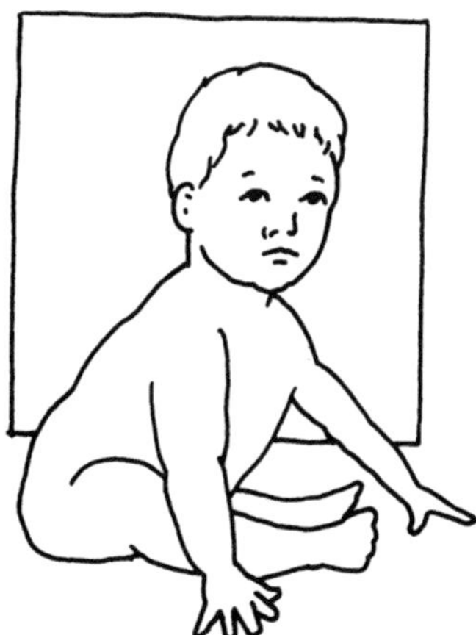

Figure 1-9 ▪ Second quarter, sitting alone propped forward on hands.

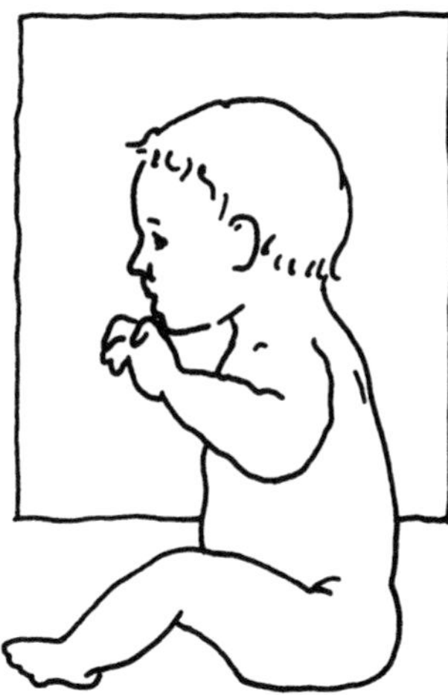

Figure 1-10 ▪ Second quarter, "high guard" independent sitting for brief periods.

the prone position (compare Figs. 1-7 and 1-9). In both the prone push-up and the propped sitting positions, the head is vertical with respect to gravity. The upper trunk is inclined forward of vertical, and weight is born on the hands. In propped sitting, the legs are commonly held in a ring position, with the hips abducted and laterally rotated and with the feet in opposition to each other. When given a supportive and protected environment, the infant will extend the trunk, retract the shoulder girdle, and flex the elbows to bring the arms into what is termed a "high guard" posture for brief instants of independent sitting (Fig. 1-10). During the second quarter, babies develop the capacity to sit with support for up to 15 to 20 minutes. Sustained periods of independent sitting will not be seen until the third quarter. Developing at the same time as the ability to hold the trunk steadily in the vertical position is the capacity to extend the arms down to the support surface to catch and protect the body from falling. This is termed a "parachute" or "protective extension" reaction and is characterized by abducted arms with extension of the elbows, wrists, and hands. Protective reactions are fundamental for safe, independent sitting (Fig. 1-11).

THE STANDING POSITION

During the second quarter, the infant begins again to accept weight through the lower limbs and is able to stand with support. The standing posture that follows the period of astasia is termed "secondary standing." The secondary standing posture is characterized by abducted legs, extended knees, and a plantigrade posture of the feet (Fig. 1-12). In the plantigrade pos-

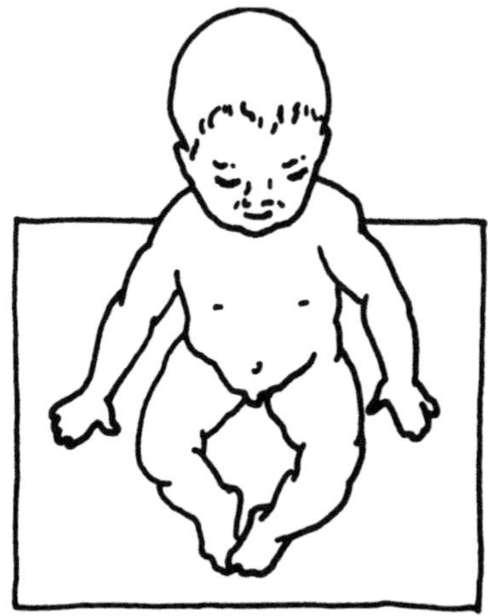

Figure 1-11 ▪ Second quarter, "parachute" or "protective extension" position as viewed from above.

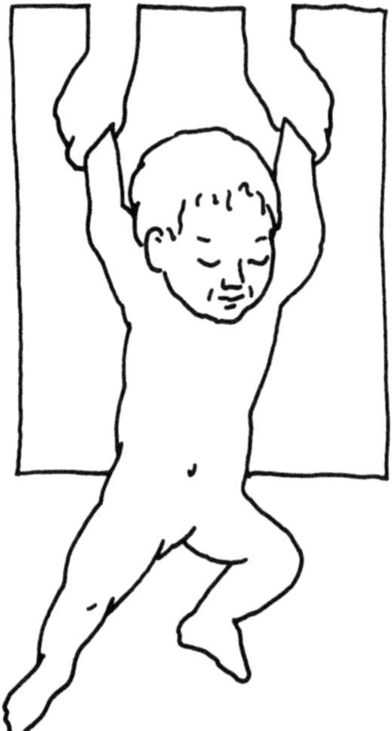

Figure 1-12 ▪ Second quarter, standing with support.

ture, the soles of the feet are in full contact with the support surface. The secondary standing posture differs from the primary standing seen during the first quarter. During primary standing, the feet are often crossed, and the infant will commonly stand on the toes, with the ankles plantar-flexed. In contrast, secondary standing is characterized by abducted lower limbs and a plantigrade posture of the feet.

Activity in standing increases across the second quarter. When supported under the arms, the child will first bounce up and down while standing; later in the quarter, the infant will begin to shift weight from side to side, picking up and stamping first one leg and then the other.

SUMMARY

The accomplishments of the second quarter are impressive: moving across the support surface by bridging or crawling, sitting with support, getting up on hands and knees, and standing with support. The infant is gaining control of the body in fundamental postures that will lead to a greater range of mobility. A supportive environment allows the infant opportunities to explore the body and conquer the force of gravity evidenced by increasingly elevated and vertical postures.

The Third Quarter: Constant Motion

During the third quarter, the infant becomes mobile and develops the ability to move about the environment. Exploration becomes a paramount activity. The drive to move up against the force of gravity seems to strengthen so that, by the end of the third quarter, babies are able to pull themselves up to standing. The world awaits discovery.

THE SUPINE POSITION

Preference for the supine position is decreasing, particularly as the infant develops the capacity to roll from supine into prone. The first roll is often accomplished with either a strong pattern of head and upper trunk extension and rotation with arm reaching up and over the shoulder (Fig. 1-13), or with a bilateral flexion pattern of the lower limbs, carrying the legs up and over to one side (Fig. 1-14). Some infants will stop in the side-lying position before completing the roll to prone. Some spend a great deal of time side lying, with the upper leg moving from be-

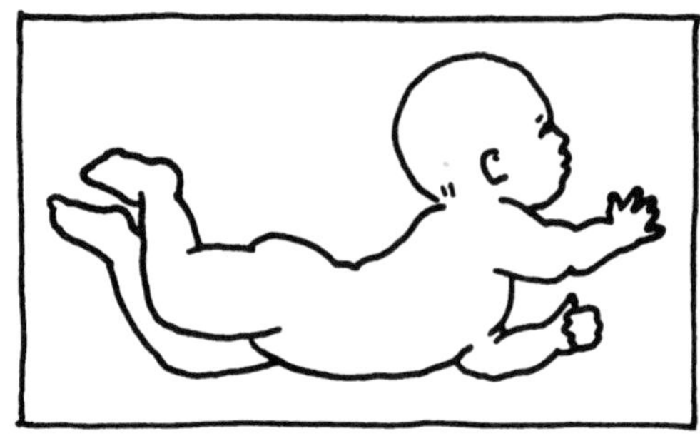

Figure 1-13 ▪ Third quarter, rolling with head and upper trunk extension.

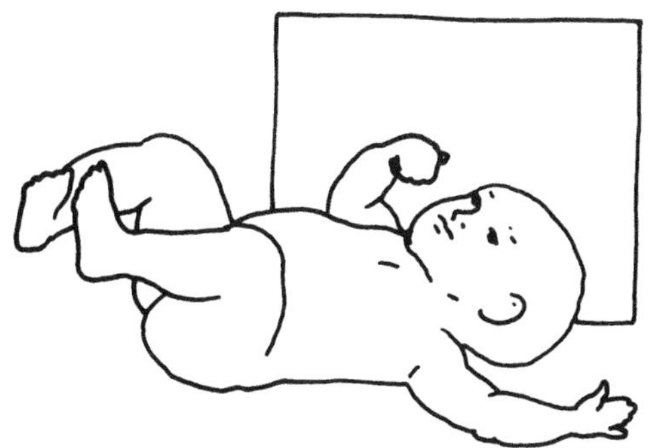

Figure 1-14 ▪ *Third quarter, initiating rolling using flexed legs.*

hind the body to a position in front of the body. It is as though the baby is learning to balance in the side-lying position. Some infants will use rolling as a means of locomotion, but more commonly, creeping is seen.

THE PRONE POSITION

The third quarter begins with the child in a prone position, pivoting in circles on the stomach. The prone position has become a very stable one for the baby. As a result of this increased stability, the baby can use more dissociated upper and lower extremity patterns of movement when playing in the prone position. Lateral flexion through the trunk is a strong component of movement, and the baby may play in a side-lying position.

THE SITTING POSITION

Maintaining an unsupported sitting position is now accomplished with ease. The posture is steady and erect (Fig. 1-15) with the baby sitting erect for as long as half an hour. The child will occasionally lean forward on the hands for support. The hands are more typically engaged in a variety of play activities: reaching out and grasping objects, banging them together, and bringing them to the mouth for exploration.

The baby plays in a sitting position, using both hands to manipulate a toy. If the toy drops out of reach, the baby will shift his or her weight laterally in an attempt to retrieve the toy. Adequate mobility of the hips may be lacking, however, thus preventing the baby from moving into a side-sitting position. The lower extremities may still be used for stability, which is shown by the baby's use of a wide-based, ring-sitting position.

Some children will "hitch" or "scoot" in sitting. The child leans on one hand and laterally rotates the leg on that side down onto the support surface while the other leg is elevated with the foot in a plantigrade posture. Next, the child steps out with the elevated leg, plants that foot and, simultaneously pushing with the other leg, slides the buttocks across the floor.

QUADRUPED POSITION

By the end of the third quarter, moving from sitting into the hands-and-knees position is also accomplished with ease. By making use of the upper limb movement pattern that also serves as the protective extension or parachute reaction, the child reaches out to the side with the arms

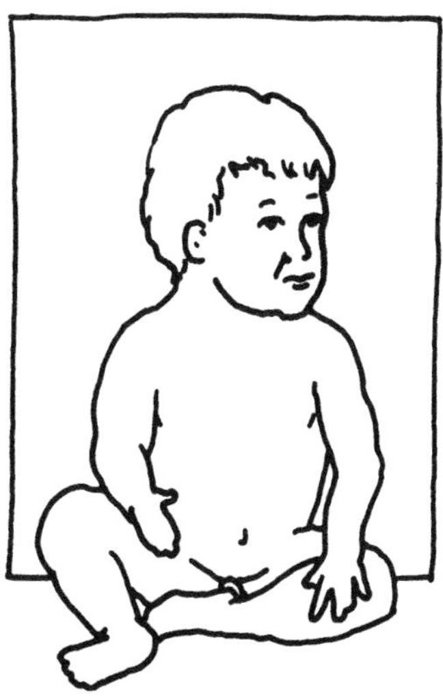

Figure 1-15 ▪ *Third quarter, unsupported sitting.*

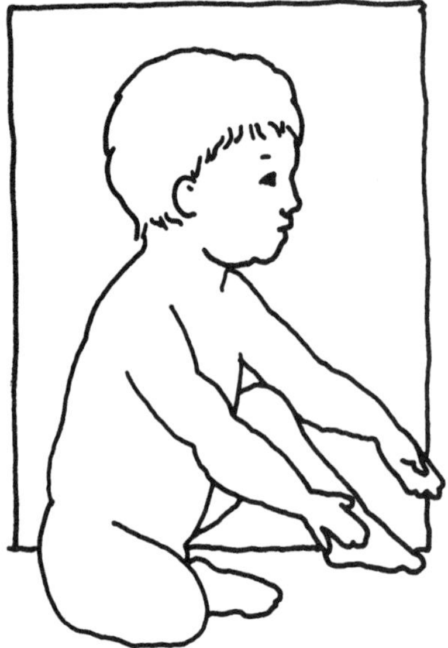

Figure 1-16 ■ Third quarter, transferring weight from buttocks to hands.

and transfers weight from the buttocks to the hands (Fig. 1-16). The lower trunk and buttocks are then raised off the support surface and rotated from the side into a symmetric hands-and-knees posture.

The child will assume a quadruped position (hands and knees) during the third quarter and will probably engage in a great deal of rocking behavior. Rocking provides intense sensory input to the upper and lower extremities and also to the vestibular apparatus. Some children assume a position resembling that of a bear walking (feet and hands), which requires greater control of the hip musculature. A child in this position can use his or her head as a stabilizer while reaching for a toy with one hand.

THE STANDING POSITION

The standing position is a favorite of babies during the third quarter. They are so captivated by this posture that they spend a great deal of time and effort pulling into kneeling and then standing positions (Fig. 1-17). Initially the standing posture is characterized by a flexed and unstable position of the hips. Later, the hips are drawn forward under the shoulders, and the standing posture is increasingly stable. Initially the child has no ability to get back down from standing. It is possible to find the child crying over the dilemma of how to get down from standing. The child will eventually discover how to fall by thrusting the buttocks backward and sitting down.

The baby will also practice pulling into kneeling and standing positions. Because extension of the hips is not a strongly developed muscular component for this child, strength in the upper extremities becomes important when the child tries to elevate. The activities of pulling to kneel or stand and playing with movement into and out of a sitting position provide a great deal of sensory input through

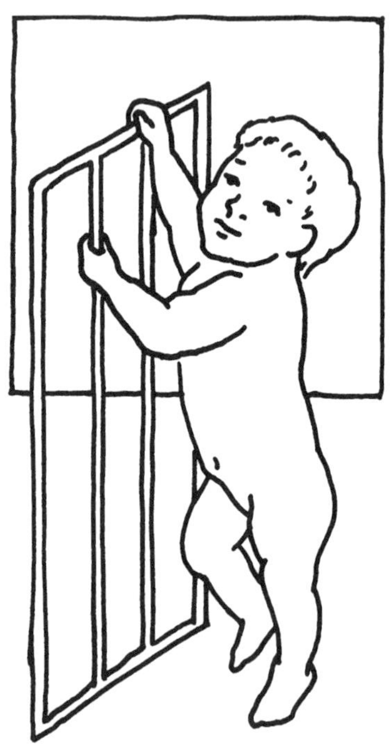

Figure 1-17 ■ Third quarter, pulling to stand.

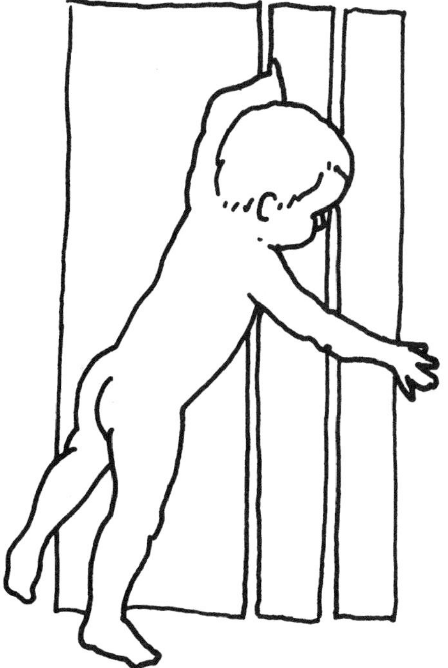

Figure 1-18 ▪ Third quarter, "cruising" along a railing.

the upper extremities and the shoulder girdle. The baby uses the upper extremity strength to propel and protect its body, while continuing to develop further mobility and control through the pelvis and hips.

After pulling up, the child spends great energy bouncing and actively disturbing balance. This up and down bouncing gradually gives way to shifting of the weight from side to side and taking steps beside the furniture. This is termed *cruising* and is the first form of independent walking (Fig. 1-18). Toward the end of this quarter, the child may begin to climb onto a low step, thus taking advantage of the increased ability to flex the hip and the ability to free one lower extremity from weight.

When supported in a standing position, the baby may bear weight on flat feet; however, when standing with the support of furniture and when cruising, the center of gravity is often thrown anteriorly, causing the baby to bear weight on the toes. The baby alternately uses flat feet and a plantar-flexed posture of the foot when moving around.

The Fourth Quarter: Walking at Last

THE SUPINE AND PRONE POSITIONS

When the baby is awake, the prone and supine positions have become primarily transitional postures. The child spends so little time in them, they seem primarily to be passing points of stability on the way to more upright postures.

The hands-and-knees posture is the basis for creeping. This locomotor pattern comprises alternate action of the opposite arms and legs in forward mobility. Some infants become quite skillful creepers and prefer this form of locomotion for months. Even the onset of walking will not preclude some children's preference for creeping.

Plantigrade creeping becomes a part of the child's repertoire. This form of locomotion involves creeping on extended arms and legs, with the feet in the plantigrade posture (Fig. 1-19).

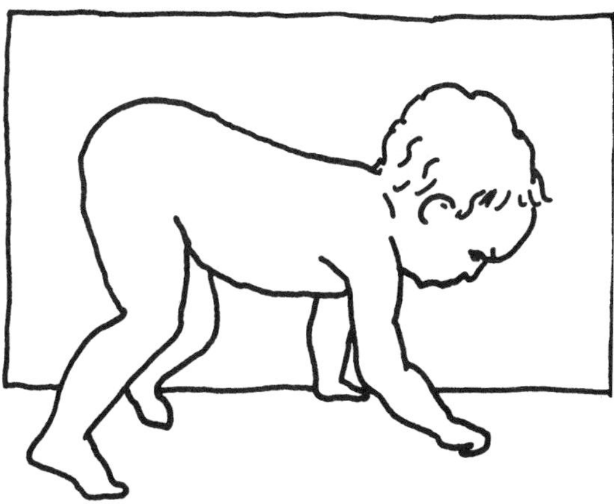

Figure 1-19 ▪ Fourth quarter, "creeping" on extended arms and legs.

Plantigrade creeping is the next step in the gradual elevation of the trunk against the force of gravity. Full extension of the upper limbs led to the hands-and-knees posture, and now extension of the lower limbs leads to a plantigrade creeping position.

THE SITTING POSITION

Sitting is a very functional position at this time. The ease with which the child moves into and out of the sitting posture is quite remarkable whether moving from sitting to the hands-and-knees posture, or pulling from sitting to kneeling and then standing. Balance abilities become very well developed in sitting. The child will often pivot around in circles while sitting, using the hands and feet for propulsion. The child sits easily and comfortably in a high chair with the legs flexed onto the foot rest. The child can move to prone from sitting in the process of play or as a part of the movements used to stand up from the floor. In addition, the increased mobility and balance affords the child the opportunity to use various sitting positions such as side-sitting and "W" sitting.

THE STANDING POSTURE

Standing is a preferred posture for most infants during the fourth quarter. Pulling to a standing position with the support of furniture leads to cruising along the edge of furniture while holding on. The ability to move back down to sitting from standing is developed early in this quarter, and later in the quarter, the ability to move down to a squat-sitting posture from standing appears (Fig. 1-20). Children climb onto furniture from the standing position. They often can get up on chairs or low tables without difficulty by the end of the fourth quarter.

Stepping begins in a diagonally forward and sideward direction. This early stepping pattern can be seen in the first steps the child takes with the hands held (Fig. 1-21). Parents who walk children from behind with two hands held are in the best position to observe this diagonal stepping pattern, which leads the child first to one side and then to the other. Only with time do leg movements correct to a more forward direction. The child progresses from walking with two hands held to walking with just one hand for support. With encouragement, the child lets go eventually and steps out alone. The first independent steps are also diagonal in nature, leading to a wide base of support.

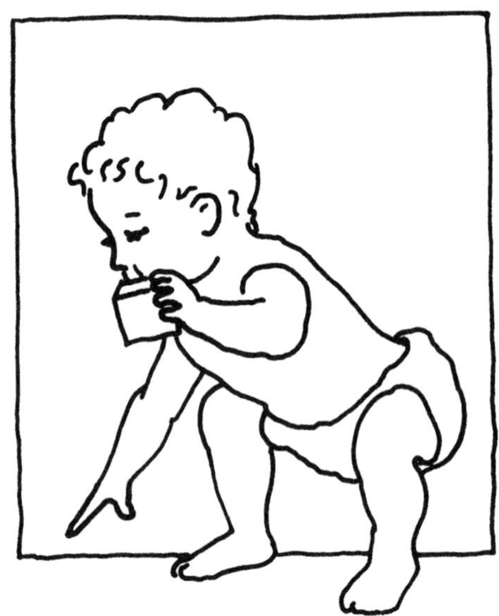

Figure 1-20 ▪ Fourth quarter, moving from standing back down to sitting.

During early attempts at cruising and walking, the child may have been on the toes with little or no true contact of the heels with the floor. The baby walks with a more flat-footed posture while using exaggerated back stepping in an attempt to maintain balance. The pattern of gait is still immature, with the tendency to laterally flex the trunk in order to advance the leg rather than using a mature pattern of shifting the weight. The arms are held in "high guard" (Fig. 1-22), which helps maintain stability and control. The child has greater difficulty

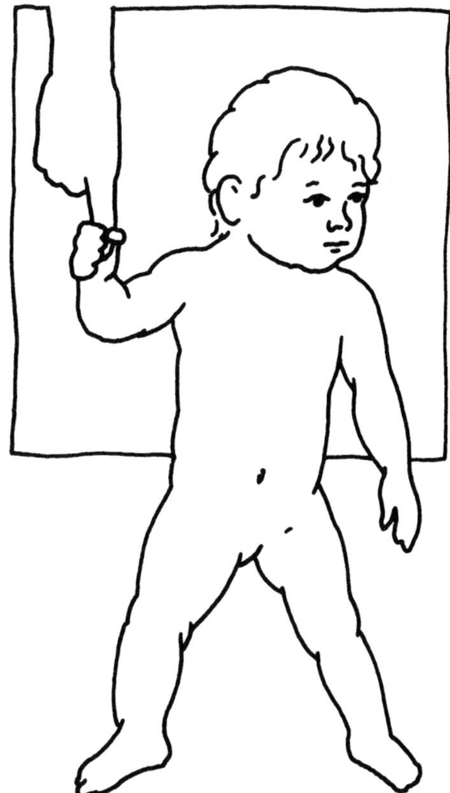

Figure 1-21 ■ Fourth quarter, forward and sideward stepping pattern.

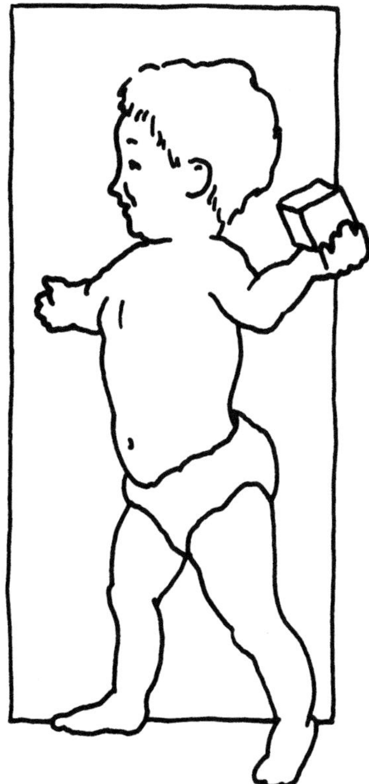

Figure 1-22 ■ Fourth quarter, independent steps with hands in high guard position.

with balance when attempting to carry a toy in one hand. A child at this age will find it impossible to use two hands to carry an object because of the need to use the upper extremities for stabilization. When the child attempts to carry an object, there is often a shift back toward toe-walking in an attempt to increase support and stability. The toe-walking pattern displaces the body weight anteriorly, which enables the child to use a more immature, stiff pattern that provides greater stability. Once the upper extremities are again available, the child returns to the flat-footed position. The independent upright position has become a consistent feature in the child's motor repertoire, thereby causing more falls but the child learns to quickly and skillfully recover to resume the previous activity.

A striking increase in stability and control occurs toward the end of the first year. The high-guard position and external support are less necessary. The child can carry toys more easily while walking, stoop to retrieve a toy from the floor without external support, and may attempt to stand on toes to reach a high object. When pushed backward, maintenance of balance without the back-stepping noted previously is more likely. In addition to rising on the toes and squatting, the child can lift one leg as if to step up. This act involves excessive flexion of the hips and a lateral shift in weight that may combine to cause a loss of balance and makes the child reach for support.

Whereas early attempts at walking show the precarious balance of the baby, the accomplishments of the first postnatal year are, nonetheless, quite remarkable. In very short order, the infant has moved from helplessness to independent mobility and active exploration of the world. Walking will progress to become smooth and coordinated. One can observe a progressively narrowing base of support, and forward-directed steps with a heel-toe pattern of foot contact. The arms move down from high, to middle, and finally to low guard, with a natural alternate-arm swing eventually appearing. With the onset of improved skill in walking and climbing, even more of the world is within reach.

Within a few short months after the onset of walking, the child will gain the ability to rise independently by rolling prone, getting onto hands and knees, assuming the plantigrade posture, and then pushing up with the arms to achieve independent standing. Climbing on and off objects, and creeping up and down stairs become routine.

SUMMARY

The transition from helplessness and physical dependence to independence during the first year after birth is very important to the child and family. As the infant gains control over the body and is able to resist the force of gravity, new worlds open up for exploration, and the baby is less dependent on parents to be held and carried. Antigravity controls begins with lifting and aligning the head during the first quarter. It then proceeds from the head down to the upper thoracic region, with the arms extending against the force of gravity and supporting the weight of the upper trunk in the second quarter. The lower trunk extends, and the child seeks the vertical posture of sitting during the third quarter. Gradually the lower limbs are extended as the child achieves a plantigrade creeping posture and pulls to standing. With increasing time spent in standing, the child develops the ability to balance in the posture and will let go of support to step out and walk. The cephalocaudal progression of antigravity extension to move into a vertical posture and the accompanying development of balance in the progressive series of postures represents an important pattern of accomplishment that leads to physical independence.

Motor Behavior During Early Childhood

Early childhood is the period from 2 to 6 years. To this point in the chapter, most of the discussion has focused on the acquisition of new motor skills. Motor development during early childhood leads to the attainment of new skills but not necessarily new patterns of movement. It is as though the child has acquired all the fundamental movement patterns but is now learning to put them to use in meaningful activity.

Development of Locomotor Skills

The child continues to practice and refine many of the motor skills acquired during the first year of life. The standing position has become more erect. Squatting can be performed for longer periods, although a wide base of support may be used. Climbing stairs on hands and knees becomes an easier task, and many children enjoy jumping. In early childhood, the locomotor pattern of walking is refined and new locomotor skills are added, including running, hopping, jumping, and skipping. These skills require increasing degrees of balance and control of force for successful performance. The development of ability within each skill appears to depend on a combination of practice, growth of the body, and maturation of the CNS. The more refined the skill, the more practice must be devoted to develop the control needed.

Children require opportunities to exercise their developing abilities within fundamental motor skills. Running is usually acquired between the ages of 2 and 4 years. Running differs from walking, specifically because of the "flight phase," during which there is no support of the body. The flight phase comes about by strong but careful application of propulsive force during the stance phase of the gait pattern. However, it is not until the age of 5 or 6 years that a degree of control in running is achieved: the ability to start, stop, and change direction with ease. Jumping first develops as the ability to jump down from heights. The child will first jump down off a box approximately 1 foot in height at about the age of 22 months. This skill is more characteristic of a stepping-down pattern than an actual jump with two feet off the ground simultaneously. With time, the ability to jump to reach an object overhead emerges and later, the ability to jump for distance emerges. Across childhood, the height and distance jumped increases. In addition, the form of the movements used to jump becomes more efficient. Primitive jumpers demonstrate a very shallow preparatory crouch, whereas advanced jumpers demonstrate deep crouches. Initially, the arms appear to move to a high guard position in young jumpers, whereas in older and more experienced jumpers, the arms tend to be used to create momentum, being thrust up and overhead while jumping. Young and inexperienced jumpers demonstrate flexed heads and trunks during the jump. By contrast, older, more experienced jumpers utilize head and trunk extension during jumping actions.

Hopping seems to be an extension of the ability to balance while standing on one leg. Hopping is defined as elevation of the body off the ground and subsequent landing using a single foot. Hopping appears at about the age of $2\frac{1}{2}$ years, but is not well performed until the child is approximately 6 years of age, when a series of about 10 hops can be strung together. After a series of hops can be performed, children tend to incorporate them into games, such as hopscotch or dancing steps.

Skipping is a complex locomotor pattern that involves a step and a hop on one leg, followed by a step and a hop on the other leg. Skipping is not achieved by most children until they are 6 years old. As with many of the locomotor skills, practice seems to be a significant factor in the acquisition of the skill. Older individuals who have not had the opportunity to practice the skill often are unable to demonstrate some of the more sophisticated locomotor patterns.

Other Fundamental Skills of Childhood

Throwing and striking are two additional skills that undergo developmental change during early childhood. Although throwing is a skill that is typically acquired during the first year of life, skillful throwing is still developing during early childhood. Sequences of change in movement patterns used to perform both throwing and striking tasks have been outlined for the trunk and lower limbs. Different steps in movement pattern development have been described for the action of the arms in throwing and striking. Across childhood, the distance of the throw becomes greater. The increase in distance is likely attributable to the emergence of movement patterns that more efficiently apply force to the object being thrown or struck. Catching and kicking are two additional skills that have been studied from a developmental perspective.

Catching begins to develop at about 3 years of age. The child initially holds the arms extended in front of the body without adjusting the arms to account for the direction or speed of the object to be caught. Eventually, the arms are used to scoop the object in toward the body, and gradually, the child can be seen to move and adjust the position of the body to intercept the object being thrown. With age and experience, the child anticipates the flight of the object, moves to arrive in time to intercept it, and uses the hands to catch with a "give" that absorbs the force of the object.

Kicking requires balancing on one foot while transferring force to an object, such as a soccer ball. Early in the development of this skill, there is little preparatory backswing or follow-through in the kicking leg. With time, a backswing appears, first at the knee, and later, involving the hip. Gradually, follow-through and a forward lean of the trunk become a part of the kicking action. These characteristics are typically seen in children at about the age of 6 years.

Performance Changes in Skills Acquired in Infancy

Age-related change in movement patterns used to perform skills first acquired during infancy continues during early childhood and into later childhood and adolescence. A series of studies has documented the movement patterns expected in tasks, such as rolling from supine to prone, moving from sitting on a chair to standing, and rising from supine to standing.

ROLLING FROM SUPINE TO PRONE

During early childhood, the movement patterns used to roll from supine to prone are age related. If the child were to roll from supine to prone over the left side, the roll would be characterized by several patterns. The child pushes with the right lower limb, leading with the right side of the pelvis, and lifts and reaches up with the right upper limb above the level of the left shoulder.

RISING FROM A CHAIR

When rising from a chair, the young child first lifts the legs up off the chair seat and then places them down on the floor. The trunk flexes forward until the buttocks are raised off the chair, at which time head and trunk extension begin to bring the child to the vertical standing posture. In children younger than 6 years of age, pushing off of the chair seat would be expected but older children more commonly use their arms to push on the legs as they rise.

RISING FROM A SUPINE POSITION

Young children rise to standing by coming forward from supine using a pattern of flexion with rotation of the head and trunk. One arm reaches forward while the other pushes against the support surface and the lower limbs assume a wide-based, medially rotated squat position. From squatting, the child extends to the vertical. This pattern of rising reaches a peak frequency at about the age of 7 years and then gradually declines in frequency during later childhood.

Motor Skill Development During Later Childhood and Adolescence

Later childhood is typically the period from 7 to 10 or 12 years of age. During later childhood, adolescence, and throughout the rest of the human life span, changes in the form of movements are related to age. It appears that the individual is constantly seeking the most efficient form of movement within skills that have already been attained, as growth and the individual's lifestyle changes.

Children have strong drives to develop self-esteem, to be accepted socially, to become skillful, and to explore the limits of their physical being. In school and in various recreational activities, the child moves into situations in which competition and cooperation are strong components of physical activity. Later childhood is a time of slow but steady physical growth that allows gradual mastery of motor skills. Skills are perfected and stabilized prior to adolescence. Preferences for various sports and athletic activities emerge.

Boys and girls tend to socialize differently to physical activity. Despite changes in school curricula over the last two or three decades that provide increasing opportunity for girls to participate in physical activities, boys still have greater opportunities available to pursue an active lifestyle. However, both boys and girls are more likely to be active if parents provide more occasions for them to be physically active. Both boys and girls demonstrate improved performance within all fundamental skills throughout early childhood. However, boys typically demonstrate greater speed and strength at all ages when compared with girls.

Adolescence begins with the physical changes that hallmark puberty and ends when physical growth has ceased. The age of onset of adolescence is approximately 11 to 12 years in girls and 12 to 13 years in boys. Growth spurts occur that likely lead to the emergence of new patterns of movement within the skills already acquired. Even though the process of age-related change in motor behavior continues throughout adolescence and adulthood, the motor skills that permit physical independence are acquired primarily during the first year after birth. Later periods of development seem to provide opportunities for further refinement and development of control and coordination, leading to improved performance within skills.

Contemporary Issues in Motor Development

Physical therapists' concepts of development have undergone great change over the past 10 to 15 years. We view developmental sequences quite differently now. We no longer regard reflexes as the building blocks of motor behavior, and we look to patients to assume increasingly active roles in determining the goals and outcomes of physical therapy. New theories are emerging that offer different explanations of the process of development.

Developmental Sequences

For a number of years, physical therapists viewed the process of motor development as a simple reflection of maturation of the nervous system. The order of development of skills during the first year of life was believed to be inherently determined and could not be changed. This affected the way in which therapists assessed and treated individuals with developmental disabilities. Through an examination, the individual's developmental level was determined and treatment was planned that would replicate the order of development of skills leading to the ability to walk independently. The sequence of development was used as a prescription for progressing patients to independence. It was believed that each skill in the sequence was a necessary precursor to the next skill, and that no step could be skipped if independence was to be achieved. This somewhat restrictive view of the developmental sequence is being replaced with a less strict interpretation.

Currently, therapists view the developmental sequence as a guide for understanding the general process by which one attains the ability to control the body against the force of gravity. Age-appropriate skills are of greater concern than replication of the sequence of accomplishments during infancy. For example, creeping is a locomotor pattern that is most common during infancy and early childhood. In the past, creeping was viewed as a precursor to walking, and individuals of all ages who were unable to walk would be taught to creep as a natural step in the progression to walking. Currently, therapists are increasingly concerned with age-appropriate skills. Beyond the period of infancy and early childhood, in our culture, creeping is less commonly used as a form of locomotion. As a result, therapists today are less likely to require older individuals to creep as a prerequisite to walking than were therapists a generation ago.

Reflexes as Fundamental Building Blocks of Motor Behavior

The discussion of the emerging motor behavior of the fetus provides an excellent example of the change in thinking regarding reflexes. Until recently, reflexes were viewed as the fundamental units of motor behavior, from which volitional movements and skilled actions evolved. Milani-Comparetti's work interpreting the spontaneous movements of the fetus while in utero represents an increasing tendency to reject models of human development that do not recognize the primary and fundamental capacity of the individual to generate behavior. This recognition of the self-generation of movement is termed an *active organism* concept. It replaces the traditional view that the fetus and infant are incapable of generating movement and rejects the theory that the young individual is a reflexive being, dependent on external stimuli to activate the motor system—a *passive organism.*

The passive organism concept has permeated many treatment theories in physical therapy, with facilitation and inhibition of reflexes as outgrowths of this concept. For many years, facilitation procedures were the primary tools therapists used to remediate movement disorders. Recently, however, therapists have been attaching increased importance to patient-generated movements. An emphasis on teaching and learning motor skills is replacing traditional facilitation approaches. Learning requires the individual to be an active participant, receiving and interpreting feedback and generating corrective action.

Coupled with the recognition of the patient's role in generating activity has been the increased recognition of the patient's role in determining the goals and outcomes of physical therapy. For young children, this translates to families assuming a greater role in determining the goals of treatment and carrying out treatment procedures for their child. Those receiving treatment are less passive and more active now than they were expected to be in years past.

New Theory of Motor Development

Contemporary theories do not rest as strongly on the CNS as the cause of motor development. Other body systems, such as the musculoskeletal system and the cardiorespiratory system, are also assumed to play a role in the process of motor development. Further, the environment represents a significant source of systematic change that influences motor development. Rather than simple singular causes of change, systems theories recognize the complex multiple causes of development. Although one factor might be found to be a catalyst for change, it is now recognized that no single agent is "the cause" of motor development. All systems are seen as undergoing constant change and are, therefore, dynamic. It is the interaction of these dynamic systems that promotes development of motor skills.

Therapists who formerly looked to the nervous system as the controller of motor skill development are now recognizing the influence of other factors, such as body size, motivation, and the environmental context in which skills occur, as important agents of developmental change. Systems theories are becoming increasingly well known and are beginning to guide research by physical therapists. This switch to new theories promises to lead to a greater understanding of how motor skills evolve, not only during infancy but also during childhood and adolescence.

BIBLIOGRAPHY AND RECOMMENDED READINGS

Albinson IG, Andrew GM, eds. *Child in Sport and Physical Activity.* Baltimore: University Park Press; 1976.

Asher C. *Postural Variations in Childhood.* Boston: Butterworths; 1975.

Bayley N. *Bayley Scales of Infant Development.* New York: Psychological Corp; 1969.

Bly L. *Motor Skills Acquisition in the First Year.* Tucson: Therapy Skill Builders; 1994.

Bobath B. *Abnormal Postural Reflex Activity Caused by Brain Lesions.* London: Wm Heinemann Medical Books Ltd; 1965.

Campbell SK. Understanding motor performance in children (section one). In: Campbell SK, ed. *Physical Therapy for Children.* Philadelphia: WB Saunders; 1994.

Caplan F. *The First Twelve Months of Life.* New York: Bantam; 1995.

Casaer P. *Postural Behavior in Newborn Infants.* Philadelphia: JB Lippincott; 1979.

Cech D, Martin ST. *Functional Movement Development Across the Life Span.* Philadelphia: WB Saunders; 1995.

Corbin CB. *A Textbook of Motor Development.* Dubuque, IA: Little, Brown & Co; 1973.

Espenschade AS, Eckert HM. *Motor Development.* 2nd Ed. Columbus, OH: Charles E. Merrill Publishing Company; 1980.

Falkner F. *Human Development.* Philadelphia: WB Saunders; 1966.

Gallahue DL. *Understanding Motor Development in Children.* 3rd Ed. Dubuque, IA: Wm C. Brown Pub.; 1997.

Gesell A. The ontogenesis of infant behavior. In: Carmichael L, ed. *Manual of Child Psychology.* 2nd Ed. New York: John Wiley & Sons; 1954.

Gesell A, Ames LB. The ontogenetic organization of prone behavior in human infancy. *J Genet Psychol* 1940;56:247–263.

Haywood K. *Life Span Motor Development.* 2nd Ed. Urbana, IL: Human Kinetics; 1993.

Holt KS. *Child Development: Diagnosis and Assessment.* Woburn, MA: Butterworth-Heinemann Medical Books Ltd; 1991.

Hooker D. *The Origin of Overt Behavior.* Ann Arbor: University of Michigan Press; 1944.

Humphrey T. Postnatal repetition of human prenatal activity sequences with some suggestions of their neuroanatomical basis. In: Robinson RJ, ed. *Brain and Early Behavior. Development in the Fetus and Infant.* New York: Academic Press; 1969.

Jacobs MJ. Development of normal motor behavior. *Am J Phys Med.* 1967;46:41–51.

Kugler PN, Kelso JAS, Turvey MT. On the control and coordination of naturally developing systems. In: Kelso TAS, Clark JE, eds. *The Development of Movement Control and Coordination.* New York: John Wiley & Sons; 1982.

Levine MD, et al, eds. *Developmental Behavioral Pediatrics.* 2nd Ed. Philadelphia: WB Saunders; 1992.

Lowry GH. *Growth and Development of Children.* 8th Ed. Chicago: Yearbook Medical Publishers; 1986.

MacDonald J. *Developmental Ordering of the Movement Patterns in Infants Rolling Supine to Prone.* Richmond: Virginia Commonwealth University, 1988. Thesis.

McGraw MB. *The Neuromuscular Maturation of the Human Infant.* New York: Hafner; 1963.

Milani-Comparetti A. Pattern analysis of normal and abnormal development: The fetus, the newborn, the child. In: Slaton DS, ed. *Development of Movement in Infancy.* Chapel Hill, NC: University of North Carolina, Division of Physical Therapy; 1981.

Payne VG, Issacs LD. *Human Motor Development: A Lifespan Approach.* 3rd Ed. Mountain View, CA: Mayfield Publishing Co; 1994.

Roberton MA, Halverson LE. *Developing Children—Their Changing Movement.* Philadelphia: Lea & Febiger; 1984.

Saint-Anne Dargassies S. *The Neuro-motor and Psycho-affective Development of the Infant.* New York: Elsevier; 1986.

Shirley MM. *The First Two Years: A Study of Twenty-five Babies.* Minneapolis: University of Minnesota Press; 1931.

Short-Deraff MA. *Human Development for Occupational Therapists: Conception through Adolescence.* Baltimore: Williams & Wilkins; 1988.

Smolak L. *Infancy.* Englewood Cliffs, NJ: Prentice-Hall; 1986.

Stockmeyer S. An interpretation of the approach of Rood to the treatment of neuromuscular dysfunction. *Am J Phys Med.* 1967;46:900–956.

Tanner JM. *Fetus into Man: Physical Growth from Conception to Maturity.* 2nd Ed. Cambridge, MA: Harvard University Press; 1990.

Touwen B. *Neurological Development in Infancy.* London: Wm Heinemann Medical Books Ltd; 1976.

Van Sant AF. Life-span motor development. In: Lister M, ed. *Contemporary Management of Motor Control Problems.* Alexandria, VA: Foundation for Physical Therapy; 1991:77–84.

Voss, DE. Proprioceptive neuromuscular facilitation. *Am J Phys Med.* 1967;46;83–98.

Wickstrom RL. *Fundamental Motor Patterns.* 3rd Ed. Philadelphia: Lea & Febiger; 1983.

Wyke B. The neurological basis of movement: A developmental review. In: Holt K, ed. *Movement and Child Development.* Philadelphia: JB Lippincott; 1975.

Assessment and Testing of Infant and Child Development

Susan K. Brenneman

Physical therapists are important members of the professional team working with disabled children. They must have the skill and knowledge to contribute to the assessment of children, as the assessment process is a professional responsibility that serves the purpose of keeping the therapist's work current. *Assessment* is a continuing process of collecting and organizing relevant information in order to plan and implement effective treatment. It is important for therapists to base their treatment recommendations on appropriate tools of assessment.

A broad view of the child's difficulty and its functional significance is the most important aspect of the assessment. Children may present with a wide variety of behavioral difficulties, and the physical therapist must determine how best to help them function to their fullest potential. Although some aspects of the disability may be better dealt with by other disciplines, whereas other aspects are best handled by physical therapists, rigid division of labor among professionals is unwise. Depending on training and competence, the traditional roles of physical therapist, occupational therapist, and speech therapist may overlap. Most physical therapists, however, will be concerned mainly with the child's basic gross motor adaptation to the environment.[1]

The challenge for the physical therapist is to assess accurately and comprehend the significance of any delay that falls outside the limits of normal variability. Knowledge of the normal, orderly sequence of developmental achievement and patterns of integration is the basis upon which significant deviation in maturation is gauged.[2] The physical therapist, therefore, must be knowledgeable about normal development, as presented in Chapter 1. Understanding this broad developmental scope forms the basis for therapeutic intervention. Developmental milestones present the major clinical parameter of progressive growth and integration in the central nervous system (CNS). It is important to focus on those aspects of motor behavior that are of greatest concern. Because of the focus of their education, most physical therapists' emphasis is on muscles and joints, rather than on total patterns of motor behavior. However, it is not acceptable to deal with isolated parts, such as a foot, gait, or the spine.[1]

A battery of tests is required to assess a child adequately. Developmental assessment tests are only one type of test used. Another category of assessment that is addressed in this chapter is that of functional capabilities. Subsequent chapters will address assessments that are unique to a particular disability, completing the total assessment for the child with that disability.

Purposes of Developmental Testing

Use of developmental tests as screening tools promotes early intervention for deviations from normal growth and development in young children. Early identification of deviations facilitates the provision of anticipatory advice to parents, clinicians, and caregivers for future planning. Early recognition and a focused plan for intervention may prevent severe disability.

Developmental tests can assist in determining a diagnosis. Comprehensive scales, such as the Gesell scale,[3] specify problem areas and indicate whether a developmental problem is likely to include all areas of development or one focal area, such as gross motor development.

Developmental tests also facilitate the planning of a treatment program. Developmental scales provide valuable information about the level of operation of the child or the milestones reached. Developmental tests indicate where treatment should begin, and they provide information by which the progression of a therapeutic regimen can be guided. An explanation of developmental tests and their results may help parents understand the child's limitations—what can and cannot be expected—making it possible to establish common goals and to plan for the future. The results of developmental testing may reveal specific areas of deficit that require additional evaluation to discover the underlying cause of the delay.

Subsequent assessments will reveal the rate and trend of development of a child. After determining goals for the child, tests can be used to monitor progress and determine whether and when the child has achieved the goals. Therapists involved in research rely on developmental assessments to evaluate strategies for treatment and means of intervention. Research continues to evaluate the assessments themselves to ensure their reliability and validity. Developmental assessments, as well as being used as a clinical research tool, can also be used for evaluation of a program.

The ways in which test data are to be used should be determined before testing so that one can avoid the collection of superfluous data and so that all necessary information is obtained. It is a waste of time and effort to perform extensive tests just to be thorough, unless all the information gained will be used. As a therapist becomes skilled in the administration of developmental assessments, the ability to test what is appropriate will improve.

Basic Methods of Assessment

Decisions regarding intervention are usually based on information from various resources. Several basic methods are used to collect information about a child. A questioning mind is important in this process. Therapists must know what questions to ask both of themselves and of others. Guiding questions during clinical observation provides the foundation for all further screening or formal evaluation.

Among the most valuable skills a therapist can possess are the abilities to observe, to be flexible and spontaneous, and to be creative with play and other activities that foster intrinsic motivation in children.[4] Different methods and adaptations must be used for assessment because children are different from adults.

Orientation of the child and the parents to the environment is crucial. Both parent and child must feel comfortable with the therapist and the setting. This orientation is often best achieved by proceeding with the evaluation at a slow pace, and by adapting one's approach according to the reaction of the child.

During the assessment, the therapist needs to take a broad view of the child, whatever the disability. The child should not merely be labeled a "crutch walker," a "hemi," or "clumsy." Rather, the child is a person with a suspected disability, and the therapist's initial task is to be thorough and sensitive in discovering whether a disability or sensori-motor delay exists and what can be done to reduce the effects of the disability.[4]

Interview

An interview with the child and the parents provides important information about the development of the child. In many cases because of the young age of the child, the interview will be conducted exclusively with the parents. An interview should be friendly and informal rather than impersonal and inquisitive. The purpose of the interview should be clear, and the interviewer should know specifically what information is desired. A skillful and well-directed interview will help fill in the gaps of an assessment. The therapist should be able to determine the area of greatest concern to the parents, and should note the age and circumstances in which the problem was first discovered.

History

A review of the child's developmental and medical history provides valuable information. A developmental history can be obtained through a questionnaire or an interview. The possible lack of reliability and bias of the parent should be considered in assessing the information gained in the history.

The medical records of a child may provide information regarding precautions, patient health status, previous medical history, suspected diagnosis, prognosis, medications, and other factors impacting on the child's health. The therapist should obtain information about the family and its genetic history; the pregnancy, labor, and delivery of the child; and the perinatal and neonatal events. This information will be useful in performing a comprehensive assessment.

Clinical Observation

Assessment begins by observation of the child at rest in various positions and during unstructured movement, as presented in Chapter 4. The therapist should also observe the child interacting with the environment, the child's social responses and communication, and the child's cognition. This observation can be done in a nonthreatening manner while the therapist is talking with the parents and establishing rapport with the child.

Tools for Assessment

After interviewing and observing the child, the administration of standardized and criterion- and norm-referenced assessments will yield an overall picture of the child's level of functioning. Tests of developmental assessment will help identify which specific tests of functioning (e.g., goniometry, manual testing of muscles, or assessment of activities of daily living [ADLs]) are needed. Those specific tests and methods used to evaluate disabilities in childhood are reviewed in subsequent chapters.

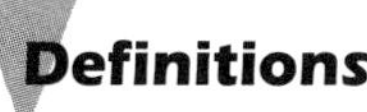

Definitions

Terms for Understanding Standardized Assessments[5]

An *age-equivalent score* is the mean chronologic age represented by a certain test score. For example, a raw score of 52 on the Bayley Mental Scales represents an age equivalent of 4½ months. Age-equivalent scores may be especially useful with developmentally delayed children for whom it may be impossible to derive a meaningful developmental index. Age-equivalent scores are easy for parents to understand, but they must be interpreted carefully because they can be misleading. Usually these children have qualitative differences in their behaviors, as well as a wide mixture of successes and failures on developmental tests.

The *criterion-referenced test* is one in which scores are interpreted on the basis of absolute criteria (e.g., the number of items answered correctly) rather than on relative criteria, such as how the rest of the normal group performed. Such tests are usually developed by the teacher or researcher and can be used for research involving a comparison of groups, just as norm-referenced tests are used. Criterion-referenced tests are used to measure a person's mastery of a set of behavioral objectives. The tests represent an attempt to maximize the validity or appropriateness of the content based on that set of objectives. The *developmental quotient* is the ratio between the child's actual score (developmental age) on a test and the child's chronologic age. An example is motor age/chronologic age equal to the motor quotient (MQ).

Norm-referenced or *standardized tests* use normative values as standards for interpreting individual test scores. The purpose of standardized tests is to make a comparison between a particular child and the "norm" or "average" of a group of children. Norms describe a person's test score relative to a large body of scores that have already been collected on a defined population. Examples of norm-referenced tests include the Bayley Scales of Infant Development,[6] the Denver II Screening Test,[7] and the Gesell Developmental Scales.[3]

The *percentile score* indicates the number of children of the same age or grade level (or whatever is used for a source of comparison) who would be expected to score lower than the child tested. For example, a child who scores in the 75th percentile on a norm-referenced test has done better than 75% of the children in the norm group.

A *raw score* is the total of individual items that are passed or correct on a particular test. On many tests, this will require establishing a basal and ceiling level of performance. The number of items required to achieve a basal or ceiling level varies from one test to another.

Reliability refers to consistency or repeatability between measurements in a series. Types of reliability include interobserver and test–retest. Interobserver reliability describes the relationship between items passed and failed, or the percentage of agreement, between two independent observers. Simply stated, interobserver reliability is an index of whether two different testers obtain the same score on a test. Test–retest reliability is the relationship of a person's score on the first administration of the test to the score on the second administration. Simply stated, this type of reliability determines whether the same or similar scores are achieved when the test is repeated under identical conditions.

Standard error of measurement (SEM) is a measure of reliability that indicates the precision of an individual test score. The SEM gives an estimate of the margin of error associated with a particular test score. For example, a Mental Development Index (MDI), from the Bayley Developmental Scales, at 12 months has an associated SEM of 6.7 points. This SEM means that one is 67% certain that the child's true MDI falls within 6.7 points of the obtained score.

Standard scores are expressed as deviations or variations from the mean score for a group. Standard scores are expressed in units of standard deviation. When using standard scores, information is needed concerning the mean and standard deviation of the standard score.

Validity is an indication of the extent to which a test measures what it purports to measure. *Construct validity* is an examination of the theory or hypothetical constructs underlying the test. *Content validity* assesses the appropriateness of the test or how well the content of the test samples the subject matter or behaviors about which conclusions must be drawn. The sample situations measured in the test must be representative of the set from which the sample is drawn. There are two types of *criterion-related validity*. *Concurrent validity* relates the performance on the test to performance on another well-known and accepted test that measures the same knowledge or behavior. *Predictive validity* means that the child's performance on the test predicts some actual behavior.

Sensitivity can be defined as the ability of a test to identify correctly those who actually have a disorder. High sensitivity results in few false-negative scores.

Specificity refers to the ability of the test to identify correctly those who do not have the disorder. High specificity results in few false-positive scores.

The *positive predictive value* of a test is defined as the proportion of true positives among all those who have positive results. The *negative predictive value* is the proportion of true negatives among all those who have negative screening results.

Guidelines for Selection of Tests

There is no lack of tests that purport to measure motor abilities of children. The problem is not quantity but quality.[8] Careful and knowledgeable selection of tests is, therefore, important. If evaluators are unaware of the strengths, weaknesses, limitations, and restrictions of the tests being used, there is a high probability that an inappropriate test could be used, thus resulting in inaccurate or misinterpreted information.[9] Most published tests have some limitations or restrictions to their use, particularly regarding the ages and populations for whom they were developed and on whom they were standardized. The result of disregarding these restrictions could be the misuse of the test or misinterpretation of the outcomes.

In order to choose an appropriate test, some guidelines by which to evaluate a test are needed. Stangler and associates[10] have proposed six criteria for evaluating a screening test that can be applied to any assessment test: (1) acceptability; (2) simplicity; (3) cost; (4) appropriateness; (5) reliability; and (6) validity. Every test may not fulfill each criterion; however, the test may be used knowledgeably if a therapist is aware of the limitations.

Acceptability is defined as acceptance to all who will be affected by the test, including the children and families screened, the professionals who receive resulting referrals, and the community. *Simplicity* is the ease by which a test can be taught, learned, and administered. *Appropriateness* of screening tests is based on the prevalence of the problem to be screened and on the applicability of the test to the particular population. *Cost* includes the actual cost of equipment, preparation and payment of personnel, the cost of inaccurate results, personal costs to the person being screened, and the total cost of the test in relation to the benefits of early detection.[10] In addition, tests must show both *reliability* and *validity*, as discussed previously.

Using Questions as Guidelines

A therapist can further ensure appropriate selection of the test by posing several questions regarding the test:

1. *For what purpose will the test be used?*
   - For diagnosis
   - For program planning
   - For research
2. *Who is the child?*
   - Age
   - Suspected diagnosis
   - Presenting disability
3. *What content areas need to be assessed?*
   - Gross motor
   - Fine motor
   - Speech
   - Muscle strength
   - Comprehensive assessment of functional capabilities
4. *What are the constraints for the examiner?*
   - Time
   - Training
   - Space and equipment
   - Money

Test Analysis Format

The Test Analysis Format developed by Clark and associates is another method for evaluating a test[4] (Display 2-1). An adapted version of this format is used to review the assessment tools in this chapter. After careful consideration of the aforementioned questions and criteria, the therapist should consult sources, including catalogs, books, and other therapists, to locate possible

DISPLAY 2-1

Test Analysis Format*

Title and authors:

What the test proposes to measure:

Population for whom the test was developed:

Test format

A. Type of instrument
B. Content of test
C. Administration
D. Scoring
E. Interpretation

Include information about the basic type of instrument that is begin used—for example, interview, criterion-referenced or standardized test. Briefly discuss the basic guidelines for administration that pertain to the entire test. For example, is information obtained by a report from parents or by presenting tasks to children? How is the test set up? In general, are there time limits for items? Include basic information about procedures for scoring and interpretation.

Advantages of the test:

Disadvantages of the test:

Purchasing information:

References:

*Adapted by permission from Pratt PN, Allen AS: *Occupational Therapy for Children*, 2nd Ed. St. Louis: CV Mosby; 1989.

choices. The therapist should be sure to review several manuals thoroughly, to learn the tests and use them, and to evaluate the results.

Overview of Tests

Assessment may be considered in several broad categories. Screening tests are used to identify deficits in a child's performance that indicate the need for further services. Assessments of component functions address specific areas of functioning (e.g., gross motor ability or reflex status). Comprehensive developmental scales evaluate all areas of development. Functional assessments evaluate the essential skills that are required in the child's natural environments of home and school.

The rest of the chapter reviews selected tests that are available. Some of the more widely known standardized evaluative procedures are presented, as are some tests that are not standardized but that have proven useful in clinical practice. The categories just mentioned are used for organization.

Screening Tests

Screening tests are intended to differentiate between those persons who are normal and healthy in a particular respect from those who are not.[9] These tests typically raise more questions than answers, but the questions raised can be used to guide the selection of formal measures for evaluation.

Milani-Comparetti Motor Development Screening Test

The Milani-Comparetti Screening Test was developed by Italian neurologists Milani-Comparetti and Gidoni.[11] The original score form was modified by the staff at Meyer Children's Rehabilitation Institute, University of Nebraska Medical Center.[12] The current test manual, which is in its 3rd edition,[13] was written to provide additional clarification of the testing and scoring procedures, to document reliability data, and to revise the developmental milestones of the original score form to reflect a normative sample.

TEST MEASURES AND TARGET POPULATION

Motor development is evaluated on the basis of a correlation between the functional motor achievement of the child and the underlying reflex structures.[11] The appropriate population for testing comprises children from birth to approximately 2 years of age.

TEST CONSTRUCTION

The items included on the chart were not randomly selected or based on the statistical difference between normal and abnormal. Rather, Milani-Comparetti selected a parameter for study that involved items that were interrelated. This interrelatedness is described by a correlation between functional motor achievement and underlying reflex structures. The parameter chosen is called "standing," and is better translated from Italian to English to mean antigravity control of the body axis. This control includes head control and control while sitting, as well as control while standing. "Standing" was found to be a suitable parameter because it includes as essential and significant components a limited number of specific reactions, such as righting, parachute, and tilting reactions.[11] The original chart used in administering the test was developed after 5 years of experience in a child welfare clinic.

TEST FORMAT

Type. The test is criterion-referenced, and the 3rd edition of the test manual provides normative data.[13] The examiner physically manipulates the child for a particular motor response. Parents can provide information if the child is uncooperative.

Content. The illustrated manual developed by Meyer Rehabilitation Center provides instructions for test administration and scoring. The score chart can be reused at successive examinations (Fig. 2-1).

Administration. The original scoring chart developed by Milani-Comparetti has been revised to permit smoother, more rapid administration of the test. All of the original test procedures and scoring mechanisms are retained in the revision; they are simply placed in a different order for more efficient testing.[13] The chart integrates spontaneous behavior and evoked responses in a manner that is easy to follow and is based on the examination sequence. The child should be positioned for only the test items relevant to a particular age, expressed in months. Experienced observers can give the test in 4 to 8 minutes.

Scoring. The chart is a shaded graph indicating the time span during which a reflex or reaction is expected to be present. The child's age in months is used to score each item tested and is placed on the age line at which the child performs. Responses are judged as being either absent or present. Completion results in a graphic profile of the child's motor development (see Fig. 2-1). A narrative summary of additional observations may be included.

Interpretation. Age levels for stages of development are inherent in the test. Normal results are shown by a vertical alignment of notations that are consistent with the child's chronologic age. Motor retardation usually appears as a homogeneous shift of notations toward the left side of the graph, but the vertical alignment is maintained. A wider scattering of findings usually indicates a more severe, or possibly more specific, motor dysfunction, such as cerebral palsy.

RELIABILITY AND VALIDITY

Interobserver reliability results of one study[14] showed a high percentage of agreement, ranging from 79% to 98%. The most consistently high level of agreement was noted for active movement and postural control items. Overall, equilibrium reactions demonstrated lower levels of agreement, with standing equilibrium being the lowest scored item at 79%. Test–retest reliability results[14] showed percentages of agreement ranging from 82% to 100%.

ADVANTAGES

This screening test is practical and useful. It can be given quickly and does not require any special equipment or setting. The test can be learned quickly and is easily scored. By providing a developmental profile, it can provide early evidence of neuromotor delay or deficits, possibly indicating a need for further evaluation. The test relies on objective observations, rather than reports by the parents. Normative data have been provided with the 3rd edition.

Denver II

The Denver Developmental Screening Test (DDST),[15] developed by Frankenburg and Dodds in 1967, has been widely used by health care providers to screen for developmental delays. It has been adapted for use and restandardized in many countries. Both despite and because of its widespread usage, there have been many criticisms of this tool, prompting a major revision and restandardization of the test. The result is the Denver II test.[7,16]

The reasons for updating the DDST included: (1) the need for additional language items; (2) questionable appropriateness of 1967 norms for 1990; (3) changes in items that were difficult to administer or score; (4) appropriateness of the test for various subgroups and for predicting later performance in children; and

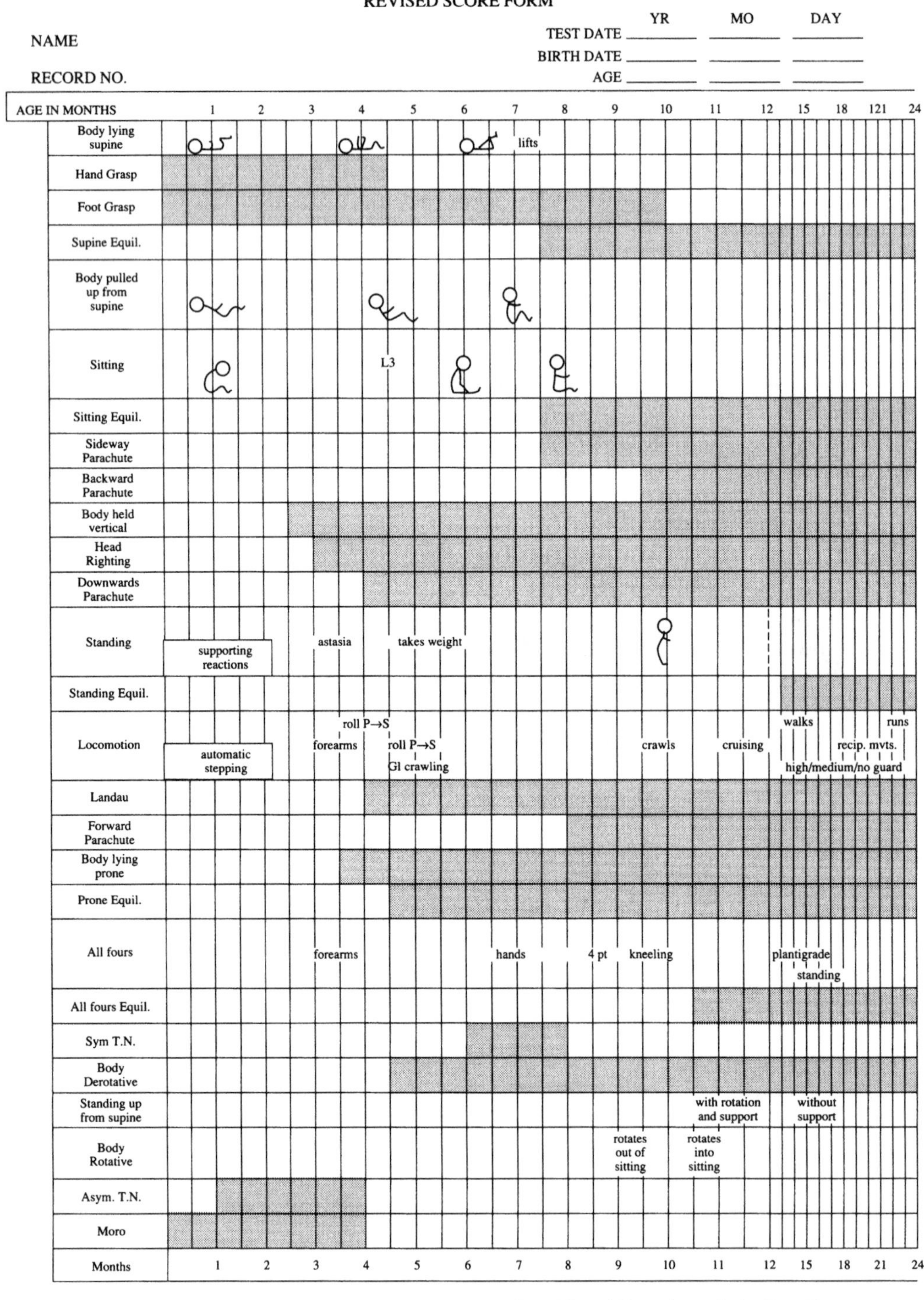

MILANI-COMPARETTI MOTOR DEVELOPMENT SCREENING TEST
REVISED SCORE FORM

NAME

RECORD NO.

	YR	MO	DAY
TEST DATE			
BIRTH DATE			
AGE			

AGE IN MONTHS: 1 2 3 4 5 6 7 8 9 10 11 12 15 18 121 24

Item	Entries printed in row
Body lying supine	lifts
Hand Grasp	
Foot Grasp	
Supine Equil.	
Body pulled up from supine	
Sitting	L3
Sitting Equil.	
Sideway Parachute	
Backward Parachute	
Body held vertical	
Head Righting	
Downwards Parachute	
Standing	supporting reactions; astasia; takes weight
Standing Equil.	
Locomotion	automatic stepping; roll P→S; forearms; roll P→S; Gl crawling; crawls; cruising; walks; runs; recip. mvts.; high/medium/no guard
Landau	
Forward Parachute	
Body lying prone	
Prone Equil.	
All fours	forearms; hands; 4 pt; kneeling; plantigrade; standing
All fours Equil.	
Sym T.N.	
Body Derotative	
Standing up from supine	with rotation and support; without support
Body Rotative	rotates out of sitting; rotates into sitting
Asym. T.N.	
Moro	
Months	1 2 3 4 5 6 7 8 9 10 11 12 15 18 21 24

Tester: __________ *Record General Observations on Back of Score Form

CRI-71 (1/88)

Figure 2-1 ▪ Revised scoring chart used for the Milani-Comparetti Motor Development Screening Test. (Stuberg W. *The Milani-Comparetti Motor Development Screening Test.* 3rd ed. Appendix B. Omaha: University of Nebraska Medical Center; 1992.)

(5) new methods for ensuring accurate administration and scoring of the test.[17]

The major additions to and differences between the Denver II and the DDST are (1) an 86% increase in language items; (2) two articulation items; (3) a new age scale; (4) a new category of item interpretation to identify milder delays; (5) a behavior rating scale; and (6) new training materials.[17]

TEST MEASURES AND TARGET POPULATION

The Denver II screens general development in four areas:

1. Personal-Social: Getting along with people and caring for personal needs
2. Fine Motor-Adaptive: Eye-hand coordination, manipulation of small objects, and problem-solving
3. Language: Hearing, understanding, and use of language
4. Gross Motor: Sitting, walking, jumping, and overall large muscle movement

Also included are five items documenting "test behavior" to be completed after administration of the test.

The Denver II is not an IQ test, nor is it designed to generate diagnostic labels or predict future adaptive and intellectual abilities. The test is best used to compare a given child's performance on a variety of tasks to the performance of other children of the same age.

The appropriate population for the test are children between birth and 6 years of age who are apparently well.

TEST CONSTRUCTION AND STANDARDIZATION

The Denver II was developed by administering 326 potential items (including several modifications of the original 105 DDST items) to more than 2000 children who were considered to be representative of demographic variables within the Colorado population. Each item was administered an average of 540 times. Composite norms for the total sample and norms for subgroups (based on gender, ethnicity, maternal education, and place of residence) were used to determine new age norms. The *Denver II Technical Manual*[17] contains details of the standardization process.

TEST FORMAT

Type. The test is norm-referenced, with data presented as age norms, similar to physical growth curve.[16] Subnorms for various subgroups that differ in a clinically significant manner from norms depicted on the reference chart are presented in the technical manual.[17]

Content. The Denver II has 125 items arranged on the test form in four sections: Personal-Social, Fine Motor-Adaptive, Language, and Gross Motor (Fig. 2-2). Age scales across the top and bottom of the test form depict ages, expressed in months and years, from birth to 6 years. Each test item is represented on the form by a bar that spans the ages at which 25%, 50%, 75%, and 90% of the standardization sample passed that item.[7] A standardized test kit, forms, and manuals are purchased to administer the Denver II.

Administration. This test generally depends on the examiner's observation of the child. Although certain items may be scored based on the verbal report of a parent (as indicated on the test form by an "R"), observation of the particular task is a more reliable method of scoring. Correct calculation of the child's age is important because correct interpretation of test results depends on accuracy of the age. Although the order of presenting the test items is flexible, the items must be given in the manner specified in the manual. The number of items given varies with the age and abilities of the child. The examiner should begin by administering

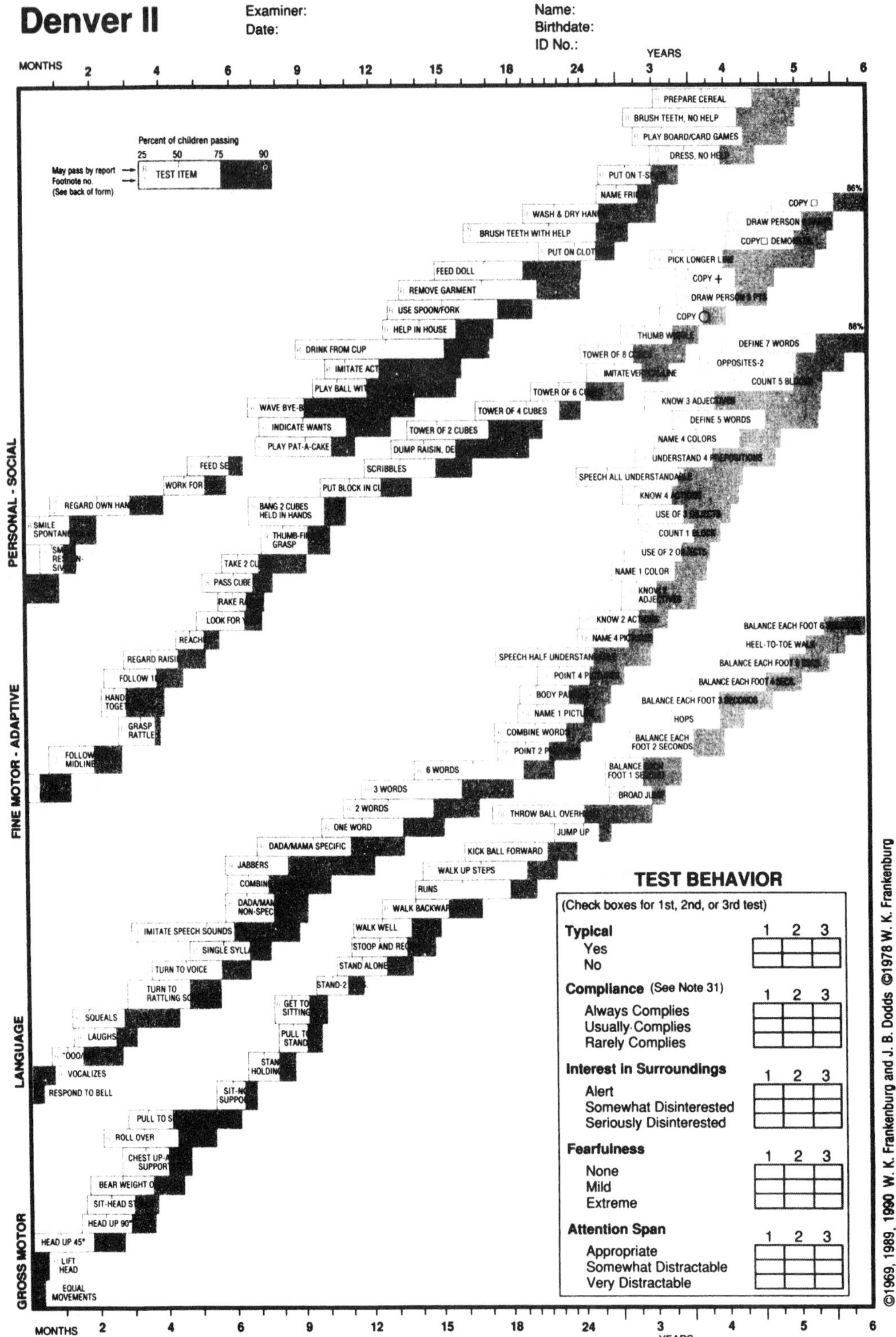

Denver II

Examiner:
Date:

Name:
Birthdate:
ID No.:

MONTHS 2 4 6 9 12 15 18 24 YEARS 3 4 5 6

Percent of children passing
25 50 75 90
May pass by report
Footnote no.
(See back of form)
TEST ITEM

PERSONAL - SOCIAL
PREPARE CEREAL
BRUSH TEETH, NO HELP
PLAY BOARD/CARD GAMES
DRESS, NO HELP
PUT ON T-SHIRT
NAME FRIEND
WASH & DRY HANDS
BRUSH TEETH WITH HELP
PUT ON CLOTHING
FEED DOLL
REMOVE GARMENT
USE SPOON/FORK
HELP IN HOUSE
DRINK FROM CUP
IMITATE ACTIVITIES
PLAY BALL WITH EXAMINER
WAVE BYE-BYE
INDICATE WANTS
PLAY PAT-A-CAKE
FEED SELF
WORK FOR TOY
REGARD OWN HAND
SMILE SPONTANEOUSLY
SMILE RESPONSIVELY
REGARD FACE

FINE MOTOR - ADAPTIVE
COPY □
DRAW PERSON 6 PARTS
COPY □ DEMONSTRATED
PICK LONGER LINE
COPY +
DRAW PERSON 3 PTS
COPY ○
THUMB WIGGLE
TOWER OF 8 CUBES
IMITATE VERTICAL LINE
TOWER OF 6 CUBES
TOWER OF 4 CUBES
TOWER OF 2 CUBES
DUMP RAISIN, DEMONSTRATED
SCRIBBLES
PUT BLOCK IN CUP
BANG 2 CUBES HELD IN HANDS
THUMB-FINGER GRASP
TAKE 2 CUBES
PASS CUBE
RAKE RAISIN
LOOK FOR YARN
REACH
REGARD RAISIN
FOLLOW 180°
HANDS TOGETHER
GRASP RATTLE
FOLLOW TO MIDLINE

LANGUAGE
86%
DEFINE 7 WORDS
OPPOSITES-2
COUNT 5 BLOCKS
KNOW 3 ADJECTIVES
DEFINE 5 WORDS
NAME 4 COLORS
UNDERSTAND 4 PREPOSITIONS
SPEECH ALL UNDERSTANDABLE
KNOW 4 ACTIONS
USE OF 3 OBJECTS
COUNT 1 BLOCK
USE OF 2 OBJECTS
NAME 1 COLOR
KNOW 2 ADJECTIVES
KNOW 2 ACTIONS
NAME 4 PICTURES
SPEECH HALF UNDERSTANDABLE
POINT 4 PICTURES
BODY PARTS-6
NAME 1 PICTURE
COMBINE WORDS
POINT 2 PICTURES
6 WORDS
3 WORDS
2 WORDS
ONE WORD
DADA/MAMA SPECIFIC
JABBERS
COMBINE SYLLABLES
DADA/MAMA NON-SPECIFIC
IMITATE SPEECH SOUNDS
SINGLE SYLLABLES
TURN TO VOICE
TURN TO RATTLING SOUND
SQUEALS
LAUGHS
"OOO/AAH"
VOCALIZES
RESPOND TO BELL

GROSS MOTOR
BALANCE EACH FOOT 6 SECONDS
HEEL-TO-TOE WALK
BALANCE EACH FOOT 5 SECONDS
BALANCE EACH FOOT 4 SECONDS
BALANCE EACH FOOT 3 SECONDS
HOPS
BALANCE EACH FOOT 2 SECONDS
BALANCE EACH FOOT 1 SECOND
BROAD JUMP
THROW BALL OVERHAND
JUMP UP
KICK BALL FORWARD
WALK UP STEPS
RUNS
WALK BACKWARDS
WALK WELL
STOOP AND RECOVER
STAND ALONE
STAND-2 SECS
GET TO SITTING
PULL TO STAND
STAND HOLDING ON
SIT-NO SUPPORT
PULL TO SIT-NO HEAD LAG
ROLL OVER
CHEST UP-ARM SUPPORT
BEAR WEIGHT ON LEGS
SIT-HEAD STEADY
HEAD UP 90°
HEAD UP 45°
LIFT HEAD
EQUAL MOVEMENTS

TEST BEHAVIOR
(Check boxes for 1st, 2nd, or 3rd test)

	1	2	3
Typical			
Yes			
No			
Compliance (See Note 31)			
Always Complies			
Usually Complies			
Rarely Complies			
Interest in Surroundings			
Alert			
Somewhat Disinterested			
Seriously Disinterested			
Fearfulness			
None			
Mild			
Extreme			
Attention Span			
Appropriate			
Somewhat Distractable			
Very Distractable			

MONTHS 2 4 6 9 12 15 18 24 3 YEARS 4 5 6

Figure 2-2 ▪ Test form for the Denver II Screening test. (Frankenburg WK, Dodds J, Archer P, et al. *Denver II Training Manual.* Denver, CO: Denver Developmental Materials, Inc.; 1992.)

every item intersected by the age line and at least three items nearest to and totally to the left of the age line. Continued testing depends on whether the goal is to identify developmental delays or the relative strengths of the child.[7] "Test Behavior" ratings are scored after the completion of the test.

Scoring. Each item given should be scored on the bar at the 50% hatch mark. Items are scored as a pass (P), failure (F), no opportunity (N.O.), or refusal (R).

Interpretation. The Denver II identifies the child whose development appears to be delayed in comparison to that of other children and identifies changes in development within one child over time. Individual items should be interpreted first, with the entire test being interpreted last.

Individual items are interpreted as "advanced," "normal," "caution," "delayed," or "no opportunity." The entire Denver II test is interpreted as "normal," "suspect," or "untestable." A child whose scores are interpreted as suspect or untestable on the first test should be screened again before referral for further diagnostic evaluation.

The *Denver II Technical Manual* contains data regarding the results that might be expected so that, in cases when marked deviation is noted, the evaluator may compare with other experiences.

RELIABILITY AND VALIDITY

Thirty-eight children from 10 age groups were tested twice on each of two occasions separated by an interval of 7 to 10 days. The mean examiner-observer reliability was found to be 0.99, with a range of 0.95 to 1.00 and a standard deviation of 0.016. The mean 7- to 10-day test–retest reliability for the same items was 0.90, with a range of 0.50 to 1.00 and a standard deviation of 0.12.[17]

The validity of the Denver II rests on its standardization, not on its correlation with other tests, as all tests are constructed slightly differently.[17]

ADVANTAGES

Administration and scoring is done quickly, and the test is acceptable to both children and parents. The *Denver II Training Manual*[7] gives detailed instructions for proper administration and interpretation of the tests. The *Denver II Technical Manual*[17] contains information on training personnel in the administration of the test and on the establishment of a community screening program. A videotaped instructional program and proficiency test have also been developed for the Denver II. This test is excellent for identifying children who are at risk for developmental problems and for monitoring a child longitudinally.

The authors of the Denver II stress that care should be taken not to use the test to generate diagnostic labels. Rather, it is more appropriately used as a "first step in tackling the problems of early detection, diagnosis, and treatment of developmental deviations in children."[17]

Tests of Motor Function

The physical therapist is concerned primarily with motor behavior. A large number of assessment tools are available that examine gross and fine motor function. The Movement Assessment of Infants, the Alberta Infant Motor Scale, the Test of Infant Motor Performance, Gross Motor Function Measure and Gross Motor Performance Measure, Peabody Developmental Motor Scales, and Bruinicks-Oseretsky Test of Motor Proficiency are described.

Movement Assessment of Infants

The Movement Assessment of Infants (MAI) test was developed by Chandler and associates in response to the need for a systematic approach to the evaluation of motor function in infants who had been treated in a neonatal intensive care unit.[18]

TEST MEASURES AND TARGET POPULATION

The test evaluates muscle tone, primitive reflexes, automatic reactions, and volitional movement in the first year of life. The MAI test, when given to infants at 4 months of age, provides an assessment of risk for motor dysfunction. According to the authors, the purposes of the test are to (1) identify motor dysfunction in infants up to 12 months of age; (2) establish the basis for an early intervention program; (3) monitor the effects of physical therapy on infants and children whose motor behavior is at, or below, 1 year of age; (4) aid in research on motor development by using a standard system of assessment of movement; and (5) teach skillful observation of movement and motor development through an evaluation of normal and handicapped children.[18] The test should not be used to identify the cause of any delay or to make a diagnosis.

The appropriate population for testing using the MAI are children ages birth through 12 months.

TEST CONSTRUCTION AND STANDARDIZATION

The MAI test was created because of a need for a uniform approach to the evaluation of the high-risk infant. Over a period of 5 years of development and use, the MAI test was constantly modified and refined in order to improve its accuracy. When initially available, the test was still being developed and was distributed with a request by the authors for more research and revisions. Subsequent research studies[19–23] continue to refine and suggest revisions for the MAI.

TEST FORMAT

Type. The test is criterion-referenced. Results are obtained by direct handling and observation.

Content. The test includes 65 items divided into four subtests: muscle tone, primitive reflexes, automatic reactions, and volitional movement. Muscle tone refers to the readiness of muscles to respond to gravity. Primitive reflexes are evaluated from fully integrated to reflex domination of movement. Automatic reactions include righting reactions, equilibrium reactions, and protective extension reactions. Volitional movement includes response to visual and auditory stimuli, production of sound, and typical motor milestones, such as hands to midline, fine grasp, rolling, and walking.

Administration. The MAI test is designed for use by physical and occupational therapists, physicians, nurses, psychologists, and others who have experience in the development of infants. Formal training is recommended for examiners using the MAI test in research projects. A pleasant room with open space is needed, but little special equipment is required. The test manual describes the specific equipment needed. The MAI test requires 90 minutes for testing and scoring.

There is no particular order for giving items in the test. Items should be grouped by position in the test, by the amount of concentration required, and by the amount of distress. Observation of spontaneous activity and handling to assess postural tone and evoked behaviors are techniques used in testing.

Scoring. Numeric rating scales, which indicate the expected sequence of development, have been designed for each subtest. Each item has its own set of scoring criteria. Scoring should be done only by applying the criteria for the specific item. Scoring of all items must be based on the performance actually observed by the examiner.

INTERPRETATION. At this point in the development of the MAI test, no method is available for calculating a developmental score. A profile of a typical 4-month-old child is presented by the authors. This profile can be used for a comparison with the scores received by another child. An overall score indicating "degree of risk" of deviance from the norm is computed. At the 4-month examination, the potential scores range from 0 to 48, with higher sores indicating greater deviance. The MAI authors suggest that children with total-risk scores of greater than 7 be identified as "at risk" in terms of motor development. Recent data on full term 4-month-old infants indicate a normal range of 0 to 13, with a mean of 6.0 and one standard deviation of 3.[21] An 8-month profile[23] and a 6-month profile[24] have been developed by additional researchers.

RELIABILITY AND VALIDITY

The test authors found an interobserver reliability of more than 90%.[18] Another study by Harris and associates showed an interobserver reliability of 0.72 and a test–retest reliability of 0.76.[25] Swanson and colleagues established interobserver reliability at a level of 0.90 agreement.[23] Subsequent reliability study of the standard and revised version of the 4-month MAI resulted in excellent interrater and test–retest reliabilities on both the standard (0.91 and 0.79, respectively) and revised (0.93 and 0.83, respectively) MAI.[26]

Harris and associates studied the predictive validity of the MAI test by comparing test scores in infants at 4 months with specific diagnoses at 12 months of age.[27] They found an 11% rate of over-referrals and no under-referrals based on the MAI test scores at 4 months. Swanson and coworkers found strong correlations between MAI scores at 4 and 8 months and performance on the Bayley Scales at 18 months.[23] Sensitivity of the MAI was 83% at 4 months and 96% at 8 months. The specificity of the MAI at 4 months was 78%; this decreased to 65% at 8 months.

When working with at-risk infants, the most relevant information is afforded by the positive and negative predictive values of the test, which indicate the likelihood of normal or abnormal outcomes. The negative predictive value of the MAI is 85% and 91% at 4 and 8 months, respectively. The positive predictive value is 59% and 52% at 4 and 8 months, respectively, but is increased to 70% with sequential examinations.[23]

ADVANTAGES

The MAI test is a comprehensive and qualitative test of motor development. It is one of few assessment tools that consider the quality of movement. Recent studies show a high predictive validity for the MAI.

DISADVANTAGES

The MAI test is lengthy to administer and requires extensive handling of the infant. Normative data are required to strengthen the ability to interpret and score the results. Studies have reported that numerous items have questionable reliability[19,21,25]; therefore, continued reliability and validity studies are needed to improve the usefulness of the MAI as a clinical tool.

Test of Infant Motor Performance

The Test of Infant Motor Performance (TIMP) developed by Campbell and colleagues[28] was developed for use by physical and occupational therapists for the purpose of capturing the components of postural and selective control of movement that are important for function in early infancy.

TEST MEASURES AND TARGET POPULATION

The test was constructed to assess specifically the postural control and alignment needed for age-appropriate functional activities involving movement in early infancy. These functions include changing positions and moving against the force of gravity, adjusting to handling, self-comforting, and orienting the head and body for looking, listening, and interaction with caregivers. The items in the test were designed to reflect the full range of motor maturity from 32 weeks' gestational age to 3.5 months after full-term delivery.

TEST CONSTRUCTION AND STANDARDIZATION

The TIMP was initially developed by Girolami for use in a controlled clinical trial assessing the efficacy of neurodevelopmental treatment in promoting motor development in prematurely born high-risk infants from 34 to 35 weeks' postconceptual age.[29] A revised research version of the TIMP was reviewed by 21 experts in early infant motor development, who suggested additional revision of item descriptors and rated each item for ability to assess developmental change and effects of therapeutic intervention. After administration to a population of 76 infants, including both prematurely born and full-term infants, the data were analyzed for conformity to a Rasch model, resulting in minor changes to the examination. Subsequent research continues to refine and suggest revisions for the TIMP.

TEST FORMAT

Type. The test is criterion-referenced. Results are obtained by direct handling and observation.

Content. The current version of the TIMP has 27 observed items and 25 elicited items, six of which are repeated on both sides of the body. The items in the test emphasize the development of head and trunk control, use of handling techniques for precocious elicitation of postural control, and observation of spontaneously emitted behaviors, such as isolated movements of the hands and feet, antigravity movements, and the ballistic and oscillatory movements indicative of developing coordination of activity in muscle synergists and antagonists. According to the test authors, the processes tested by the items include:

1. The ability to orient and stabilize the head in space and in response to auditory and visual stimulation in supine, prone, side-lying, and upright positions, and during transitions from one position to another
2. Body alignment when the head is manipulated
3. Distal selective control of the fingers, wrists, hands, and ankles
4. Antigravity control of arm and leg movements

Administration/Scoring. The test takes from 25 to 40 minutes to administer, depending on the child's abilities, behavioral state, physiologic stability, and level of cooperation. Observed items are rated *present* or *absent* on the basis of continuous observation of spontaneously emitted behaviors throughout the course of the examination, including brief periods when the child is observed without handling. These items were designed to represent skills that should be present in a majority of normal full-term infants. Elicited items are administered according to standardized instructions and involve direct handling of the infant. Responses to these items are scored on 5- or 6-point scales that describe specific behaviors to be noted, ranging from less mature or minimal response to mature or full response, as defined individually for each test item.

INTERPRETATION. Preliminary analysis, using a Rasch model, of the items on the TIMP demonstrates that a hierarchy of difficulty exists and adequately separates infants by ability. The scale reflects both maturational level of subjects and degree of medical risk for mortality and morbidity across the range of age from 32 weeks' postconceptional age to 3.5 months postterm.

RELIABILITY AND VALIDITY

According to the test author, items are internally consistent (0.97). Intra- and interrater reliabilities are high, as demonstrated by Rasch model assessment of 5% or fewer misfitting ratings by each of five experienced examiners on 14 videotaped tests.[30] Construct validity was assessed by determining the test's sensitivity for assessing age-related changes in motor skill and correlation with risk for developmental abnormality. The correlation between postconceptual age and TIMP performance measures was 0.83. Risk and age together explained 72% of the variance in TIMP performance (r = .85, $p < .00001$).[31]

ADVANTAGES/DISADVANTAGES

Development of the TIMP has followed recommended procedures for assessing reliability and validity properties. Interested users of the test are encouraged to obtain the published reports of these issues and make informed decisions as to the appropriateness of the test for their population.

Alberta Infant Motor Scale

The Alberta Infant Motor Scale (AIMS),[32] an observational assessment scale, was constructed by Piper and associates to measure gross motor maturation in infants from birth through independent walking. The overall objectives of the AIMS are to (1) identify infants whose motor performance is delayed or aberrant relative to a normative group; (2) provide information to the clinician and parent(s) about the motor activities the infant has mastered, those currently developing, and those not in the infant's repertoire; (3) measure motor performance over time or before and after intervention; (4) measure changes in motor performance that are quite small and thus not likely to be detected using more traditional motor measures; and (5) act as an appropriate research tool to assess the efficacy of rehabilitation programs for infants with motor disorders.

TEST MEASURES AND TARGET POPULATION

The test is an assessment of gross motor performance designed for the identification and evaluation of motor development of infants from term (40 weeks postconception) through the age of independent walking (0 to 18 months of age). The focus of the assessment is on the evaluation of the sequential development of postural control relative to four postural positions: supine, prone, sitting, and standing.

TEST CONSTRUCTION AND STANDARDIZATION

Test items were obtained through an exhaustive review of existing instruments and descriptive narratives of early motor development. Content validation of the instrument was accomplished through meetings with and a mail survey of Canadian pediatric physical therapists and consultation with an international panel of experts. A total of 58 items were included in the provisional test for reliability and validity testing. Five hundred and six infants, age-stratified from birth through 18 months, participated in the reliability and validity testing of the AIMS. Scale properties were examined using the following techniques: multidimensional scaling, item response theory, and Guttman scaling. In addition, 20 infants who were experiencing abnormal motor development and 50 infants at risk for motor disorders were assessed and compared with the results of the full-term sample. The establishment of norms for the AIMS involved data collection on 2200 Albertan infants stratified by age and sex.[33]

TEST FORMAT

TYPE. The test is criterion-referenced with normed percentile ranks to allow for the determination of where an individual stands on the ability or trait being measure compared with those in the reference group.

CONTENT. The test includes 58 items organized into four positions: prone, supine, sitting, and standing. The distribution of these items is as follows: 21 prone, 9 supine, 12 sitting, and 16 standing. For each item, certain key descriptors are identified that must be observed for the infant to pass the items. Each item describes three aspects of motor performance—weight-bearing, posture, and antigravity movements.

ADMINISTRATION/SCORING. The administration of the test involves observational assessment with minimal handling required. The surface of the body bearing weight, posture, and movement are assessed for each item. The scoring is pass/fail. Scores in each area (prone, supine, sitting, standing) are summed to one total score of items passed.

INTERPRETATION. Age levels for stages of development are inherent in the test. Percentiles derived from the norming sample provide a comparison for monitoring a child's motor maturation over time.

RELIABILITY AND VALIDITY

The original sample consisted of 506 (285 males, 221 females) normal infants, age-stratified from birth through 18 months. One hundred twenty infants were scored on the AIMS, Peabody, and Bayley Scales for an assessment of concurrent validity and 253 infants were each scored two or three times on the AIMS to assess the interrater and test–retest reliability of the AIMS.[33]

The authors found an interrater reliability of 0.99 and a test–retest reliability of 0.99. Correlation coefficients reflecting concurrent validity with the Bayley and Peabody scales were determined to be $r = .98$ and $r = .97$, respectively.[33]

ADVANTAGES AND DISADVANTAGES

The AIMS provides the ability to detect, as early as possible, any deviations from the norm; thereby permitting early intervention to remediate or minimize the effects of dysfunction. Use of percentile ranking should be done with caution because a small change in raw score can result in a large change in percentile ranking.[34]

Gross Motor Function Measure

The Gross Motor Function Measure (GMFM),[35,36] developed by the Gross Motor Measures Group, was designed for use by pediatric therapists as an evaluative measure for assessing change over time in gross motor function of children with cerebral palsy.

TEST MEASURES AND TARGET POPULATION

The test is designed to assess motor function, or how much of an activity a child can accomplish. It is an evaluative index of gross motor function and changes in function over time, or after therapy, specifically for children with cerebral palsy (CP) or head injuries.

TEST CONSTRUCTION AND STANDARDIZATION

The GMFM was developed and tested according to contemporary principles of measurement design through a process of item selection, reliability testing, and validation procedures. The selection of items was based on a literature review and the judgment of pediatric clinicians. Items were judged to have the potential of showing change in the function of children. All items usually could be accomplished by a 5-year-old with normal motor abilities.[35,36]

TEST FORMAT

TYPE. Criterion-based observational measure.

CONTENT. The test includes 88 items that assess motor function in five dimensions: (1) lying and rolling; (2) sitting; (3) crawling and kneeling; (4) standing; and (5) walking, running, and jumping. Because the aim of treatment is to maximize the child's potential for independent function, it was considered important to determine whether a child could complete the task independently (with or without the use of aids), without any active assistance from another person.

ADMINISTRATION/SCORING. For ease of administration, the items are grouped on the rating form by test position and arranged in a developmental sequence. For scoring purposes, items are aggregated to represent five separate areas of motor function. Each GMFM item is scored on a four-point Likert scale. Values of 0, 1, 2, and 3 are assigned to each of the four categories; 0 = cannot do; 1 = initiates (<10% of the task); 2 = partially completes (10 to <100% of the task); and 3 = task completion. A one-page score sheet is used to record results. Specific descriptions for how to score each item are found in the administration and scoring guidelines contained within the test manual.[36]

INTERPRETATION. Each of the five dimensions contributes equal weight to the total score; therefore, a percent score is calculated for each dimension (child's score/maximum score × 100 percent). A total score is obtained by adding the percent scores for each dimension and dividing by five. A "goal score" can also be calculated in order to increase the responsiveness of the GMFM: For this score only those dimensions identified as goal areas by the therapist at time of evaluation are included. (For example, if standing as well as walk, run, and jump activities were treatment goals, the goal total score is calculated by adding the percent score obtained for both these dimensions and dividing by two.[35])

RELIABILITY AND VALIDITY

The test authors found intraobserver reliability for each dimension and the total score to range from 0.92 to 0.99 and interobserver reliability to range from 0.87 to 0.99 (ICC[2,1]).[35] A subsequent study using videotapes resulted in ICCs of 0.75 to 0.97.[36]

Construct validity was assessed by establishing the GMFM responsiveness to change over time.[35] Four hypotheses were tested: (1) that if the measure were responsive, it should be capable of detecting change in children judged by their parents and therapists; (2) that children with "mild" CP should show more change per unit of time than age-matched children with "severe" CP; (3) that younger children with CP should change more than older children in the same time period; and (4) that children recovering from acute head injury should show more change than children with CP. The scale was applied to 140 children of various ages with a wide range of neuromotor disabilities and to 30 healthy preschool-aged children on two occasions separated by a 3- to 6-month interval.

To address the concern of reliable use of the GMFM, the effects of training pediatric developmental therapists to administer and score the GMFM were examined.[36] The authors found that clinicians who attended a 1-day GMFM training workshop improved their scoring reliability significantly when tested using videotaped assessments. To make training more accessible to therapists who are unable to attend a workshop, the Gross Motor Measures Group has developed a videodisc training package that contains videotape examples of children similar to those used for a workshop, along with a written commentary.

ADVANTAGES/DISADVANTAGES

The GMFM is based on comprehensive development and testing and continues to be refined as it is used and studied. Clear administration and scoring guidelines are available, as well as training workshops and videotapes. It is designed to assess function in a quantitative manner, without regard to the quality of performance; therefore, it is likely that the changes detected by the GMFM reflect only part of the "real" change in motor behavior over time. For that reason, the Gross Motor Measures Group developed the Gross Motor Performance Measure.

Gross Motor Performance Measure

TEST MEASURES AND TARGET POPULATION

The Gross Motor Performance Measure (GM PM)[37–39] was developed to evaluate the quality of movement of children with cerebral palsy (CP). This measure was developed to be used in conjunction with the Gross Motor Function Measure (GMFM). The distinction between the two measures is that the GMFM measures how much a child can do, whereas the GMPM measures quality of performance, or how well a child performs a subset of the same gross motor tasks.

TEST CONSTRUCTION

Principles of contemporary test construction were used in the development of the GMPM: (1) a collaborative multicenter and multidisciplinary approach; (2) use of standard methodologic steps in instrument development; and (3) use of consensual methods with therapists and experts.[37] After reviewing the literature relative to attributes of gross motor performance, definitions were written for 33 attributes. Through nominal groups process meetings the number of attributes were reduced to five and attribute scales were developed. An international panel of experts provided the basis for content validity of the GMPM. Assessment of construct validity and reliability were performed.[38,39] The authors state that further work is required to add to the evidence of the validity and reliability of the GMPM.

TEST FORMAT

Type. The GMPM is a criterion-referenced observational instrument.

Content. The measure consists of 20 items derived from the GMFM, each of which is matched with three designated attributes of performance. Possible attributes to be assessed include (1) alignment; (2) stability; (3) coordination; (4) weight shift; and (5) dissociation. Definitions are provided for each of the attributes.

Administration/Scoring. The instrument can be administered with a minimum of equipment in less than 1 hour, depending on assessor skill, developmental stage, and cooperation of the child. Children are assessed only on items in which they can achieve at least a partial GMFM score, meaning that they can initiate an activity, thereby allowing an assessment of motor quality. Some children have motor performance assessed on all 20 items, whereas others are assessed on as few as two or three items.

A five-point scale (1 = severely abnormal, 2 = moderate abnormal, 3 = mildly abnormal, 4 = inconsistently normal, and 5 = consistently normal) is used to score each attribute.[37–39] In total, a maximum of 60 GMPM items (three attributes for each of 20 GMFM items) can be scored. The mean score obtained for each attribute is calculated and converted to a percentage. This is referred to as the attribute percent score. The mean of the five attribute percent scores is then computed to give a total percent score.

INTEPRETATION. Scores are used to track change over time and as a result of therapeutic intervention. At this stage of development, the GMPM scores have been correlated with therapists' global ratings of change and with varying severity of disability.

RELIABILITY AND VALIDITY

During development testing the ICCs [2,1] for the total percent scores varied from 0.92 to 0.96 for intrarater, interrater, and test–retest reliability. The ICCs for the five attribute percent scores varied from 0.90 to 0.97 for intrarater reliability, from 0.84 to 0.94 for interrater reliability, and from 0.89 to 0.96 for test–retest reliability.[38]

Concurrent and construct validity and responsiveness of the GMPM were investigated.[39] Five hypotheses were tested: (1) that children will show different change according to diagnosis; (2) that children with CP will show different change according to severity classification; (3) that younger children with CP will show more change than older children; (4) that GMPM scores will correlate with GMFM scores; and (5) that change scores on the GMPM will correlate with therapist ratings of change. A measure of responsiveness was obtained by relating the variability in test scores of stable children to the scores of children who were identified as changing.

Results show that the GMPM is sensitive to diagnostic differences and severity of CP differences. Correlation between GMFM and GMPM was inconsistent across age groups and diagnoses. Differential change according to age was not supported, nor was the relationship between GMPM scores and therapist ratings of change. Responsiveness to change was supported with changes in GMPM total scores accurately reflecting therapist judgments of overall change in performance in children with CP.

ADVANTAGES/DISADVANTAGES

The GMPM represents an important attempt to construct and validate an observational measure of quality of movement for use with children with CP. According to the authors, there are advantages in utilizing an existing measure of gross motor function as a source of observable activities. There are also difficulties, however, for observers to distinguish between motor function and performance in scoring activities.[39] The authors state that "future work may involve refinement of the GMPM measure as a clinical tool and evaluation of observer training techniques to ensure that potential users are capable of learning and applying the instrument to the complex patterns of motor behavior in children with CP."[39] Therefore, the reader who is interested in this instrument should obtain the original reports and contact the authors directly for the most current edition.

Peabody Developmental Motor Scales

The Peabody Developmental Motor Scales (PD MS) and Activity Cards[26] represent a comprehensive program combining in-depth assessment with instructional programming. The test was developed by Folio and Fewell between 1969 and 1982.

TEST MEASURES AND TARGET POPULATION

The PDMS provides a comprehensive sequence of gross and fine motor skills from which the therapist can determine the relative developmental skill level of a child, identify skills that are not completely developed or not in the child's repertoire, and plan an instructional program to develop those skills.[40]

Children from birth through 83 months of age are candidates for the text. The PDMS can be used with both able-bodied and disabled children.

TEST CONSTRUCTION AND STANDARDIZATION

The PDMS was developed to improve on the existing instruments used for motor evaluation. Test items were obtained from validated motor scales, and new items were created based on studies of children's growth and development. The test was standardized on a sample of 617 children considered to be representative of the American population by geographical region, race, and sex.

TEST FORMAT

TYPE. The PDMS is an individually administered test. Instructions are provided that enable examiners to give the test to groups of children in a station-testing format. Although the PDMS is norm-referenced, it can be used as a criterion-referenced measure of motor patterns and skills.

CONTENT. The PDMS is divided into two components: the Gross Motor Scale and the Fine Motor Scale. The Gross Motor Scale contains 170 items divided into 17 age levels. The items are divided into five categories of skills, including reflexes, balance, nonlocomotor, locomotor, and receipt and propulsion of objects.

The Fine Motor Scale contains 112 items divided into 16 age levels. The items are classified into four skill categories that include grasping, use of hands, eye-hand coordination, and manual dexterity. Norms are provided for each skill category at each age level, as well as for total scores.

ADMINISTRATION. Both scales can be given to a child in approximately 45 to 60 minutes. Basal (item preceding earliest failure) and ceiling (item representing the most difficult success) rules are provided to eliminate unnecessary administration of items, thereby reducing the time taken for testing.

No specialized training is required to administer the scales and implement the activities, although the examiner should be thoroughly familiar with and have had practice in giving the test. In order to use the PDMS, norms for valid interpretation of a child's performance, the scales must be given exactly as specified, including the presentation of materials, verbal instructions to the child, and adherence to basal and ceiling rules.[40] When instructional programming is the main purpose for testing, the directions can be adapted to fit the child's handicapped condition while retaining the intent of the item.

SCORING. The norms of the PDMS are based on scoring each item as 0, 1, or 2. Specific criteria are given for each item, as are the general criteria for the numeric scores. Scores are assigned as follows:

0. The child cannot or will not attempt the item.
1. The child's performance shows a clear resemblance to the item criterion but does not fully meet the criterion. (This value allows for emerging skills.)
2. The child accomplishes the item according to the specified item criterion.

INTERPRETATION. Raw scores are determined and can be converted, by using the norms tables, to normative scores, which included percentile rank scores, standard scores, age-equivalent scores, and scaled scores. After the standard scores have been determined, they may be plotted on the Motor Development Profile. This profile provides a means of visually comparing performance on the Gross Motor Scale and Fine

Motor Scale and on the skill categories in each scale.

RELIABILITY AND VALIDITY

Test–retest reliability for the total score is 0.99 for both scales. The test–retest reliability is 0.95 for items given on the Gross Motor Scale and 0.8 for the Fine Motor Scale.[40] Interobserver reliability for total scores is 0.99 for both scales. When calculated on an item-by-item basis, the reliability coefficients are 0.97 for the Gross Motor and 0.94 for the Fine Motor Scale.[40] Subsequent research has shown similar results for interobserver reliability.[41] The strong reliability data indicate that PDMS is a highly stable assessment instrument.

According to the authors, the content validity of PDMS is based on established research on normal children's motor development and on other validated tests assessing motor development.[40] All of the data related to construct validity indicate that PDMS is a valid instrument for assessing motor development and that PDMS can discriminate motor problems from normal developmental variability.[40]

ADVANTAGES

The PDMS is a standardized, reliable, and valid assessment tool that is both norm-referenced and criterion-referenced and that allows the scales to meet the needs of various users. The three-point scoring system enables examiners to identify emerging skills and to measure progress in children who are slow in acquiring new skills. The scales are translated into a specific instructional program—the activity cards. Administration can be adapted for disabled children.

DISADVANTAGES

Several drawbacks of the PDMS have been identified by its researchers and users.[41,42] The Peabody kit does not provide all of the items necessary for administration of the Fine Motor and Gross Motor scales, thus threatening standardization. The test manual does not provide clear criteria for each item for assigning a score of 1, thereby leaving the raters to decide whether there is a resemblance to the criteria needed for a successful performance.

Bruininks-Oseretsky Test of Motor Proficiency

The Bruininks-Oseretsky Test (BOT) of Motor Proficiency was developed by Dr. Robert H. Bruininks and is based partly on the American adaptation of the Oseretsky Tests of Motor Proficiency.[43] Although some similarity exists between the items in the two tests, the revised test reflects important advances in content, structure, and technical qualities.[43]

TEST MEASURES AND TARGET POPULATION

The BOT is designed to assess gross and fine motor functioning in children so that a decision can be made about appropriate educational and therapeutic placement. The Complete Battery—eight subtests comprising 46 separate items—provides a comprehensive index of motor proficiency, as well as separate measures of both gross and fine motor skills.

This test is appropriate for children from 4 ½ to 14 ½ years of age. This test is designed for use with normal and developmentally disabled populations.

TEST CONSTRUCTION AND STANDARDIZATION

Development and evaluation of the BOT has been extensive. The test has been standardized on a sample of 765 children who were carefully selected on the basis of age, sex, size of their community, and geographic location based on the 1970 census in the United States.

TEST FORMAT

TYPE. The BOT is norm-referenced, and it involves individually administered tasks with direct observation and assessment of a child in a structured environment.

CONTENT. Each of the eight subtests is designed to assess an important aspect of motor development. The fine motor tests include coordination of the upper limbs, speed of response, visuomotor control, and speed and dexterity of the upper limbs. The subtests for gross motor skills assess speed and agility while turning, balance, bilateral coordination, and strength. The relationship of the eight subtests to the composites is shown in Figure 2-3.

ADMINISTRATION. The entire battery can be given in 45 to 60 minutes. Two short testing sessions are recommended for young children. A large area, relatively free from distraction, is required. Examiners do not need special training, but they must be familiar with the directions for giving the test. Procedures for administration and scoring of the test are well written and are shown in the manual. All of the materials needed to administer the BOT are provided in the standardized test kit.

SCORING. The person's raw scores are recorded during the administration of the test and are converted first to point scores, then to standard scores and approximate age equivalents (see Fig. 2-4 for a sample record form).

INTERPRETATION. Tables of norms are provided, and by comparing derived scores with the scores of subjects tested in the standardization program, users can interpret a person's performance in relation to a national reference group.

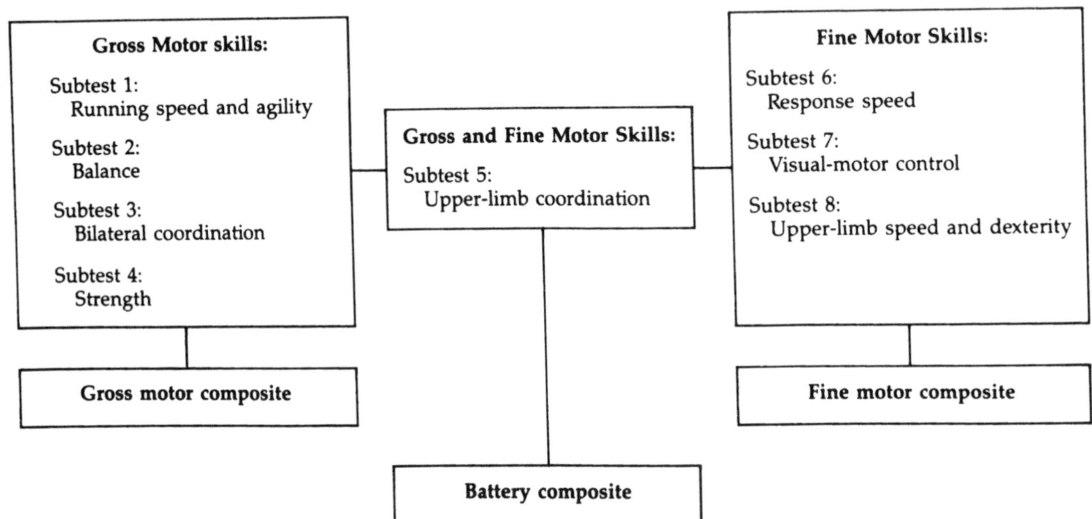

Figure 2-3 ▪ Relationship of the eight subtests of the Bruininks-Oseretsky Test of Motor Proficiency to the composite test. (Adapted from Bruininks RH: *Examiner's Manual for Bruininks-Oseretsky Test of Motor Proficiency,* Circle Pines, MN: American Guidance Service; 1978:12.)

SUBTEST 1: Running Speed and Agility

RECORD POINT SCORES FOR COMPLETE BATTERY | RECORD POINT SCORES FOR SHORT FORM

1. **Running Speed and Agility**[SF*]

TRIAL 1: 8.7 seconds TRIAL 2: 7.5 seconds

Raw Score	Above 11.0	10.9-11.0	10.5-10.8	9.9-10.4	9.5-9.8	8.9-9.4	8.5-8.8	7.9-8.4	7.5-7.8	6.9-7.4	6.7-6.8	6.3-6.6	6.1-6.2	5.7-6.0	5.5-5.6	Below 5.5
Point Score	0	1	2	3	4	5	6	7	8	9	10	11	12	13	14	15

Point score: 8

POINT SCORE SUBTEST 1 (Max: 15)

SUBTEST 2: Balance

1. **Standing on Preferred Leg on Floor** *(10 seconds maximum per trial)*

TRIAL 1: 10 seconds TRIAL 2: ______ seconds

Raw Score	0	1-3	4-5	6-8	9-10
Point Score	0	1	2	3	4

Point score: 4

2. **Standing on Preferred Leg on Balance Beam**[SF] *(10 seconds maximum per trial)*

TRIAL 1: 2 seconds TRIAL 2: 4 seconds

Raw Score	0	1-2	3-4	5-6	7-8	9	10
Point Score	0	1	2	3	4	5	6

Point score: 2

3. **Standing on Preferred Leg on Balance Beam—Eyes Closed** *(10 seconds maximum per trial)*

TRIAL 1: 2 seconds TRIAL 2: 5 seconds

Raw Score	0	1-3	4-5	6	7	8	9	10
Point Score	0	1	2	3	4	5	6	7

Point score: 2

4. **Walking Forward on Walking Line** *(6 steps maximum per trial)*

TRIAL 1: 6 steps TRIAL 2: ______ steps

Raw Score	0	1-3	4-5	6
Point Score	0	1	2	3

Point score: 3

5. **Walking Forward on Balance Beam** *(6 steps maximum per trial)*

TRIAL 1: 2 steps TRIAL 2: 4 steps

Raw Score	0	1-3	4	5	6
Point Score	0	1	2	3	4

Point score: 2

6. **Walking Forward Heel-to-Toe on Walking Line** *(6 steps maximum per trial)*

TRIAL 1: [1|0|0|0|1|0] = 2 steps TRIAL 2: [1|1|0|0|1|0] = 3 steps

Raw Score	0	1-3	4-5	6
Point Score	0	1	2	3

Point score: 1

7. **Walking Forward Heel-to-Toe on Balance Beam**[SF] *(6 steps maximum per trial)*

TRIAL 1: [1|0|0|0|0|0] = 1 steps TRIAL 2: [1|1|0|0|1|0] = 3 steps

Raw Score	0	1-3	4	5	6
Point Score	0	1	2	3	4

Point score: 1

8. **Stepping Over Response Speed Stick on Balance Beam**

TRIAL 1: Fail (Pass) TRIAL 2: Fail Pass

Raw Score	Fail	Pass
Point Score	0	1

Point score: 1

Total: 16

POINT SCORE SUBTEST 2 (Max: 32)

*SF and the box in left-hand margin indicates short form.

Figure 2-4 ■ Recording form for the eight subtests of the Bruininks-Oseretsky Test of Motor Proficiency. (Adapted from Bruininks RH: *Examiner's Manual for Bruininks-Oseretsky Test of Motor Proficiency.* Circle Pines, MN: American Guidance Service; 1978:37.)

RELIABILITY AND VALIDITY

Test–retest reliability scores average 0.87 for the complete battery. Interobserver reliability is excellent, with the results of two studies showing a reliability of 0.98 and 0.90.[43]

The validity of the BOT, according to Bruininks, "is based on its ability to assess the construct of motor development or proficiency."[43] In terms of motor proficiency, as measured by the performance of a particular child on a particular day, the BOT is a valid test.[8] The tests discriminate well between nonhandicapped populations and children learning who are disabled or mentally retarded.

ADVANTAGES AND DISADVANTAGES

The testing procedure is standardized and scores are normed. This is an excellent instrument for evaluating school-aged children who show motor problems but who do not have an obvious physical handicap. The test is valuable as a research tool because of the ability to differentiate between populations.

One of the potential disadvantages of this test is that the space required to administer the BOT may limit its usefulness.

Comprehensive Developmental Scales

A basic component of any physical therapy assessment is a developmental evaluation. Developmental testing looks at the whole child, across all areas of development. These developmental areas include language, personal-social, fine motor, gross motor, self-help, and cognitive development. By using a comprehensive assessment, the therapist can develop strategies for treatment that address the whole child.

Gesell Developmental Schedules

The Gesell Developmental Schedules were developed by Arnold Gesell and his associates beginning in the 1920s. The original test items and procedures have been modified and updated through the years.[3] The Gesell schedules are the basis for future developmental scales.

TEST MEASURES AND TARGET POPULATION

The test assesses behavior in the areas of adaptive, gross motor, fine motor, language, and personal-social development. It can be used to identify even minor deviations in children, and to determine the maturity and integrity of an individual's CNS.

The test is appropriate for children of ages 4 weeks to 36 months. Additional schedules are available to test children up to 60 months of age.

TEST CONSTRUCTION AND STANDARDIZATION

During years of studying a large number of normal children, Gesell mapped the development of fetal, infant, and early behavior in children. The schedules have been standardized by Gesell and associates.

TEST FORMAT

Type. The Gesell test is norm-referenced and involves direct assessment and observation by the examiner of the quality of and integration of behaviors.

Content. Standardized materials can be obtained, or substitutes can be made according to the directions provided.[3] Developmental schedules show the behavioral characteristics of a key age and its two adjacent ages in three vertical columns. The key age occupies the central position (see Fig. 2-5 for an example of the key age

H = History
O = Observation

	12 Weeks	KEY AGE: 16 Weeks	20 Weeks
Adaptive	Dangling Ring: prompt midline regard (*16w) Dangling Ring: follows 180° Rattle: glances at in hand Cube, Cup: regards more than momentarily	Dangling Ring, Ra: regards immediately Dangling Ring, Rattle, Cube, Cup: arms activate (*24w) Dangling Ring, Rattle: regards in hand Dangling Ring: to mouth D. Ring: free hand to midline (*28w) Tabletop: looks down at table top or hands Cube, Cup: looks from hand to object (*20w) Pellet: regards recurrently	Rattle, Bell: 2-hand approach (*28w) Rattle, Dangling Ring: grasps only if near hand (*24w) Rattle: visual pursuit lost rattle Cube: holds 1st regards 2nd Massed Cubes: grasps 1 on contact (*24w)
Gross Motor	Supine: head predominantly half side (tonic-neck-reflex) (*16w) Supine: midposition head and symmetric postures seen Sit: head set forward, bobs (*16w) Stand: small fraction weight briefly Stand: lifts foot (*28w) Prone: head Zone II, sustainedly Prone: on forearms (*20w) Prone: hips low, legs flexed (*40w)	Supine: midposition head predominates Supine: symmetric postures predominate Supine: hands engage (*24w) Sit: head steady, set forward (*20w) Prone: head Zone III, sustainedly Prone: legs extended or semi-extended (*40w) Prone: verge of rolling (*20w)	Pull-to-Sit: no head lag Sit: head erect, steady Prone: arms extended
Fine Motor	Supine: hands open or loosely closed Rattle: holds actively Cup: contacts	Dangling Ring: retains Supine: fingers, scratches, clutches (*24w)	Prone or Tabletop: scratches tabletop or platform (*28w) Cube: precarious grasp (*24w)
Language	Vocalization: coos (*36w) Vocalization: chuckles Social: vocal-social response	Expressive: excites, breathes heavily (*32w) Vocalization: laughs aloud	Vocalization: squeals (*36w)
Personal-Social	Social: vocal-social response Supine: regards examiner predominantly Play: hand regard (*16w) Play: pulls at dress (*24w)	Social: spontaneous social smile Social: vocalizes or smiles, pulled to sitting (*24w) Feeding: anticipates food on sight Play: sits propped 10-15 minutes (*40w) Play: hand play, mutual fingering (*24w) Play: pulls dress over face (*24w)	Social: smiles at mirror image Feeding: pats bottle, both hands (*36w)

Figure 2-5 ▪ Key Age chart from the Gesell Developmental Schedules for a 16-week-old child. (Knobloch H. Pasamanick B. *Gesell and Armatruda's Developmental Diagnosis.* 3rd Ed. Philadelphia: JB Lippincott; 1974:42.)

of 16 weeks). Horizontally, the characteristics of behavior are grouped according to the five major behavioral fields.

ADMINISTRATION. As far as is possible, the standard sequences should be followed in the administration of the examination. The standard sequence differs depending on the maturity and age of the child. Examination procedures used in administering the individual items are well described and should be given in the prescribed, standardized manner[3] (Display 2-2).

SCORING. Two columns are provided on the developmental schedules for scoring: H for history, and O for observation. Some information is available only by report, particularly when it concerns language and personal-social behavior. A minus sign (−) indicates that the behavior does not occur, a plus sign (+) signifies the behavior occurs. And a plus-minus (±) notation is made if the behavior is just emerging but has not yet been fully integrated. A double plus sign (++) is recorded if a more mature pattern is observed.

INTERPRETATION. The final estimate of developmental maturity is based on the distribution of pluses and minuses. This estimate is not merely achieved by adding the pluses and minuses but by determining how well a child's behavior fits one age level rather than another. In

DISPLAY 2-2

Prescribed and Standardized Examination Sequence for the Administration of Test Items for the Gesell Developmental Schedules*

Age: 12–16–20 Weeks	Situation No. (Appendix A-4)
Supine	1
Dangling ring	2
Rattle	3
Social stimulation	4
Bell ringing	5
Pull-to-sitting	6
Sitting supported	50
Chair—table top	
Cube 1,(2)	7,8
Massed cubes	11
(Cup)	16
Pellet	18
(Bell)	22
Mirror	24
Standing supported	51
Prone	52

Note: Italicized items appear for the first time in this sequence. Items in parentheses refer to situations sometimes omitted for special reasons.

Normative behavior characteristic of the *key age: 16 weeks* and adjacent age levels is codified by the Developmental Schedule.

*Adapted from Knobloch H, Pasamanick B. *Gesell and Armatruda's Developmental Diagnosis,* 3rd ed. Philadelphia: JB Lippincott: 1974:43.

any field of behavior, the child's maturity level is that point at which the aggregate of plus signs changes to an aggregate of minus signs.[3] The examiner assigns a representative age to each of the four areas, as well as an overall age. The ages can then be used to work out a developmental quotient (DQ), which is the age of maturity divided by the chronologic age.[44]

RELIABILITY AND VALIDITY

Knobloch and Pasamanick reported that, on more than 100 clinical observations, a correlation of 0.98 was found between the DQs assigned by 18 pediatricians and those assigned by their instructor.[3] Test–retest reliability is reported to be 0.82 for 65 infants examined within 2 to 3 days of the initial date of testing.[3]

Correlations between infant and later examinations range from 0.5 to 0.85.[27]

ADVANTAGES AND DISADVANTAGES

The test's reliability and validity are generally excellent, and it is a good diagnostic tool. Testing procedures are standardized. This test is especially useful in research.

One disadvantage of the test is that the directions for testing are quite involved and require extensive practice and use in order to ensure valid results.

Bayley Scales of Infant Development

The Bayley Scales of Infant Development (BSID) were devised by Nancy Bayley and associates and are essentially a revision of Bayley's earlier work.[6]

TEST MEASURES AND TARGET POPULATION

The Bayley Scales are a comprehensive means of evaluating a child's current developmental status at a particular age. The scales are composed of three parts, each of which is designed to assess a separate component of the child's total development. The Mental Scale is designed to assess sensory-perceptual acuities, discrimination, and the ability to respond to these; the early acquisition of object constancy, as well as memory, learning, and problem-solving ability; vocalization and the beginnings of verbal communication; and early evidence of the ability to form generalizations and classifications, which is the basis for abstract thinking. The Motor Scale is designed to provide a measure of the degree of control of the body, and coordination of the large muscles and finer manipulatory skills of the hands and fingers. The Infant Behavior Record assesses the nature of the child's social and objective orientations toward the environment as expressed in attitudes, interests, emotions, energy, activity, and tendencies to approach or withdraw from stimulation.

The appropriate population for the BSID includes infants and toddlers between the ages of 1 and 30 months.

TEST CONSTRUCTION AND STANDARDIZATION

The current scales represent the culmination of more than 40 years of research and clinical practice with small children.[6] The test has been standardized on a sample of 1262 children, distributed in approximately equal numbers among 14 age groups ranging from 2 to 30 months. The sample was selected to be representative of the population in the United States, as described in the 1960 United States Census of Population.

TEST FORMAT

Type. The test is norm-referenced. Information is obtained by direct observation and interaction with the child.

Content. All materials needed for the test are included in the test kit except for stairs and a balance board. Materials have been selected carefully, and casual substitutions are discouraged. A manual describes the procedures and progression of the test.

Administration. The time required for administration of the BSID varies with the number and complexity of items that must be presented. An average testing time for the Mental and Motor Scales is approximately 45 minutes, with some children occasionally requiring 75 minutes or more. After the child leaves, the researcher completes the Infant Behavior Record.

Changes may be made in the order of presentation, but no changes should be made in the specified manner of presenting test stimuli, as any such change would invalidate scoring. The Mental Scale is usually administered before the Motor Scale because the change in pace from sitting to moving about is the preferred sequence.

Scoring and Interpretation. Individual record forms are used to record a response on the test. For each item, the child is graded as follows: pass (P), fail (F), omit (O), refuse (R), or reported by mother (RPT). Only those items noted as passed are credited in scoring the test, but other results are useful in reviewing the adequacy of the test as an accurate measure of the child's performance. A basal level (item preceding earliest failure) and a ceiling level (item representing the most difficult success) are determined. The raw scores are changed to the Mental Development Index (MDI) and the Psycho-motor Development Index (PDI) by consulting the norms for the child's particular age as derived by Bayley. An intelligence quotient should not be computed, because there is no evidence to support the interpretation of a figure of this kind derived from the BSID.[6]

RELIABILITY AND VALIDITY

The reliability of the 1958 to 1960 version of the Mental and Motor Scales, the immediate predecessor of the current version of the BSID, was assessed by Werner and Bayley. Interobserver reliability rates for the Mental Scale and the Motor Scale were 89.4% and 93.4%, respectively. Test–retest reliability was 76.4% for the Mental Scale and 75.3% for the Motor Scale.

The correlation between results derived from the BSID and the Stanford-Binet Scale has ranged from minimal to moderate. Because the scales have limited value as predictors of future abilities, they are most useful in ascertaining the developmental status of a particular child at a particular age.

ADVANTAGES

Collectively, the BSID probably represent the best standardized techniques for behavioral assessment available for infants. These scales have been used extensively as an instrument for research, and are helpful in determining the developmental status of infants at a particular age.

DISADVANTAGES

To administer the Bayley Scales, one must undergo training sessions and be validated as an examiner. The Bayley Motor Scale contains a small number of items for each level of development and omits stages that are generally accepted in the motor developmental sequence. For example, the Bayley Scales contain no items for running or kicking, and a single item incorporates all methods of the progression to walking. The Bayley Motor Scales, therefore, do not provide in-depth motor assessment nor do they delineate gross and fine motor development.[45]

Bayley II

After 24 years of use, the Bayley Scales of Infant Development (Revised Edition) were revised. The changing nature of child care and the accumulation of information regarding children's abilities led to the revision. The *Bayley II*[46] reflects current norms and allows diagnostic assessment at an earlier age.

The fundamentals of the test remain unchanged. It is a norm-referenced, standardized, three-part evaluation of the developmental status of children. The three parts are the Mental Scale, the Motor Scale, and the Behavior Rating Scale (formerly the Infant Behavior Record).

The revisions include (1) revised norms; (2) age range extended downward to 1 month and upward to 42 months; (3) new items measuring a broader skill range; (4) updated stimulus materials that are more attractive and durable; (5) improved psychometric properties, and improved clinical utility; and (6) new scoring procedures.

STANDARDIZATION

The *Bayley II* has been renormed on a stratified random sample of 1700 children (850 boys and 850 girls) ages 1 month to 42 months, grouped at 1 month intervals. The children came from all four geographic regions of the U.S. and closely parallel the 1988 U.S. Census statistics on the variables of age, gender, region, ethnicity, and parental education. These normative data enable the clinician to compare the infant's performance with same age peers and, if needed, help initiate intervention.

CLINICAL VALIDITY

The Bayley Scales were originally designed to assess normal development in infants and young children. Because the primary use of developmental scales today is with children who are at risk or suspected of bring at risk, an effort was made to gather more information about the use of the test with clinical samples.

The *Bayley II Manual* contains data for the following groups of children: children who were born prematurely, have the HIV antibody, were prenatally drug exposed, were asphyxiated at birth, are developmentally delayed, have frequent otitis media, are autistic, and/or have Down syndrome.

ADMINISTRATION AND SCORING

Although the fundamentals of the test remain unchanged, there have been some changes that facilitate the administration of the test. A second level of scoring was developed that is facet-based to match the content areas of cognition, language, person/social, and motor development. A developmental age for each facet can be obtained. This complements the traditional Mental/Motor Scale scoring.

Neonatal Behavioral Assessment Scale

The Neonatal Behavioral Assessment Scale (NBAS), 3rd edition,[47] was first developed by T. Berry Brazelton and published in 1973[48] with the help of many people who collaborated directly and indirectly. The second edition contains some additions and a few revisions designed to allay some of the criticisms of the first edition, as well as to restate some of the original purposes of the scale.

TEST MEASURES AND TARGET POPULATION

The NBAS closely approximates a developmental evaluation of the neonate. It is intended to be a means of scoring interactive behavior rather than a formal neurologic evaluation, although the neurologic implications of such a scale make inclusion of some basic neurologic items necessary. The evaluation is primarily behavioral and is an attempt to score the infant's available responses to the environment and, indirectly, the infant's effect on the environment.[47]

The NBAS is appropriate for the testing of children ages newborn to 1 month of age. It has been used to study both normal and premature infants, as well as infants from different national and ethnic groups.

TEST CONSTRUCTION AND STANDARDIZATION

No formal standardization sample has been used in the development of the NBAS. As yet, the normative base for the NBAS is relatively limited.[47] Researchers using the scale have provided their own normative data with the population for which they were using the NBAS.

TEST FORMAT

CONTENT. The score sheet includes 28 behavioral items and nine supplementary items (Display 2-3) that assess the neonate's capacity to organize states of consciousness, habituate reactions to disturbing events, attend to and process simple and complex events in the environment, control motor activity and postural tone while attending to these environmental events, and perform integrated motor acts.[47,49] The supplementary items have been developed for use with preterm, sick, fragile, and stressed infants, as well as to capture some of the more general characteristics of the infant's behavior in addition to the response of the examiner to the infant.[47] The test also includes 20 elicited (neurologic) responses (Display 2-4) that are based on Prechtl and Beintema's neurologic assessment of the infant.[50]

ADMINISTRATION. An important consideration throughout the tests is the state of consciousness or "state" of the infant,[47] classified according to six stages: (1) deep sleep; (2) light sleep; (3) drowsy or semidozing; (4) alert; (5) active; and (6) crying. The examiner attempts to bring the baby through an entire spectrum of states in each examination.

The examination usually takes 20 to 30 minutes and involves about 30 different tests and maneuvers. The examiner tries to elicit the best performance rather than an average performance from the infant; therefore, the examiner attempts to verify that the infant is incapable of

DISPLAY 2-3

Neonatal Behavioral Assessment Scale (NBAS)*

1. Response decrement to light (1,2)
2. Response decrement to rattle (1,2)
3. Response decrement to bell (1,2)
4. Response decrement to tactile stimulation of foot (1,2)
5. Orientation-inanimate visual (4,5)
6. Orientation-inanimate auditory (4,5)
7. Orientation-inanimate visual and auditory (4,5)
8. Orientation-animate visual (4,5)
9. Orientation-animate auditory (4,5)
10. Orientation-animate visual and auditory (4,5)
11. Alertness (4 only)
12. General tonus (4,5)
13. Motor maturity (4,5)
14. Pull-to-sit (4,5)
15. Cuddliness (4,5)
16. Defensive movements (3,4,5)
17. Consolability (6 to 5,4,3,2)
18. Peak of excitement (all states)
19. Rapidity of build-up (from 1,2 to 6)
20. Irritability (all awake states)
21. Activity (3,4,5)
22. Tremulousness (all states)
23. Startle (3,4,5,6)
24. Lability of skin color (from 1 to 6)
25. Lability of states (all states)
26. Self-quieting activity (6,5 to 4,3,2,1)
27. Hand-to-Mouth facility (all states)
28. Smiles (all states)

Supplementary Items

29. Alert responsiveness (4 only)
30. Cost of attention (3,4,5)
31. Examiner persistence (all states)
32. General irritability (5,6)
33. Robustness and endurance (all states)
34. Regulatory capacity (all states)
35. State regulation (all states)
36. Balance of motor tone (all states)
37. Reinforcement value of infant's behavior (all states)

*The behavior scale of the NBAS identifies the items examined and, in parentheses, the numbers of the appropriate states in which the assessment of each item on the scale can be made.

a better response. The examiner must be flexible in the sequence of item administration to allow most of the items to be given at a time when the best performance will be achieved. Use of the NBAS requires direct training by experienced examiners. There are seven established reliability training centers.[47]

SCORING. Most of the items are scored at the end of the examination. The elicited neurologic items are scored on a three-point scale designating low, medium, or high intensity of response. Asymmetry of response can also be noted. The behavioral items are each rated on a nine-point scale, with most of the items rated as optimal at the midpoint of the scale. A nine-point scale allows for a range of behavior that can bring out subtle differences among different groups of babies.

INTERPRETATION. The NBAS does not yield an overall score for an infant. Rather the results of the test are the scores for each of the items. The mean is related to the expected behavior of an "average" full-term, normal, white infant weighing 7 lb or more whose mother has not received more than 100 mg of barbiturates and 50 mg of other sedative drugs before delivery, whose Apgar scores were no less than seven at 1 minute, eight at 5 minutes, and eight at 15 minutes after delivery, who needed no special care after delivery, and who had an apparently normal intrauterine experience.[48]

DISPLAY 2-4

Elicited Responses of the Neonatal Behavioral Assessment Scale*

1. Plantar grasp
2. Hand grasp
3. Ankle clonus
4. Babinski's response
5. Standing
6. Automatic walking
7. Placing
8. Incurvatum
9. Crawling
10. Glabella
11. Tonic deviation of head and eyes
12. Nystagmus
13. Tonic neck reflex
14. Moro reflex
15. Rooting (intensity)
16. Sucking (intensity)

17–20. Passive movements: right arm; left arm; right leg; left leg

*Items the examiner attempts to elicit during the examination.

RELIABILITY AND VALIDITY

The reliability of independent testers trained at the same time is reported to range from 0.85 to 1.[20] Testers can be trained to a 0.9 criterion of reliability, and the level of reliability is still determined to be 0.9 or higher for a prolonged time.[47]

According to the author, test–retest reliability must be viewed in terms of the kinds of questions being posed when the NBAS is employed. It is clear that the standard psychometric criterion of a Pearson Product Moment Correlation Coefficient will yield low to moderate day-to-day stabilities. Conversely, an individually derived measure of day-to-day stability reveals quite a different and much more variable picture. Patterns of score changes over repeated examinations may well reveal important characteristics about individual infants and about groups of infants.[47]

In terms of validity, studies have shown that individual differences, as measured by the NBAS, are related to later individual differences.[47,48]

ADVANTAGES

The NBAS is an effective predictor of neurologic problems, as well as an effective teaching tool for parents. It is a valuable technique for differentiating the behavioral characteristics of normal neonates for research and clinical purposes.

DISADVANTAGES

Among the disadvantages of the NBAS is that it is a difficult test to learn, and the tester must guard against overinterpretation when discussing test results with physicians and parents.[20] When the time required for scoring, interpretation of the test, and writing of the report is considered, the test becomes a lengthy process. The relationship between results on the NBAS and those derived from later functional testing has yet to be demonstrated.

Early Intervention Developmental Profile

The Early Intervention Developmental Profile (EIDP) was developed by an interdisciplinary team at the University of Michigan under the direction of Schafer and Moersch.[51]

TEST MEASURES AND TARGET POPULATION

The EIDP is an infant assessment-based programming instrument made up of six scales that provide developmental norms and milestones in the following areas: perceptual or fine motor, cognition, language, social or emotional, self-care, and gross motor development. The profile should not be used to diagnose handicapping conditions, nor does it supply data that can predict future capabilities or handicaps. However, by examining a child's skills in six different areas, the profile helps describe the child's comprehensive function, identifying relative strengths and weaknesses.[51]

Designed for children from birth to 36 months, the EIDP yields information that can be used to plan comprehensive developmental programs for children with all types of handicaps who function below the 36-month level.

TEST CONSTRUCTION AND STANDARDIZATION

Test items were selected from well-known, standardized instruments for the evaluation of infants, including general developmental scales, motor scales, and language scales. Some original profile items were based on current developmental theories. The profile has not been standardized. Assignment of items to specific age ranges was based on standardizations or research from other instruments. The age-norm suggestions derived from the original source (i.e., Piaget) were used for original items.

TEST FORMAT

CONTENT. Each section of the profile is divided into age groupings, each of which covers 3 months within the first year of life and 4 months within the second and third years. No consistent attempt was made to arrange items within age ranges in a developmental sequence.

The gross motor scale reflects a body of knowledge that constitutes the basis for the current treatment of cerebral palsy in infants and young children (e.g., Bobath and Fiorentino). There is an emphasis on neurodevelopmental theories of reflex development and integration of primitive reflexes into higher order righting reactions, protective responses, and equilibrium responses.[51]

The cognitive scale reflects the theories of Piaget, whereas the social-emotional scale reflects current theory on the emotional attachment between the mother and child and the child's gradual acquisition of ego functions during the first 36 months of life.[51]

ADMINISTRATION. The profile was designed to be given by a multidisciplinary team that includes a psychologist or special educator, physical or occupational therapist, and a speech and language therapist. Each member of the team can learn to give the entire profile, rather than being limited to only certain scales by one's chosen discipline. Administration of test items is thoroughly explained in the evaluation manual. References for each item are well documented. Test items are given until the child fails either six consecutive items or all items in two consecutive age ranges. The total time required for administration of the test may vary from 30 minutes to several hours. The materials needed for administration are described in the manual and should be available.

SCORING. Items are scored as a "pass" (P) when the criteria are met; however, when the child's behavior on an item does not meet scoring criteria, it is scored as a "fail" (F). A score of "pass-fail" (PF) indicates the emergence of a skill. An item is scored as "omitted" (O) when the evaluator must exclude an item.

INTERPRETATION. Ceiling levels (the age range containing the child's highest passed item) and basal levels (the age range preceding the child's earliest failure) are determined for each section. The ceiling and basal levels define a range of items on which the child's performance is inconsistent, which will provide the focus for programming efforts. Age levels for each area of performance are recorded on a composite table to yield a profile. Each testing booklet can be used for several subsequent evaluations, with the composite profile recorded with a different color or line notation for each item to document the child's progress.

RELIABILITY AND VALIDITY

Interobserver and test–retest reliability values were assessed using small sample sizes; however, the results were generally excellent. Interobserver reliability ranged from a low of 80% to a high of 97%. Test–retest reliability ranged from 93% to 98%.[51]

Significant correlations were found between children's scores on the EIDP, the BSID, the Vineland Society Maturity Scale, and clinical motor evaluations. Thus, strong validity of content was found for the EIDP.

ADVANTAGES AND DISADVANTAGES

The combined results of the six scales provide a comprehensive record of the child's skills. Moreover, the completed profile lends itself well to the formulation of individualized objectives. The third volume of *Developmental Programming for Infants and Children: Stimulation Activities* is a comprehensive collection of sequenced activities designed to complement the Developmental Profile.[52] The EIDP reflects current developmental theory in the motor, cognitive, and social areas and is best used as a clinical instrument for interdisciplinary team planning.

The sample sizes for reliability and validity testing were small. Thus, the EIDP cannot be used for diagnosis or for predicting future capabilities or handicaps.

Assessment of Functional Capabilities

Functional capabilities are viewed as skills that are essential within the child's natural environments of home and school. According to Haley,[53] the concept of disability and functional assessment incorporates the following key concepts:

1. A child may have serious motor impairments that are not always reflected by the level of functional limitation or disability.
2. Functional deficits may or may not lead to a restriction in social activities and important childhood roles.
3. Environmental factors, family expectations, and contextual elements of functional task requirements play an important role in the eventual level of disability and handicap of the child.

Comprehensive functional assessment instruments contain mobility, transfer, self-care, and social function items; they include measurement dimensions of assistance and adaptive equipment; and they incorporate developmental stages of functional skill attainment.[54] Pediatric physical therapists have long expressed the need for a functional approach to the assessment of children with movement disorders.

Pediatric Evaluation of Disability Inventory

The Pediatric Evaluation of Disability Inventory (PEDI)[55] was developed to meet the need for a reliable, valid, and norm-referenced instrument for assessing functional status in infants and young children by physical therapists and other rehabilitation personnel. The PEDI was designed to be a comprehensive yet clinically feasible instrument that can be used for clinical assessment, program monitoring, documentation of functional progress, and clinical decision making.[56]

TEST MEASURES AND TARGET POPULATION

The PEDI measures both the capability and performance of functional activities in three content domains: (1) self-care; (2) mobility; and (3) social function. Capability is measured by the identification of functional skills for which the child has demonstrated mastery and competence (Display 2-5). Functional performance is measured by the level of caregiver assistance and environmental modifications needed to accomplish major functional activities (Display 2-6).

Children ranging in age from 6 months to 7.5 years may be tested. The PEDI is primarily designed for the evaluation of young children, but it can be used to evaluate older children whose functional abilities fall below those expected of 7.5-year-old children with no disabilities.

TEST CONSTRUCTION AND STANDARDIZATION

The content and measurement scales of the PEDI underwent numerous revisions prior to the publication of the final version. Initially, content was identified based on the available literature, previous functional and adaptive tests, and the clinical experience of the authors and consultant involved. A Development Edition was field-tested on more than 60 handicapped children and their families. The scales' comprehensiveness and representativeness was evaluated by external content experts. Revisions based on the field testing and the content validity study were then incorporated into the final PEDI items to establish the Standardization Version.

Normative data for the PEDI were gathered from 412 children and families distributed throughout Massachusetts, Connecticut, and New York. The sample closely approximated most of the demographic characteristics of the U.S. population as defined by the 1980 U.S. census data. Additionally, three groups of children (totaling 102) with disabilities composed clinical samples for validation purposes.

DISPLAY 2-5

Functional Skills Content of the Pediatric Evaluation of Disability Inventory*

Self-Care Domain	Mobility Domain	Social Function Domain
Types of food textures	Toilet transfers	Comprehension of word meaning
Use of utensils	Chair/wheelchair transfers	Comprehension of sentence complexity
Use of drinking containers	Car transfers	Functional use of expressive communication
Toothbrushing	Bed mobility/transfers	Complexity of expressive communication
Hairbrushing	Tub transfers	Problem-resolution
Nose care	Method of indoor locomotion	Social interactive play
Handwashing	Distance/speed indoors	Peer interactions
Washing body and face	Pulls/carries objects	Self-information
Pullover/front-opening garments	Method of outdoor locomotion	Time orientation
Fasteners	Distance/speed outdoors	Household chores
Pants	Outdoor surfaces	Self-protection
Shoes/socks	Upstairs	Community function
Toileting tasks	Downstairs	
Management of bladder		
Management of bowel		

*Used with permission from Haley SM, et al. *Pediatric Evaluation of Disability Inventory (PEDI): Development, Standardization and Administration Manual*, Boston; New England Medical Center Hospital and PEDI Research Group: 1992:13.

DISPLAY 2-6

Complex Activities Assessed with Caregiver Assistance and Modification Scales*

Self-Care Domain	Mobility Domain	Social Function Domain
Eating	Chair/toilet transfers	Functional comprehension
Grooming	Car transfers	Functional expression
Bathing	Bed mobility/transfers	Joint problem solving
Dressing upper body	Tub transfers	Peer play
Dressing lower body	Indoor locomotion	Safety
Toileting	Outdoor locomotion	
Bladder management	Stairs	
Bowel management		

*Used with permission from Haley SM, et al. *Pediatric Evaluation of Disability Inventory (PEDI): Development, Standardization and Administration Manual,* Boston; New England Medical Center Hospital and PEDI Research Group; 1992: 13.

TEST FORMAT

TYPE. The test is norm-referenced, and it can also be used as a criterion-referenced measure of functional status.

CONTENT. The PEDI includes three sets of measurement scales: Functional Skills, Caregiver Assistance, and Modifications. These scales are used to assess the three content areas of self-care, mobility, and social function. The *Functional Skills Scales* were designed to reflect meaningful functional units within a given activity. The *Caregiver Assistance Scales* measure disability of children with respect to the amount of help they need to carry out functional activities. The *Modifications* section is not a true measurement scale, but rather a frequency count of the type and extent of environmental modifications the child depends on to support functional performance.

ADMINISTRATION. The PEDI can be administered by clinicians and educators who are familiar with the child, or by structured interview of the parent. The PEDI's focus on typical performance requires the respondent to have had the opportunity to observe the child on several different occasions in order to gain an accurate picture of the child's typical performance.[55] Administration guidelines, criteria for scoring each item, and examples are provided in the accompanying manual. Specific training is required to ensure that examiners are knowledgeable about the item criteria used in the instrument and the methods employed in determining the child's level of assistance.

SCORING. Scores are recorded in a booklet that also contains a summary score sheet that is used to construct a profile of the child's performance across the different domains and scales. A summary of rating criteria for the three sets of measurement scales is provided in Display 2-7.

INTERPRETATION. The PEDI provides two types of transformed summary scores: normative standard scores and scaled scores. Separate summary scores are calculated for Functional Skills and for Caregiver Assistance in each of the three domains, thus yielding six normative standard scores and six scaled scores. Normative standard scores are transformed scores that take into account the child's chronological age, thereby providing an indication of the child's

DISPLAY 2-7

Rating Criteria for the Three Types of Measurment Scales*

Part I: Functional Skills	Part II: Caregiver Assistance	Part III: Modification
(197 discrete items of functional skills) Self-Care, Mobility, Social function 0 = unable, or limited in capability to perform item in most situations 1 = capable of performing item in most situations, or item has been previously mastered and functional skills have progressed beyond this level	(20 complex functional activities) Self-care, Mobility, Social function 5 = Independent 4 = Supervise/Prompt/Monitor 3 = Minimal Assistance 2 = Moderate Assistance 1 = Maximal Assistance 0 = Total Assistance	(20 complex functional activities) Self-care, Mobility, Social function N = No Modifications C = Child-oriented (non-specialized) R = Rehabilitation Equipment E = Extensive Modifications

*Used with permission from Haley SM, et al. *Pediatric Evaluation of Disability Inventory (PEDI): Development, Standardization and Administration Manual,* Boston; New England Medical Center Hospital and PEDI Research Group; 1992:16.

relative standing in relation to age expectations for functional skills and performance. Scaled scores, distributed along a scale from 0 to 100, provide an indication of the performance of the child along the continuum of relatively difficult items in a particular domain on the PEDI. Scaled scores are not adjusted for age and, therefore, can be used to describe the functional status of children of all ages. In addition, frequency totals of the four levels of modifications can be calculated. These totals provide descriptive information on the frequency and the degree of modifications a child uses.

RELIABILITY AND VALIDITY

The internal consistency reliability coefficients obtained from the normative sample range between 0.95 and 0.99. Inter-interviewer reliability in the normative sample was very high (ICCs = 0.96 to 0.99) for the Caregiver Assistance Scales. Agreement on Modifications was also quite high, except for Social Function, where it was still adequate (ICC = 0.79).[55] Further studies are planned to assess test–retest reliability and interobserver reliability between rehabilitation team members.

Content validity was examined using a panel of 31 experts[56] to validate and confirm the functional content of the PEDI. Data related to construct validity and concurrent validity[54] indicate that the PEDI is a valid measure of pediatric function. Preliminary data also support the discriminant and evaluative validity of the PEDI.[55]

ADVANTAGES AND DISADVANTAGES

The PEDI represents a standardized clinical instrument for pediatric functional assessment. Rigorous methodology during its development has resulted in an instrument that is both valid and reliable. The authors welcome input and feedback from users of the PEDI that will be useful to the authors as updated and revised versions are made available in the future.

Owing to the "newness" of the PEDI, further studies are needed to confirm its technical validity and to identify any needed changes or additions.

Functional Independence Measure for Children (WeeFIM)

The Functional Independence Measure for Children (WeeFIM) builds on the conceptual framework and is an adaptation of the Functional Independence Measure (FIM) for adults of the Uniform Data System for Medical Rehabilitation (UDS).[57] The WeeFIM was developed to assess and track development of functional independence in children with disabilities. Key characteristics of the WeeFIM are the minimal data set, emphasis on consistent actual patient performance, and use by any trained health or educational professional.

TEST MEASURES AND TARGET POPULATION

The WeeFIM consists of 18 items within six domains—self-care, sphincter control, mobility, locomotion, communication, and social cognition—and is designed for use with children between the ages of 6 months and 7 years and individuals of all ages with developmental and mental disabilities ages less than 7 years.

TEST CONSTRUCTION AND STANDARDIZATION

To develop the appropriate levels of performance of daily living tasks for children for the WeeFIM, an interdisciplinary team, knowledgeable in the use of traditional developmental scales, reviewed developmental pediatric, developmental psychological, pediatric physical, occupation, speech-language, and preschool educational scales. Pilot testing was performed with two groups of well children in Buffalo and Chicago (n = 111 and n = 170, respectively).[58] Content validity was assessed and reported by McCabe and Granger.[59] Additionally, two groups of children (totaling 58) with motor impairments and a group of 66 survivors of extreme prematurity (less than 29 weeks' gestation) composed clinical samples for validation purposes.

TEST FORMAT

TYPE. The test is criterion-based and is a descriptive measure of the caregiver and special resources that are required because of functional limitations.

CONTENT. The test consists of six domains as shown in Display 2-8.

ADMINISTRATION/SCORING. Assessment is based on direct observation of the child by an individual clinician or a team or by interviewing an informant who is knowledgeable about the usual and consistent performance of the child. Learning to use the WeeFIM correctly is important and is facilitated by a guide to its use,[57] and introductory videotape,[60] and training workshops. Performance of the child on each of the items is assigned to one of seven levels of an ordinal scale that represents the range of function from complete and modified independence (levels 7 and 6) without a helping person to modified and complete dependence (levels 5 to 1) with a helping person (Display 2-9).

INTERPRETATION. The WeeFIM measures disability, not impairment. The focus of the assessment is on the impact that a disorder has on the degree of independent performance of daily living tasks. The WeeFIM is a minimum data set and is not intended to supplant detailed clinical assessment of component parts of motor, sensory, cognitive, or communicative abilities. It is designed to track functional status and out-

DISPLAY 2-8
WeeFIM Domains

Self-care
1. Eating
2. Grooming
3. Bathing
4. Dressing—upper body
5. Dressing—lower body
6. Toileting

Sphincter Control
7. Bladder management
8. Bowel management

Mobility
9. Transfer chair, wheelchair
10. Transfer toilet
11. Transfer tub

Locomotion
12. Crawl/walk/wheelchair
13. Stairs

Communication
14. Comprehension
15. Expression

Social Cognition
16. Social interaction
17. Problem solving
18. Memory

comes over time both in preschool years and in the early elementary school years.

RELIABILITY AND VALIDITY

The test–retest reliability coefficients (Pearson's correlation) for the 6 domains range from r = 0.83 for sphincter control to r = .99 for mobility, communication, and social cognition. Interrater reliability coefficients (Pearson's correlation) range from 0.74 for mobility to 0.96 for communication and social cognition. Test–retest

DISPLAY 2-9
Levels of Function for the WeeFIM

No Helper
7 = Complete independence (timely, safely)
6 = Modified independence (device needed)

Helper
Modified dependence
5 = Supervision
4 = Minimal assist (child = 75%–99%)
3 = Moderate assist (child = 50%–74%)
Complete dependence
2 = Maximal assistance (child = 25%–49%)
1 = Total assistance (child = 0–24%)

and interrater reliability for the total WeeFIM are 0.99 and 0.95, respectively. Data related to construct and discriminative validity[57] indicate that the WeeFIM is a valid measure of disability related to functional independence. Additional work (5–10) with the WeeFIM including a normative sample (n = 413) and samples of children with a variety of developmental disabilities contribute to the validation of the measure.[61–66]

ADVANTAGES AND DISADVANTAGES

The WeeFIM can be used by health and educational providers, resulting in a common language to describe the child's ability to cope with daily living tasks and to set habilitation goals across health, educational, and community settings.

Integration of Information

Throughout the process of evaluation, physical therapists compile extensive information concerning their young clients. The final component of a thorough assessment is to organize, synthesize, and use the data to guide intervention. There are four possible uses for the information gained from evaluation.[67]

1. To plan a treatment program
2. To identify areas of progress or lack of progress
3. To identify or rule out the existence of a specific problem
4. To provide diagnostic information

Physical therapists are primarily involved with the first two areas. The way in which test data are to be used should help determine the data needed, thus ensuring the collection of necessary data while avoiding superfluous information. As a result of the procedure for assessment, the physical therapist identifies specific areas of dysfunction in a particular child. Program goals and objectives can then be developed to address these areas of dysfunction. *Program goals* describe long-term expectations of treatment and relate to general areas of development. *Objectives* are short-term accomplishments, written in behavioral terms, which enable the child to progress toward achievement of the long-term goals. A program for therapy is designed to meet the objectives identified by focusing on the activities required for the child to achieve the objectives.

The assessment process can be seen as an ongoing cycle. The information gathered from the formal assessment is used in the development of goals and objectives that guide the treatment program. Reassessments are periodically performed to review the appropriateness of the treatment program and to monitor the progress of the child. Reports of physical therapy assessments are usually presented in narrative form. The purposes of a report are to clarify what has been heard and observed, to give the data on which recommendations for treatment are based, and to transmit this information in a clear and understandable way to others. Certain information is included for all patients, but each child's report should provide a specific description of the distinctive abilities and disabilities of that child.[3] An outline of a narrative report is given in Display 2-10.

DISPLAY 2-10

Suggested Outline for a Narrative Report on the Results of Development Testing

1. Identification information: child's name, date of birth, current age, date of evaluation
2. Reason for evaluation and source of referral
3. History
   A. Perinatal history
   B. Significant medical history
   C. Developmental history as presented by parents or other historian
4. Clinical observations
   A. Neurologic development: reflex development, muscle tone, equilibrium, and protective responses
   B. Musculoskeletal status: range of motion, manual muscle test, anthropometric measurements
   C. Sensory status: results of sensory testing, visual ability, and auditory ability
   D. Functional abilities: daily activities (e.g., feeding, toileting, dressing), assistive devices
5. Results of developmental assessments: include developmental age
6. Summary of findings
7. Recommendations

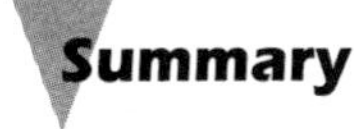

Summary

Several clinically useful and commonly used tools for assessment have been described, among them screening tests, tests of motor function, and comprehensive developmental assessments. The information gained from these assessments, when combined with the information obtained from an interview, medical and developmental history, and clinical observation, completes the comprehensive evaluation of a child. The guidelines presented for the selection of specific tests will aid the therapist in choosing the test most appropriate for the population to be assessed. The therapist should remember that a questioning attitude, based on and supported by knowledge of human growth and development, is necessary for a comprehensive evaluation.

REFERENCES

1. Semans S. Specific tests and evaluation tools for the child with central nervous system deficit. *Phys Ther.* 1965;45:456–462.
2. Scherzer AL, Tscharnuter I. *Early Diagnosis and Therapy in Cerebral Palsy.* New York: Marcel Dekker; 1982.
3. Knobloch H, Pasamanick B, eds. *Gesell and Armatruda's Developmental Diagnosis: The Evaluation and Management of Normal and Abnormal Neuropsychologic Development in Infancy and Early Childhood.* Hagerstown, MD: Harper & Row; 1974.
4. Clark PN, Coley LI, Allen AS, et al. Basic methods of assessment and screening. In: Clark PN, Allen AS, eds. *Occupational Therapy for Children.* St. Louis: CV Mosby; 1985.
5. Connolly B, Harris S. Survey of assessment tools. *Totline.* 1983;9:8–9.
6. Bayley N. *Bayley Scales of Infant Development.* New York: The Psychological Corporation; 1969.
7. Frankenburg WK, Dodds J, Archer P, et al. *Denver II Training Manual.* Denver, CO: Denver Developmental Materials, Inc; 1992.
8. Gallahue D. Assessing child's motor behavior. In: *Understanding Motor Development in Children.* New York: John Wiley; 1982.
9. Lewko JH. Current practices in evaluating motor behavior of disabled children. *Am J Occup Ther.* 1976;30:413–419.
10. Stangler SR, Huber CJ, Routh DK. *Screening Growth and Development of Preschool Children: A Guide for Test Selection.* New York: McGraw-Hill; 1980.
11. Milani-Comparetti A, Gidoni EA. Routine developmental examination in normal and retarded children. *Dev Med Child Neurol.* 1967;9:631–638.
12. Trembath J, Kliewer D, Bruce W. *The Milani-Comparetti Motor Development Screening Test.* Omaha, NE: University of Nebraska Medical Center; 1977.
13. Stuberg WA, et al. *The Milani-Comparetti Motor Development Screening Test.* 3rd Ed rev. Omaha, NE: University of Nebraska Medical Center; 1992.
14. Stuberg WA, White PJ, Miedaner JA, et al. Item reliability of the Milani-Comparetti Motor Development Screening Test. *Phys Ther.* 1989;69:328–335.
15. Frankenburg WK, Dodds JB, Fandel AW. *Denver Developmental Screening Test Manual.* Denver, CO: LADOCA Project & Publishing Foundation; 1973.
16. Frankenburg WK, Dodds J, Archer P, et al. The Denver II: A major revision and restandardization of the Denver Developmental Screening Test. *Pediatrics.* 1992;89:1.
17. Frankenburg WK, Dodds J, Archer P. *Denver II Technical Manual.* Denver, CO: Denver Developmental Materials, Inc; 1990.
18. Chandler LS, Andrews MS, Swanson MW. *Movement Assessment of Infants—A Manual.* Rolling Bay, WA: Chandler, Andrews, and Swanson; 1980.
19. Haley SM, Harris SR, Tada WL, et al. Item reliability of the movement assessment of infants. *Phys Occup Ther Pediatr.* 1986;6(1):21–38.
20. Harris SR. Early neuromotor predictors of cerebral palsy in low birthweight infants. *Dev Med Child Neurol.* 1987;29:508–519.
21. Schneider JW, Lee W, Chasnoff IJ. Field testing of the Movement Assessment of Infants. *Phys Ther.* 1988;68:321–327.
22. Piper MC, Pinnell LE, Darrah J, et al. Early developmental screening: Sensitivity and specificity of chronological and adjusted scores. *Dev Behav Pediatr.* 1992;13:95–101.
23. Swanson MW, Bennett FC, Shy KK, et al. Identification of neurodevelopmental abnormality at four and eight months by the Movement Assessment of Infants. *Dev Med Child Neurol.* 1992;34:321–337.
24. Washington K, Deitz JC. Performance of full-term 6-month-old infants on the movement assessment of infants. *Pediatr Phys Ther.* 1995;7(2):65–74.
25. Harris SR, Haley SM, Tada WL, Swanson MW. Reliability of observational measures of the Movement Assessment of Infants. *Phys Ther.* 1984;64:471–475.
26. Brander R, Kramer J, Dancsak, et al. Inter-rater and test-retest reliabilities of the movement assessment of infants. *Ped Phys Ther.* 1993;5(1):9–15.
27. Harris SR, Swanson MW, Andrews MS, et al. Predictive validity of the movement assessment of infants. *J Dev Behav Pediatr.* 1984;5:336–343.
28. Campbell SK, Osten ET, Kolobe THA, et al. Development of the Test of Infant Motor Performance. *Phys Med Rehab Clin North Am.* 1993;4(3):541–550.

29. Girolami GL, Campbell SK. Efficacy of a neurodevelopmental treatment program to improve motor control in infants born prematurely. *Pediatr Phys Ther.* 1994;6(4):175–184.
30. Campbell SK. The child's development of functional movement. In: Campbell SK, ed. *Physical Therapy for Children.* Philadelphia: WB Saunders; 1994.
31. Campbell SK, Kolobe TH, Osten ET, et al. Construct validity of infant motor performance. *Phys Ther.* 1995;75(7):585–596.
32. Piper MC, Darrah J. *Alberta Infant Motor Scale.* Philadelphia: WB Saunders; 1995.
33. Piper MC, Pinnell LE, Darrah J, et al. Construction and validation of the Alberta Infant Motor Scale (AIMS). *Can J Public Health.* 1992;83(Suppl 2):S46–50.
34. Fetters L, Tronick EZ. Neuromotor development of cocaine-exposed and control infants from birth through 15 months: poor and poorer performance. *Pediatrics.* 1996;98(5):938–943.
35. Russell DJ, Rosenbaum PL, Cadman DT, et al. The Gross Motor Function Measure: A means to evaluate the effects of physical therapy. *Dev Med Child Neurol.* 1989;31:341–352.
36. Russell DJ, Rosenbaum PL, Lane M, et al. Training users in the Gross Motor Function Measure: Methodological and practical issues. *Phys Ther.* 1994;74(7):630–636.
37. Boyce WF, Gowland C, Hardy S, et al. Development of a quality-of-movement measure for children with cerebral palsy. *Phys Ther.* 1991;71(11): 820–828.
38. Gowland C, Boyce WF, Wright V, et al. Reliability of the Gross Motor Performance Measure. *Phys Ther.* 1995;75(7):597–602.
39. Boyce WF, Gowland C, Rosenbaum PL, et al. The Gross Motor Performance measure: Validity and responsiveness of a measure of quality of movement. *Phys Ther.* 1995;71(7):603–613.
40. Folio MR, Fewell PR. *Peabody Developmental Motor Scales and Activity Cards Manual.* Allen, TX: DLM Teaching Resources; 1983.
41. Stokes NA, Deitz JL, Crowe TK. The Peabody Developmental Fine Motor Scale: An interrater reliability study. *Am J Occup Ther.* 1990;44:334–340.
42. Harris SR, Heriza CB. Measuring infant movement: Clinical and technological assessment techniques. *Phys Ther.* 1987;67:1877–1880.
43. Bruininks RH. *Bruininks-Oseretsky Test of Motor Proficiency: Examiners' Manual.* Circle Pines, MI: American Guidance Services; 1978.
44. Self PA, Horowitz FD. The behavioral assessment of the neonate: An overview. In: Osofsky JD, ed. *Handbook of Infant Development.* New York: Wiley; 1979.
45. Palisano RJ. Concurrent and predictive validities of the Bayley Motor Scale and the Peabody Developmental Motor Scales. *Phy Ther.* 1986;66: 1714–1719.
46. Bayley Scales of Infant Development, 2nd Ed. *The Bayley II.* The Psychological Corporation. San Antonio, TX: Harcourt Brace & Co; 1993.
47. Brazelton TB. Neonatal Behavioral Assessment Scale. *Clin Dev Med.* 1984:88.
48. Brazelton TB. Neonatal Behavioral Assessment Scale. *Clin Dev Med.* 1973:50.
49. Stengel TJ. The Neonatal Behavioral Assessment Scale: Description, clinical uses, and research implications. *Phys Occup Ther Pediatr.* 1980;1:39–57.
50. Prechtl HFB, Beintema B. The neurological examination of the full-term infant. *Clin Dev Med.* 1964:12.
51. Rogers SJ, D'Eugenio DB. Assessment and application. In: Schafer DS, Moersch MS, eds. *Developmental Programming for Infants and Young Children.* Vol I. Ann Arbor, MI: The University of Michigan Press; 1977.
52. Brown SL, Donovan CM. Stimulation activities. In: Schafer DS, Moersch MS, eds. *Developmental Programming for Infants and Young Children.* Vol 3. Ann Arbor, MI: The University of Michigan Press; 1977.
53. Haley SM: Motor assessment tools for infants and young children: A focus on disability assessment. In: Forssberg H, Hirschfeld H, eds. *Movement Disorders in Children.* Basel: S. Karger, AG; 1992: 278–283.
54. Feldman AB, Haley SM, Coryell J. Concurrent and construct validity of the Pediatric Evaluation of Disability Inventory. *Phys Ther.* 1990;70:602–610.
55. Haley SM, et al. *Pediatric Evaluation of Disability Inventory (PEDI): Development, Standardization and Administration Manual.* Boston: New England Medical Center Hospitals and PEDI Research Group; 1992.
56. Haley SM, Coster WJ, Faas RM. A content validity study of the Pediatric Evaluation of Disability Inventory. *Pediatr Phys Ther.* 1991;3:177–184.
57. Data Management Service of the Uniform Data System for medical Rehabilitation and the Center for Functional Assessment Research: Guide for Use of the Uniform Data System for Medical Rehabilitation, Including the Functional Independence Measure for Children (WeeFIM), State University of New York at Buffalo, 82 Farber Hall, SUNY South Campus, Buffalo, version 1.5, July 1991.
58. Msall ME, DiGaudio KM, Duffy LC. Use of assessment in children with developmental disabilities.

Phys Med Rehab Clinics North Am. 1993;4(3): 517–527.

59. McCabe MA, Granger CV. Content validity of a pediatric functional independence measure. *Appl Nurs Res.* 1990;3:120–122.
60. Msall ME, Braun S, Granger CV. Use of the functional independence measure for children (WeeFIM: An interdisciplinary training tape [abstract].) *Dev Med Child Neurol.* 1990;62:46.
61. Msall ME, Braun SL, Duffy L, et al: Normative sample of the Pediatric Functional Independence Measure: A uniform data set for tracking disability [abstract]. *Dev Med Child Neurol.* 1992;66:19.
62. Msall ME, Heffner H, DiGaudio K, et al. Functional independence in school age children with lower extremity neurological impairment: Use of WeeFIM in spastic diplegia and paraplegia [abstract]. *Dev Med Child Neurol Suppl.* 1992;66:21.
63. Msall ME, Monti DA, Duffy LC, et al. Measuring functional independence in children with spina bifida [abstract 60]. *Pediatr Res.* 1992;31:12A.
64. Msall ME, Roehmholdt SJ, DiGaudio KM, et al. Functional independence of school age children with Down syndrome [abstract 61]. *Pediatr Res.* 1992;31:13A.
65. Msall ME, Rogers BT, Buck GM, et al. Functional status of extremely preterm infants at kindergarten entry. *Dev Med Child Neurol.* 1993;35:312–320.
66. Msall ME, Rosenberg S, DiGaudio KM, et al. Pilot testing of the WeeFIM in children with motor impairments [abstract]. *Dev Med Child Neurol Suppl.* 1990;32:41.
67. Stockmeyer S. A pattern for evaluation in the assessment of motor performance. *Phys Ther.* 1965; 45:453–455.

The High-Risk Infant

Mary Soltesz Sheahan and Nancy Farmer Brockway

Recent advances in neonatology have reduced significantly the morbidity and mortality rates for high-risk infants. Premature infants, however, are at greater risk than infants born at term for developmental deficits and handicapping conditions. As a result of this risk, pediatric therapists have become increasingly involved in providing intervention in the neonatal intensive care unit (NICU). These therapists advocate early detection and remediation of neuromotor deficits to minimize or prevent further disabilities that emerge as compensations for initial movement disorders.[1]

The pediatric therapist's role in the NICU requires a good understanding of the medical needs of high-risk neonates. The ability to assess thoroughly the physiologic status of the neonate is crucial for successful implementation of developmental intervention. Therapists initially entering the NICU setting need close supervision from an experienced clinician. Advanced training in normal and abnormal development is also strongly recommended.

The chapter examines the role of the pediatric therapist working with high-risk infants in the NICU. A basic description of the high-risk infant is given and appropriate intervention techniques are presented. The term *high-risk infant,* as used in the context of this chapter, refers to those infants whose perinatal medical course might contribute to motor, cognitive, or social deficits. Some of the most common medical problems associated with the high-risk infant are described.

The Environment of the Neonatal Intensive Care Unit

A comparison between the intrauterine and NICU environment is necessary in order to appreciate the complexities of the problems faced by the neonate who is at high risk. The intrauterine environment is ideally suited for the development of the fetus for a variety of reasons. In utero, the fetus receives muted sounds generated by the mother, including rhythmic heartbeats, respiratory sounds, and voice. Although sounds from the external environment are heard by the fetus, those sounds are dampened. Intrauterine visual input is limited to a dim red glow. The amniotic fluid provides an optimal environment for the elimination of gravity to provide for random movement, and the boundaries of the uterine wall provide deep proprioceptive input as the fetus moves. Maternal movement provides additional proprioceptive and vestibular input to the fetus. Fetal thermoregulation is controlled well in the intrauterine environment.

In stark contrast, the NICU environment is characterized by bright light and constant and offensive noise produced by medical equipment, voices, telephones, radios, alarms, and closing of incubator doors. The medically unstable infant experiences adverse tactile input from necessary invasive medical intervention. Gravity makes movement into flexed positions difficult for the often hypotonic neonate. The previous intrauterine boundaries are now absent and proprioceptive feedback changes. Postnatally, the infant is subjected to thermoregulatory problems.

Neonatal Development

A basic understanding of the development of the premature and full-term infant is necessary in order to appreciate the rationale behind developmental intervention in the nursery. This section of the chapter provides a comparison of the development of a premature infant and that of a full-term infant. A complete discussion of normal development is found in Chapter 1.

The premature infant characteristically displays global hypotonia.[2] The level of hypotonia is related to the degree of prematurity.[3] For example, the infant of 28 weeks' gestation shows greater range of motion and flexibility in the shoulders, elbows, hips, and knees than infants born at later gestational ages. The extremities of the premature infant are typically postured in extension and abduction, with decreased flexor patterns and midline orientation. The reduced timespan spent in the tightly packed uterine environment contributes to the premature infant's lack of physiologic flexion. The force of gravity against weak muscle groups further reinforces the extended posture in premature infants. Primitive reflexes may be absent, reduced, or inconsistent, and spontaneous movement is minimal.[2] Infants maintained for long periods with mechanical ventilation may show increased hypertension of the neck, scapular elevation, retraction of the shoulders and upper extremities, arching of the trunk, and immobility of the pelvis.[4]

By contrast, the full-term infant displays strong physiologic flexion. The 40 weeks spent in utero allows for full development of flexor muscle tone. The tightly compacted uterine posture causes mild flexor contractures in the elbows and knees. These contractures are gradually reduced. Flexion of the wrist and dorsiflexion of the ankle increase in the full-term infant. At term, the infant's extremities are generally flexed and adducted. Spontaneous movements can be limited by the strong physiologic flexion.[2]

As the premature infant develops, flexor muscle tone increases in a caudocephalic direction.[5] The premature infant usually does not achieve the full degree of flexor muscle tone seen in the full-term infant.[3] Therefore, the premature infant lacks the counterbalance of flexor tone to offset the normal progression of extensor muscle tone, thereby causing an imbalance between extensor and flexor groups. This imbalance may interfere with development of midrange control of the head, sitting balance, reaching skills, and bilateral coordination. Secondary to the decreased midline and reaching skills, body image and exploratory skills may be adversely affected (Table 3–1).[6]

Synactive Model of Infant Behavior

A synactive model of infant behavior has been postulated by Als and is based on a hierarchical interaction of four subsystems: (1) autonomic; (2) motor; (3) state; and (4) attentional/interactive, as described in Table 3–2.[7] Stability or equilibrium of the lower subsystems is required for the maturation and expression of the higher subsystems, but the expression of higher level subsystems can jeopardize the equilibrium or stability of the lower level subsystems. For example, an infant struggling to maintain cardiorespiratory homeostasis will find it difficult or impossible to assume an alert state and to interact with the environment. Conversely, alertness and responses to environmental events may contribute to instability of the autonomic,

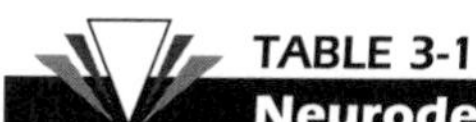

TABLE 3-1
Neurodevelopmental Profile of the Fetus and Premature Neonate*

1 Week

Implementation into the uterine wall

3 Weeks

Beginning of heart contractions

3–6 Weeks

Nonnervous (aneural) muscular activity
Spontaneous contractions of skeletal muscles are more pronounced cephalad than caudal

4 Weeks

Heart pulsation and pumping of blood
Formation of backbone and spinal canal
Beginning of formation of digestive system
Length of 3/4 inch

8–9 Weeks

Continuous trembling secondary to autonomous muscle contraction without organization
Generalization avoidance reflexes resulting from stimulation around lips and nose with a fine hair
Limbs that are beginning to show divisions (thigh, knee, calf, foot)
Formation of umbilical cord
Disappearance of tail-like process
Length of 1 1/8 inches
Weight of 1/30 oz

9–12 Weeks

Primitive palmar grasp reflex
Mouth opening elicited by stimulation of lower lip area
Mouth opening, but not sucking, elicited by stimulation of both lips
Global flexion and extension
Formation of nails on digits
External ears present
Almost full development of the eyes but persistent fusion of eyelids
Length of 3 inches
Weight of 1 oz
Brain weight of 10 g

16 Weeks

Increased frequency of fetal propulsion—head rotation with thrusting

(continued)

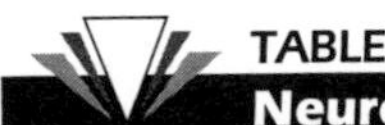

TABLE 3-1

Neurodevelopmental Profile of the Fetus and Premature Neonate* (Continued)

16 Weeks

Respiratory movements—mouth opening and head extension with inspiration
Skin—bright pink and transparent; covered with a fine, down-like hair
Length of 6 1/2 to 7 inches
Weight of 4 oz

17 Weeks

Initial appearance of sucking reflex

20 Weeks

Fully developed repertoire of movement patterns
Isolated, independent movements of the extremities and head
- Opens hands with extension of digits to explore surrounding surfaces
- Opens mouth; sucking and swallowing present
- Uses facial expressions—grimaces, wrinkles forehead

Protective or avoidance light reflex—turns away from light even though eyes are closed
Length of 10 to 12 inches
Weight of 1/2 lb to 1 lb

22 Weeks

Initial myelination of the CNS and peripheral nervous system

24 Weeks

Lungs have matured to the degree that viability is possible
Length of 11 to 14 inches
Weight of 1 1/4 to 1 1/2 lb
Brain weight of 150 g

28 Weeks

Appearance of alert state—able to respond to stimuli
Remains dominant by sleep state
Movement
- Tremulous, random movements
- Slow, global movements with rapid, jerky, segmental movements

Muscle tone
- Moderate hypotonia segmentally and axially
- Extreme passivity, which is greater in the upper extremities than in the lower extremities
- Excessive mobility—more pronounced in proximal segments

Length of 14 to 17 inches
Weight of 2 1/2 to 3 lb

32 Weeks

Spontaneous appearance of an alert state that may not correlate with motor activity
More pronounced state differentiation
Movement
- Bursts of movement when in an awake state
- Movement dominated by trunk
- Creeping in isolette, especially to sides
- Marked decrease in tremulousness and clonic movements
- Attempted hand-to-mouth movements

Muscle tone
- Noted decrease in lower extremity hypotonia to hip joint
- Increased strength of weight bearing
- Ability to attempt to straighten head (life-saving reactions)

36 Weeks

Vigorous, sustained cry
Continued improvement in behavioral state differentiation
Movement
- Spontaneous movement that is more limited and less varied in the upper and lower extremities
- Increased cocontraction of agonist/antagonist muscle groups causing a restraining quality

Muscle tone
- Hypotonia of the upper extremities and upper trunk in comparison to the lower trunk and lower extremities (frog-like position)

40 Weeks

Sustained periods of a quiet-alert state
Improved state of differentiation
Movement
- Less disorganizing and more uniform spontaneous movement

Muscle tone
- Diminished hypotonia in the upper extremities and upper trunk

---

*Information has been compiled from the following sources: Comparetti AM. *Prenatal and Postnatal Development of Movement: Implications for Developmental Diagnosis.* Arlington, VA, 1982; Forslund M, Bjerre I. Neurological assessment of preterm infants at term conceptual age in comparison with normal full-term infants. *Early Hum Develop.* 1983;8:195–208. Piper M, Byrne P, Pinnell L. Influence of gestational age in early neuromotor development in the preterm infant. *Am J Perinatol* 1989;6:405–411; and Saint-Anne Dargassies S. Neurological maturation of the premature infant of 28 to 41 weeks gestational age. In: *Human Development.* Philadelphia: WB Saunders; 1966.

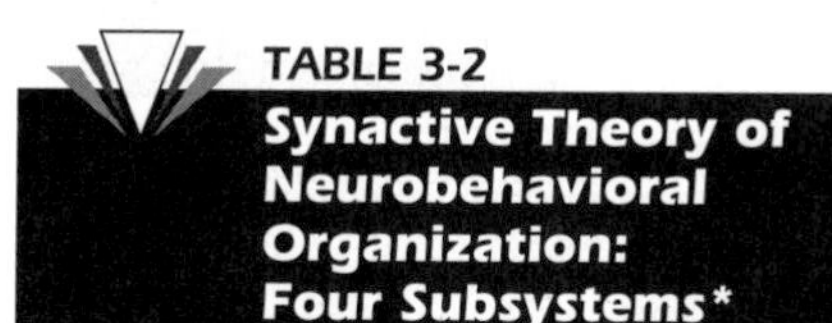

TABLE 3-2
Synactive Theory of Neurobehavioral Organization: Four Subsystems*

Autonomic: Includes patterns of respiration, heart rate, thermoregulation, and digestion.

Motor: Includes posture, tone and activity of the trunk, extremities, and face. The infant's active movements can contribute to instability in the autonomic system.

State: This includes the range of states available to the infant, the transitions from one state to another, and the clearness and differentiation of states.

Attention/Interactive: This includes the infant's ability to assume and maintain an alert state, and take in and respond appropriately to environmental input, including social cognitive, and emotional input.

*From Als H, Leter BM, Tronick EZ, Brazelton TB. In: Fitzgerald H, et al., eds. *Theory and Research in Behavioral Pediatrics.* Vol 1. New York: Plenum; 1982 and 1985.

motor, or state subsystems. As a result, the infant might have reactions, such as apnea, bradycardia, or loss of muscle tone. When interacting with the environment, the infant strives to regulate its responses to maintain a balance among the four subsystems.[7,8]

Als and associates have documented neonatal behavioral cues that act as indicators of either stress or stability (Table 3–3).[7,8] Physical therapists must be able to recognize these signals and modify treatment in response to these cues. Additionally, parents and all caregivers should be educated about appropriate responses to these infant cues.

Risk Factors

Neurologic Conditions

ASPHYXIA

Asphyxia is the result of an inadequate exchange of oxygen and carbon dioxide and can have many causes.[9,10] Events occurring during pregnancy

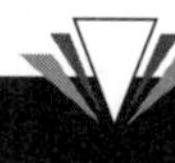

TABLE 3-3
Behavioral Indicators of Stress and Stability*

- Signs of Stability or Approach Signals
  - Smooth respiration
  - Pink, stable color
  - Animated facial expression
  - Brightening of the eyes
  - "Oh" face
  - Cooing
  - Smiling
  - Hand-to-mouth activity
  - Well-regulated muscle tone
  - Smooth body movements, minimal movement
- Signs of Stress
  - Physiologic indicators
    - Color changes
    - Circumoral cyanosis
    - Skin mottling
    - Change in respiratory rate or rhythm
    - Change in heart rate
    - Coughing
    - Sneezing
    - Yawning
    - Vomiting
    - Bowel movement
    - Hiccups
  - Motor indicators
    - Sudden change in muscle tone
    - Flaccidity (truncal, extremities, facial)
    - Stiffness
      - Leg bracing
      - Opisthotonos
      - Finger splaying
      - Facial grimacing
      - Tongue extension
      - Hyperflexion
    - Alterations in the quality of movement
      - Disorganized movement
      - Jitteriness
      - Squirminess
  - Behavioral Indicators
    - Irritability (crying, inconsolability)
    - Staring
    - Gaze aversion
    - Hyperalertness
    - Roving eye movements
    - Glassy-eyed appearance
      - Sleeplessness and restlessness

*Als H, Lester BM, Tronick EZ, Brazelton TB. Manual for the Assessment of Preterm Infants' Theory and Behavior (APIB). IN: Fitzgerald H, et al., eds. *Theory and Research in Behavioral Pediatrics,* Vol I. New York: Plenum; 1982;65–132.

and at the time of delivery can contribute to asphyxia. The impact of an episode of asphyxia on a neonate's brain is called *hypoxic-ischemic encephalopathy* (HIE). Hypoxia and ischemia usually occur concurrently or serially.[11,12] The major factors contributing to neonatal asphyxia are interference with umbilical blood flow and poor gas exchange from the mother's circulation through the placenta to the fetus. Failure of the infant's lungs to inflate, which can be caused by many factors, results in persistent fetal circulation (pulmonary hypertension), which may either contribute to, or be secondary to, neonatal asphyxia.[9] Hypoxic-ischemic injuries are the most common cause of severe, nonprogressive neurologic defects caused by perinatal events. Mental retardation, spasticity, choreoathetosis, ataxia, and seizure disorders are associated with asphyxia in the neonate.[12,13]

Cerebral ischemia refers to decreased blood flow to the brain and is typically related to systemic hypotension and decreased cardiac output.[3,5] *Hypoxemia,* or decreased arterial oxygen concentration, can result from perinatal asphyxia, recurrent apnea, or severe respiratory disease. Additionally, fetal hypoxemia depresses the myocardium, causing neonatal bradycardia and hypotension, which lead to further systemic ischemia. In particular, systemic ischemia affects the kidneys, liver, lungs, and gastrointestinal tract. Altered vascular autoregulation in the neonate increases the infant's vulnerability to ischemic injury.[14] When an asphyxial event occurs, the physiologic systems offer the greatest protection to the brain. Systemic complications may occur even though the central nervous system (CNS) is spared. Asphyxia leads to metabolic disturbances, including hypoglycemia, hypocalcemia, and hyperkalemia.[9,10] Hypoglycemia generates lactic acid, which adds to the brain damage incurred by asphyxia. Lactic acid can then cross the blood–brain barrier, which can be beneficial for a short period but subsequently has serious deleterious effects, including brain damage.[13]

When the infant is traumatized by severe HIE at birth, immediate stupor or coma occurs after birth, often requiring mechanical ventilation. Seizures and severe apnea may occur within the first 12 to 24 hours after birth. Severe hypotonia and absence of spontaneous movement will be seen. Neonatal reflexes are absent or greatly reduced. Brain stem–mediated ocular reactions may be disturbed. Mortality among these infants is high, and survivors have a high incidence of significant neurologic impairment.[11,12,15] Stupor or coma is associated with bilateral hemispheric disturbances. Recovery from the stupor may occur 12 to 24 hours after birth. At that time, seizures frequently increase in severity.[12] At 24 to 72 hours of age, the infant may reenter a stuporous or comatose state. Mortality of asphyxiated infants is highest at this stage. The most common causes of death after severe asphyxia are hypoxemia caused by pulmonary hypertension; intraventricular or intracerebral hemorrhage; disseminated intravascular coagulation (DIC) that causes uncontrolled hemorrhage, particularly in the lungs; arrhythmias or inadequate cardiac output caused by myocardial failure; and renal failure.

Infants who suffer moderate HIE at birth are usually lethargic and difficult to arouse during the first 12 hours of life. These infants have a history of acidosis and hypotension at delivery. They often require resuscitation at delivery and commonly need assistance to establish adequate respiration. Mechanical ventilation is usually short-term. Seizures and apnea are less likely to occur in those infants with moderate HIE than in those with the severe form. Infants with moderate HIE are often hypotonic with weak proximal musculature. Their muscle tone and level of arousal may improve within 2 to 3 days. They are at much less risk of mortality and long-term neurologic sequelae than are infants with severe HIE.[11,15] Necrotizing enterocolitis (NEC) and acute renal problems are among the significant risks for the moderately involved group.

Mild HIE is usually the result of asphyxia occurring immediately before delivery. Affected infants usually recover well and require minimal resuscitation. Acidosis and hypotension are less severe in this population. Reactions to mild HIE peak during the first 24 hours of life. Characteristically, these infants have a brief period of lethargy shortly after birth. Later, they may display jitteriness, hyperalertness, irritability, and exaggerated responses to stimulation. The Moro response may be hyperactive and easily elicited, or it may occur spontaneously, without an antecedent stimulus. Muscle tone and strength are likely to be normal, although deep tendon reflexes may be slightly hyperactive. Associated transitory hypoglycemia may be present and occasionally causes seizures. Infants with mild HIE do not incur long-term neurologic impairment.[9,16] Rapid recovery from a state of reduced consciousness and quick recovery of spontaneous respirations are associated with a more optimistic outcome.[9,12]

LESIONS ASSOCIATED WITH HYPOXIC-ISCHEMIC ENCEPHALOPATHY

Lesions associated with HIE include selective neuronal necrosis, status marmoratus of the basal ganglia and thalamus, parasagittal cerebral injury, and periventricular leukomalacia (PVL).[17] Selective neuronal necrosis of the cerebral cortex, diencephalon, basal ganglia, cerebellum, and especially the brain stem in a characteristic but widespread distribution is a common result of a hypoxic-ischemic episode. As a result of neuronal necrosis, the gyri may decrease in size, and glial fibers may replace gray and white matter. Myelination of white matter may be sparse. Associated disorders include mental retardation, hypertonicity, and seizures. Ataxia associated with spasticity is related to cerebellar lesions.[17]

Status marmoratus is characterized by a marbled appearance of the thalamus and basal ganglia. Neuronal loss, gliosis, and hypermyelination typify the pathology found with this defect.[18] Hypoxemia contributes to the cause of status marmoratus. Extrapyramidal disturbances, including choreoathetosis and rigidity, accompany the condition. The abnormalities in tone tend to be symmetric, thus reflecting the symmetry and bilaterality of this lesion.[12]

Parasagittal cerebral injury (watershed infarcts) is mainly the result of decreased cerebral blood flow. The areas in which the lesions occur are associated with the peripheral branches of the major cerebral arteries. Although such lesions are bilateral, they may be asymmetric. Decreasing systemic blood pressure makes the parasagittal areas highly vulnerable to damage, and the posterior aspects of the cerebral hemispheres are even more susceptible to injury. The full-term infant is most likely to be affected by the watershed phenomenon. Clinical features related to parasagittal injury include spastic quadriplegia, delays in language, and visuospatial deficits.[13,15]

Unlike full-term infants, premature infants typically exhibit PVL as a result of decreased blood flow. PVL refers to necrosis of white matter in areas surrounding the lateral ventricles. Intraventricular hemorrhage and ventricular dilatation often accompany this defect. PVL may be transitory, although white matter lesions often reduce to cystic cavities and are highly correlated with cerebral palsy. Spastic diplegia is the most common form of cerebral palsy resulting from PVL owing to the proximity of the ventricular system of descending motor fibers that innervate the lower extremities.[12,19]

INTRAVENTRICULAR HEMORRHAGE

Intraventricular hemorrhage (IVH) is the most common brain lesion seen in infants younger than 32 weeks of gestation and occurs in approximately 40% of all premature infants.[10] Infants with a low birth weight and those with a more complicated medical course are at greatest risk. Unstable respiratory status, especially when complicated by pneumothorax and hypoxemia, and difficult deliveries, especially breech presentation, are factors thought to contribute strongly to IVH. IVH also occurs as a result of frequent swings in blood pressure that cause alternating ischemia followed by reperfusion and hyperemia. The fragile cerebral vasculature of the premature infant is poorly supported in the gelatinous subependymal germinal matrix in the periventricular region. As a result, the swings in blood pressure and perfusion put stress on the fragile vasculature to the point of rupture. Hemorrhages usually originate in arterioles in the germinal matrix near the caudate nucleus. IVH may occur suddenly, or it may evolve and expand slowly for 1 to 3 days. Because blood has a higher acoustic impedance than cerebrospinal fluid and brain matter, IVH can be detected easily by a neurosonogram through the anterior fontanelle.[17,20] The extent of bleeding shown by the neurosonogram is graded as described in Table 3-4.

Neurologic outcome has been correlated with the severity of the hemorrhage. Infants with grades I and II IVH are considered to be at minimal risk for developing a long-term neurologic deficit. However, IVH of grades III and IV is associated with a significantly higher incidence of neurologic deficits, including hydrocephalus, cerebral palsy, and mental retardation.[21]

TABLE 3-4
Grades of Intraventricular Hemorrhage*

Grade	Extent of Hemorrhage
I	Isolated germinal matrix hemorrhage
II	Intraventricular hemorrhage with normal ventricular size
III	Intraventricular hemorrhage with ventricular dilation
IV	Intraventricular dilation with parenchymal hemorrhage

*Adapted from Papile L. Munsick-Bruro G. Shaefer A. Relationship of cerebral intraventricular hemorrhage and early childhood neurologic handicaps. *J Pediatr.* 1983;103:273–277.

Respiratory Conditions

RESPIRATORY DISTRESS SYNDROME

Respiratory distress syndrome (RDS), also called hyaline membrane disease (HMD) because of the appearance of the lungs at autopsy, is characterized by clinical signs that include chest wall retractions, cyanosis, expiratory grunt- ing, flaring of the nares, and tachypnea. Apnea, hypotension, and pulmonary edema are also associated with RDS. Premature infants born at less than 37 weeks of gestation are most commonly affected.[22] RDS is a leading cause of death in premature neonates, but medical advances, especially the recent introduction of exogenous surfactant, have led to a significant reduction in morbidity and mortality.[23]

A decreased production of chemically mature levels of surfactant is associated with RDS. This lack of adequate levels of surfactant causes a reduced alveolar surface tension, which causes alveolar collapse on expiration. This atelectasis, which occurs repeatedly, requires a massive increase in work of breathing as the infant tries to reinflate the lungs. Eventually, the infant suffers from decreased oxygenation, asphyxia, metabolic acidosis, and acute respiratory failure, any one of which can be fatal.[22]

BRONCHOPULMONARY DYSPLASIA

Bronchopulmonary dysplasia (BPD) is a chronic lung disease of infancy. The specific pathogenesis of BPD is controversial, but most neonatologists believe that iatrogenic factors, such as barotrauma associated with mechanical ventilation, elevated concentrations of administered oxygen, and endotracheal intubation, play a significant role in the development of BPD. Other factors, such as air leaks, patent ductus arteriosus, and fluid overload, are known to increase the likelihood of BPD.[24]

The process of BPD begins with the destruction of the respiratory tract cilia. Ciliary destruction is followed by necrosis of the cells of the respiratory epithelium as distal as the bronchioles. Capillary endothelial cells and cells lining the alveolar sacs may also be damaged. Pulmonary interstitial fibrosis may occur as early as 2 to 3 days in infants born between 25 to 26 weeks of gestation.[24] Recovery from the pulmonary damage of BPD is a slow process, with pulmonary impairment persisting for up to 1 year or longer.[25,26] The chronic lack of oxygenation in these babies often impairs neuromotor development.

MECONIUM ASPIRATION

In some cases, the fetus aspirates with its initial breath the thick meconium that it passed in utero. This meconium aspiration causes airway obstruction that can produce respiratory distress with chest wall retraction, grunting, tachypnea, and cyanosis. Infants born at term, or postterm, are at greatest risk. The incidence of meconium aspiration is approximately 5% to 15% of all live births.[27]

Metabolic Conditions

METABOLIC ACIDOSIS

Metabolic acidosis results from increased production or inadequate excretion of hydrogen ions, which form acid, or from excessive loss of basic material, such as bicarbonate ions, in the urine or stools. The result of either is a reduction of pH in the body.[27]

HYPERBILIRUBINEMIA

Hyperbilirubinemia (jaundice) is the accumulation in the blood of excessive amounts of bilirubin. Causes include Rh factor or ABO factor incompatibility of blood, physiologic jaundice, reabsorption of blood, and infection. Physiologic jaundice is commonly seen in premature infants who have a limited ability to excrete bilirubin from their systems. Excessive hemolysis of red blood cells can lead to excessive amounts of bilirubin and occurs with maternal–fetal blood group incompatibility. This type of hyperbilirubinemia has been the leading contributor to neurologic sequelae of all the causes of jaundice. Recent prevention of Rh sensitization of mothers, as well as improved management of Rh incompatibility, has almost eliminated the disease and its neurologic consequences.[22]

Kernicterus, or yellow staining of the brain, is caused by the deposition in the brain of unconjugated bilirubin. Most frequently, damage caused by kernicterus occurs in the basal ganglia and hippocampus. The mortality rate of affected infants is high. Long-term neurologic sequelae include choreothetosis, rigidity, hypotonia, high-frequency deafness, and mental retardation.

Recent evidence indicates that decreased levels of bilirubin in the very preterm infant may have subtle effects on learning and development.[9,22,28] Psychomotor delays may occur even in the absence of overt kernicterus.[11,22]

Congenital Heart Disease

Although there is no physical therapy intervention specifically directed at the effects of the various congenital heart diseases, these malformations with their physiologic disorders are very prevalent and worthy of note. Physical therapy for infants and children with congenital heart defects usually entails immediate preoperative and postoperative care and rehabilitation following the acute effects of surgery. The estimated incidence has been noted as high as 1:170 live births. In addition, congenital heart diseases commonly accompany other disorders commonly seen by the physical therapist including Down syndrome, fetal alcohol syndrome, and Marfan syndrome to name but a few.[29]

Congenital heart defects can be classified loosely into those that usually result in cyanosis and those that are acyanotic.

ACYANOTIC CONGENITAL HEART DISEASES

Patent Ductus Arteriosus. In utero, the ductus arteriosus is a normal vascular connection that shunts blood from the pulmonary artery to the descending aorta, thereby shunting blood away from the lungs, which do not participate in gas exchange during fetal life. The ductus arteriosus normally closes shortly after birth. Failure to close can result in a range of problems from congestive heart failure with pulmonary vascular obstructive disease with a large patent ductus to asymptomatic situation with a small, insignificant patent ductus.[30]

Atrial Septal Defect. Abnormal communication between the atria is the hallmark of an atrial septal defect, one of the most common congenital heart defects. The disorder is associated with a left-to-right shunt through the abnormal communication that may lead to pulmonary vascular obstructive disease and associated pulmonary hypertension. Prognosis is related to the extent of defect, and a large percentage of these communications will close spontaneously during the first 3 years of life. Surgical closure of the defect with suturing or insertion of a patch is usually performed by 4 or 5 years of age and earlier if symptoms dictate.[31]

Ventricular Septal Defects. Ventricular septal defects are the most common structural cardiac disorders and exist commonly as isolated defects and as part of a large constellation of abnormalities such as tetralogy of Fallot. Hemodynamic changes typically include left-to-right shunt at the site of the abnormal communication between the ventricles. As with atrial septal defect, the range of severity is from small asymptomatic defects to larger defects associated with pulmonary hypertension and right ventricular hypertrophy. If the right ventricular hypertrophy becomes great, the left-to-right direction of shunting can reverse as the right ventricular pressure overcomes the left ventricle.[32] In instances of right-to-left shunt the disorder commonly results in cyanosis that is not seen with less severe forms of this defect. Ventricular septal defects can also close spontaneously, but large defects in which symptoms are early and severe will be treated surgically.

CYANOTIC CONGENITAL HEART DISEASES

Tetralogy of Fallot. This most common of all cyanotic defects is characterized by four major abnormalities, hence the name *tetra*logy. The defects include ventricular septal defect, pulmonary artery stenosis, right ventricular hypertrophy, and an aorta that overrides the interventricular septum. Hemodynamic abnormalities include a right-to-left shunt into the ascending aorta thereby bypassing the pulmonary circulation and resulting in inadequate oxygenation with resultant cyanosis and associated dyspnea and syncopal episodes. As with other congenital heart defects, there is a range of severity, with the more severely involved children also suffering height and weight retardation. Surgical approaches may include palliative surgery that improves the hemodynamic status of the more severely involved infant or corrective surgery to completely repair the anatomical defect.[33]

Anomalous Pulmonary Venous Return. This condition occurs when all (total) or part (partial) of the pulmonary venous circulation enters the right atrium rather than the left atrium. Drainage of the pulmonary veins into the right atrium occurs by virtue of direct connection to the atrium or anastomosis with systemic veins. The condition results in excessive volume entering the right atrium, followed by right ventricular hypertrophy. Systemic oxygen desaturation may also be present. Prognosis and treatment are predicated on the degree of anomalous return and varies from asymptomatic to early congestive right heart failure in infants with total anomalous pulmonary venous return. Surgical correction attempts to connect the pulmonary veins to the left heart.[32,33]

TRANSPOSITION OF THE GREAT VESSELS. Transposition is seen when the aorta arises from the right ventricle and the pulmonary artery runs from the left ventricle. The resulting hemodynamic abnormality is severe in that the systemic circulation receives only deoxygenated blood from the right heart (aorta), whereas the pulmonary circulation receives fully oxygenated blood from the left heart (pulmonary trunk). This disorder is incompatible with life if untreated. Early treatment involves attempting to maintain a patent ductus arteriosus, the normal fetal opening between the atria, which can be done medically by administering prostaglandins and surgically via a balloon septostomy. Correction of the defect employs an "arterial switch" procedure that attempts to move the aorta to the left ventricle and the pulmonary artery to the right ventricle.[34]

Viral Infections of the Fetus and Neonate

The developing brain is highly susceptible to injury as a result of viral infection acquired in intrauterine or early neonatal life when cell structures are organizing and myelinating and the vascular system is proliferating. The result of these infections may be malformations or impeded growth of the brain. Viral infections may persist in the infant's system for an extended time and may cause further neurologic impairment. Common nonbacterial agents affecting the neonate have been reported to cause so-called TORCH infections. These include toxoplasmosis (T) and other (O) infections, such as syphilis, rubella (R), cytomegalovirus (C), and herpes simplex (H). As additional microorganisms have been identified, the TORCH group actually represents only one subgroup of congenital infections.

Various neurologic sequelae are associated with congenital infections. Psychomotor retardation, microcephaly, learning disability, seizures, blindness, sensorineural hearing loss, and hydrocephalus are examples of these sequelae.[35]

Human immunodeficiency virus (HIV) has quickly become a major public health problem.[36] Of those children with acquired immunodeficiency syndrome (AIDS), 80% contracted the virus in utero via transplacental transfer.[37,38] Intravenous drug use is the major risk factor associated with mothers who give birth to HIV-infected infants. Maternal antibodies to the virus cross the placenta, and infants of infected mothers will have HIV antibodies whether or not the infants are infected.[38] Infants diagnosed with AIDS usually have specific clinical features, including opportunistic infections; interstitial pneumonitis with respiratory distress resulting from lymphocytic interstitial pneumonitis, microcephaly, and other neurologic abnormalities; and recurrent bacterial infections.[38] Infants with AIDS present a major challenge to the rehabilitation field, as more than 90% of these young patients show signs of static or progressive encephalopathy.[39,40] Therapists working in the NICU, as well as those in all areas of rehabilitation, must be informed of and adhere strictly to infectious disease control policies.

In Utero Substance Exposure

FETAL ALCOHOL SYNDROME

Fetal alcohol syndrome (FAS) occurs in infants whose mothers consume more than 1 to 2 oz of alcohol a day during their pregnancy.[17] The likelihood of the infant developing FAS increases if the mother smokes and drinks.[41]

The incidence of FAS is 1 in 750 live births.[42] FAS is the most common cause of birth defects that is completely preventable. Characteristics that babies with FAS demonstrate include poor motor control, tremulousness during the newborn period, mental retardation, facial dysmorphism, prenatal and postnatal growth deficiency, congenital hip dislocation, abnormalities of the joints, and attention deficit disorders.[4,13]

COCAINE EXPOSURE; MATERNAL COCAINE ABUSE

The recent epidemic of cocaine abuse, in all its various forms, including crack cocaine, has resulted in large numbers of infants being born after in utero exposure to cocaine. Serious effects of cocaine exposure have been reported in neonates. These effects include low birth weight, intrauterine growth retardation, reduced head circumference, preterm birth, hemorrhagic infarctions, cystic lesions, and congenital anomalies and malformations.[43–48] Additionally, increased obstetric complications, especially placenta abruptio, have been reported.

Infants exposed to cocaine in utero may demonstrate withdrawal symptoms characterized by irritability, jitteriness, and vigorous sucking.[43,49] When the Neonatal Behavioral Assessment Scale (NBAS) has been used to assess these neonates, they have shown deficits in the areas of orientation, motor ability, and regulation of state, including a low threshold for overstimulation.[44,50] In addition, abnormal reflex behavior and autonomic instability have been documented.[47] Diminished scores for orientation have been attributed to the infant's inability to attain an alert state.[44]

NEONATAL DRUG WITHDRAWAL SYNDROME

Infants born to mothers who abused narcotics during pregnancy may show symptoms of withdrawal when they are deprived of the drug after birth. Low birth weight has been reported in 50% of infants born to mothers addicted to heroin. Symptoms of withdrawal increase in infants if the maternal dosage is high, if the mother's last dose was within 24 hours of delivery, or if the maternal addiction is longstanding. Symptoms of withdrawal from heroin typically appear within the first 4 days of life, whereas withdrawal from methadone may appear slightly later.[17,51]

The classic symptom of withdrawal from heroin in a neonate is jitteriness, which is further delineated as being stimulus-sensitive, rhythmic, and easily stopped by passive flexion of the extremities.[17] Other common signs and symptoms include hyperirritability, increased activity, hypertonicity, and reduced sleep. There is frequently a high-pitched cry and excessive sucking behavior. These infants are commonly poor feeders despite their tendency toward a strong sucking pattern. Gastrointestinal complications, including regurgitation and diarrhea, are common. Seizures are uncommon with withdrawal from heroin but are more likely to occur with withdrawal from methadone.[39]

Necrotizing Enterocolitis

Necrotizing enterocolitis is a pathologic condition of the gastrointestinal tract that often occurs during the first 6 weeks of life in premature infants weighing less than 2000 g.[52,53] These infants have also suffered perinatal insults, such as asphyxia, sepsis, hypoxia, or respiratory distress. The disease process leads to intestinal mucosal ulceration and hemorrhage, necrosis, and epithelial sloughing. Intestinal perforation may occur.[54]

Retinopathy of Prematurity

Retinopathy of prematurity (ROP) is the main cause of childhood blindness and is a process by which abnormal growth of blood vessels occurs in the immature part of the retina in some premature infants. The cause of this abnormal vascular growth is not fully understood. High levels of administered oxygen are believed to have a detrimental effect on the infant's vulnerable intraocular vasculature. There is an increased incidence of ROP in low-birth-weight infants who have numerous medical complications during hospitalization in the NICU.

In most infants with ROP, the abnormal blood vessels heal by themselves during the first year of life and cause little or no visual impairment. Nearsightedness or strabismus will be the result in many of the patients in whom healing is incomplete. Scarring of the retina may also occur in patients who have only partial healing and who may have visual problems that cannot be corrected completely. In the most severe cases, retinal blood vessels continue their abnormal development and form scar tissue that may cause retinal detachment. Retinal detachment causes severe visual impairment and, occasionally, complete blindness. Only a small percentage of premature infants develop the severe form of the disease. ROP is graded according to its severity (Table 3-5).

Prevention of prematurity is the only effective prophylaxis for ROP. Cryotherapy is effective in arresting many moderately severe cases (designated as Zone 1 or 2 and Stage 3 or 4+). Although cryotherapy does not always prevent retinal detachment, it decreases the incidence of poor outcome from 55.5% to 33.9% based on visual acuity and from 47.4% to 25.7% based on anatomic outcomes.[55]

TABLE 3-5
Stages of Retinopathy of Prematurity

Stage	Characteristics
I	Normal newborn eye demonstrating incomplete vascularization of the peripheral temporal retina
II	Active stage: early vascularization with engorged arterioles and venules
III	Advanced active phase: more advanced venules with vitreous proliferation and organization, as well as retinal traction
IV	Cicatricial phase: localized retinal detachment and severe retinal traction with "temporal dragging" of the macula vessels

From Eden R, et al. *Assessment and Care of the Fetus.* Norwalk: Appleton Lange, 1990.

Neonatal Orthopedic Problems

BRACHIAL PLEXUS INJURY

Brachial plexus injuries are classified as those injuries involving the upper plexus, Erb palsy, and those involving the lower plexus, Klumpke paralysis. Brachial plexus injuries occur in approximately 0.25% of all deliveries.[56]

Erb palsy involves the fifth and sixth cervical roots and accounts for most brachial plexus injuries.[56] Erb palsy occurs most frequently following difficult breech or forceps delivery. Spontaneous recovery is often seen within a few days or weeks. When recovery is delayed, contractures can occur at the shoulder or elbow, and atrophy is common in the affected muscle groups.[57] The infant will have weakness in external rotation, extension, and abduction at the shoulder; elbow flexion, forearm supination; and wrist extension.

A pediatric therapist usually instructs the parents to position the involved upper extremity in a neutral position by pinning the sleeve of the baby's tee shirt to the diaper. This position protects against further injury to the plexus and prevents overstretching of flaccid muscles, tendons, and ligaments. Although this pinned position may reinforce adduction and internal rotation of the shoulder, contractures can usually be prevented with gentle range of motion (ROM) exercises. A 2-week recovery period prior to rehabilitation is usually prudent.

CONGENITAL DISLOCATION OF THE HIP

Congenital dislocation of the hip (CDH) is an abnormality in the relationship between the femoral head and the acetabulum. Subluxation occurs if the two structures are in partial contact, whereas dislocation occurs when there is complete loss of contact. The femoral head is usually displaced in a lateral, posterior, or superior direction owing to the pull of the major muscle groups. Seventy percent of cases occur in females. The incidence increases in breech deliveries. Dysplasia of the femoral head and acetabulum increases with growth.

Because successful correction of the deformity depends on treatment within the first 3 months of life, all neonates should be screened routinely for CDH. The Barlow maneuver, in which medial-to-lateral pressure on the proximal femur is used to test the stability of the hip joint, is the preferred method of screening. Treatment becomes more complicated and invasive if CDH is not detected until later in infancy or early childhood. If hip dysplasia or CDH is diagnosed within the first 3 months of life, it can be treated effectively with dynamic splinting that maintains the hip in a flexed, abducted position with the femoral head seated in the acetabulum. Some of the most commonly used splints were designed by Pavlic, Ilfeld, and Von Rosen. Subluxation may be treated by using double or triple diapers on the infant or by using a Frejka pillow.[58–60]

TALIPES EQUINOVARUS (CLUBFOOT)

Talipes equinovarus, a foot deformity, has three components. Plantar flexion (equinus) occurs at the joint where the talus articulates with the distal tibia and fibula. Inversion (varus) occurs primarily at the subtalar, talocalcaneal, talonavicular, and calcaneocuboid joints. Supination occurs at the midtarsal joint. All three components must be present for the diagnosis of classic talipes equinovarus.[61]

The incidence of talipes equinovarus is approximately 1 in 800 to 1000 live births. Approximately 10% of cases are associated with a hereditary pattern. The deformity is often associated with a neuromuscular disorder (e.g., myelomeningocele). When clubfoot is detected, the infant should be examined carefully for other anomalies, particularly those involving the spine.

Talipes equinovarus can be corrected most rapidly if the treatment is begun shortly after birth, while the foot is still malleable. Treatment consists of manipulation with gentle stretching of the contracted muscle tissues of the medial and posterior aspects of the foot. Manipulation and exercise is often followed by splinting to maintain the desired position, or serial casting. If treatment is delayed, surgery may be necessary to lengthen the tightened soft tissue structures of the foot.[60]

METATARSUS VARUS

Metatarsus varus consists of adduction of the forefoot, which occurs primarily at the midtarsal joint (the talonavicular and calcaneocuboid joints). The severity of this deformity depends on the relative flexibility or rigidity of the joint. A more rigid deformity, unable to be manually corrected past midline, may be treated with serial casting. Passive ROM exercise may be adequate for a more flexible deformity. The role of the pediatric therapist will often include instruction in proper exercise technique for the infant's caregiver.[61]

TIBIAL TORSION

Tibial torsion, often described as "toeing in," consists of excessive internal rotation of the tibia. The problem is more pronounced in premature infants who have low muscle tone. Prone positioning may exacerbate tibial torsion. This deformity is often corrected by using an external rotation splint that is worn at night.

Laxity of the ligaments of the knee in young children may also cause tibial torsion.[61,62]

Neonatal Assessment

A thorough assessment of the infant's neurodevelopmental and behavioral status is the initial step in establishing an intervention program for the infant. Neurologic development of both the premature and full-term infant occurs in a predictable sequence. This sequence provides expectations of an infant's performance at various gestational and corrected ages.

The authors of the first neurologic assessments of the neonate, including Amiel-Tison, Prechtl, and Saint-Anne Dargassies, mainly examined muscle tone and reflex development as manifestations of neurologic function.[63–65] Assessment of behavior as a reflection of more complex neurologic function has now been included in evaluations of the newborn infant. The therapist can draw from various tools of assessment to conduct a comprehensive neurodevelopmental evaluation. Special emphasis is given to muscle tone, development of reflexes, the quality of motor responses, and state organization.

Some general guidelines should be remembered when initiating the assessment process. First, it is important to capture the infant's optimal performance during the assessment.[66] This necessitates flexibility in scheduling. Periods of assessment should be scheduled midway between the infant's feedings. The schedule for other medical procedures, such as heel sticks for blood samples, should be considered when planning a schedule for assessing the infant. A knowledge of the effects on the infant's performance of medications and the overall medical condition are essential for accurate interpretation of assessment procedures. For example, some recovery of asphyxiated infants is expected for up to 2 weeks after birth. Assessment before the end of this recovery period must take into account the neurologic delay associated with asphyxia in order not to underestimate the capabilities of these infants.

Age corrected for prematurity is appropriate when interpreting the results of a neurodevelopmental assessment. Full-term gestation is considered to be 40 weeks. Infants are considered to be premature if they are born before the completion of 37 weeks of gestation.[22] The corrected age is established by subtracting the estimated number of gestational weeks less than 40 from the chronologic age. For example, 4 weeks after birth, an infant born at an estimated 32 weeks of gestation, or 8 weeks earlier than 40, has a corrected age of 36 weeks (4 weeks chronologic age minus 8 weeks equals 36). The same infant, 24 weeks after birth, is corrected to 24 weeks minus 8 weeks, which equals 16 weeks, or 4 months.

Use of corrected age for interpreting assessment procedures in both the neonatal period and throughout infancy varies among institutions. Our policy is to correct ages until the chronologic age of 18 months; however, this interpretation can artificially inflate assessment scores, thus disguising developmental delays. The experienced therapist must be aware of the quality of movement patterns and must look for subtle signs of neurologic deviations.

A brief discussion of the most commonly used neonatal assessments follows. Several of these tools require additional training in their administration and interpretation. In all cases, supervised experience is suggested to improve reliability. A detailed discussion of assessment tools can be found in Chapter 2.

Apgar Score

The Apgar score is a quantitative assessment of the neonate's medical status that is usually performed at 1 and 5 minutes of age and, occasionally, at 10 and 15 minutes of age as well. A score of eight or more at 1 minute of age means that the baby will not require extensive resuscitation. A score of zero to two indicates severe asphyxia and may indicate the need for intubation and cardiac massage. Scores of five to seven may indicate a need for less intense resuscitation, such as vigorous stimulation and administration of supplemental oxygen (Table 3-6).[42,52,67,68]

Clinical Assessment of Gestational Age in the Newborn Infant

The Clinical Assessment of Gestational Age in the Newborn Infant, developed by Dubowitz, Dubowitz, and Goldberg, is the most widely used and accepted scale for determining gestational age.[69] The scale involves evaluating 11 external characteristics or 10 neurologic criteria. These characteristics appear predictably with gestational age. The results of this assessment are then compared to obstetric records and prenatal sonograms to establish the gestational age. The determined gestational age is then plotted against the infant's height and weight to determine whether intrauterine growth was adequate or retarded.

Neonatal Behavioral Assessment Scale

The Neonatal Behavioral Assessment Scale (NBAS),[69] designed by Brazelton, permits the examiner to measure an infant's ability to respond to environmental events. Intrinsic to this assessment is the concept that the neonate is a complex organism capable of protecting itself from negative environmental stimuli while still being able to respond to positive input. The neonate also has the capacity to elicit responses from people in the environment. Despite the inclusion of some neurologic items, Brazelton does not consider the tool to be a formal neurologic evaluation. Brazelton was a pioneer in establishing the need to elicit an infant's best performance, rather than relying on average performance. The examiner is responsible for altering the infant's environment to attain an optimal response to a stimulus. Ideally, the examiner brings the infant through various behavioral states beginning with the infant in light sleep, progressing to an alert state, then to an active and crying state, and then back to a quieter state. This tool was developed for use with

TABLE 3-6
Apgar Score for Condition of the Newborn Baby*

Sign	Score 0	Score 1	Score 2
Heart rate	Absent	Slow (<100 bpm)	>100 bpm
Respiratory effort	Absent	Slow, irregular	Good, crying
Muscle tone	Limp	Some flexion of extremities	Active motion
Reflex irratability			
Response to catheter in nostril	No response	Grimace	Cough or sneeze
Response when feet are stimulated	No response	Some motion	Cry
Color	Blue, pale	Body pink, extremities blue	Completely pink
			Total score

*From Apgar V. Proposal for new method of evaluation of newborn infant. *Anesth Analg.* 1953;32:269; Avery G, ed: *Neonatology, Pathophysiology and Management of the Newborn.* Philadelphia: JB Lippincott; 1975:117.

infants between 36 and 44 weeks' gestational age. Reliability in administering and scoring the NBAS is achieved through specific training and supervised practice.

Assessment of Preterm Infant's Behavior

Adapted from the NBAS, the Assessment of Preterm Infant's Behavior (APIB) evaluates the developing behavioral organization of the premature infant.[7] The APIB is based on the synactive model of newborn behavioral organization discussed earlier. This assessment uses graded maneuvers to assess the functioning and interplay of five subsystems, including physiologic, motor, state, attentional-interactive, and self-regulatory. Like the NBAS, reliability in administering and scoring the APIB depends on the extensive training and supervised practice.[8]

Neurologic Assessment of the Full-Term and Preterm Newborn Infant

The Neurologic Assessment of the Full-term and Preterm Newborn Infant[70] investigates the infant's capabilities for habituation, movement and muscle tone, reflexes, and neurobehavioral responses. It provides diagrams in chart format for recording, and is based on a five-point scale for categorizing results. The tool was designed to meet four specific requirements. First, minimal training in neonatal neurology is required to administer this test. Second, it assesses both premature and full-term infants. Third, there is high test–retest reliability. Finally, administration of the assessment takes no longer than 10 or 15 minutes. The authors of the test have correlated results of assessments with the development of IVHs. The ability of this assessment device to document progression or resolution of neurologic abnormalities raises the possibility that this tool may be used to predict prognosis.

Morgan Neonatal Neurobehavioral Examination

The Morgan Neonatal Neurobehavioral Examination is divided into three sections: tone and motor patterns, primitive reflexes, and behavioral responses. Similar to the Dubowitz Neurologic Assessment, the Morgan examination is provided in chart format to expedite recording. Each of the three sections has nine items that are scored based on the level of maturity of a normal response or on the abnormality of a response. This assessment is applicable for infants between the ages of 34 and 44 weeks' gestation or corrected age. A numeric quotient, which Morgan has correlated with developmental outcome, can be obtained from the assessment (Table 3-7).[71]

Movement Assessment of Infants

Movement Assessment of Infants (MAI) provides a uniform approach to the evaluation of high-risk infants. It is used for infants between the ages of birth and 12 months. This assessment requires extensive handling of the infant, which makes the MAI very time-consuming.[72]

Milani-Comparetti Motor Development Screening Test

The Milani-Comparetti motor assessment test is used to test reflexes and motor milestones of infants from birth to 2 years of age. This assessment is relatively easy to administer and has a high reliability.[73]

Developmental Intervention

Numerous theories of intervention have been proposed by various experts who work in NICUs. Neurodevelopmental and sensorimotor

TABLE 3-7

Morgan Neonatal Neurobehavioral Examination*

Name______________

Date of Birth______________ Gestational Age______________

Date of Exam______________ Chronological Age______________

Timing of Exam______________ Corrected Age______________

STATES

1. Deep sleep, no movement, regular breathing
2. Light sleep, eyes shut, some movement
3. Dozing, eyes opening and closing
4. Awake, eyes open, minimal movement
5. Wide awake, vigorous movement
6. Crying

Tone and Motor Patterns	1 (<32 Wks)	2 (32–36 Wks)	3 (>36 Wks)	A (Abnormal)
Posture Predominant	Total extension	LE flexed, UE extended	Total flexion	Opisthotonus Tonic extension
Arm recoil Infant supine. Take arms and extend parallel to the body; hold several seconds and release.	No flexion within 5 sec	Partial flexion at elbow >100° within 4–5 sec	Arms flex at elbow to <100° within 2–3 sec	Difficult to extend Jerky flexion
Scarf Infant supine, head in midline. Bring arm across chest until resistance is met.	No resistance	Limited resistance past midline	Resistance at or before midline	Tonic flexion Shoulder retraction
Popliteal angle Infant supine. Approximate knee and thigh to abdomen; extend leg by gentle pressure with index finger behind ankle.	180°–135°	90°–135°	90°–60°	<60°
Ankle dorsiflexion Infant supine. Flex foot against shin until resistance is met.	Limited 60°–90°	Partial 30°–60°	Complete <30°	Equinus > 90°

A. Tone and motor patterns______________
   Abnormal patterns______________

B. Primitive reflexes______________
   Abnormal patterns______________

C. Behavioral responses______________
   Responsiveness______________
   Temperament______________
   Equilibration______________

Prone suspension Hold infant in ventral suspension, observe curvature of back and relation of head to trunk	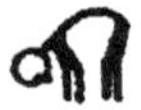 Complete	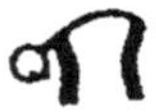 Partial	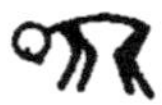 Near horizontal	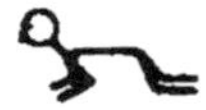 Tonic extension
Slip-through Hold infant in vertical suspension under axillae. Observe the amount of support required to prevent infant from "slipping."	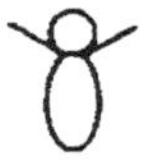 Complete	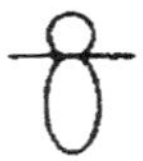 Partial	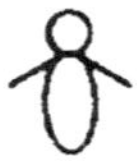 None	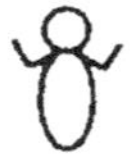 Shoulder retraction
Pull-to-sit Pull infant toward sitting posture by traction on both arms	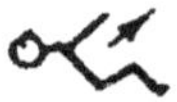 Complete head/leg	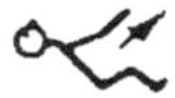 Partial flexion	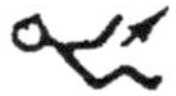 Occasional alignment	Tonic extension Shoulder retraction
Head righting Place infant in sitting position, allow head to fall forward, then wait 30 seconds	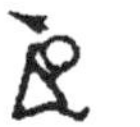 No attempt to raise head	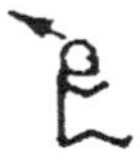 Unsuccessful attempt to raise head upright	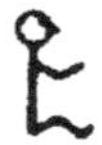 Occasional alignment	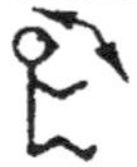 Head cannot be flexed forward
Primative Reflexes				
Root	Absent	Mouth opening, partial head turning	Full head turning with mouth opening	Tongue thrust
Suck	Weak	Inconsistent, irregular	Strong regular sucking in bursts if 5 or more movements	Clenching-tonic bite
Grasp	Absent	Sustained flexion	Traction	Thumb adduction
Positive support	Astasis	Inconsistent, partial	Full extension	Equinus
Walking	No response	Some effort, but not continuous with both legs	At least two steps	Scissoring
Crossed extensor	No response	Withdrawal and flexion	Flexion and extension	Tonic extension
Moro	No response	Abduction only	Abduction and adduction	Tremor only
Tonic neck	No response	Legs only	Arms and legs respond	Obligate
Cry	Absent	Whimpering	Sustained cry	High pitched

(continued)

SCORING

1. Total responses to the 9 items in each area; A scored as 1
2. Behavioral subtest scored 3, if 2 of three items are scored 3
3. Behavioral subtest scored 1, if 2 of three items are scored 1
4. Behavioral subtest scored 2 if neither of the above criteria are met
5. Score number of abnormal patterns

TABLE 3-7

Morgan Neonatal Neurobehavioral Examination* (Continued)

Tone and Motor Patterns	1 (<32 Wks)	2 (32–36 Wks)	3 (>36 Wks)	A (Abnormal)
Behavioral Responses				
Responsiveness/alertness	1 (<32 wks) Inattentive or brief responsiveness (4 or less)		2 (32–36 wks) Moderately sustained alertness; may use stimulation to come to alert state (5,6)	3 (>36 wks) Sustained and continuous attentiveness (7–9)
Orientation to face and voice	Does not focus or follow stimulus, brief following (4 or less)		Inconsistent or jerky following horizontal 30° (5,6)	Sustained, smooth following 60° horizontally and occasionally vertically (7–9)
Defensive reaction to cloth over face	No response, nonspecific activity with long latency (1–3)		Rooting, head turning (5,6)	Swipes with arms (7–9)
Temperament	I-Flat	I-Labile		
Irritability	No cry (1)	Cries to 6 stimuli (7–9)	Cries to 4 or 5 stimuli (5,6)	Cries to 1–3 stimuli (2–4)
Peak of excitement	Low level of arousal never > state 3 (1,2)	Insulated crying in response to stimuli (8,9)	Predominantly state 4—may reach state 5 with stimulation (3,4)	Predominantly state 5; reaches state 6 with stimulation (5–7)
Cuddliness	No moulding (3)	Resists, arches (1,2)	Molds with movement and handling (4,5)	Molds and nestles spontaneously (6–9)
Equilibration				
Self-quieting	Cannot quiet self (1–3)		Occasional success (4–6); no sustained crying	Quiets self on two or more occasions (7–9)
Consolability	Inconsolable (1)		Consoles with holding and rocking (2–5) consoling not needed	Consoles with talking or handling in crib (6–9)
Tremors	Tremors in all states (8,9)		Tremors occasionally with aversive stimuli (6,7)	No tremors or tremors only with crying (1–5)

*After Morgan A: *Neuro-Developmental Approach to the High-Risk Neonate* (Notes from a seminar). Williamsburg, VA, Nov 3–4 1984.

LE, lower extremities; UE, upper extremities.

approaches are the bases for most interventional programs implemented by physical and occupational therapists. Both approaches take into account the fact that infant neuromotor development is a unique and individualized process. Treatment, therefore, is designed to meet the specific problems and needs of each infant.

Neurodevelopmental treatment, as designed by Bobath, uses handling to inhibit abnormal responses while facilitating automatic reactions.[74] Handling techniques are used with the neonate to provide normal sensory and motor experiences that will provide the basis for motor development. Movement experience is frequently limited or disturbed in the premature or medically unstable infant. Disruptions and abnormalities of the normal patterns of movement may interfere with the development of head control, trunk stability, oculomotor coordination, eye-hand coordination, and social interaction.

With sensorimotor approaches, specific sensory input is administered to elicit a desired motor or behavioral response. Sensory integration techniques, originally developed for treatment of learning disabled children, are sometimes incorporated into sensorimotor programs. Sensorimotor intervention can be applied to the high-risk infant in various ways (e.g., linear rocking on a small beach ball might be used to stimulate the vestibular system and promote an alert state). If an infant is tightly swaddled, deep tactile and proprioceptive input can promote calming and self-regulating behavior.

Common goals of developmental intervention in the NICU include the following:

1. To promote state organization
2. To promote appropriate parent–infant interaction
3. To enhance self-regulatory behavior through environmental modification
4. To promote postural alignment and more normal patterns of movement through therapeutic handling and positioning
5. To enhance oral-motor skills and assist with oral feedings
6. To improve visual and auditory reactions
7. To prevent iatrogenic musculoskeletal abnormalities
8. To provide appropriate remediation of orthopedic complications
9. To provide consultation to team members, including the nursing staff and parents, regarding developmental intervention
10. To participate in interagency collaboration in order to facilitate transition to the home environment.

Success of intervention depends on individualization of treatment techniques to meet the infant's specific needs. The suggestions that preceded and that follow are not a "cookbook" to be used for solutions to particular problems. No activity is appropriate for all infants, and all activities must be adapted to respond to the infant's unique reactions to handling. For best results, therapeutic handling must be incorporated into routine care activities, such as rolling the infant or lifting and carrying the infant.

As previously emphasized, the therapist must have a complete understanding of normal and abnormal development before entering the NICU. When handling, positioning, or feeding an infant, the therapist must be aware of the signs of physiologic stress (see Table 3-3). Therapy must be modified or deferred if signs of stress are noted. Periodic rest breaks during the treatment session may help the infant to maintain physiologic homeostasis.

Therapeutic Handling

The primary goals of therapeutic handling in premature infants are to decrease hyperextension of the neck and trunk, reduce elevation of the shoulders, decrease retraction of the scapula, and reduce extension of the lower extremities. Activation of the primary flexor muscle groups must occur simultaneously.

In the supine position, neck and trunk hyperextension can be reduced by gently flexing the hips and knees. Extreme care must be taken with this activity to avoid hyperflexion of the neck, which can cause airway obstruction and pulmonary compromise in premature infants. Elevation of the shoulders can be reduced in the supine position by bringing the infant's hands toward the buttocks. With the lower extremities flexed and the hands on the buttocks, weight bearing through the shoulder girdle can be introduced, as can subtle weight shifts. Alignment of the head and trunk should be maintained, especially during weight shifts (Fig. 3-1).

The side-lying position is advantageous for accomplishing several therapeutic goals. Neck and trunk hyperextension can be reduced in side-lying, and deep proprioceptive input can be applied through the shoulders and hips to promote postural stability. Additionally, scapular protraction (abduction) and upper extremity midline activities can be enhanced in the side-lying position (Fig. 3-2*A*). Weight bearing through the shoulders, hips, and feet provides proprioceptive input that may promote the development of more normal muscle tone and increase proximal stability (Fig. 3-2*B*).

Several therapeutic goals can be achieved using a technique called hammock handling. This handling technique is used to activate flexor muscle groups, facilitate head righting, and facilitate alerting. A hammock-like sling is made with a doubled blanket whose sides have been rolled toward the infant for stability. The infant is placed in the hammock in a supine position and is elevated slowly to a semi-sitting position, after which the infant is lowered back to a supine position. This activity must be done slowly to fully elicit the desired head righting reactions. Promotion of an alert behavioral state through stimulation of the vestibular system is an additional benefit of the linear rocking that occurs with raising and lowering. A desired response to the hammock activity is activation of anterior neck and abnormal musculature to promote flexion. In addition, scapular retraction and shoulder elevation can be reduced, and

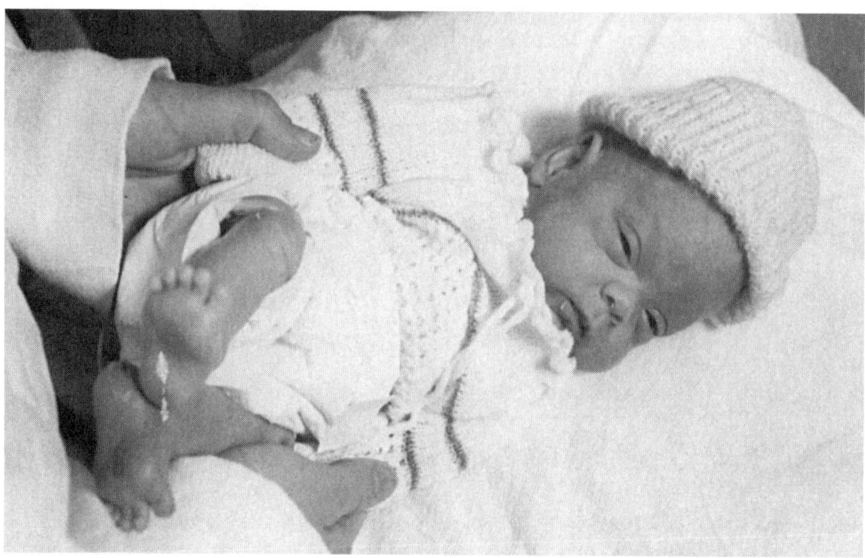

Figure 3-1 ■ Weight bearing through the shoulder girdle to promote proximal stability. Lateral weight shift provides a valuable sensorimotor experience.

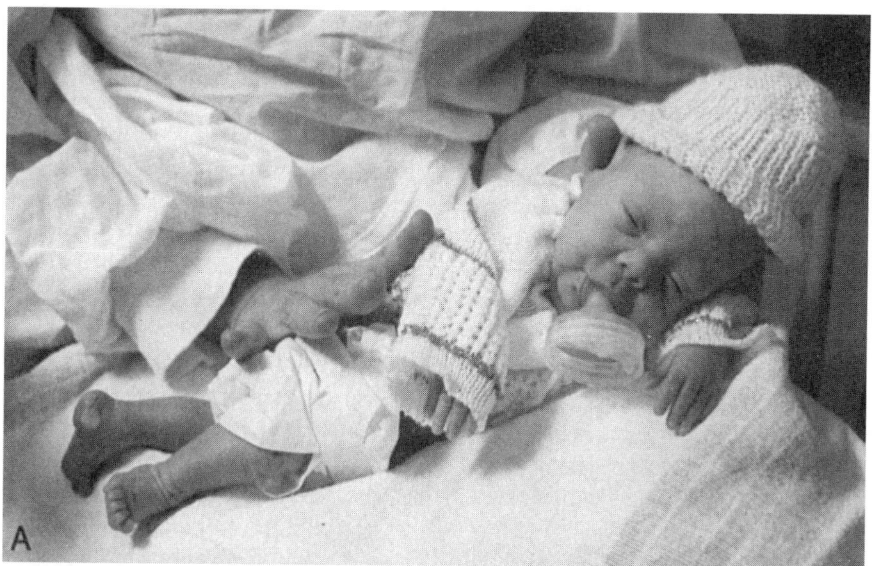

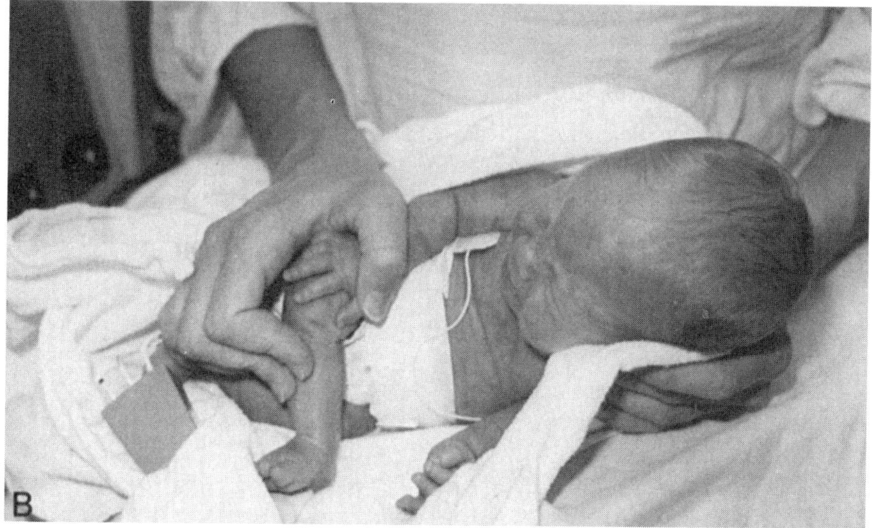

Figure 3-2 ▪ (**A**) In a side-lying position, disassociation not only between shoulder and pelvic girdles, but also between the lower extremities, can be achieved. (**B**) Incorporation of weight bearing through the foot helps reduce tactile hypersensitivity of the foot.

upper extremity midline skills can be increased with this activity (Fig. 3-3).

By placing the infant in a prone position, weight bearing and weight shifting can be introduced. The upper extremities of the infant should be held near the body in a flexed posture. The lower extremities should be flexed and adducted at the hip in order for the knees to be placed in position under the abdomen. By using this position, the infant's center of gravity is

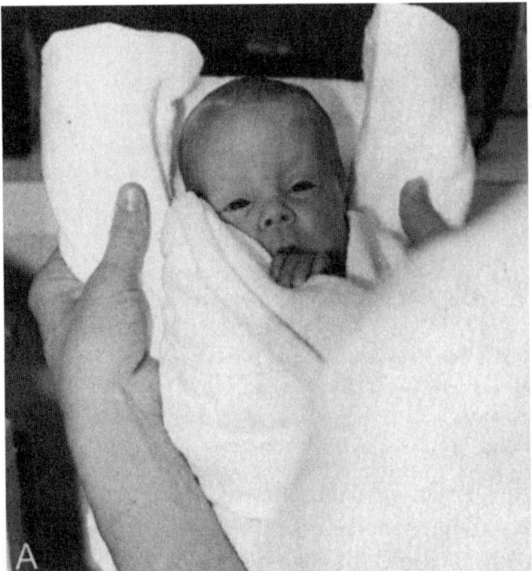

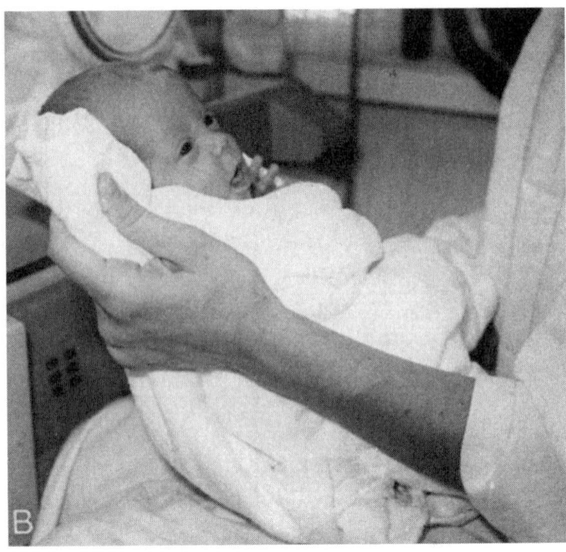

Figure 3-3 ■ (**A**) and (**B**) Hammock handling to improve head-righting reactions and to increase flexor responses. Vestibular input facilitates alert behavior state (origination of this technique is unknown to these authors).

placed forward at a point near the cheek, similar to that of a full-term infant. The therapist's hands are placed along the infant's trunk to provide important tactile and proprioceptive cues that reinforce symmetry and facilitate graded extension of the neck and trunk. Subtle shifts in weight in lateral and anterior or posterior directions can be facilitated by the therapist, who should hold the infant on his or her lap while gently raising and lowering his or her own legs. Downward pressure through the infant's shoulders serves to elongate the cervical musculature. Stroking of the cervical extensor muscle groups promotes head-turning reactions. If hyperextension of the neck or trunk or increased elevation of the shoulder is elicited in this position, handling must be altered to incorporate a greater degree of flexion into the infant's posture.

Supported sitting offers an opportunity to increase the infant's ability to assume and maintain an alert state. The upright or semi-upright position, because of vestibular input, encourages arousal and alert behaviors. This allows the infant to begin to interact with the environment, and may improve visual and auditory responses. Again, it must be stressed that coming to an alert state may contribute to loss of stability in the motor and autonomic subsystems. Therefore, the infant must be monitored closely. Adequate support of the trunk during supported sitting is essential to help prevent the elevation or retraction of the scapula, which is often seen in infants in an attempt to compensate for poor control of the head.

Head righting may become a realistic goal for more long-term hospitalized infants and can be facilitated with work in prone and supported sitting. In a supported sit, extension of the trunk may be facilitated through subtle lateral shifting of weight over the ischial tuberosities. The trunk must be erect and aligned with the head before attempts are made to facilitate trunk extension. Anterior flexion of the neck can be stimulated by slowly shifting the infant's weight in a posterior direction, whereas extension of the neck can be achieved by anteriorly shifting the infant's weight.

Premature infants often show hypersensitivity to tactile input. The oral motor area, the palms of the hands, and the soles of the feet are especially prone to tactile hypersensitivity. Essential but aversive medical intervention, such as prolonged intubation, repetitive gavage feedings, and frequent heel sticks, may contribute to the infant's hypersensitivity. Various methods can be used to decrease the neonate's hypersensitivity. Deep rhythmic tactile and proprioceptive input, rather than light touch when handling the infant, will effectively reduce defensive behaviors. Light touch tends to be disorganizing and may elicit a sympathetic nervous system response ("fight or flight"). Conversely, deep and rhythmic tactile sensation provides the discriminative tactile input and tends to be more organizing.[75]

Early deep stroking of the perioral area may be appropriate even if the infant is being mechanically ventilated. Stroking, for example, can be done from the temporomandibular joint toward the mouth, and deep pressure can be applied to the upper lip. Infants have a variable tolerance to this technique and should be monitored closely. Weight bearing and other forms of deep proprioceptive input also may help normalize the neonate's tactile system. Deep pressure to the soles of the feet assists in reducing hypersensitivity in that area. Lotions and oils are usually contraindicated during tactile activities because they may irritate the skin.

In some instances, an infant's stay in the NICU may extend well past the neonatal stage. It may then become necessary to address higher level motor, cognitive, and social skills. For example, in the 4- to 6-month-old infant (adjusted age), the therapist might introduce counterrotation of the shoulder girdle and pelvic girdle in sidelying, as this improves coordination between flexor and extensor muscle groups. Similarly, the counterrotation provides the infant with early sensorimotor experience in dissociation between the shoulder and pelvic girdles and dissociation between the lower extremities. These experiences provide the infant with a foundation for higher level, more complex motor skills (see Fig. 3-2*A*).[76]

Infants who have deficits in state and behavioral organization are frequently referred for therapy. Infants included in this group of referrals may be lethargic or hyperirritable, such as those infants suffering from drug withdrawal syndrome. Calming techniques, such as tight swaddling and slow, rhythmic rocking, have been effective in soothing hyperirritable infants. Deep proprioceptive input may also promote calming. A pacifier can be soothing for infants, and its use is recommended, particularly for infants addicted to drugs. Techniques to increase the alertness of lethargic infants may include carefully graded, but arrhythmic vestibular input, such as bouncing, light tactile input to the face and body, and upright positioning. Modulated stimulation may be indicated for all sensory systems. The infant's response must always be monitored carefully to avoid overstimulation.

Therapists rarely need to be concerned about the development of contractures in infants in the NICU. Ligamentous laxity in newborn infants typically protects them from permanent loss of joint mobility. Sloughing of skin and soft tissue that is the result of an infiltrated intravenous site, however, may cause contractures if located directly over a joint. Gentle ROM exercise can be provided to minimize contractures. The integrity of the area of sloughing must be respected during exercise. Infants who receive medications to cause paralysis (e.g., those receiving mechanical ventilation) will require ROM exercises if the medication is used for a long time. In order to minimize the number of different people handling the critically ill infant, the physical therapist may instruct the nursing staff in proper exercise techniques.

Therapeutic Positioning

Proper positioning of the high-risk and premature infant reinforces the therapist's goals to enhance flexor patterns, increase midline orientation, and promote state organization. Positions are changed frequently to offer the infant various sensorimotor experiences. The infant's medical status determines both the readiness for certain positions and the tolerance for a change of position. Careful attention must be given to protect the respiratory capacity of the infant. Hyperflexion of the neck and trunk, for example, can compromise both upper airway patency and diaphragmatic descent. Depending on the specific needs of the infant, individualized instructions in positioning should be made easily accessible to the infant's primary caregivers (Fig. 3-4).

The side-lying position has been strongly recommended for the infant in the NICU. In side-lying, the effects of gravity are reduced, thus promoting midline and flexor responses. Blanket rolls, bags of intravenous fluid, and sandbags can help provide stability for the infant. Symmetric development can be enhanced by using alternate right and left side-lying. The infant should be placed on the right side to facilitate gastric emptying after feeding (Figs. 3-5 and 3-6).

The desired flexor response can also be reinforced with the infant in a prone position. A small washcloth or diaper roll placed under the pelvis and below the abdomen increases flexion of the hip and knee to approximate the posture of a full-term infant. This position also minimizes excessive abduction and external rotation of the hip. Iatrogenic changes in the lower extremity, arising from extended abduction and external rotation of the hip, are also reduced. Rolls placed along the infant's sides help rein-

PROBLEM: Preterm infants lack sufficient muscle tone to maintain symmetrical, flexed body posture.
SOLUTION: Assist developing tone with proper positioning.

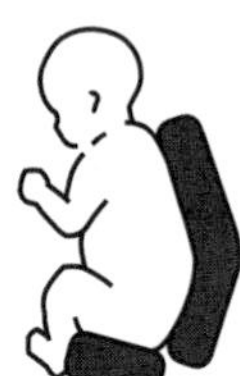

SIDE-LYING #1
Place sandbag or rolled cloth diaper at infant's back from shoulder level to buttocks. Round pelvis and buttocks forward.

A second roll is placed below buttocks to support hips and legs into a more flexed position.

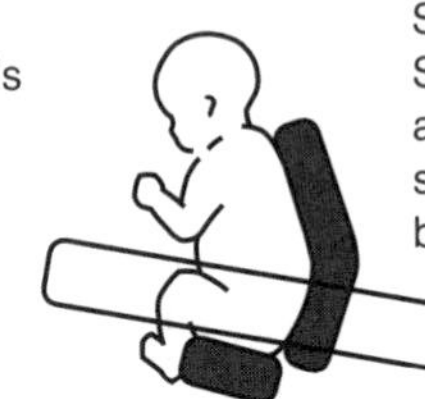

SIDE-LYING #2
Support rolls as described at left. Fold a cloth diaper diagonally into a narrow strip. Tuck one end under mattress, bring across infant's hips until taut and tuck remaining free end under mattress on other side.

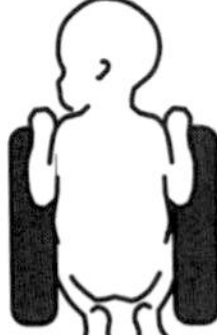
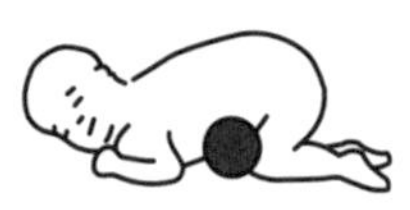

PRONE
Roll a Chux pad or diaper into tight roll and place under infant's abdomen so pelvis is raised up. Bend infant's legs up under pelvis. Place sand bags or blanket rolls on either side of infant to maintain flexion and keep arms and legs close together.

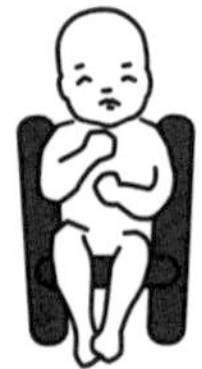

SUPINE
Place tightly rolled cloth diapers on either side of infant to support arms and legs in flexion and toward midline of body.

A smaller roll is then placed below the buttocks to reinforce flexion of legs, rounding forward of pelvis.

Figure 3-4 ■ Primary caregivers should receive individualized instructions for positioning an infant.

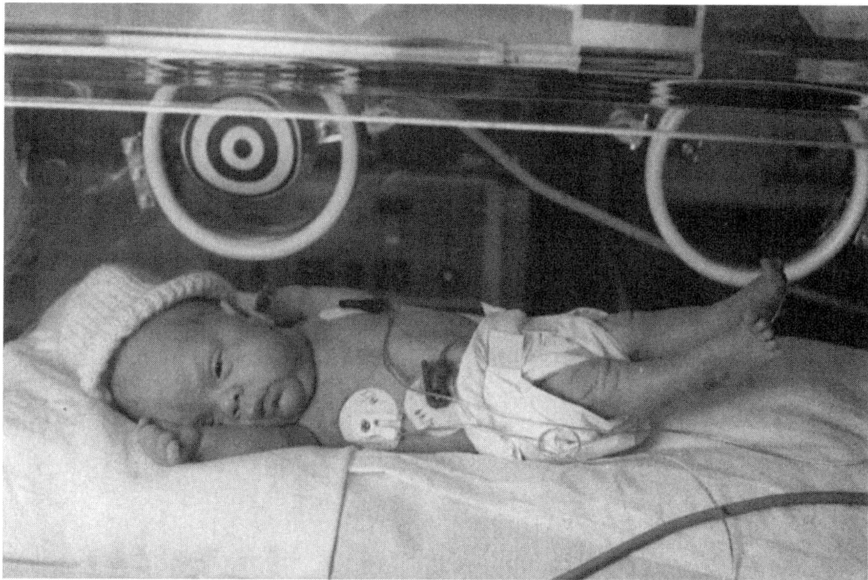

Figure 3-5 ▪ Infant shows the excessive extensor posturing that is commonly seen in premature infants. The influence of the asymmetric tonic neck reflex is apparent in the upper extremities.

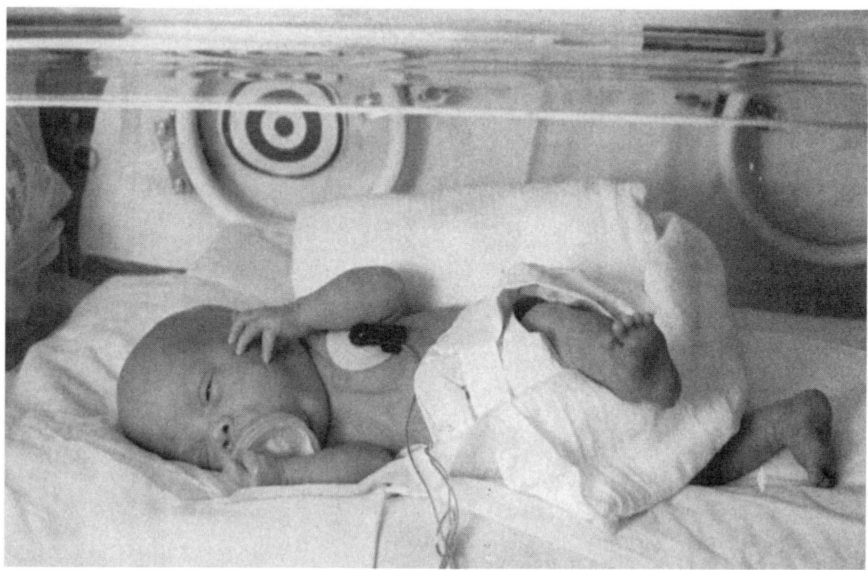

Figure 3-6 ▪ Positioning the infant in a side-lying position using diaper and blanket rolls for support reduces extensor posturing and encourages flexion and midline orientation.

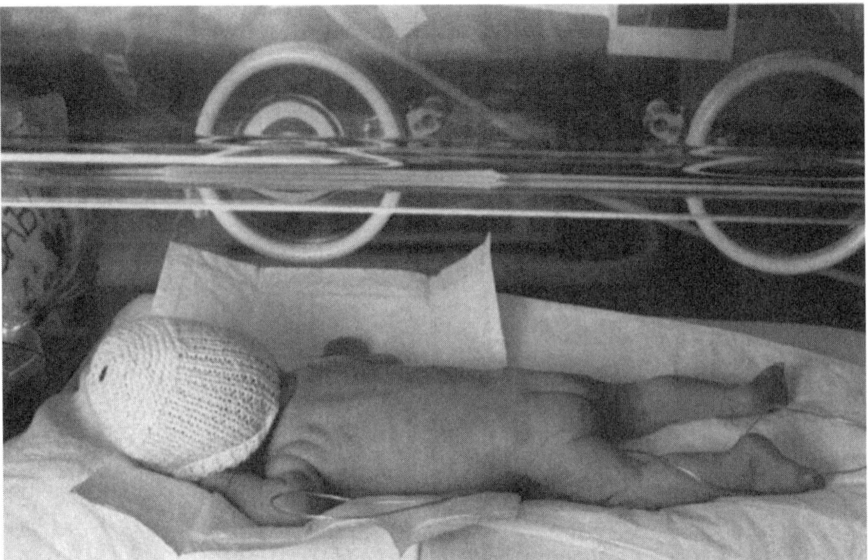

Figure 3-7 ▪ Extensor patterns continue to predominate in the posture of the premature infant in the prone position.

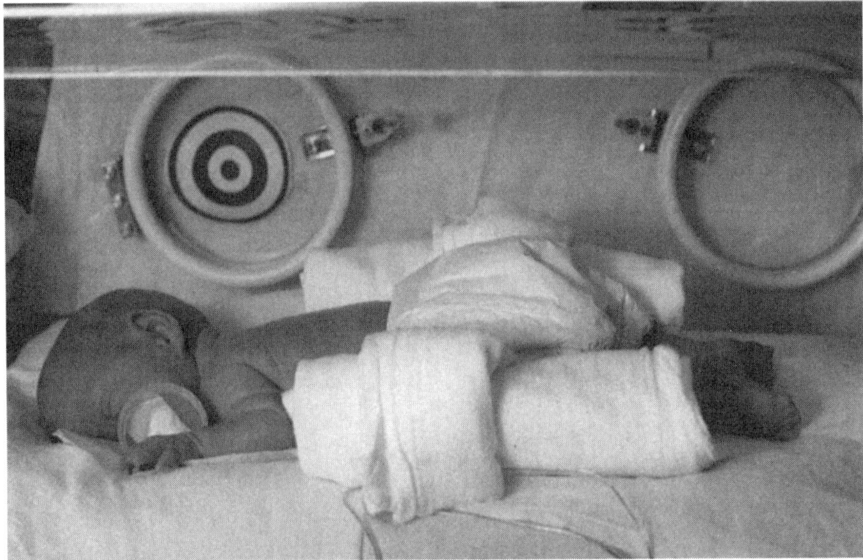

Figure 3-8 ▪ Flexor tone and symmetry are promoted through the use of small rolls placed under the pelvis and along the infant's sides.

force symmetry (Figs. 3-7 and 3-8). The premature infant tends to be more organized, shows improved regulation of sleep and wake patterns, and demonstrates better self-calming skills in the prone position.[77]

The medically unstable infant is often placed in a supine position for better accessibility for medical procedures. With the infant in a supine position, the force of gravity strongly enhances extensor postures and impedes random flexor movements. By placing blanket rolls along the infant's sides and under the shoulder girdles for support, antigravity flexor patterns are fostered in the upper extremities. Another roll under the knees helps increase flexion of the hip and knee. Care must be taken to ensure that the airway stays open (Figs. 3-5 and 3-9).

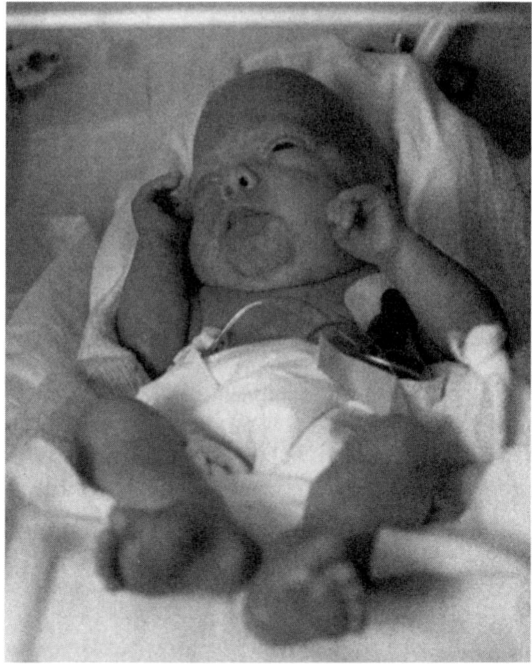

Figure 3-9 ▪ Rolls placed along the infant's sides, below the scapulae, and under the knees encourage flexion, symmetry, and an alert state of behavior.

Infant seats provide experience in the upright position, which helps promote an alert state. Adaptations of the seat are usually necessary to accommodate the low-birth-weight infant and to increase flexor positioning. Infant seats made for dolls can be effective for low-birth-weight babies, and they often fit into the isolette. Various commercial positioning devices are also available.

Feeding

The pediatric therapist plays a crucial role in evaluating oral-motor skills, neurobehavioral readiness to feed, and establishment of successful feeding programs. The suck-swallow reflex emerges by 28 to 30 weeks of gestation. At this early stage, the reflex is weak, poorly coordinated, and lacks rhythmicity. Nippling at this time is unsafe.[2] Usually not until 33 to 35 weeks estimated gestational age has there occurred sufficient coordination of suck, swallow, and breathing to initiate oral feedings.

The therapist should do a comprehensive assessment of the infant's readiness to feed before oral feedings begin. An assessment of oral-motor reflex development is crucial. The presence of an effective gag reflex, which is a primary defense against aspiration, must be ascertained. The gag reflex is often either hyperactive or hypoactive as a result of prolonged endotracheal intubation and repetitive gavage feedings. The infant may not accept the nipple if a hyperactive gag reflex is present.[78]

Additional reflexes that should be assessed before feeding include rooting and suckling. Depending on the infant's gestational age, these reflexes may be absent, depressed, or incomplete. A feeding assessment also includes an evaluation of oral-motor muscle tone; tongue configuration; coordination of suck, swallow, and breathing; and excursion of the jaw. Because a quiet, alert state is optimal for effective feeding, the infant's state should also be considered in the assessment of feeding.

Feeding skills of premature infants are adversely affected by decreased flexor and proximal muscle tone, decreased buccal fat pads, limited endurance, and a low state of arousal. Infants who are mechanically ventilated tend to display high arched palates that further impede their ability to express liquid from the nipple. Tactile hypersensitivity in the oral motor area is commonly observed.

Preparation for oral feeding can begin soon after birth through graded tactile stimulation. This procedure can be begun even with the infant who is mechanically ventilated. Nonnutritive sucking, when encouraged during gavage feeding, has been shown to facilitate earlier oral feeding and weight gain.[79]

Therapeutic positioning and handling are used to enhance development of normal oral-motor skills. Placing the infant in an upright position with the neck elongated is encouraged. Hyperflexion of the neck must be avoided because occlusion of the infant's airway will be the result. Positioning and handling during feeding should provide for depression of the shoulder and should encourage midline orientation. Specific oral-motor techniques can be used to facilitate closure of the lips, stability of the jaw, suckling, and swallowing (Fig. 3-10). The infant's respiration, heart rate, color, and other physiologic signs should be monitored constantly during feeding. When first attempting oral feeding, the infant's nurse and suctioning equipment must be nearby.

Various nipples are available for use with premature infants and infants with structural problems of the mouth, such as cleft palate. Some of these nipples are shown in Figure 3-11. Selection of the proper nipple depends on the infant's ability to suck, strength of sucking, endurance, and preference. Nipples vary in firmness, size, and the rate of flow. Occupational therapists and/or speech pathologists may be consulted for oral-motor and feeding intervention.

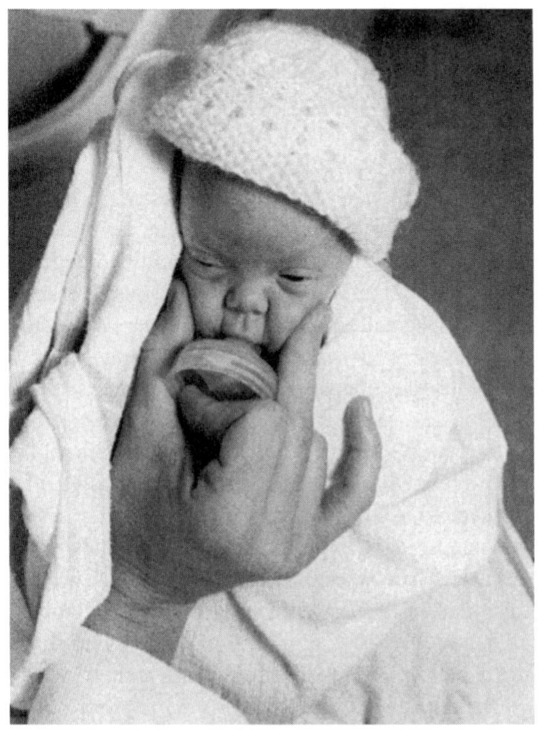

Figure 3-10 ▪ External support to the infant's cheeks increases the strength of the infant's ability to suck and encourages greater approximation of the lips. Pressure is applied downward and forward toward the mouth.

Parent Education

Parent education is an essential component of developmental intervention in NICU. Enactment of the amendments of the Education of the Handicapped Act (P.L. 99-457) has changed the focus of infant intervention from infant-centered to family-centered care.[80] The therapists now view parents as team members, and encourage participation to the extent the family wishes to participate in their infant's care. The therapist needs to be sensitive to variations in a family's ability or willingness to share in their infant's care, and must maintain a nonjudgmental attitude. Additionally, diversities in culture, values,

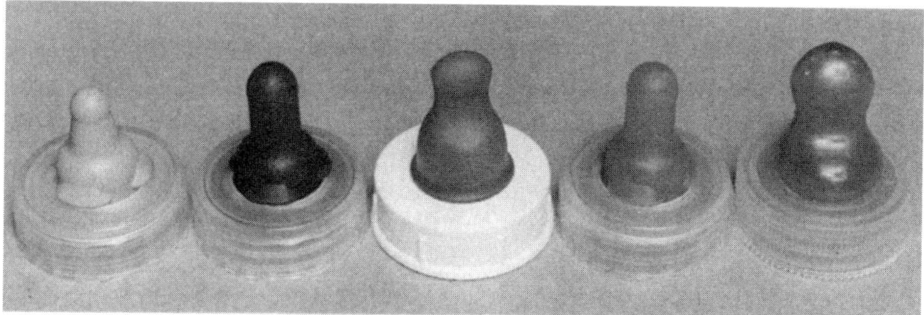

Figure 3-11 ▪ *Available nipples vary in size, shape, firmness, and rate of flow.*

and background must be respected. The major goals of parent education are to strengthen the parents' feelings of competency and to improve parent–infant interactions.

Open communication with the family is essential and can be facilitated using verbal and written means. Some therapists have found it useful to attach a communication booklet to the isolette in order to share information with parents who may visit after usual treatment hours. This may also serve to maintain an updated Individualized Family Service Plan (IFSP) as required by P.L. 99-457. Personal contact and telephone calls will keep parents informed of the infant's progress or developmental changes. The therapist involved in the NICU may need to consider flexible work schedules to guarantee family contact.

To improve parent–infant interaction, it is essential that the family be informed of the infant's behavioral cues and signs of stress. Showing the family techniques to foster alertness as the infant's medical and behavioral stability increases is recommended. The parents may be shown positions that enhance social interaction, such as holding the infant in a semireclined, face-to-face position. Parent education can be enhanced with the use of commercially available literature designed for family use.

Emphasis is placed on instruction in therapeutic positioning and handling techniques, rather than on specific exercise regimens. The positioning and handling techniques can be incorporated into daily caregiving activities. By alerting the parents to the differences between desired and unwanted postures, the therapist can facilitate the parents' implementation of the various therapeutic techniques; furthermore, parents can become creative and inventive in analyzing and responding to the infant's motor needs. The parents, for example, must understand the objectives of each of the various recommended positions; thus, if an infant is arching into trunk extension in the side-lying posture, the parent will realize that extension is an unwanted position and will modify the position to better facilitate flexion. If parents do not understand the objectives, the fact that side-lying is a recommended position may be considered more important than the infant's arching into extension, and the position may be maintained, thereby reinforcing extension.

Parents spend many hours holding and carrying their infants. Therapeutic goals can be reinforced through proper carrying techniques. A parent will foster flexion and midline orientation by cradling the infant in the crook of the arm (Fig. 3-12). One of the infant's arms is often allowed to wrap around the body of the parent. This position of the upper extremity reinforces scapular retraction and should be discouraged. The infant should be carried on alter-

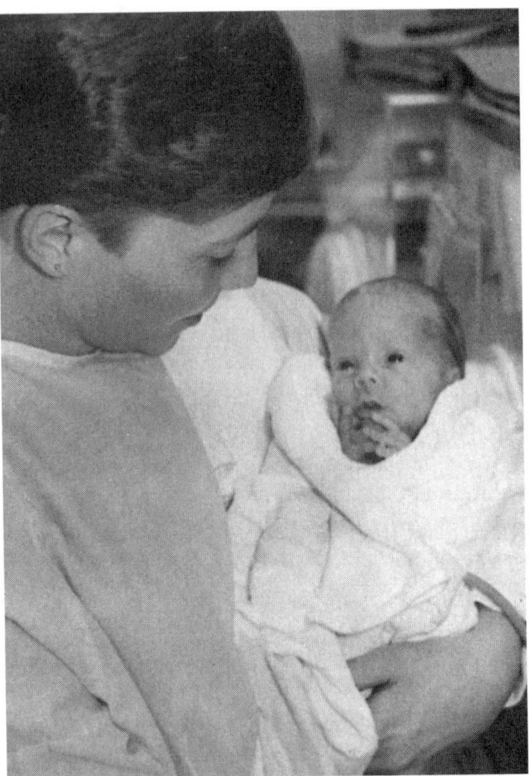

Figure 3-12 ▪ Parents are encouraged to cradle infants in a flexed and upright position. Swaddling promotes an organized and alert state of behavior. Infants are swaddled with the hands toward midline and the lower extremities flexed.

nating sides of the parent's body to foster symmetric development. Parents commonly hold infants against their chest in a posture of total extension. This position should be modified to incorporate some components of flexion.

If specific exercises are recommended, they should be done only by persons who have been instructed by the therapist. Parents and others instructed in exercises must also be instructed in the recognition of signs of infant distress and signs of good tolerance. Discretion must be used by therapists because not all parents can successfully interpret and replicate the exercise regimen suggested. The skilled and sensitive therapist should be aware of the parent's level of understanding and responses and proceed accordingly. Instruction may be limited in some instances to rolling the infant from a prone to a supine position, or to picking up the infant. Written instructions with diagrams should facilitate both understanding and follow-through with the program.

The therapist should explain to the parents the difference between chronologic age and corrected age. This knowledge may help the parent establish realistic expectations about he infant. For example, knowing that their 8-week-old premature infant will perform, at 6 months of age, more like a 4-month-old baby, may help relieve the anxiety of a parent.

The NICU Team

Optimal care is facilitated by a coordinated team approach. Team members may include the parents, physicians, nurse practitioners, nurses, physical therapists, occupational therapists, speech pathologists, respiratory therapists, social workers, infant educators, and child life specialists. Communication among team members is essential for successful team interactions.

Staff education and training is an integral part of the role of the physical therapist in the NICU. Education can be achieved through formal in-service programs, direct and indirect consultation, and informal communication. In order for the therapist's program to be effective, staff support is essential to assist in carrying out the program. Frequently, owing to the fragility of the infant, specific handling performed by the therapist may be limited to 10- or 15-minute sessions. This minimal time is inadequate to achieve most therapeutic goals. The therapist must rely on the nursing staff to incorporate therapeutic positioning and handling into their routine care activities. General recommendations regarding development can benefit all infants in the NICU, even those who are not receiving direct physical therapy and occupational therapy services.

In-service training for the nursing staff regarding infant development and the goals of therapeutic intervention better enables the nurses to incorporate therapeutic goals into their care of all premature and high-risk infants. The nursing staff must be informed about the benefits of proper positioning. Members of the nursing staff must also be aware of the impact that their interventions may have on the infant's behavioral organization, as well as the effects of the infant's behavioral organization on his or her physiologic system.

A system of primary care nursing has been established in many NICU settings. An infant's primary care nurse not only provides most of the care, but is responsible for facilitating communication between staff and family members. Maintaining good, open communication with the primary care nurse is effective in integrating the therapeutic program into the nursery setting.

Another major role for the therapist is increasing the awareness of neonatologists, pediatricians, resident physicians, and nursing staff to the role of physical therapists in the NICU. This process should include educating the nurse and physicians as to the criteria and procedure for referring infants for physical therapy. Some criteria for referral are suggested in Table 3-8.

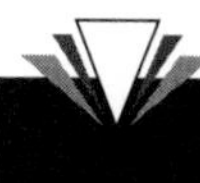

TABLE 3-8
Criteria for Referral for Physical Therapy Intervention in the Neonatal Intensive Care Unit

Birth weight ≤ 1500 g

Gestational age ≤ 32 weeks

Severe perinatal asphyxia with Apgar scores of 5 or less at 5 minutes of age

Evidence of intraventricular hemorrhage, intracranial hemorrhage, or periventricular leukomalacia

Hydrocephalus or microcephalus

Dystonia (hypertonia, hypotonia, asymmetry)

Recurrent neonatal seizures (5 or more)

Intrauterine growth retardation or small for gestational age (two standard deviations below the mean in growth charts corrected for gestational age)

Peripheral nerve injury (injuries to the brachial plexus)

Musculoskeletal abnormalities (arthrogryposis, congenital hip dislocation, congenital torticollis, talipes equinovarus)

Myelodysplasia (spina bifida)

Neuromuscular diseases (Werdnig-Hoffmann disease, myotonic dystrophy)

Symptomatic neonatal drug withdrawal

Persistently poor nipple feedings

Chromosomal abnormalities affecting development (trisomy 21)

Abnormal behavior persisting for longer than 48 hours and suggestive of disturbances in the central nervous system (irritability, tremor, lethargy)

Failure to thrive

Discharge Planning and Developmental Follow-up

To facilitate a smooth transition to home, it is essential that all members of the team coordinate discharge plans. Some nurseries provide rooming-in arrangements for parents prior to hospital discharge to allow them to begin to assume care of their infant. A home visit by a discharge planning nurse may be helpful prior to discharge.

Close developmental follow-up may be warranted depending on a variety of risk factors, including neurologic and social risk factors. An infant's neurodevelopmental status at discharge may necessitate continuation of ongoing direct therapeutic intervention. Both public and private resources for payment for therapy should be researched and taken into account when referrals are made.

Developmental follow-up programs are often available through the discharging NICU. Additionally, comprehensive developmental programs may be available through local counties and university-affiliated programs. Developmental programs are designed to supplement, but not supplant, the medical care provided by the infant's primary physician.

Summary

This chapter has discussed major disorders affecting infants in the NICU. Guidelines and specific tests of assessment have been described. Goals for developmental intervention have been presented, and numerous therapeutic techniques have been discussed. Therapeutic handling, positioning, and feeding are reviewed as they relate to the goals for developmental intervention. The importance of parent and staff education and training, as well as team collaboration, has been emphasized. The need for well-coordinated discharge planning and developmental follow-up has also been emphasized. The NICU offers a major challenge to the physical therapist. The morbidity and mortality rates of these fragile infants are constantly being improved through advances in medical technology.

REFERENCES

1. Salek B. Sensorimotor pathology in infancy and early childhood. In: Braun MA, Meyer-Palmer M, eds: *Detection and Treatment of the Infant and Young Child with Neuromuscular Disorders.* New York: Therapeutic Media; 1983.
2. Saint-Anne Dargassies, S. *Neurological Development in the Full-Term and Premature Neonate.* Amsterdam: Excerpta Medica; 1977.
3. Carter RE, Campbell S. Early neuromuscular development in the premature infant. *Phys Ther.* 1975;55:1339.
4. Anderson J, Auster-Liebhaber J. Developmental therapy in the neonatal intensive care unit. *Phys Occup Ther Pediatr.* 1984;4:100.
5. Amiel-Tison C, Grenier A. *Neurological Assessment during the First Year of Life.* New York: Oxford University Press; 1986.
6. Scherzer AL, Tscharnuter I. *Early Diagnosis and Therapy in Cerebral Palsy: A Primer on Infant Developmental Problems.* New York: Marcel Dekker; 1982.
7. Als H, Lester BM, Tronick EZ, Brazelton TB. Manual for the Assessment of Preterm Infants' Theory and Behavior (APIB). IN: Fitzgerald H, et al., eds. *Theory and Research in Behavioral Pediatrics,* Vol I. New York: Plenum; 1982;65–132.
8. Als H, Lester BM, Tronick EZ, Brazelton TB. Toward a research instrument for the assessment of preterm infants' behavior (APIB). In: Fitzgerald H, et al., eds. *Theory and Research in Behavioral Pediatrics.* Vol I. New York: Plenum; 1982:35–61.
9. Fenichel G. *Neonatal Neurology.* New York: Churchill Livingstone; 1985.
10. Phibbs R. Delivery room management of the newborn. In: Avery G, ed. *Neonatology: Pathophysiology and Management of the Newborn.* Philadelphia: JB Lippincott; 1981:182–201.
11. Volpe J. In: Avery E, ed. *Neonatology: Pathophysiology and Management of the Newborn.* Philadelphia: JB Lippincott; 1981.
12. Fitzhardinge P, Pape K. Follow-up studies of the high-risk newborn. In: Avery E, ed. *Neonatology: Pathophysiology and Management of the Newborn.* Philadelphia: JB Lippincott; 1981.
13. Menkes J. *Textbook of Child Neurology.* Philadelphia: Lea & Febiger; 1985.
14. Lou HC. Perinatal hypoxic-ischemic brain damage and periventricular hemorrhage. In: Harel S, et al., eds. *The At-Risk Infants.* Baltimore: Paul H. Brookes; 1985:153–157.
15. Volpe JJ. *Neurology of the Newborn.* Philadelphia: WB Saunders; 1987.
16. Robertson C, Finer N. Term infants with hypoxic-ischemic encephalopathy: Outcome at 3–5 years. *Dev Med Child Neurol.* 1985;27:473–484.
17. Malamud N. Status marmoratus: A form of cerebral palsy following either birth injury or inflammation of the central nervous system. *J Pediatr.* 1950;37:610.
18. Bozynski ME, Nelson MN, Matalon TAS, et al. Cavitary periventricular leukomalacia: Incidence and short-term outcome in infants weighing less than 1200 grams at birth. *Dev Med Child Neurol.* 1985;27:572–577.
19. McMenamin JB, Shackelford GD, Volpe JJ. Outcome of neonatal intraventricular hemorrhage with periventricular echodense lesions. *Ann Neurol.* 1984; 15:285–290.

20. Bjar R, Coln R. *Brain Insults in Infants and Children*. Orlando, FL: Grune & Stratton; 1985.
21. Papile L, Munsick-Bruno G, Schaefer A. Relationship of cerebral intraventricular hemorrhage and early childhood neurologic handicaps. *J Pediatr.* 1983;103:273–277.
22. Evans HE, Glass L. *Perinatal Medicine*. Hagerstown, MD: Harper & Row; 1976.
23. Corbet AJ, Bucciarelli R, Goldman S, Mammel M, Wold D, Long W. Decreased mortality rate among small premature infants treated at birth with a single dose of synthetic surfactant: A multicenter controlled trial. *J Pediatr.* 1991;118:277–284.
24. Singer D. Morphology of hyaline membrane disease and its pulmonary sequelae. In: Stern L, ed. *Hyaline Membrane Disease*. Orlando, FL: Grune & Stratton; 1984:81–83.
25. Reid L. Bronchopulmonary dysplasia—pathology. *J Pediatr.* 1979;95:836–841.
26. Vohi BR, Bell EF, Vih W. Infants with bronchopulmonary dysplasia: Growth patterns and neurologic and development outcome. *Am J Dis Child.* 1982;136:443–447.
27. Behrman RE, Vaughan VN. *Textbook of Pediatrics*. 13th Ed. Philadelphia: WB Saunders; 1987.
28. Scheidt PC, Mellits ED, Hardy JB, et al. Toxicity to bilirubin in neonates: Infant development during the first year in relation to maximal neonatal serum bilirubin concentration. *J Pediatr.* 1977;91:292.
29. Riopel DA. The Heart. In: Stevenson RE, Hall JG, Goodman RM, eds. *Human Malformations and Related Anomalies*. Vol. II. New York: Oxford University Press; 1993.
30. Mullins CE. Patent ductus arteriosus. In: Garson A Jr, Bricker JT, McNamara DG, eds. *The Science and Practice of Pediatric Cardiology*. Philadelphia.: Lea & Febiger; 1990.
31. Kopf GS, Laks H. Atrial septal defects and cor triatriatum. In: Baue AE, Geha AS, Hammond GL, et al., eds. *Glenn's Thoracic and Cardiovascular Surgery*, 5th Ed. Norwalk, CT: Appleton & Lange; 1991.
32. Approach to Examination of the Heart. In: Romero R, Pilu G, Jeanty P, et al. eds. *Prenatal Diagnosis of Congenital Anomalies*. Norwalk, CT: Appleton & Lange; 1988:142.
33. Howell BA. Thoracic Surgery. In: Campbell SK, ed. *Physical Therapy for Children*. Philadelphia: WB Saunders; 1994.
34. Freed M, Fyle DS. Cardiology. In: Avery ME, First LR, eds. *Pediatric Medicine*, 2nd Ed. Baltimore: Williams & Wilkins; 1994.
35. Griffith JF. Nonbacterial infections of the fetus and newborn. *Clin Perinatol.* 1977;4:117–130.
36. Prose NS. HIV infection in children. *J Am Acad Dermatol.* 1990;22:1223.
37. Grossman M. Children with AIDS. *Infect Dis Clin North Am.* 1988;2:533.
38. Pahwa S. Human immunodeficiency virus infection in children: Nature of immunodeficiency, clinical spectrum, and management. *Pediatr Infect Dis J.* 1988;7:S61.
39. Curless RG. Congenital AIDS: Review of neurologic problems. *Child Nerv Syst.* 1989;5:9.
40. Diamond GW. Developmental problems in children with HIV infection. *Ment Retard.* 1989;27:213.
41. Wright JT, et al. Alcohol consumption, pregnancy, and low birth weight. *Lancet.* 1983;1:663.
42. Silk A (Fair Oaks Hosp, VA). Personal communication, July 1992.
43. Bingol N, Fuchs M, Diaz V. Teratogenicity of cocaine in humans. *J Pediatr.* 1987;110:93.
44. Chasnoff IJ, Griffith DR, MacGregor S, Dirkes K, Burns KA. Temporal patterns of cocaine use in pregnancy. Perinatal outcome. *Am Med Assoc.* 1989; 261:1741.
45. Chouteau M, Namerow PB, Leppert P. The effect of cocaine abuse on birth weight and gestational age. *Obstet Gynecol.* 1988;72:351.
46. Dison S, Bejar R. Echoencephalographic findings in neonates associated with maternal cocaine and methamphetamine use: Incidence and clinical correlates. *J Pediatr.* 1989;115:770.
47. Eisen L, Field T, Bandstra E. Perinatal cocaine effects on neonatal stress behavior and performance on the Brazelton Scale. *Pediatrics.* 1991;88:427.
48. Little BB, Snell LM, Klein VR, Gilstrap LC III. Cocaine abuse during pregnancy: Maternal and fetal implications. *Obstet Gynecol.* 1989;73:157.
49. Van der Bor M, Walther FJ, Sims M. Increased cerebral blood flow velocity in infants of mothers who abuse cocaine. *Pediatrics.* 1990;85:733.
50. Lane SJ. Prenatal cocaine exposure: A role for occupational therapy. *Devel Disabil Special Interest Section Newslett.* June 1992;15:1–2.
51. Zelson C, Rubio E, Wasserman E. Neonatal narcotic addiction: 10-year observation. *Pediatrics.* 1971;48:178.
52. Lake AM, Walker WA. Neonatal necrotizing enterocolitis: A disease of altered host defense. *Clin Gastroenterol.* 1977;6:463–480.
53. Touloukian RJ. Neonatal necrotizing enterocolitis: An update on etiology, diagnosis, and treatment. *Surg Clin North Am.* 1976;56:281–298.
54. Neu J. Gastrointestinal problems and nutrition in neonatal and pediatric intensive care. In: Vidyasagar D, ed. *Neonatal and Pediatric Intensive Care*. Boston: PSG Publishing; 1985;299–300.

55. Fanaroff A, Martin R. *Neonatal-Perinatal Medicine.* St. Louis: Mosby–Year Book; 1992.
56. Eng GD. Brachial plexus palsy in newborn infants. *Pediatrics.* 1974;48:18.
57. Nellhaus D, et al. Neurologic and muscular disorders. In: Kempe CH, ed. *Current Pediatric Diagnosis and Treatment.* Los Altos: Appleton and Lange; 1982:615.
58. Coleman SS. *Congenital Dysplasia and Dislocation of the Hip.* St Louis: CV Mosby; 1978.
59. Weiner D, et al. Congenital dislocation of the hip: The relationships of premanipulation, traction, and age to avascular necrosis of the femoral head. *J Bone Joint Surg.* 1977;59A:306.
60. Gartland J. *Fundamentals of Orthopedics.* Philadelphia: WB Saunders; 1974.
61. Hoppenfeld S. *Physical Examination of the Spine and Extremities.* New York: Appleton-Century-Crofts; 1976.
62. Kempe CH, et al. *Current Pediatric Diagnosis and Treatment.* Los Altos, CA: Lange Medical Publications; 1982.
63. Amiel-Tison C. Neurological evaluation of the maturity of newborn infants. *Arch Dis Child.* 1968; 43:89–93.
64. Prechtl H. *The Neurological Examination of the Full-term Newborn Infant.* 2nd Ed. Philadelphia: JB Lippincott; 1977. Clinics in Developmental Medicine, No. 63.
65. Andre-Thomas CY, Saint-Anne Dargassies S. *The Neurological Examination of the Infant.* London; National Spastics Society; 1960. Little Club Clinics in Developmental Medicine, No. 1.
66. Brazelton TB. *Neonatal Behavioral Assessment Scale.* 2nd Ed. Philadelphia: JB Lippincott; 1984.
67. Apgar, V. Proposal for a new method of evaluation of newborn infant. *Anesth Analg.* 1953;32:260.
68. Drage JS, Berendes H. Apgar scores and outcome of the newborn. *Pediatr Clin North Am.* 1966;13:635.
69. Dubowitz LMS, Dubowitz V, Goldberg C. Clinical assessment of gestational age in the newborn infant. *J Pediatr.* 1970;77.
70. Dubowitz L. Neurological assessment of the full-term and preterm newborn infant. In: Harel S, Anastasiow N, eds. *The At-risk Infant.* Baltimore: Paul H. Brookes; 1985;185–196.
71. Morgan A. *Neuro-Developmental Approach to the High-Risk Neonate.* (Notes from a seminar presented in Williamsburg, VA; Nov 3–4, 1984.
72. Chandler LS, et al. *Movement Assessment of Infants: A Manual.* Rolling Bay, WA: Chandler LS, et al.; 1980.
73. Milani-Comparetti A, Gidoni EA. Routine developmental examination in normal and retarded children. *Dev Med Child Neurol.* 1967;9:631.
74. Bobath K. *A Neurophysiological Basis for the Treatment of Cerebral Palsy.* Philadelphia: JB Lippincott; 1980.
75. Ayres AJ. *Sensory Integration and Learning Disorders.* Los Angeles: Western Psychological Services; 1972.
76. Gilfoyle EM, Grady AP, Moore JC. *Children Adapt.* Thorofare, NJ: Charles B. Slack; 1981.
77. Als H. Lecture notes. George Washington University, Washington, DC: Feb 21, 1985.
78. Evans MS, Stockdale WS. Problems of cerebral palsy and oral-motor function. In Wilson JM, ed. *Oral-Motor Function and Dysfunction in Children.* Chapel Hill: University of North Carolina at Chapel Hill Division of Physical Therapy; 1977: 163–166.
79. Field T, et al. Nonnutritive sucking during tube feedings: Effects on preterm neonates in an intensive care unit. *Pediatrics.* 1982;70:381–384.
80. The Education of the Handicapped Act Amendments of 1986. Public Law No. 99–457 (1986).

Physical Therapy for the Child with Cerebral Palsy

Jane Styer-Acevedo

Definition

"Cerebral palsy is not a disease, but is, rather, a category of disability including patients with one kind of problem: chronic nonprogressive disorders of movement or posture of early onset. The anatomic sites of involvement, degree of motor disability, associated dysfunctions, and cause are heterogeneous."[1] "Cerebral palsy is often associated with other neurologic difficulties, including mental retardation."[2]

Incidence

The United States Collaborative Perinatal Project conducted by the National Institute of Neurologic and Communicative Disorders and Stroke included a study of 54,000 pregnant women from 12 urban teaching hospitals in the United States between 1959 and 1966.[3] Of the women in the study, 46% were white, 46% were black, and most of the rest were Puerto Rican. The socioeconomic status of the sample was lower than that of the general population. The children born to these women had a regular schedule of examinations, including a general physical examination and a neurologic examination at both 1 and 7 years of age. Among the 38,533 children whose outcome was known at 7 years of age, 202 met criteria for cerebral palsy (CP). Of the 202 children, 24 (12%) children had an acquired motor deficit secondary to a variety of factors in the early developing years, rather than congenital motor deficits occurring as a result of in utero factors or events at the time of labor and delivery. Infectious meningitis and trauma were the most common causes of acquired CP. In addition to the 202 children with CP who were alive at 7 years of age, 24 children with CP, most commonly with spastic quadriplegia, had died before 7 years of age. The following figures indicate the prevalence of CP based on the National Collaborative Perinatal Project:

5.2:1000—diagnosed as having CP
4.6:1000—when acquired cases of CP are excluded
2.6:1000—excluding mildly afflicted children. (This figure more closely represents the prevalence of handicapping congenital CP.)

Further study of the population in the United States Collaborative Perinatal Project indicated that there are "relatively low risks for cerebral palsy (1.3–2.9 per 1000) among children who had no abnormal signs, whether or not they had low 5-minute Apgar scores or whether or not they had seizures in the nursery period."[4] Other authors have found the incidence of CP to be 2 per 1000 infants in the United States.[5–7]

The Metropolitan Atlanta Developmental Disabilities Surveillance Program monitors the prevalence of four serious developmental disabilities, including cerebral palsy. For the reporting period January 1991 to December 1991, the overall crude rate of cerebral palsy was 2.4 per 1000 children. The rate among black children was found to be 3.1 per 1000 children as compared to 2 per 1000 for white children.[6] These rates were not adjusted for possible confounding factors.

Etiology

Despite a marked increase in perinatal intervention aimed at reducing intrapartum asphyxia in recent years, CP rates have not shown a consistent decrease either in the United States or in Australia.[1] There has been a reduction in the perinatal mortality rate over the past decade owing to improvements in obstetric management, but this reduction has not been accompanied by a decrease in the prevalence of CP. In an effort to confirm the study regarding perinatal asphyxia by Ellenberg and Nelson,[4] the California Child Health and Development Studies group monitored 19,044 pregnancies to evaluate their long-term outcome. The children underwent follow-up for 5 years. Forty-one (0.2%) were found to have CP that was not the result of a progressive disease or a neural tube defect. Thirty-two (78%) of the children with CP did *not* have birth asphyxia, and the 22% who had asphyxia had other perinatal risk factors that may have compromised their recovery. Of the control infants, 2.9% had birth asphyxia but recovered without neurologic damage. The authors believed that the strongest predictors of CP were the presence of a congenital anomaly, low birth weight, low placental weight, and an abnormal fetal position. All of these conditions are antecedents to the birth process and strong indicators of a fetus who is compromised prior to labor or delivery.[8] Melone and associates, in another study, confirmed that the intrapartum period is an infrequent source of CP.[5]

Others have investigated several areas in both full-term and premature infants in an attempt to identify the risk factors and sources for CP. Their findings include, but are not limited to, abnormal neonatal signs[9]; hypoxia or ischemia[1,8,10,11]; chronic lung disease requiring 28 days or more of supplemental oxygen[12]; low Apgar scores[2,13]; neurosonographic abnormalities, such as severe intracranial hemorrhage,[12,13] increased periventricular leukomalacia,[14] increased periventricular echogenicity,[15,16] and periventricular cysts[14–16]; the need for mechanical ventilation[15,16] and prematurity/gestational age.[15,17]

Blitz et al. assessed the outcome of 100 extremely low birth weight (ELBW; i.e., <1001 g) infants born in Maryland in 1990. When assessed at 1 year corrected age, they found that 51% had abnormal or suspect neurologic examinations and 24% had CP. There was no single cause or constellation of factors noted; however, this study shows that ELBW infants are at risk for significant developmental problems.[18]

Predicting the long-term outcome of infants in the neonatal period continues to be difficult based upon the available data. In general, the higher the risk associated with a characteristic, or constellation of characteristics, the lower the prevalence of that characteristic or constellation.[4]

Classification

Scherzer and Tscharnuter describe how the motor pattern type of CP may take several forms.[17]

> The spastic variety is most common and indicates a fixed lesion in the motor portion of the cerebral cortex. Athetosis or dystonia reflects involvement in the basal ganglia. Athetosis frequently involves intermittent tension of the trunk or extremities and a variety of uninhibited movement patterns—sometimes a basis for confusion in classification. Ataxia refers to a cerebellar lesion. Mixed types are also common. These may include combinations of spasticity with athetosis or ataxia. Rigidity suggests a severe decerebrate lesion.[17]

Scherzer and Tscharnuter have included in their work the definitions that are in common use for various clinical neurologic lesions.[17]

Monoplegia—involvement of one extremity
Hemiplegia—upper and lower extremity involvement on one side
Paraplegia—involvement of both lower extremities
Quadriplegia—equal involvement of upper and lower extremities
Diplegia—quadriplegia with mild involvement of the upper extremities

These authors further state that "Type, distribution, and severity are essential aspects of the cerebral palsy diagnosis. They give meaning and direction to treatment and management of the patient."[17]

The Bobaths'[19] description of the distribution of the various types of CP is similar to that of Scherzer and Tscharnuter,[17] but includes the trunk in the description of motor involvement. Molnar[20] identifies several major groups of children with CP based upon clinical signs. *Spastic CP* includes hemiparesis, diplegia, and quadriparesis. *Dyskinetic forms* include *athetosis* (slow, writhing movements of the face and extremities, particularly affecting the distal musculature), *dystonia* (rhythmic, twisting distortions and changes in tone involving primarily the trunk and proximal extremities and causing slow, uncontrolled movements with a tendency toward fixed postures), *choreiform movements* (rapid, irregular, jerky motions most commonly seen in the face and extremities), *ballismus* (coarse flailing or flinging motion of the extremities characterized by a wide amplitude of motion), and *tremor* (fine shaking motion of the head and extremities). Rarer types of CP include ataxia, rigidity, and atonia. Clinical types of CP with mixed neurologic signs typically involve spastic athetosis spastic ataxia, or spastic rigidity.[20]

Associated Problems

Frequently the child with cerebral palsy will have a sensory processing dysfunction. Three sites of central nervous system damage result in primary sensory processing dysfunctions and are often associated with CP.[21]

1. The cerebellum is a major sensory processing center, and when impaired, it will result in ataxia.
2. The cortical-basal ganglia-thalamic loop is a sensory and motor feedforward and feedback circuit and when impaired, results in athetosis.
3. The cerebral cortex and pyramidal tracts, when impaired, result in spasticity as the pyramidal system plays an important role in regulating sensory information.[21]

The sensory deficits in children with CP may be primary or secondary and should always be addressed in the treatment program. Cooper et al. found significant bilateral sensory deficits in children, with hemiplegia with stereognosis and proprioception the chief modalities affected bilaterally.[22]

Strabismus is present in 20% to 60% of children with CP; the highest incidence is in the diplegic and quadriplegic populations. *Esotropia,* deviation of the eyes toward the midline, is more prevalent than exotropia. Homonymous hemianopsia occurs in 25% of children with hemiplegia.[20,23] Nystagmus is most common in children with ataxia. Mental retardation is more common in children with CP than in normal children. Of children with CP, 40% to 60% have some degree of retardation, with the highest proportion of severe deficits seen in children with quadriplegia, rigidity, and atonia.[20] Seizure disorders occur in as many as 50% of children with CP, with the severity and incidence varying across the different types of CP.[20] Significant communication disorders may be present in children with CP. These disorders may be secondary to poor oral-motor control of speech, central language dysfunction, hearing impairment, or cognitive deficits. Growth disturbances in both longitudinal and cross-sectional directions have been shown in the involved limbs of children with hemiplegia. Disturbances in longitudinal growth were greatest in the radius, followed by the humerus and tibia. Cross-sectional area of the involved limb segments was decreased by 16% to 19%. Limb muscle atrophy increased with age. Although these findings are well documented, the causes, which may include neurotrophic and vascular changes, are obscure.[24–26]

Older individuals with athetoid CP are at risk for acquiring devastating neurologic deficits owing to disc degeneration and instability in their cervical spines. After radiologic study of 180 patients, Harada and associates found that disc degeneration occurred earlier and progressed more rapidly in subjects with athetoid CP than in those without CP. Advanced disc degeneration was found in 51% of those studied, which is eight times the typical frequency.[27] Individuals with athetosis typically initiate and attempt control of movement with the jaw or head. This eventually causes the musculoskeletal changes noted on radiographic studies.

Assessment of the Child with Cerebral Palsy

In this era of high technologic intervention, it is essential that therapists become very sensitive to the possible neurologic deficits in any infant or child with developmental delay or behavioral difficulties. According to Kitchen, 10% of very low birth weight (VLBW) infants weighing between 500 and 1500 g can be expected to develop CP. Kitchen further states that there may be a high rate of fetal aberration associated with the abnormal event of premature birth.[28] Several authors suggest that infants who are at increased risk for the development of CP can be predicted through the use of ultrasonography of the head.[14–16,29–32] Cystic lesions found in the occipital region confer a very high risk of severe CP.[31] Periventricular cystic lesions probably reflect damage to the white matter fibers of the cerebral corticospinal tracts and may appear clinically as spasticity (Fig. 4-1).[29,31] When findings cited earlier are noted in an infant in the nursery, they should be used to guide the discharge plan for the infant and family. The goal of this early diagnosis is to provide early therapeutic intervention for the child with CP. This intervention should be in the form of developmentally based therapy, including physical, occupational, and speech therapies. Many practitioners recommend that graduates from neona- tal intensive care units (NICUs) who have the neurologic signs just mentioned should be closely monitored after discharge. Of course, normal findings in an evaluation can be very reassuring for parents and caregivers alike. However, abnormal neonatal examination results cannot be used to diagnose CP definitively in the neonatal period. Rather, the results should be used to identify infants who are at increased risk for later developmental disability and who will require closer monitoring and possibly, early intervention programs.[33]

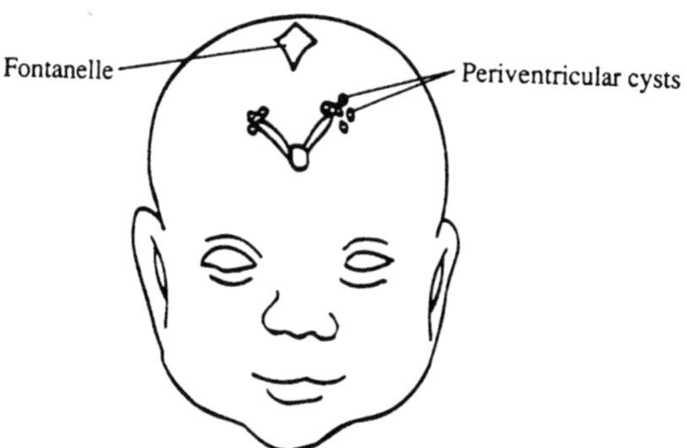

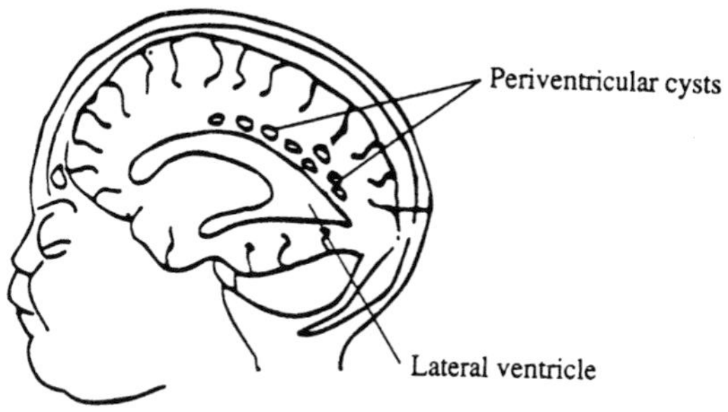

Figure 4-1 ▪ Location of periventrical cysts, which are thought to affect the corticospinal tracts and cause spasticity. (Compliments of Leonard Graziani, MD.)

There is disagreement in the literature and in practice regarding how early an infant can be diagnosed with CP. Burns and colleagues believe that a diagnosis of very mild CP should be possible at 8 months of age.[34] Identification depends on a combination of suspicious and abnormal signs revealed during comprehensive assessment of motor attainments, neurologic signs, primitive reflexes, and postural reactions.

Children with persistent subtle or mild signs should be monitored closely until the possible outcome is clear.[34] Harris, using the Movement Assessment in Infants (MAI), found that certain items can help distinguish the infant with CP from the nonhandicapped infant at 4 months of age.[35] Items of diagnostic value include neck hyperextension and shoulder retraction, ability to bear weight on the forearms while prone, ability to maintain a stable head position in supported or independent sitting, and the infant's ability to flex the hips actively against gravity.[35,36] Seven of the 17 MAI items that Harris found to be highly significant predictors are observational items. Both Harris and Milani-Comparetti found that watching the infant move against gravity is of greater diagnostic value than intrusive handling or attempts to stimulate a response.[35,36] Harris compared the diagnostic value of the MAI with the Bayley Scales in infants at 4 months of age and found that the MAI was more sensitive than the Bayley Scales.[35] However, the Bayley Motor Scale was extremely sensitive at 1 year of age. Nelson and Ellenberg[37] studied children who were diagnosed with CP at 1 year of age who subsequently "outgrew the cerebral palsy." They found that children with mild motor impairment at 1 year of age and those thought to have CP were all free of CP by the age of 7 years. However, all who were diagnosed with severe CP, and many with moderate CP, still carried the same diagnosis at the age of 7 years. Those who "outgrew" the CP were likely to have neurologic problems, such as mental retardation, nonfebrile seizures, or difficulty with speech articulation.[37] These findings substantiate the fact that any infant or child who demonstrates neurologic or behavioral abnormalities should undergo follow-up until early school age.

In order to understand the atypical movement and motor control that occurs in children with CP, the therapist must understand the acquisition of motor control against gravity, the development of postural control, and the musculoskeletal development in typically developing children. This information can be found in Chapter 1. Atypical development has been described by many authors, including numerous sources cited in this chapter.[17,20,38–52]

The purpose of the assessment is to discover the functional abilities and strengths of the child, determine the primary and secondary impairments (compensations used because of the primary impairments), and discover the desired functional goals of the child and/or family. The therapist must use an organized approach to the observation of, interaction with, and handling of the child in order to get an accurate baseline of the child's functional abilities. Display 4-1 is a suggested organization for an assessment utilizing the S.O.A.P. (Subjective-Objective-Assessment-Plan) format to document the assessment and use a multisystem approach.

Assessment of Movement

Much of the information about a child's movement and posture can be gathered by an observant therapist who watches the child entering the treatment area. The child can also be observed while the therapist is taking a history and discussing with the parents the various concerns that have brought them to a habilitation program.

Observation of the baby or young child being held in the arms or lap of the parent or caregiver can reveal important information. The following questions may be answered through observation:

1. How does the mother hold the baby? Does she support the head and trunk, or does she hold the baby at the pelvis?
2. Are the baby's head and trunk rotated or collapsed consistently to one side?
3. Do the baby's arms come forward to hold the mother or play with a toy in midline? Are the arms held behind the body with the

DISPLAY 4-1

S.O.A.P Outline for Assessment of the Child with Cerebral Palsy

Subjective
Objective
- Brief history
- Functional level—gross motor
- Neuromotor status
  - Stiffness—degree, area, symmetry
  - Coactivation (muscles on both sides of the joint are activated) reciprocal inhibition (muscles on one side of joint are more activated)
  - Initiation/sustain/termination—of muscle action
  - Concentric/eccentric/isometric—contractions
  - Agonist/antagonist
    - Flexion/extension
    - Lateral weight shifts
    - Rotation
  - Synergies—functional muscle groups
- ROM/musculoskeletal
- Strength
- Sensory/perceptual
  - Vision
  - Auditory
  - Vestibular
  - Proprioception/kinesthesia
  - Body awareness
  - Tactile
- Respiratory/endurance
- Cardiovascular
- Skin
- Other: posture, social-emotional, behavior, etc.

Assessment
- Strengths
- Areas of concern (impairments: primary then secondary)
- Long-term goals
- Short-term goals

Plan
- Mini-goal
- Treatment

scapulae adducted, or are the arms flexed and adducted against the trunk?

4. While being held, does the baby thrust backward into trunk extension or collapse forward into trunk flexion?
5. How are the lower extremities held: Are they adducted tightly in extension or are they floppy in flexion and abduction?
6. Is there isolated movement at the toes or ankles, or are the ankles held in plantar flexion or dorsiflexion? Is the foot everted or inverted, and are the toes held loosely or tightly curled?

This type of observational analysis is not limited to the child held in the parent's arms. When the child arrives at the physical therapy department in a wheelchair, there are additional questions that may add to the baseline information.

1. Did the child independently propel the wheelchair, or did someone help him or her?
2. In addition to mobility, does the wheelchair provide total postural support for major segments of the body? If the segments are free of support from the wheelchair, do those segments of the body seem in good postural alignment and do they move freely?
3. Does the child tend to thrust backward in the chair into trunk extension? Is the pelvis positioned in a posterior tilt? If the child does behave in this manner, is there similar thrusting and tightness in the extremities?
4. Is the child seated in a reasonably symmetric position or are there significant asymmetries in the posture?
5. Does the child seem comfortable in the chair?

Children with less severe movement disorders may ambulate into the department. Another group of questions will be helpful in assessing the movement of the ambulatory child.

1. Did the child ambulate with or without an assistive device, such as a walker, cane, or crutches?
2. Did the child need physical assistance from another person while ambulating?
3. Is the child's gait pattern stable, and is the child safe?
4. When assessing temporal parameters, such as length of step, stance time, swing time, or base of support, is the gait pattern grossly symmetric or asymmetric?
5. Does the child's trunk collapse into lateral flexion on weight bearing on one or both legs, or is the trunk maintained in proper antigravity extension?
6. Does the child have a heel-toe gait pattern? Does the child stand on the balls of the feet?
7. Are the hips and knees extended during stance phase, or are they flexed with the child in a crouched position?

In addition to the gross observational assessment described, the therapist should examine individual aspects of motor function as part of the overall evaluation of the child. The therapist should begin with the level of function appropriate to the child's age and functional ability. The following list of positions provides a guideline by which to assess functional antigravity control:

Prone
Supine
Side-lying
Sitting—short sit, long sit, side sit, ring sit
Quadruped
Kneeling
Half-kneeling
Standing
Walking

If the child possesses higher level skills the evaluation should be extended to include the following:

Climbing stairs
Navigating ramps or curbs
One-foot stance
Tandem gait
Running
Jumping
Hopping
Skipping

The child who functions from a wheelchair should be evaluated in terms of the following parameters:

Alignment and mobility of body
Shifting of weight
Propulsion of wheelchair
Management of wheelchair and its parts
Transfer to and from wheelchair

Assessment of Postural Control

Historically, posture was defined through reflex terminology and facilitated through controlled sensory feedback.[53] Infants were evaluated for the presence or absence of and the strength of primitive reflexes. The reflexes were thought to "integrate" as the infant developed. Therapists utilized stimulation of and feedback from: optical righting, labyrinthine righting, neck righting, body righting on the head and body righting on the body, to facilitate normal righting and equilibrium responses in the clients.[53] In treatment, lower level reflexes were inhibited to decrease the abnormal sensory feedback and facilitate the emergence and integration of the righting responses and equilibrium reactions.

According to more recent motor science studies, the human system is no longer thought to function via a hierarchical model. Various systems models are used currently to describe the organization and functions of the nervous system.[53]

In assessing postural control of the child with CP, it is important to understand several concepts. Postural activity is noted when the child has muscle activation against the supporting surface.[54] An example would be the infant, at 7 to 9 months of age, who has just learned how to gain stability in sitting by pushing his or her legs into the floor. The arms and hands are now free to explore toys and play as they are no longer needed for propping. Postural preparations are strategies that the child uses well before a functional movement and increase stability by changing the base of support or increasing muscle activation around joints.[54] These changes are in anticipation of a specific task that has been learned previously. The child received sensory input (feedback) from having completed the task previously and makes the necessary postural adjustments to complete the task in the most efficient, effective way. For example, the infant, sitting on the floor, sees a toy to the side and tries reaching for it. If it is too far outside the base of support, the infant may fall in attempting to grab the toy. On the next try, the infant will make adjustments to the base of support and/or muscle activation in the attempt to grasp the toy without falling over.

Feedforward is identified in postural preparations for movement. It occurs as a result of learning through experience.[53] Postural setting is the muscles getting active around a joint or joints, without obvious movement, in anticipation of the task. Current motor sciences endorse the importance of anticipation (feedforward) in movement and postural control.[54] Feedforward is learned through trial and error practice as the example illustrates and must be client-generated and be goal- or task-oriented. Postural control is learned specific to a task and in a variety of environmental conditions.[54] Motor learning occurs when the child is actively involved in the session and advances from using only the feedback responses to feedforward control.[53] For example, the child experiences the tactile and proprioceptive properties of objects (feedback) when handling and playing with toys. This helps in preshaping of the hand in preparation for more refined reach and grasp tasks in the future.

When assessing the infant/child's postural control, find answers to the following questions:

- Does the child have a variety of ways to transition between postures or only stereotypic choices?
- Does the child actively push into the supporting surface with the pelvis or extremities?
- Is the child able to repeat movements or tasks and make small changes in its motor performance?

Assessment of Postural Tone

The clinical term "tone" describes the impairments of spasticity and abnormal extensibility. Abnormally high tone may be caused by spasticity, a velocity-dependent overactivity that is proportional to the imposed velocity of limb movement.[55]

Clinicians tend to use the word *tone* to describe how a muscle or group of muscles feel under their hands when the joints of a body part are moved through a particular range. The sense of abnormally high tone can result from hypoextensibility of the muscle because of abnormal mechanical characteristics.[55] These same muscles can have increased stiffness if they require greater force to produce a change in length than is typically expected. Some clinicians use the terms tone and stiffness interchangeably. Here, the word stiffness describes the resistance to movement felt when joints are moved in space.

In assessing the child's stiffness, it is necessary to describe the relative amounts of stiffness in the head, neck, trunk, and extremities. For example, the child with classic spastic diplegia will typically demonstrate early decreased stiffness in the neck and trunk while having increased stiffness in both legs. Frequently, one can observe stiffness while watching the child play. However, for detailed accurate information, it is necessary to feel the child transition between postures and move its limbs through space. The clinician may recognize that stiffness increases while working with the child. This response is typical as the child expends greater effort to perform a task or as the child brings its center of mass higher off the support surface. The level of stiffness should decrease when the clinician uses inhibitory techniques with the child.

It is necessary to distinguish between stiffness that is a primary impairment (a loss or abnormality at the organ or organ system level of the body)[56] and stiffness that is compensatory (used by the child to compensate for a primary impairment). Treatment is most effective when aimed at changing the primary impairments as the secondary compensations may be reduced or eliminated in this situation.

It is important to identify compensatory stiffness. Focusing on the child with spastic diplegia again, the level of stiffness may increase in the upper extremities when the child is seated on a bench secondary to the low level of stiffness noted in the trunk. The child may elevate its shoulders and attempt to use the scapulae in adduction and arms in humeral hyperextension with elbow flexion as an assist to sitting erect because it is unable to maintain an erect trunk. The stiffness in the arms and shoulder girdle is considered compensatory stiffness.

Signs of increased stiffness include distal fixing (toe curling or fisting), difficulty moving a body segment through a range, asymmetric posture, retracted lips and tongue, and so on. Signs of decreased stiffness include excessive collapse of body segments, loss of postural alignment, and inability to sustain a posture against gravity. A child may also have fluctuating levels of stiffness, which is noted as signs of both increased and decreased levels of stiffness. Two more commonly known types are athetosis and ataxia.

Musculoskeletal Assessment

Persistent shortening of a muscle or group of muscles without adequate activation of antagonists—resulting from spasticity, increased or decreased stiffness, weakness, or static positioning—places the child at risk for soft tissue contractures and, over time, bony deformity. With an awareness of the sequence usually seen in atypical motor development and with knowledge of the postural and movement consequences, the therapist must be alert for areas at risk for contracture and deformity.

GONIOMETRIC MEASUREMENTS

Range of motion (ROM) should be measured with a goniometer at joints with limited motion. The results should be documented clearly for later comparison. Muscles whose influence is exerted across two joints should be examined and elongated over both joints when measurements are taken. Move the child's limb slowly through the range to avoid eliciting a stretch reflex.

EVALUATION OF THE SPINE

Mobility of the spine in all planes is necessary for correct alignment, for smooth, symmetric movements of the spine, and for full ROM of the extremities. Evaluation of the child's passive and active movement of the trunk is an essential part of the evaluation. Passive spinal flexion can be evaluated with the child in supine and rounding the spine by putting the child's knees up to their chest. Look for the spinous processes to be showing evenly down their spine. This is smooth flexion of the spinal column. If an area is flattened—without the spinous processes showing—it is indicative of a decrease in spinal flexion. Spinal extension, lateral flexion, and rotation are most easily assessed in sitting. The pelvis must be stabilized by the child or the therapist and the trunk taken through the various movements. Note the smoothness of the movement, the end range and end feel, the symmetry in the trunk, and the amount of movement at each joint in the spinal column. Children with CP often have tightness and limitation in cervical and capital flexion, thoracic extension, lateral flexion, and lumbar flexion.

The therapist must document any deviation from normal in the spinal curves. Note scoliosis and excessive kyphosis and lordosis, and whether the curves are structural or functional.

THORACIC MOVEMENT

An area of special concern for the child with CP is the coordinated motion of the thorax that occurs during the breathing cycle. In normal babies younger than 6 months of age, there is an approximate 90-degree angle between the ribs and the spine. As control of the head and trunk develops typically, and as the baby begins to develop a more upright posture, there is a change in this 90-degree relationship. Owing to both gravity and the forces of the axial musculature in resisting gravity, there is a posterior to anterior downward slant to the ribs. As a result of this slant, there is an increased ability to expand the diameter of the thorax in both an anterior-posterior (pump-handle motion) and lateral direction (bucket-handle motion). In addition to this ability to change the inspired volume, the thoracic (external intercostal) and abdominal (obliques) muscles act to fix the rib cage. This fixation facilitates more complete contraction of the diaphragm, thus increasing lung volume. Children with CP typically have low levels of stiffness proximally. They also tend to have decreased active balance of trunk flexors and extensors when in an upright position with difficulty sustaining muscle activation. As a result, there are differences in motion of the chest wall during inspiration. First, the downward slant of the ribs never fully develops, thus minimizing the mechanical advantage of the pump-handle and bucket-handle motions of inspiration. Second, without the muscle tone necessary to fix the rib cage, the diaphragmatic fibers, particularly the sternal fibers, serve an almost paradoxical function—that is, they cause depression of the xiphoid process and the sternum during inspiration. The lack of thoracic expansion, in conjunction with the sternal depression, causes shallow respiratory efforts. Vocalizations will be of short duration and will be low in intensity because of poor breath support. Examination of the respiratory excursion of the thorax is a critical portion of the motor assessment for the child with CP. Respiratory function should be assessed with the child in various functional positions. It may be useful to assess thoracic excursion in a young child while the child is crying. The "crying vital capacity" is a reasonable index of lung expansion in the infant.[50] The therapist should develop interventions aimed at increasing postural control throughout the trunk. The therapist must specifically facilitate antigravity control of both axial extensor and flexor muscles, particularly the oblique abdominal muscles that aid in the forceful expiration needed for coughing and sneezing.

EVALUATION OF THE SHOULDER GIRDLE AND UPPER EXTREMITY

The child with CP with excessive axial extension and poor activation of cervical and capital flexors and abdominal muscles will likely demonstrate tightness and limitation of the shoulder girdle. Tightness of the pectoralis major, especially the sternal portion, tends to occur once the child assumes or maintains a sitting position. Poor extension of the trunk in a sitting position causes the child to collapse into gravity, with resultant rounding of the thoracic spine and tightness of the pectoralis major and rectus abdominus muscles. Dynamic scapular stability fails to develop, and the scapulae become fixed in downward rotation and a forward-tipped position. These fixed positions will restrict motion at the sternoclavicular and acromioclavicular joints.[43] Full shoulder motion cannot be achieved with these limitations. The child with CP is likely to be limited in passive flexion, abduction, and external rotation of the shoulder. Elevation of the shoulder, which is used to stabilize the head, may produce limitations in scapulothoracic movement needed for depression of the shoulder. Moving distally, the therapist often finds limitations in extension of the elbow, supination of the forearm, and extension of the wrist and fingers.

EXAMINATION OF THE HIP AND PELVIS

The child with CP, typically with spastic diplegia or quadriplegia, commonly has tightness in the hip flexors, adductors, and internal rotators with resultant limitation in hip extension, abduction, and external rotation. The Thomas test is used to identify a flexion contracture of the hip. Abduction and adduction of the hip should be assessed with the hip and knee extended. Internal and external rotation of the hip should be measured while the child is prone with the hips extended and the knees flexed.

Subluxed or dislocated hips can occur in children with very tight hip flexion, adduction, and internal rotation. The subluxed or dislocated hip has limited abduction. The Ortolani click test is used to help determine whether a hip is congenitally dislocated. The child is supine, and both hips are flexed to 90 degrees. The hips are abducted and externally rotated, with the examiner's first two fingers placed over the lateral hip and the infant's knees in the examiner's palms. If the hip is dislocated, the femoral head can slide over the acetabular rim, reducing the hip and producing a palpable, and sometimes audible, click.[57] An older child in the same position will be evaluated by the apparent length of the femur. A subluxed or dislocated hip is suggested by a shorter femoral length.

FEMORAL ANTEVERSION

Femoral anteversion is a torsion or internal rotation of the femoral shaft on the femoral neck. Other terms that may be synonymous with femoral anteversion include fetal femoral torsion and persistent fetal alignment of the hip.

At birth, an infant has approximately 40 degrees of femoral anteversion, as measured by the angle between the transcondylar axis of the femur and the femoral axis of the neck. The neonate also has 25 degrees of flexion contracture of the hip owing to intrauterine positioning and physiologic flexor tone. In the progression of normal development, hip flexors lengthen as the result of gravitational pull while the child is lying in either a prone or supine position. Active extension and external rotation of the hip tighten the anterior capsule of the hip joint, thus producing a torque or torsional stress that decreases the anteversion that is present from birth.[51] In addition to the effects of the tightened hip capsule, the hip extensors and external rotators insert near the proximal femoral growth plate. When activated, the extensors and external rotators pull on the plate and help decrease the torsion on the femur. The result of the various forces is that the adult value of 15 degrees of femoral anteversion is reached by 16 years of age.[52,58] Femoral anteversion is determined by biplane roentgenograms. Anteversion may be suspected on the basis of a simple clinical test. Internal and external rotation of the hip are tested with the hip in a position of extension (i.e., with the child in a prone position with knees flexed). Femoral anteversion may be suspected when external rotation at the hip is substantially less than internal rotation.

The child with CP often has overactivity and shortening of the flexors of the hip and poor control of extensors and of external rotators of the hip. Beals, in 1969, studied 40 children with CP and found that the degree of femoral anteversion was normal at birth.[59] However, this study also revealed that the amount of anteversion did not decrease over the first few years of life, as occurs with typically developing children. After 3 years of age, there was no significant change in anteversion with either age or ambulation status. The sample of children with CP had a mean of 14 degrees greater anteversion than the children without CP.[59]

Staheli and associates found greater angles of anteversion of the femur in the involved lower extremity of a group of children with CP than was found in their uninvolved limb.[25] Children with hemiparesis also commonly show poor activation of extensors and external rotators of the hip, with or without flexion contractures of the hip.

EXAMINATION OF THE KNEE

The child with CP may have limited knee flexion or extension as a result of inadequate length of the quadriceps or hamstrings. Length of the medial and lateral hamstrings and the rectus femoris, all of which cross two joints, should be assessed by elongating the muscle over the knee and the hip. Passive straight leg raising or measurement of the popliteal angle will indicate the degree of hamstring tightness. If hamstring tightness is excessive, the child may be unable to sit on the ischium with 90 degrees of flexion of the hip, and stride length may be limited during ambulation.

Tightness of the quadriceps, which limits flexion of the knee, can be identified by looking for a patella that is located more superiorly than normal and by assessing the degree of flexion of the knee with the child a prone position.

TIBIAL TORSION

Tibial torsion (tibial version) describes a twist of the tibia along its long axis so that the leg is rotated internally or externally. The specific angle of torsion is determined by the intersection of a line drawn vertically from the tibial tubercle and a line drawn through the malleoli.

Like the femur, the tibia undergoes developmental torsional changes. The malleoli are parallel in the frontal plane at birth. During infancy and early childhood, the tibia rotates externally, which places the lateral malleolus in a posterior position relative to the medial malleolus. Normal values for this gradual rotation are presented in Table 4-1.

TABLE 4-1
Normal Values for External Rotation of the Tibia

Age	Degree of External Rotation
0–3 months	4
3–6 months	6
6–12 months	7
2 years	11
9 years	13
10 years–adult	14

Engle, gu, Staheli, LT. The natural history of torsion and other factors influencing gait in childhood. *Clin: Orthop.* 1974; 99:12.

The "unwinding" of the tibia, or the progression from relative internal to external tibial torsion, is attributable to changes in force on the tibia arising from the decrease in femoral anteversion that occurs as the child grows.

EXAMINATION OF THE FOOT

Dorsiflexion of the ankle is often limited in the child with CP because of spasticity affecting the plantar flexors, mainly the gastrocnemius. Dorsiflexion of the ankle should be assessed with the subtalar joint maintained in a neutral position. Neutral alignment will prevent hypermobility of the forefoot while ensuring excursion of the hindfoot.[60]

Midtarsal movement can be assessed by stabilizing the hindfoot with one hand while passively supinating and pronating the forefoot with the other. Toes should be straight and mobile with approximately 90 degrees of extension available at the first metatarsophalangeal joint.

With the child standing, the calcaneous should be vertical or slightly inverted in relation to the lower one third of the leg. Children should begin to show a longitudinal arch at 3 ½ to 4 years of age. Depression of the medial longitudinal arch is caused by adduction and plantar flexion of the talus with relative eversion of the calcaneous. These deformities are also associated with internal rotation of the lower extremity. Another mechanism for malalignment during standing occurs in children with extensor spasticity who have tightness of the plantar flexors. Their calcaneous is often maintained in some degree of plantar flexion and does not truly participate in weight bearing. The talus stays plantar-flexed with "apparent full weight bearing," with pronation achieved through hypermobility into extension through the midtarsal joint.[60,61] These two mechanisms must be examined carefully when considering an orthosis for standing or ambulation.

DISCREPANCY IN LEG LENGTH

Measurement of leg length should be done in supine with the pelvis level in all planes, the hips in neutral rotation and abduction or adduction, and the knees fully extended. Measurements are taken from the anterosuperior iliac spine to the distal aspect of the medial malleolus.

Staheli and associates studied the inequality in the leg lengths in 50 children with spastic hemiparesis.[25] Of the 16 children who were older than 11 years of age, 70% had a significant discrepancy in leg length. Ten children had a discrepancy of 1 cm or more, and two children had discrepancies of greater than 2 cm between the involved and uninvolved limbs.

Correction of a discrepancy in the leg length by using a shoe lift is not advocated by some sources.[51] However, children with CP who have asymmetry in tone, muscle activation, posture, and movement are placed at even greater risk for muscle shortening and scoliosis when a discrepancy in leg length exists. Such a child will try to equalize the length by ambulating with the shortened limb in plantar flexion with the heel off of the floor, thus maintaining muscles with increased tone—the plantar flexors—in a continually shortened position. When a full-length shoe lift is used to correct the discrepancy in length, the child should be assessed in a standing posture for symmetry of the posterior iliac spines, anterior superior iliac spines, and the iliac crests. When the child wears an orthosis, the shoe-lift thickness must take this added measurement into account. Shoe lifts can be applied to shoes and sneakers in an attractive way at a minimal cost.

Evaluation of Gait

A baby prepares for ambulation by acquiring antigravity movement components of the neck, trunk, and extremities while in prone, supine, and side-lying positions. These movement components are also practiced by the baby in higher level positions against gravity (i.e., sitting, quadruped, kneeling, and standing). Stability of the joints increases as strength is gained in the surrounding musculature. Weight shifting has been practiced by the baby and is mastered in all directions.

From the onset of independent ambulation until approximately 3 years of age, the young child's gait pattern will continue to change with the acquisition of mature components in gait. An early, immature gait pattern is characterized by the following:

- Uneven length of step
- Excessive flexion of the hip and knee during swing phase
- Immobility of the pelvis without pelvic tilting or rotation
- Abduction and external rotation of the hips throughout swing phase
- Base of support that is wider than the lateral dimensions of the trunk
- Pronation of the foot as a consequence of the wide base
- Contact with the floor that is made with the foot flat
- Hyperextension of the knee throughout stance phase
- Upper extremities in a high-,medium-, or low-guard position[62]

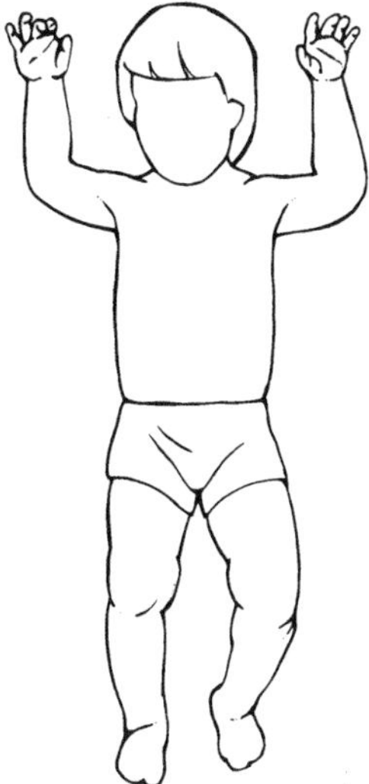

Figure 4-2 ■ *Child ambulating with the upper extremities in a high-guard position.*

Sutherland[63] and colleagues described five kinematic gait characteristics that change in normal childhood development during the ages of 1 to 7 years:

1. The duration of single-limb stance increases with age (especially up to the age of 2.5 years).
2. Walking velocity increases steadily (especially up to the age of 3.5 years).
3. Cadence (and its variability) decreases with age.
4. Step length increases (especially until the age of 2.5 years).
5. The ratio of body width to stride width (computed from the "pelvic span," which is measured from the level of the anterosuperior iliac spines, and the "ankle spread," which is the distance between left and right ankle centers during double-limb support) increases rapidly until the age of 2.5 years. It then increases more slowly until the age of 3.5 years, and then plateaus.

Furthermore, the *step factor* (step length divided by limb length) increases during the first 4 years of life and is suggested as a measure of neuromuscular maturation.[64]

Thelen and Cooke maintain that there is "a gradual evolution from the simple pattern generation of the newborn period," and that "an essential process is the individuation of joint action from the obligatory synergy of the newborn period."[65] In an earlier publication, Thelen also states that "Learning to walk is a complex, gradual process of maturation of motivation, the integration of subcortical pattern-generating centers with neural substrate for control of posture and balance, and important changes in body proportions and tone and muscle strength."[64]

To gain the stability not yet available at the trunk and pelvis, an early ambulator maintains a certain degree of scapular adduction, either bilaterally or unilaterally. The high-guard position (Fig. 4-2) consists of adduction of the scapulae; extension, abduction, and external rotation of the shoulder; and flexion of the elbow. This position affords the greatest stability by maintaining maximal scapular adduction, leading to strong extension of the trunk with an anterior, immobile pelvis. A medium-guard position (Fig. 4-3) reduces the degree of scapular adduc-

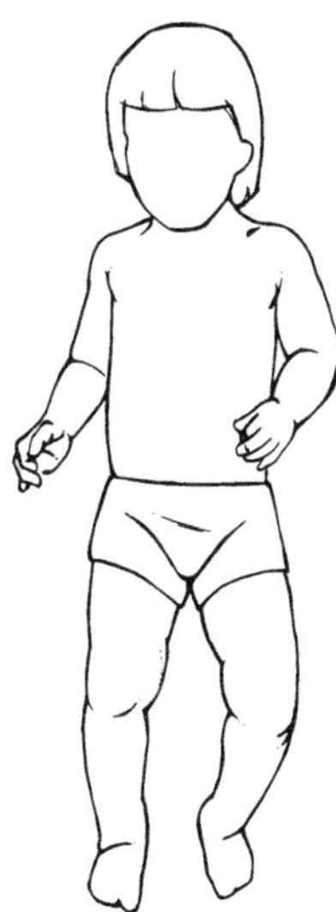

Figure 4-3 ■ *Child ambulating with the upper extremities in a medium-guard position.*

tion. Shoulders continue to be held in extension, abduction, and external rotation, and elbows are flexed with forearms pronated. The low-guard position (Fig. 4-4) consists of scapular adduction with the arms at the sides.

The mature components of gait provide a useful framework for evaluating the gait of a child with CP.[66]

1. *Pelvic tilt.* A downward tilt of the pelvis from the horizontal plane occurs on the non--weight-bearing side. This tilt allows the center of gravity to be lowered as the body passes over the stance limb, thus reducing vertical oscillations of the body.
2. *Pelvic rotation.* Transverse rotation of the pelvis in an anterior direction occurs with internal rotation of the lower extremity at the end of the swing phase. This rotation contributes to a narrowing of the base of support and changes the distribution of weight during stance phase to the lateral border of the foot.
3. *Knee flexion at midstance.* This position permits a more fluid, smoother gait pattern.
4. *Heel strike.* Ankle dorsiflexion near the end of the swing phase readies the foot for contact with the floor made at the heel.
5. *Mature mechanism of the foot and knee.* These mechanisms consist of an extension of the knee just before or at heel strike, flexion of the knee in a midstance position, and extension of the knee at heel-off.
6. *Mature base of support.* The base of support narrows to within the lateral dimensions of the trunk.
7. *Synchronous movement of the upper extremities.* Arm swing achieves a reciprocating movement with the lower extremities. Movements of the upper extremities balance out the leg advance and pelvic rotation that produce angular momentum to the lower body.[66]

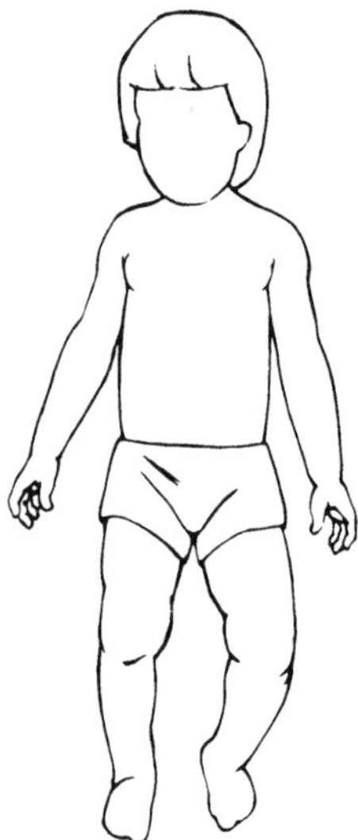

Figure 4-4 ■ Child ambulating with the upper extremities in a low-guard position.

GAIT IN CEREBRAL PALSY

One of the most frequently asked questions from parents and caregivers upon being told their child has CP is, "When will my child walk?" This prediction can be very difficult and should be approached with caution. Watt and coworkers attempted to determine the usefulness of early prognosis.[67] They discovered that predictions made at 1 year of age were the least useful, and that predictions made at 3.5 years of age did not significantly increase in accuracy over the information that was available at 2 years of age. They found that the age at which the child sat, the type of CP, certain reflexes (tonic labyrinthine, ATNR, symmetrical tonic neck, and Moro), and two postural reactions (foot placement and parachute) all had a statistically significant correlation with ambulation at 8 years of age. However, no absolute value could be placed on the items.[67]

In 1987, Bleck reviewed 423 patients with cerebral palsy and found 66% to fit in the classification of spastic diplegia. Of those, 79% were independent ambulators, 19% ambulated with external assistance, and 2% were non-ambulators.[7]

There are several classic gait patterns that are characteristic of the different types of CP. Variations do exist within each type, however. The classic gait patterns are described in the following section.

Many children with spastic diplegia have limited mobility in their lumbar spine, pelvis, and hip joints and show limited asymmetric pelvic tilt or pelvic rotation during gait.[42] In an effort to compensate for the lack of mobility of the lower body, these children shift their weight and maintain balance by using excessive mobility through the head, neck, upper trunk, and upper extremities. Their hips stay flexed during stance, and full extension of the hip is never achieved. Excessive adduction and internal rotation of the hip are frequently found; in severe cases, the medial aspect of the knees may approximate. Depending on the function of the pelvic, lumbar, and ankle musculature, the knees may be either flexed or hyperextended during stance. The feet may be in valgus outside the lateral dimensions of the trunk, or they may be close together in a narrow base of support in plantar-flexion with the heels off of the floor. There can be concern and confusion regarding the differentiation between idiopathic toe walking and spastic diplegic CP. Hicks et al.[68] found that idiopathic toe walkers typically have heel cord contracture but minimal or no hamstring tightness, along with increased knee extension in stance and increased external rotation of the foot with increased plantar flexion. Conversely, they found that children with CP had an essentially normal gait pattern with the exception of sustained knee flexion at terminal stance and initial contact.[68] Although children with more severe involvement may require an assistive device for ambulation, many children ambulate without any devices, or with only a shoe insert or orthosis. Generally, children with spastic diplegic CP ambulate at about half the speed of children without CP, and the self-selected velocity is usually the most efficient rate of ambulation.[69]

Asymmetry is the most obvious feature of the gait of a child with hemiplegia, with most of the body weight borne on the uninvolved lower extremity. Shifting of weight to the involved side is brief and incomplete. Limbs on the involved side are retracted or rotated posteriorly, when compared with the shoulder and pelvis on the contralateral side. Arm swing occurs only on the uninvolved side, with the involved upper extremity held in shoulder hyperextension and elbow flexion as part of an associated reaction. The lower extremity can vary between stiffness in extension to greater mobility with flexion. Almost all children with spastic hemiplegia ambulate without assistive devices, but many use a shoe insert or an orthosis.

Children with milder cases of athetosis without significant spasms have underlying low postural stiffness that fluctuates to high stiffness. The gait pattern in the lower extremity is poorly graded and in total patterns of movement. The lower extremity is usually lifted high into flexion and placed down in stance into extension with adduction, internal rotation, and plantar flexion. The hips stay slightly flexed, the lumbar spine is hyperextended, the thoracic spine is excessively rounded, and the cervical spine is hyperextended with the chin jutting forward.[42]

Assessment of Fine Motor and Adaptive Skills

Assessment of the fine motor and adaptive skills of the child with CP is traditionally one of the main areas of concern for the occupational therapist, as well as for the physical therapist. If a treatment center or a school does not have an occupational therapist available, the physical therapist should have the basic skills to assess this area of movement and development. Questions to the parents, caregivers, or teachers that may alert the therapist to the need for intervention relate to the child's functional abilities during feeding, dressing, toileting, bathing, and prehensile and manipulation skills for play and school function. Additional firsthand information may be obtained by having the child undress and dress (including shoes, socks, and shirt) independently before and after the assessment session. As the child moves to attempt these tasks, the therapist can evaluate sitting balance, pelvic weight shifting, and righting actions of the head and trunk. Other parameters that can be evaluated as the child removes clothes include the ability to reach as well as various modes of grasp—depending on the object, the ability to release an object, and bimanual skills, such as buttoning and unbuttoning. During the evaluation process, the therapist should ascertain the following:

1. How the particular skill is accomplished
2. The degree of assistance required
3. At what point in the task assistance was necessary
4. *Why* the assistance was necessary
5. Does the child accomplish the task using compensatory movement that will lead to structural changes and potential deformity?

Consideration of Speech and Language Abilities

A comprehensive assessment of speech and language is not within the scope of practice of the physical therapist. However, the physical therapist can offer important information to the speech and language pathologist regarding the speech and language abilities and quality of respiration of the child based on observations made during physical therapy assessment and treatment. In obtaining this information, the physical therapist should consider the following questions:

- Did the child appear to hear your voice or other environmental sounds by becoming quiet or looking in the direction of the stimulus?
- Did the child understand questions asked during the evaluation, and did he or she follow step-by-step directional commands?
- Did the child vocalize or verbalize during the assessment? What types of sounds were made? Did the child repeat or appear to stutter speech sounds?
- If the child was verbal, were the words intelligible? Was breath support adequate for speech, or was the child able to speak in only one- or two-word utterances owing to poor control of respiration? Do the expressive language skills appear to be delayed for the child's chronologic age?
- If the child was nonvocal, was there another means of communication used (i.e., gestures, manual language board, electronic communication system)? Did the child use eye localization, pointing, or another means within this alternate system?
- Was the child's communication at a functional level?

The therapist should also ask if the parents have noted any problems with the child's speech or related functional areas, such as difficulty sucking, swallowing, chewing, feeding, or drinking.

These observations and questions can assist in making an informed referral to a speech and language pathologist who will perform a more detailed assessment. If appropriate, the speech and language pathologist can institute a therapeutic program that can be augmented during physical therapy sessions.

A comprehensive assessment of the thorax can be very beneficial to the child and can assist the speech and language pathologist in attaining the goals established for the child. The mobility of the vertebral column and the rib cage has a great impact on the effectiveness of respiration and breath support for vocalization. It also has an impact on pulmonary hygiene, as improved rib cage mobility and deeper respirations help air to flow in the lungs and can prevent or help cure pneumonia. Rib cage mobility and abdominal support provide a good basis for speech control and voice quality. Cotreatment with the speech and language pathologist can be very beneficial to the child, often resulting in more rapid progress. Addressing the child's musculoskeletal problems can assist the speech and language pathologist in planning therapy for communication and respiration issues.

Establishing Goals of Treatment

The therapist's assessment of the child should yield a list of strengths, those things the child can do and likes to do; those functional tasks that are difficult for the child to do, his/her functional limitations; the primary and secondary (compensations) impairments; and the child's or family's desires for the child's function. This information will lead the therapist to establishing functional goals for the child that correlate with the family's needs and desires.

Long-term and short-term goals are written for each child. The duration for achievement of these goals varies with the setting in which the child is being seen. In a school setting, the long-term goals are generally the length of the school year, and the short-term goals are between 3 and 6 months. In a hospital setting, the long-term goals are typically written for the date of the anticipated discharge, and the short-term goals are written weekly. In an outpatient setting, the long-term goals are typically of 6 months' duration and the short-term goals for 1 to 2 months' duration. Short-term goals are not necessarily direct components of the long-term goal.

Stamer[70] has stated clearly the requirements for writing acceptable goals in a variety of situations. The following items should be part of every goal:

1. Subject
2. An observable action verb
3. An observable functional performance with a beginning and an end point
4. Conditions under which the performance will be met (conditions describe the circumstances and environment)
5. Criteria, or how well the client performs this function[70]

Each goal must have each part to be observable and measurable. A goal guides the therapist in the treatment of the child towards a functional task.

Following is a list of examples of acceptable long-term goals (LTG) and short-term goals (STG) for various children and their situations.

Mary, 8 Years Old with Spastic Diplegia

LTG (to be achieved in 6 months)

1. Mary will ascend 10 of the 13 8-inch rise steps in the household staircase leading to the second floor using a step-to-step pattern and leading with either leg while her right hand is on the railing and the left hand at her side; she will require standby supervision only and complete this task four of five trials in a 1-week period of time.

STG (to be achieved in 2 months)

1. Mary will safely ascend and descend a 6-inch curb from her sidewalk to the street using forearm crutches and require standby assist only for 100% of 5 trials.
2. Mary will walk independently without assistive device while wearing her articulating MAFOs for 4 feet between the kitchen cupboard and the refrigerator, keeping her head and trunk erect over her vertical pelvis and her arms free to swing at her sides in three out of five trials.

Emily, 3 Years Old with a Diagnosis of Moderately Severe Spastic Quadriplegic CP

LTG (to be achieved in 6 months)

1. Emily will sit in a ring sit on the the carpeted floor with her head in midline with a chin tuck and an erect spine over a vertical pelvis and her eyes looking downward to the toy held in her hands, given support at her pelvis for 2 minutes, two of three trials in a single session.

STG (to be achieved in 2 months)

1. Emily will prop on her extended arms with hands open and wrists in at least 45 degrees extension when placed in prone on the floor, keep her head in a vertical position in relationship to the floor to visually scan the environment, and hold the position for 45 seconds given moderate assistance for stability through her pelvis in two out of three trials.
2. Emily will sit in an adapted chair with tray in place in the therapy room with her hips, knees, and ankles at 90 degrees; her feet touching the floor, head erect, and both arms on the tray for manipulation of a toy appropriate for her cognitive level and functional abilities; and sustain postural control for 10 minutes one time during the therapy session.

Therapeutic Intervention

The therapeutic team should consist of the child, the family, the medical staff, and allied health professionals and paraprofessionals based on the child's functional abilities and needs (both in the medical model and the school system). The child and family are the core of the team with the emphasis placed on function in the home and function in the community (including school, church, recreation, etc.). Documenting and quantifying outcomes for the child is critical to physical therapy. Several authors discuss the need for outcome research and efficacy studies.[71–73] The need for physical therapy has come under scrutiny both in the medical model and in early intervention, which forces the physical therapist to provide the most efficacious intervention with

Teddy, 6 Years Old with a Diagnosis of Athetoid CP of Moderate Severity

LTG (to be achieved in 6 months)

1. Teddy will ambulate 30 feet using a posterior walker (independently propelling the walker) and wearing his DAFOs, with therapist providing minimal compression through the stance leg from behind, in a hallway with minimal obstacles and/or few people, while sustaining midline head control with thoracic extension and soft lumbar lordosis, four out of five trials.

STG (to be achieved in 2 months)

1. Teddy will independently cruise to both sides along a support surface of 36 inches in height and 8 feet in length, using bilateral hand support on the surface, keeping his head in neutral extension/flexion position with active rotation to scan the environment, with abduction of the advancing leg in the coronal plane, in his classroom of peers at least two times per day, five out of 5 days.
2. Teddy will independently raise his left hand to 80 degrees of shoulder flexion, hand toward the ceiling in 90 degrees of external rotation, shifting his base of support through his pelvis; while sitting in his classroom chair with his legs in 90 degrees of hip and knee flexion, both feet flat on the floor with his head, neck, and trunk held in balanced flexion and extension, in response to the teacher's question, three out of three trials.

careful documentation addressing the areas of need and expected outcome in functional terms. For example, physical therapy can minimize the need for or postpone orthopedic surgery, thereby reducing the number of surgeries a child may need.[74] To consider when physical therapy is the most beneficial, it is necessary to look at the child in terms of his or her current function, prognosis for acquiring new functional skills, "windows of opportunity" when the child may make the greatest gains in the shortest period of time, the child's growth spurts, recent surgery, the family's ability to manage a home program at each level of the child's progress, and the child's level of comfort in terms of pain and deformity. A burst of physical therapy is essential after neurosurgery and orthopedic surgery, after growth spurts that impact the biomechanics of the child's movement, and whenever the child is in a "window of opportunity." Intensive therapy may be required for shorter periods of time to accomplish specific tasks. Formal physical therapy should be supplemented in early adolescence and adulthood in those with mild to moderate impairment by alternative activities such as recreational pursuits.[74,75] With the child's age and functional abilities in mind, consider extracurricular activities such as therapeutic or adaptive swimming; hippotherapy; and dance, tumbling, or music lessons. Frequently, participation in these activities with the child's family or peer group will motivate the child and will assist in the acquisition of new skills.

Therapists must be very clear about the frequency and duration of service required for the child to make functional gains. According to Fetters, we need a new way to look at treatment, and we need ecologically valid movement goals to guide treatment of motor dysfunction, as well as research in motor control.[76] The parameters that therapists have been using to guide their treatment sequences may need to be altered to achieve documented quality improvement in terms of functional goals. Kluzik and colleagues examined kinematic properties of reaching children with spastic quadriplegia and showed that, in using the neurodevelopmental treatment approach, the children experienced an immediate improvement in reaching at the end of the session.[77]

Kamm and colleagues address treatment from a dynamic systems approach, considering the goal of treatment to be working on the system when it is in transition.[78] According to their approach, the therapist would complete an assessment, then attempt to predict under what conditions and how patients will change. The therapist would also anticipate systemwide responses to small changes in a control parameter. For example, placing an orthotic device in a shoe may alter the pattern of weight bearing, thus influencing the posture of the knee, hip, pelvis, and trunk. "When patients are able to explore and use the limits of postures to actively engage in tasks, they are adaptive and independent."[78]

Discussions and explanations are presented in this chapter as to various methods of treatment intervention, including therapeutic exercise, Neurodevelopmental Treatment (NDT), Sensory Integration (SI), Therapeutic Electrical Stimulation (TES), equipment uses and considerations, neuromedical and neurosurgical interventions, orthopedic surgical interventions, and bracing of the lower extremity. There is no singular recommended intervention for any specific category of cerebral palsy as each child presents a unique array of functional abilities, goals, and impairments. It would be a great disservice to the reader to be limited to one or two ways to treat an individual. It is common to use various principles from a variety of approaches for a well-rounded treatment. The therapist must determine the array of methods used for each child. Displays 4-2 through 4-5 present "typical" impairments in four major classifications of cerebral palsy. They are meant to be used as references and not as the "true picture" of every child in that classification. Frequently, children will have impairments within two or more classifications. For example, a child may

DISPLAY 4-2

"Typical" Impairments of the Child with Spasticity

Increased stiffness in extremities, distal > proximal
Decreased stiffness in neck and trunk
Inability to grade between coactivation (CA) and reciprocal inhibition (RI), times with excessive amounts of either CA or RI
Difficulty initiating certain muscle groups (i.e., hip extensors, triceps)
Difficulty sustaining certain muscle groups (i.e., thoracic extensors)
Difficulty terminating certain muscle groups (i.e., hip flexors, adductors, internal rotators)
Decreased ability to use eccentric control in certain muscle groups (i.e., quadriceps)
Decreased ability to balance flexors and extensors
 Trunk activation greater in extension than flexion
 Upper extremity activation greater in flexion than extension
 Lower extremity activation greater in extension than flexion
Uses the synergy of hip flexion, adduction, and internal rotation for function
Decreased ROM
Decreased strength
Vision used more in upward gaze and asymmetrically
Decreased proprioception and kinesthesia
Decreased body awareness
Decreased ability to discriminate between diffferent kinds of touch

have spastic quadriplegia with an athetoid component that involves the upper extremities more than the lower extremities. The information included in these tables is derived from numerous sources.[19,38,39,46,79,80]

Therapeutic Exercise

Therapeutic exercise plays an important role in the habilitation/rehabilitation of the child with CP. The exercise program should be developed

DISPLAY 4-3

"Typical" Impairments of the Child with Hypotonia

Decreased stiffness in trunk and extremities
Decreased ability to coactivate muscle groups (substitutes with ligamentous support)
Initiates muscle activation in phasic bursts
Decreased ability to sustain muscle group activation
Termination of muscle activity is passive
Difficulty with concentric and eccentric muscle use
Difficulty balancing flexors and extensors in the trunk, use extension > flexion
Increased ROM
Decreased strength
Decreased proprioception and kinesthetic awareness
Decreased ability to process tactile information
Shallow respiration with increased rate

DISPLAY 4-4

"Typical" Impairments of the Child with Athetosis

Global decrease in stiffness—quite profound
Fluctuations in stiffness with high-amplitude, low-frequency oscillations
Problems with coactivation and reciprocal inhibition, resulting in extreme range of movement
Inability to grade initiation of muscle activity
Inability to sustain muscle activity
Termination of muscle activity is passive
Inability to use eccentric control
Tends toward extensor activation > flexor, becomes very asymmetric
Difficulty in selecting synergies for functional activities
Hypermobile at cervical joints: occiput on C1, C6-C7, and thoracolumbar junction
Decreased strength
Vision used in upward gaze
Problems with proprioception upper extremities > lower extremities
Decreased body awareness
Respiration fluctuates in rate and rhythm

DISPLAY 4-5

"Typical" Impairments of the Child with Ataxia

Sensory/perceptual area is the greatest problem
Relies on vision for balance and posture
Visual system demonstrates severe nystagmus
Decreased proprioception
Increased latency in processing sensory information
Severe postural insecurity—very fearful of movement
Poor vestibular system
Tactilely defensive
Difficulty generalizing sensory and motor information to perform novel tasks
Minimally decreased stiffness
Tremors of increased frequency and decreased amplitude, increase with increase in skill demanded in task
Difficulty timing and sequencing initiation/sustaining/termination of muscle activity
Difficulty grading midrange of coactivation and reciprocal inhibition
Favors flexion over extension to lower the center of mass

in relation to the assessment of the child, the identified long- and short-term goals, and the functional abilities of the child. It is similar to other forms of exercise in that the therapist must upgrade the difficulty of the program to progress the child to greater achievement in strength, endurance, and coordination. In order to increase the child's strength, the therapist has two available options: (1) progress the movement from a gravity-eliminated movement to one that is working against gravity, and (2) alter the amount of assistance given by the therapist so that the child has to use greater force and control. Increasing the number of repetitions of a movement or lengthening the time of exercise will help to improve endurance. Coordination should improve with an increase in strength and endurance, depending on the lesion.

GRAVITY

The therapist can use the effects of gravity as a force against which the child must move and function. The therapist places the child in a position so that any movement of the head and trunk, or the limbs, must be done against gravity. Of course, this technique requires that the child have postural control that is strong enough to function against gravity. The motion can be made in a position with no gravity if the child's "strength" is inadequate or if the movement is poorly coordinated. An example of progression against gravity is shown when the child attempts to progress from a sitting position to kneeling, then to standing. Each progression requires greater strength to stabilize the trunk owing to the increasing height of the center of mass from the floor.

DISSOCIATION OR DIFFERENTIATION

Therapeutic exercise should be directed toward dissociation of one extremity from the opposite limb and the limbs from the body to achieve greater muscular coordination. Emphasis should be placed on achieving greater differentiation of the joints within a limb as well.

EXTERNAL SUPPORT

The therapist's hands or a piece of equipment may be used to provide initial support to inhibit excessive stiffness, maintain alignment, initiate a weight shift, support a movement, or aid smooth transitions of movement. This external support should be altered intermittently at first to provide the child with an opportunity to practice the movement independently.

Support of the child's body to decrease stiffness and to facilitate movement can be moved from a proximal point such as the trunk, shoulder, or pelvis, which provides a greater amount of support, to a more distal point along the limb. By moving the point of support more distally, the therapist expects that the child will assume a greater degree of control over the movement at the unsupported joints.

SENSORY SYSTEMS

It is necessary to address the child's sensory system (proprioceptive, visual, tactile, vestibular, and body awareness) specifically as it affects motor function. The child with CP may have difficulty in receiving and interpreting sensory feedback and is, therefore, at a disadvantage for motor output. The therapist should provide the child with movement experiences and sensory input that will help teach the child correct interpretation of sensory stimuli. The experience should begin as exact stimulation for the child who has great difficulty interpreting or receiving sensory stimuli. The kinds of sensory stimuli can be broadened with improvement.

SECONDARY MUSCULOSKELETAL CHANGES

A child's difficulty in performing functional tasks may be attributable to changes within the musculoskeletal system. An assessment should identify which muscles are shortened, which joint capsules are tight, and where the fascia has thickened over time owing to injury or stress of movement. These areas should be addressed so that smoothly coordinated motor tasks can be accomplished. It is beyond the scope of this chapter to address myofascial release; however, once learned, it can be easily adapted to the pediatric client.

OTHER CONSIDERATIONS

The therapist should avoid prolonged holding in static positions during treatment. Smoothly graded transitions in movement with brief holding of midline or neutral alignment is more desirable than extended periods in static postures. Imposed weight shifts and transitions in movement should be varied, both in speed and range, so that the child cannot anticipate rhythmic displacements. Weight shifts and transitions in movement must be practiced in different positions for improved function. Initiation of weight shifts and transitions in movement are important parts of treatment, particularly for the child with spasticity. Active movement and much repetition are needed for a child to "learn" a movement.

Tables 4-2 through 4-4 provide examples of activities for therapeutic exercise sessions. These are to be used as guides only—not prescribed activities for a particular child with CP. There may be several different responses noted with a given activity. The therapist and child should be limited only by their own creativity.

Neurodevelopmental (Bobath) Treatment

Neurodevelopmental/Bobath Treatment (NDT) was originally developed by the Bobaths in England in the early 1940s for the treatment of individuals with pathophysiology of the central nervous system (CNS), specifically children with CP and adults with hemiplegia.[81] Dr. and Mrs. Bobath described NDT as a "living concept," and as such, it has continued to evolve over the years. "The NDT approach is not a set of techniques but more an understanding of the developmental process of motor control and the motor components which make up functional motor tasks."[80] The goal is to have effective carryover from the treatment session to real life and the following treatment sessions. Carryover is actually motor learning, "a relatively permanent change in the capability for responding."[53]

The ultimate goal of NDT is for the child to have the best possible function. Treatment sessions are goal directed toward a functional task. The process by which this is achieved includes child-initiated movement and tasks. The therapist will do preparatory work (e.g., muscle elongation) to enable the child to perform the task and may initially facilitate and guide the move-

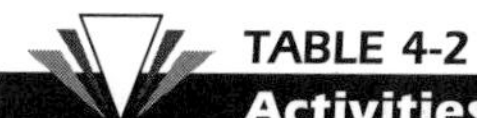

TABLE 4-2
Activities for Therapeutic Exercise Session—Example 1

Placement of Child or Stimulus	Response
1. Child side-lying, head supported on small pillow or towel; therapist's hands on child's abdominal muscles; lower extremities dissociated or symmetrically flexed; toy placed in front of child at chest level	1. Maintains head in line with trunk; sensory input to abdominal muscles; will encourage downward gaze, flexion of neck, and shoulder flexion in gravity-eliminated position; will provide a midline orientation of the body
2. From side-lying, backward weight shift into supine with buttocks maintained elevated off the support with hips and knees flexed; lower extremities just outside lateral dimensions of trunk	2. Activation of axial flexors and antigravity movement of upper extremities; elongation of axial and hip extensors
3. Hand → knees and hands → feet play in supine with buttocks elevated	3. Head in midline, chin tucked. Antigravity shoulder flexion and elbow extension
a. Right hand → right foot Left hand → left foot	a. Bilateral, symmetric activation of trunk musculature
b. Two hands → one foot	b. Bilateral, diagonal activation of trunk musculature Midline orientation of body
4. Child side-lying as described in No. 1; forward weight shift into prone position	4. Activation of axial extensors and propping on forearms requiring a balance by axial flexors
5. Propping on forearms with elbows in line with or anterior to shoulders and scapulae against thoracic wall; Hips extended with lower extremities in line with trunk Provide lateral weight shift through the pelvis	5. Balance of axial flexors and extensors; elongation of muscles between scapula and humerus; activation of serratus anterior Elongation of hip flexors and abductors Movement of body weight over extended, internally rotated hip to allow elongation of muscles on weight-bearing side. Spinal lateral flexion, lateral pelvic tilt, and dissociation of upper and lower extremities on non–weight-bearing side

ment as needed to decrease or prevent abnormal compensatory movements. Feedforward is developed as the child actually practices the skill or task with the therapist's guidance. The therapist does less and less as the child takes over and anticipates postural and motor requirements.[53]

The following is a synopsis of the current key theoretical summary statements.

1. Human behavior/function is based on the continuous interaction among the individual, the environment, and the task. The individual is comprised of many subsystems that are interactive and interdependent. The subsystems are plastic and adaptive to both internal and external changes. . . . During the acquisition of functional motor skills, the individual focuses on the goal rather than the specific movement components of the task.
2. A standard of reference for proficient human motor function is based upon the study of motor control, motor development, and motor learning. A hallmark of efficient human motor function is the ability of the individual to combine an infinite number of movements into desired functional activities under a wide variety of environmental conditions. Learning and adaptation of motor skills involve a process associated with practice and experience.

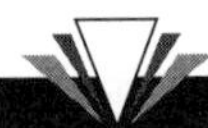

TABLE 4-3
Activities for Therapeutic Exercise Session—Example 2

Placement of Child or Stimulus	Response
1. Prone on extended arms over a ball; lower extremities in line with trunk; one leg dissociated and flexed under the trunk with the opposite leg in extension	1. Extension of trunk (cervical to lumbar) with active holding by abdominal muscles; shoulder flexion with elbow extension; slight lateral pelvic tilt; unilateral hip extension or hyperextension; full hip and knee flexion with ankle plantar flexion on contralateral side
2. Lateral displacement of ball towards extended lower extremity	2. Lateral weight shift through pelvis; increased lateral pelvic tilt (from above); lateral flexion of trunk and neck
3. Presentation of toys to side and slightly behind child's body	3. Lateral weight shift through pelvis; thoracic and lumbar extension rotation; dissociation of upper extremities for unilateral reach with shoulder extension and external rotation; elbow, wrist, and finger extension; forearm supination to neutral
4. Backward and lateral movement of the ball toward the flexed lower extremity	4. Will allow weight shift onto flexed leg and assumption of three-point or a quadruped position; requires activation of seratus anterior, shoulder flexors, elbow extensors, axial extensors with abdominal holding, hip extensors, hip abductors, hip adductors, and quadriceps
5. From a symmetric quadruped position, backward movement of the ball	5. Hip extension with abdominal holding; contraction of lumbar and thoracic extensors; greater acceptance of weight in entension on upper extremities
6. From a symmetric quadruped position, forward and lateral movement of the ball	6. Transition of movement into side sit, causing hip flexion; dissociated hip rotation, abduction, and adduction positions, and spinal lateral flexion
7. Sitting on the ball in a symmetric position; lower extremities just outside lateral dimensions of trunk; child holds a small hoop, shoulders are flexed to 90 degrees; backward displacement of ball	7. Activation of neck and trunk flexors with stabilization around hip joints

Figure 4-5 demonstrates the response as described in number 1 above. Figure 4-6 demonstrates the response as described in number 4 above. Figure 4-7 demonstrates the response as described in number 7 above.

3. Individuals with motor control problems resulting from CNS pathophysiology present with somewhat predictable primary and secondary impairments. These impairments may limit the person's ability to function.
4. The intervention process begins with the assessment of the individual's functional performance. Analytical problem solving is used to develop a treatment plan. Treatment focuses on increasing function by building on the individual's strengths while addressing the impairments. Therapeutic handling is one strategy utilized to help the individual achieve his or her functional goals.[81]

Sensory Integration

"Sensory Integration (SI) is the primary treatment approach with children who have learning disorders, attention deficits, and autism."[21] SI focuses on sensory aspects and their impact on

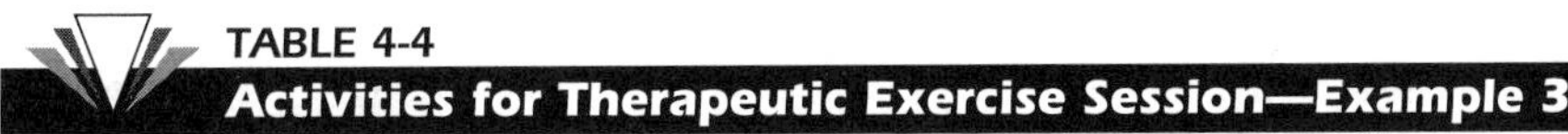

TABLE 4-4
Activities for Therapeutic Exercise Session—Example 3

Placement of Child or Stimulus	Response
1. Standing at a table higher than waist level; placement of toys out of child's reach laterally	1. Cruising to obtain toy requiring abduction and adduction of hips with extension
2. Child standing; placement of toys on small bench beside child and on floor	2. Play activities will require flexion and extension of lower extremities in varied joint ranges with muscle holding; activation of hip abductors/adductors, trunk and neck extensors and rotators. Child may work in squat position for symmetry or through 1/2 kneel for greater dissociation
3. Forward weight shift onto front leg in a step position	3. Bilateral hip and knee extension; lumbar extension with abdominal holding a. Forward stance leg—weight accepted on dorsiflexed foot with greater weight on the ball of the foot b. Rear leg—ankle plantar flexion, mobility of metatarsal-phalangeal joints allowing dissociation through the foot

Figure 4-8 demonstrates the response as described in number 3 above.

motivation, attention, movement, and socio-emotional well-being.[21]

The principles of SI treatment include:

1. Providing the opportunity to experience a variety of controlled sensory input to encourage the production of an adaptive response that includes motor behaviors, social interactions, or cognitive skills
2. Encouraging the child to utilize intrinsic motivation
3. Promoting purposeful behaviors within a meaningful activity[21]

SI can be used to obtain an optimal state of arousal and to affect the child's motivation, initiation, and purposeful interaction with the environment. This is frequently helpful for the child with low level of arousal who is difficult to encourage to interact with peers in the classroom or in a treatment session. Utilizing the techniques of SI intervention in the early part of the treatment session will prepare the child for more active participation in the session, which is necessary for carryover and learning.

As noted previously, feedforward is a vital part of functional movement. "Feedforward needs to be treated from both a sensory and motor planning point of view, as it requires sensory input to organize the actions and it requires the ability to volitionally organize the movement."[21] Many children with CP experience difficulty in processing sensory input and therefore have even greater difficulty producing a desired motor output. It is appropriate to use both an SI approach combined with a motor-based approach with these children.

Some pediatric therapists will use a combination of SI and NDT with children who require both interventions. SI focuses primarily on the sensory processing aspect of the motor act, whereas NDT focuses primarily on the motor response to the sensory input.[21] The same therapist can provide the intervention, or two separate therapists can provide the intervention in which each is skilled. Excellent communication between them is needed to most effectively treat the child. Be diligent in your observations when using SI with a child who has increased stiffness as a primary or secondary impairment. There can be an increase in the compensatory postures and movements as the linear vestibular input provided through the SI approach increases extensor tone. The use of the techniques must be well graded when used with children with CP. Children with CP often lack independent mobility in their environment, and therefore a pure SI approach is difficult and inappropriate.[21]

Therapeutic Electrical Stimulation

TES is a method of low intensity nighttime electrical stimulation for the treatment of muscle weakness in CP. It was initially developed in 1985 by K.E. Pape, MD and the research group at the Hospital for Sick Children in Toronto, Canada.[82,83] The aim of TES is to increase the rate of change; it is not in itself, used to change something (personal communication). TES differs from neuromuscular stimulation in that it employs low intensity stimulation, delivered just above the sensory threshold, and does not produce a muscle contraction.

Muscle is grown and repaired at night, during sleep. Growth hormone, the major trophic hormone in the body, is secreted predominantly at night (80% to 90%) in a single peak, approximately 2 to 3 hours after falling asleep. By applying the current during sleep, the body may be tricked into growing muscle.[82] New muscle bulk has been noted in 6 to 8 weeks of treatment.[82] This process has translated into functional use within 12 months.

TES is intended to be used as an assist to the total management of the child, not to replace primary therapeutic intervention.[83] Research has shown that the child demonstrates results faster when it is used in conjunction with hands-on therapy.[82] To ready the increased muscle bulk for functional use, it must be strengthened and integrated into the child's daily activities. The technique to use TES is taught by certified instructors in the field and is currently advertised as Therapeutic Electrical Stimulation Level One—Cerebral Palsy.

Refer to Display 4-6 for specific information in the use of TES.

DISPLAY 4-6
Therapeutic Electrical Stimulation*

Indications

1. Muscle disuse atrophy
2. Status post casting
3. Long-term bracing
4. Status postsurgical intervention

Contraindictions

1. Obesity
2. Younger than 2 years of age

Program Requirements

1. Consistent family involvment (key criterion)
2. Child/family motivation
3. Ability to carry out a home program

Program Length

1. Treat until muscles are used functionally
2. Return to treatment when child enters puberty
3. Child with mild involvment: 18 to 24 months
4. Child with moderate/severe involvment: 3 to 4 years

*Personal communication with Dr. Pape

Equipment Uses and Considerations

Equipment may be used as an aid to therapeutic intervention and handling. The therapist may use equipment to place the child in a position to enhance movement, inhibit undesirable responses, introduce instability into the context of movement, assist in controlling the amount of instability and the degrees of freedom,[78] or assist in the handling and movement of larger patients. The positions and movements available to the therapist are limited only by the therapist's creativity and handling skills.

Mats

A firm mat provides a good working surface on the floor against which the child can push or work in attempting to attain specific postures or movements against gravity. The mat provides proprioceptive and tactile feedback so that the child has better sensory information regarding movement. A softer mat will challenge the child's balance while it moves across the surface.

Benches

Benches of various heights can be used for short-sitting, tabletop activities, stepping, climbing, cruising, and so on. One bench can be adjustable in height, or the therapist may wish to have several benches of graduated height to accommodate the tabletop and climbing activities.

Balls and Bolsters

Firm balls and bolsters provide mobile surfaces that can aid the therapist in facilitating postural control and postural preparations of the child. The direction in which the ball is moved and the position of the child on the ball can be varied to facilitate movement of the head and trunk into flexion, extension, lateral flexion, and/or rotation. It is essential to remember that the ball has a curved weight-bearing surface so that lateral displacement of the ball will result in weight bearing through the ischium that is on top of the ball (the shortened side of the trunk). Varied use of the ball and its infinite possibilities for movement allows the therapist to control the degree to which the movement is assisted by or performed against gravity. Figures 4-5 through 4-8 give visual examples of ways in which such a ball can be utilized.

Adaptive Equipment

Adaptive equipment is often a necessary and useful adjunct to treatment of the child with CP. Equipment may be provided to offer postural support to the child, or it may aid functional skills and mobility. Any equipment used should be "family-friendly" (functional for the family), comfortable safe, easy to use, and attractive. Adaptive equipment and its use should coincide and reinforce therapeutic goals for the child. The equipment should be reassessed frequently and adapted as necessary based on the child's current needs.

A brief description of common items used for children with CP will be presented here. Chapter 9 deals exclusively with Adaptive Equipment and should be consulted for detailed information, including information on the appropriate use of and ordering of wheelchairs.

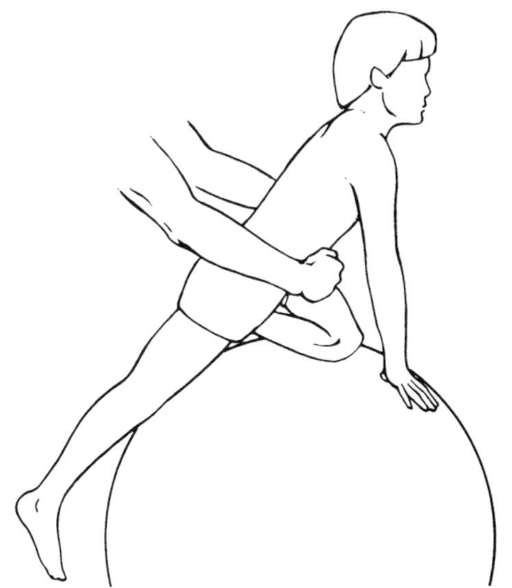

Figure 4-5 ▪ Child in the prone position being supported on a ball with lower extremities dissociated, extension throughout the spine, shoulders flexed, and elbows extended.

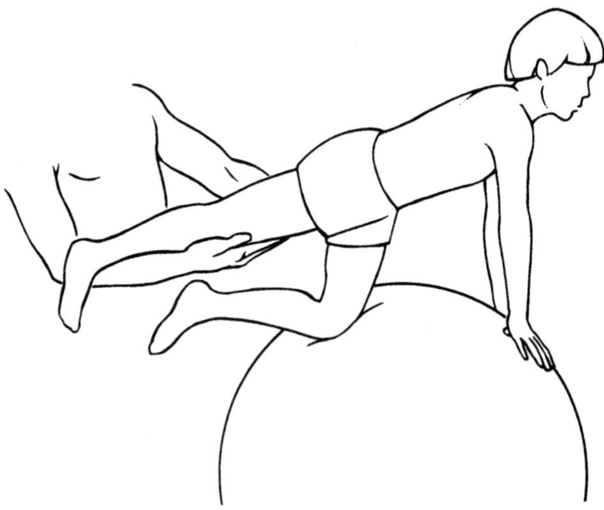

Figure 4-6 ▪ Forward weight shift onto extended upper extremities with lower extremities maintained in dissociated position. This is designed to facilitate trunk extension with abdominal holding and shoulder flexion with elbow extension without excessive extension through the lower extremities.

EQUIPMENT TO AID POSITIONING

Children with CP may lack the necessary postural control and coordination to function in a variety of positions. Children should have a variety of positions in which they can function, travel, and rest.[84] Side-lyers, adaptive seating systems, and standing systems are the more common items used by children in the classroom and in the home environment to optimize

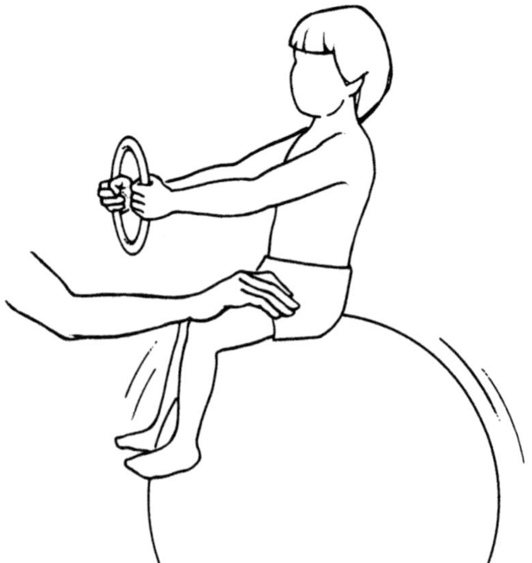

Figure 4-7 ▪ Activation of the axial flexors with posterior displacement of the ball. Active antigravity work of the shoulder girdle muscles with bilateral play activity in space.

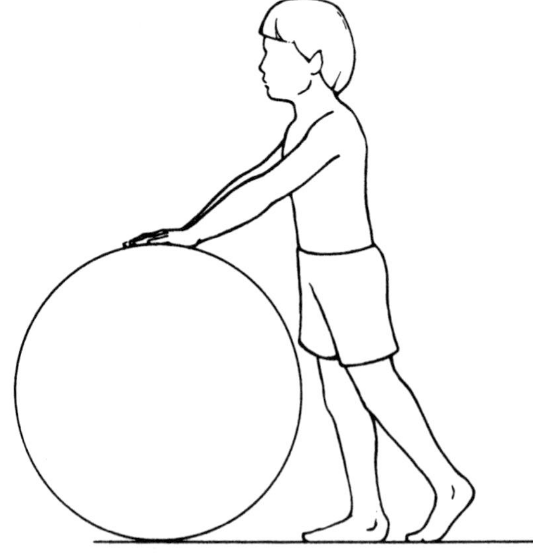

Figure 4-8 ▪ Older child assuming a forward stance position while weight bearing at a mobile surface.

function. Other equipment found to be helpful in the home for improved function and safety include tub seats, adapted potty chairs, and car seats.

Side-lying is used to promote eye-hand coordination and bilateral play skills as well as to encourage more typical development of the rib cage. Prolonged supine and prone positioning with weak trunk musculature and immobility contributes to abnormal shaping of the rib cage with a decrease in the anterior-posterior diameter. Side-lying can be achieved with towel or blanket rolls in front of and behind the child. There are also a variety of side-lyers on the market for purchase.

When assessing a child for adaptive seating, first complete your assessment out of the chair. What are the goals of the seating system? Is the child's posture fixed or flexible? Can the child sit independently without external support? Can the child sit by propping on its arms, or is the child dependent on external support to maintain an upright posture? How can the pelvis be maintained in neutral alignment with the trunk and head held in proper alignment? Consider where the child needs to be in space for optimal function. The more severely involved child may require 90 degrees of hip and knee flexion but may also need to be tilted back in space so the head has support and will not fall forward onto the child's chest, thereby overstretching the posterior neck muscles. The child may function best in a simple corner chair or bolster seat with an attached tray. Numerous commercial options offer an adjustable system to allow for high chair sitting at the dinner table and positioning to be used on the floor. Many systems also have detachable trays for positioning and play. The best option is generally the one the family finds most functional for use in the home. Carryover to the home is improved if the family finds the equipment easy to use and aesthetically pleasing.

Children with CP often have atypical methods of standing and bearing weight. The following are some typical lower extremity postures:

1. Asymmetric weight bearing
2. Hip flexion, adduction, and internal rotation with knee flexion, ankles in excessive dorsiflexion with feet pronated and forefoot abducted (crouched gait)
3. Stiff extension in legs with hips flexed, adducted, and internally rotated, ankles in equinovarus
4. Hips flexed with knees hyperextended and ankles plantarflexed (heels on floor) with pronation

For children who are unable to stand independently or for whom standing in proper alignment is indicated, standing systems can be used for external support. The child can be placed in various positions from supine or prone toward vertical, or in vertical standing, dependent on their neuromotor control and coordination. Many standers adjust to the exact position needed for good alignment. Stuberg indicates that standing is thought to reduce or prevent secondary impairments by maintaining lower extremity extensibility, by maintaining or increasing bone mineral density, and by promoting optimal musculoskeletal development.[85] Stuberg further recommends positioning in standing for 45 minutes two or three times a day to control lower extremity flexor contractures, and for 60 minutes four or five times per week to facilitate bone development.[85]

ASSISTIVE DEVICES TO AID AMBULATION

Several devices are available to assist a child in ambulation and to make ambulation as functional, energy-efficient, and least cumbersome as possible. A study by Rose et al. documented a linear relationship between oxygen uptake and heart rate throughout a wide range of walking speeds for children with and children without CP.[86] They suggested that heart rate be used to evaluate the child's fitness and to measure energy expenditure. This may be a good method to aid in the decision about which assistive device should be used for the child.

WALKERS. Traditional walkers are forward walkers, sometimes known as rollator walkers. They have two wheels in front, and the child pushes it in front of him or her. A recurrent problem with this type of walker is anterior trunk lean, so that the body's line of gravity is anterior to the feet and the hips are held in flexion.[87,88] Sometimes, vertical handles are added to facilitate more forearm supination, shoulder depression, and thoracic extension. However, posterior walkers have proven to be more energy-efficient, and have resulted in improved upright posture. The shoulders are held in greater depression with extension, the scapulae tend to be more adducted, and greater thoracic extension is noted. The posterior walker may have either two or four wheels. Logan and associates found that the posterior walker with two wheels increased stride length by 41% and decreased double limb support by 39% over anterior walkers.[87] However, Levangie and colleagues, in their comparison of posterior walkers with four wheels, posterior walkers with two wheels, and anterior walkers, found that the four-wheel posterior walker was more efficient and allowed more significant increases in the child's velocity, right and left stride length, and left step length.[88] The results obtained with anterior walkers and posterior walkers with two wheels were similar.[88]

It should be remembered that each child's ambulation abilities and deficits are unique and should be evaluated on an individual basis when determining which walker affords the greatest stability and safety while providing for the most energy-efficient gait pattern.

CRUTCHES. Axillary and forearm crutches are rarely used for the child with CP because the child's balance must be significantly better than when a walker is used. The child with improved balance often prefers using no assistive device and having the upper extremities free to assist in maintaining balance. Forearm crutches tend to facilitate rounding of the shoulders and forearm pronation with a forward leaning trunk. When excessive effort is needed to maintain balance, the lower extremities will tend to adduct and the hips will internally rotate. When combined with hip flexion, the child is at risk for hip subluxation and dislocation.

INFANT WALKERS. There is great controversy over the use of infant walkers for any infant owing to the accidents associated with their use. The Canadian Medical Association has requested that their government ban the sale of walkers. They believe that their use is too risky, recognizing that two of five children (30% to 45%) who use walkers have mishaps ranging from finger entrapment to falls down stairs.[89] Kauffman and Ridenour have shown that use of a walker enables an infant to commit substantial mechanical errors, yet succeed in bipedal locomotion.[90] Some physicians believe that walkers adversely affect muscle development, cognitive development, and coordination, which can lead to a delay in walking alone, along with other developmental problems.[91]

Infant walkers should not be used for infants with CP. Despite the fact that manufacturers are altering walkers, making them adjustable in height, and providing a more supportive seat, walkers still promote abnormal movement patterns. Walking on the toes is common for any infant while in a walker, but a child with CP is more likely to have lower extremity extension with ankle plantar-flexion. This pattern typically includes arching of the back and adduction of the scapulae with humeral extension for counterbalance. Propulsion in the walker is achieved by pushing with the feet when the body is supported by the tray or sides of the walker.[92] The infant has not acquired the motor control and balance necessary for walking and has not mastered any skill that is transferable to independent ambulation. The infant with CP may actually be reinforcing abnormal patterns of movement, which can cause further developmental delays or even lead to deformity, such as hip subluxation.

EQUIPMENT FOR MOBILITY

Infants and children have a strong desire to move through the environment. This movement allows the child to explore the surroundings, to retrieve a toy lost during play, and to interact with others for comfort and play. The child with CP may lack independent mobility, may have poor endurance in whatever means of mobility may exist, or may exert such effort as to produce an increase in tone that may limit other body functions, such as upper extremity use or vocalization. Adaptive equipment, either manual or electric, may expand the world of the child with CP and may foster independence not only in mobility but also in other areas of function. Mobility, which offers a level of control over oneself and the environment, will improve the child's self-image and lead to other positive behavioral changes.

M.O.V.E. (Mobility Opportunity Via Education) International is a program developed by Blair Learning Center in their Special Education Program in Bakersfield, CA in 1986 (Kyle Northway; Kern County Superintendent of Schools, Bakersfield, CA, 1995). M.O.V.E. develops the idea that children with severe motoric limitations should have the opportunity to make choices and to move through their environment given whatever physical assist is required. This curriculum makes use of equipment manufactured by Rifton Equipment, which offers more physical support for vertical mobility to children. The equipment typically used is called the gait trainer and the mobile prone stander.

Of course, this mobility also affords the opportunity for the child with CP to get into the same kinds of trouble and predicaments encountered by peers with typical motor abilities. Wheelchairs, tricycles, and scooters of different types can provide mobility, and their use should be considered early in the habilitative effort.

Neurologic Interventions for Children with Cerebral Palsy

Neuromedical Interventions

MUSCLE RELAXANTS

Oral medications have been used for children with CP who have spasticity, for the dampening of excessive motor activity. Black et al. indicate that there are different types of motor control problems that result from brain injury. They fall into the following categories: spasticity 60%, dyskinesia 20%, ataxia 1%, and about 20% have a combination of the preceding with one of the movement disorders being dominant.[93] Pranzatelli labels the movement disorders slightly differently as dystonia, hyperkinesias choreoathetosis, and myoclonus.[94] Com- monly used oral muscle relaxant drugs include diazepam, dantrolene, and baclofen. There has been little study of the functional effects of these drugs in children, and little is known about optimal dosing, safety, and side effects.[93] In particular, Black lists baclofen as a drug to be used with caution and the Physician's Desk Reference (Medical Economics, Montrale, NJ 07645) does not recommend its use for CP or for children under the age of 12 years.

NEUROMUSCULAR BLOCKS

Children with CP frequently have difficulty balancing the agonist with the antagonist muscle group for smooth, coordinated, efficient motor function. Instead, they frequently overuse one muscle, the agonist, and have great difficulty activating its antagonist, which may cause muscle shortening, contractures, and eventually deformity. The physical therapist must assess the joint and the muscles crossing the joint or joints carefully to determine whether a deformity is dynamic or fixed. According to Sutherland et al., a dynamic deformity results from dominance of certain agonist muscles over antagonist muscles. This muscle imbalance results in abnormal motion and function.[95] Dynamic deformity will frequently become fixed over time. The goal is to manage a dynamic deformity carefully to delay the need for surgical intervention that is often required with a fixed deformity. A dynamic deformity offers options to the child and family. Sutherland says that the ideal treatment must: (1) prevent fixed deformity; (2) be painless; (3) be cost effective; and (4) not result in any serious complications.[95]

Neuromuscular blocks, injections into the muscle to decrease its activity, are a current method of treatment for overuse of particular muscle groups. Alcohol and phenol are known to reduce muscle tone and have been used for many years in the evaluation and management of spasticity and movement disorders.[95,96] Each has the capacity to permanently damage the muscle and nerve tissues and produce scar tissue that interfere with muscle growth. Both chemicals should be used with caution, if at all, in children.[95]

Botulinum A toxin (BOTOX®) has been proven to be a useful neuromuscular blockade in the treatment of muscle imbalance.[95,97] It is an injection into the dominant agonist muscle at the nerve terminals to cause temporary paralysis of the muscle lasting 3 to 6 months. Botulinum A toxin blocks the release of acetylcholine by the synaptic vesicles. Recovery occurs by terminal sprouting of the nerves.[95] Therefore, it is necessary to continue the injections to prevent further development of muscle contractures. Sutherland adds that this is *not* a stand-alone treatment. Injections should be preceded and followed by physical therapy with the appropriate use of orthotics.[95] Both authors agree that surgery will be likely in the future and that the goal is to delay the surgery as long as possible until the child is older and at less risk of possible complications and to decrease the probability of repeated surgical intervention.[95,97]

Neurosurgical Interventions

SELECTIVE DORSAL RHIZOTOMY

Selective dorsal rhizotomy (SDR), otherwise known as selective posterior rhizotomy (SPR), is not a new surgical approach to the treatment of children with CP but has been a poorly understood procedure aimed at reducing the spasticity of children with CP.[98–101] Oppenheim, Staudt, and Peacock have provided a current explanation for the effectiveness of this intervention: ". . . it focuses on the spinal reflex arc and its modulation at the level of the anterior horn cell by supraspinal and segmental influences. Selective division of posterior spinal nerve rootlets is believed to balance the decrease of normal inhibitory influences on the motoneurons."[102] Simply removing the spasticity does not, however, produce improved motor control. The team approach is absolutely vital to this procedure, both before and after surgery.[7,102] Patient selection is critical to a good outcome as only two types of patients are appropriate candidates. The first group includes patients who are functionally limited by spasticity but who have sufficient underlying voluntary power to maintain and eventually improve their functional abilities. Keen intelligence and motivation are also helpful. The second group includes nonambulatory patients whose spasticity interferes with sitting, bathing, positioning, perineal care, classroom activities, and so on.[100,101] The surgery is typically completed across segments L2–S2[98,100] or L2–S1[101] and only a selected number of dorsal rootlets are sacrificed—those that appear to have the greatest influence on the spasticity and produce abnormal movement patterns.

Research has shown that patients who have undergone SPR have been very positive about the outcome and that the quality of life has been enhanced.[103,104] This surgical intervention has delayed orthopedic surgery by improving both passive and dynamic ROM in children, specifically in the hip adductors, hamstrings, and heelcords and preventing lateral migration of the femoral head in children with spastic quadriplegia.[105–108] Any necessary orthopedic surgery should be delayed for 6 to 12 months after SPR. Dias and Marty have found that 40% to 50% of patients who have received SPR will require further orthopedic procedures in the future.[7]

For the best surgical outcome, intensive physical therapy is recommended to address the weakness that underlies the spasticity.[98–101] The importance of strengthening and achieving improved motor control becomes apparent after the surgery.[99] There are varying approaches to physical therapy treatment after surgery. Abbott et al. advocate limiting the patient's active movements after surgery, outside of therapy, to avoid a return to the child's old patterns of limb use.[100] These researchers suggest that three components be included in the physical therapy program: (1) muscle stretching to gain joint mobility and range; (2) muscle strengthening to increase endurance; and (3) muscle reeducation to impart a better pattern of muscle use.[100] Giuliani advocates treatment aimed at strengthening the muscles and improving motor control because "treatment aimed at reducing tone and spasticity will not necessarily improve movement coordination."[99] Most recommend that therapy be continued for at least 6 to 12 months following surgery to allow optimal functional improvement.[98,100,101]

SPINAL CORD STIMULATORS

Implanting a spinal cord stimulator is a controversial treatment approach and can produce drastically different results in different children. A variety of electrodes can be used. Waltz and coworkers, for instance, prefer four electrodes over two electrodes when working with the child with athetosis.[109] Optimal frequencies vary between less than 500 Hz[109] and 500 to 1450 Hz.[110] Placement of the electrodes is typically between C2 and C4, with the pattern and the polarity of the applied field being critical to achieving a satisfactory therapeutic result.[109] In the author's experience, once optimal settings have been achieved for the greatest reduction in spasticity and abnormal movement patterns, therapy is essential to address muscle strengthening, reeducation, and acquisition of functional skills.

CONTINUOUS INTRATHECAL BACLOFEN INFUSION

Continuous intrathecal baclofen infusion (CIBI) has been evaluated for the relief of spasticity in patients with spasticity of cerebral origin. Albright et al. undertook a study of 37 patients between 5 to 27 years of age and gave them CIBI for 3 to 48 months.[111] Muscle tone was significantly decreased in both the upper and the lower extremities. They found that spasticity of cerebral origin can be effectively treated with CIBI, which can be titrated for the desired clinical response, and is quite useful for the patients who need some spasticity to stand and ambulate.[111]

Orthopedic Surgery for Children with Cerebral Palsy

Orthopedic management for children with CP is best accomplished with a team approach, including the child and family, and with ongoing care. Problems such as severe contracture, joint deformity, and scoliosis interfere with the basic requirement of comfortable seating.[112] The goal of orthopedic management is to help each individual reach optimal functional ability and prevent deformity through detection at an early stage when simple and more effective treatment options may be instituted.[113,114] The goals of surgical intervention are to improve function, decrease discomfort, and prevent structural changes that may become disabling.[113]

An understanding of atypical development and movement compensations is critical for determining how surgery will likely impact the child's future function. As Green says,

> . . . treating one problem without consideration of the others will result in unnecessary additional hospitalizations for subsequent operations. In addition, since each joint is intimately linked to another, surgical treatment of one joint problem may lead to worsening of an adjacent joint deformity unless it too is addressed. Thus, the surgical care of the lower extremities in spastic cerebral palsy requires that the entire patient be evaluated and all necessary surgical procedures be coordinated.[115]

The more common orthopedic problems that involve the lower extremities will be addressed in the following sections. General physical therapy interventions are also discussed. However, many surgeons have established their own postoperative protocols, including the prescribed period of immobilization. Therefore, the information presented here should be used only as a guide in planning and implementing a therapeutic program.

The Hip

SUBLUXATION/DISLOCATION

Hips begin to migrate laterally, or to sublux, as a result of muscular imbalance. When left untreated, the hip may continue the migration until it is dislocated. Gamble and coworkers maintain that this process occurs over a 6-year period and that there is a strong correlation between the stability of the hip and the ambulatory status of the patient.[116] Other causes of hip dislocation include persistent fetal femoral geometry, acetabular dysplasia, and flexion-adduction contractures.[116]

Conservative treatment options for the subluxated hip include passive muscle stretching of the adductors and hip flexors and splinting of the hips in abduction (generally done at night while the child sleeps). With progression of the subluxation, surgery may become necessary, in which case tenotomies or myotomies are the treatments of choice. The effectiveness of muscle transfer is controversial.[116] Dislocated hips are a more serious problem for the child, as the hip may become painful, sitting may become more difficult, decubitus ulcers may be caused by asymmetric weight bearing, nursing care may be made more difficult, and fractures are possible.[117,118] Various surgical interventions may be appropriate, including the following (listed in order of increasing complexity):

1. Soft tissue transfer and/or releases involving the adductors, iliopsoas muscle, or proximal hamstring[88,90–93,116,118–123]
2. Femoral osteotomy[88,90–92,116,118–120,124,125]
3. Pelvic osteotomies (iliac, Chiari, Salter, Steel)[116,118–120,126]
4. Combined femoral osteotomy and pelvic osteotomy (with and without soft tissue release)[124,127–130]
5. Resection of the femoral head and neck[116, 120,130–131]
6. Arthrodesis and arthroplasty[116,119]

Treatment of each child must be individualized, and every surgeon has individual surgical preferences. The decision as to whether to operate at all on the child with severe involvement,[117] or whether to perform unilateral versus bilateral surgery,[132] is the surgeon's decision, which is ideally made after receiving input from the team members.

Postoperative management should include ROM exercise of the hips to maintain or increase the range, strengthening of muscles in an effort to achieve muscle balance around the hips, and proper positioning to prevent recurrence of the dislocation. Harryman presents specific intervention following soft tissue surgery and immobilization.[133] The severity of the CP and the functional abilities of the child will dictate the treatment approach.

ADDUCTION DEFORMITY

Conservative management of the short adductors involves passive stretching and night-time bracing, with the hips in as much abduction as possible. Proper positioning in a wheelchair is essential for maintaining the integrity of the hip joints. One indication for a more aggressive approach is when the ambulatory child has severe hypertonus of the adductors, which causes scissoring of the legs during ambulation. Scissoring of the lower extremities in the severely involved child will make sitting and perineal care difficult. Three typical surgical procedures are currently performed in such cases:

1. Adductor tenotomy[119,120]
2. Obturator neurectomy[118,119]
3. Posterior transfer of the adductors (with or without iliopsoas tenotomy)[119,120,134]

In general, postoperative treatment of the child includes continued stretching, strengthening of the muscles around the hips in order to achieve muscular balance, and functional training. Harryman presents specific intervention techniques.[135] Grogan et al. have developed a removable abductor bar so that therapy, including ambulation, can commence with long-leg casts on the child, and abduction can be maintained whenever the child is not in therapy.[135]

FLEXION DEFORMITY

Hip flexion contractures interfere with function in any upright position because full hip extension becomes impossible. Compensation occurs typically at the thoraco-lumbar junction and the knees (increased flexion) so that body orientation in space can remain vertical. It is difficult to stretch the hip flexors because the pelvis tends to rock forward into anterior tilt while extension occurs at the thoraco-lumbar junction. For passive stretching to be effective, the pelvis must be stabilized in either a supine or prone position.

Surgical intervention usually includes soft tissue releases and can involve the iliopsoas muscle[118] or transection of the tensor fasciae latae muscle and aponeurosis and detachment of the heads of the rectus femoris.[119]

Physical therapy after surgery should include stretching into hip extension and strengthening of the hip extensors and abductors. Facilitation of functional skills should continue, with care taken to prevent a return to the child's previous compensatory patterns of movement.

INTERNAL ROTATION DEFORMITY

Femoral anteversion, rather than muscular action, is a consistent deformity associated with exaggerated internal rotation during gait, as previously noted. Anteversion interferes with functional ambulation by tripping the child when the toe of one shoe gets caught behind the heel of the opposite shoe. A femoral derotation osteotomy, which may include medial hamstring release, is the standard surgery performed for this deformity.[115,118,119,125]

A longer period of immobilization is necessary for bony surgery than for soft tissue releases, and the child is likely to be unable to bear weight until the casts are removed. Harryman presents specific postsurgical management protocols related to immobilization in splints/casts.[135] Rehabilitation is directed toward increasing ROM and strengthening the muscles around the hips. Unilateral hip surgery may result in leg length discrepancy, which must be considered during treatment and in consultation with the surgeon. Facilitation of functional skills is critically important to help the child learn new movement patterns and strengthen weakened muscles.

The Knee

KNEE FLEXION DEFORMITY

Knee flexion deformity is often related to spastic, shortened hamstrings and can be secondary to a hip flexion deformity. Persistent flexion of the knee can lead to a contracture of the knee joint capsule and shortening of the sciatic nerve. Serial casting of the knees is a conservative approach to the deformity that has been successful in some patients.[136] Soft splints applied at night for severe knee flexion deformities have proven to be both effective and inexpensive.[137] Hamstring lengthening is the most common surgical approach to knee flexion deformities.[115,118,138,139]

Gage presents indications for hamstring lengthening: (1) persistent knee flexion of 20 to 30 degrees during stance; (2) popliteal angle of greater than 40 to 45 degrees or straight leg raise less than 45 degrees; and (3) using gait analysis, hamstring overactivity with persistent knee flexion of 20 to 30 degrees or inadequate knee extension in terminal swing.[139] Root's goals of distal hamstring lengthening include (1) eliminate or diminish inefficient crouched gait pattern; (2) improve stride length; (3) decrease compensatory ankle equinus and hip flexion; (4) minimize internal rotation in gait; (5) improve sitting balance and posture; and (6) decrease abnormal pull that can cause hip dislocation.[138] Variations on lengthening of the hamstrings have been developed, with the medial transfer of the distal rectus femoris tendon to the sartorius or gracilis being the more successful.[122,139,140] In extreme cases of harmful spasticity, selective neurotomies have been performed on the hamstring branches of the sciatic trunk.[141]

Postoperative management should include passive and active exercise into knee extension and strengthening of both knee extensors and flexors. Because the hamstrings cross the knee and hip joints, the therapist must also emphasize ROM and strengthening exercises for the hip musculature. Nightly use of knee extension splints should be considered to help maintain muscle length, especially in children who have difficulty learning new patterns of movement. Harryman presents physical therapy intervention immediately following soft tissue surgery.[135]

The Ankle and Foot

EQUINUS DEFORMITY

Equinus, a very common foot deformity in children with CP, results from a muscular imbalance between the plantar flexors and dorsiflexors. It is manifested as toe-walking in the ambulatory child. Children with more severe involvement may have difficulty with foot placement on the pedals of the wheelchair, assisted stand-pivot transfers, and donning of shoes. Conservative management includes passive stretching, with care taken to "lock" the subtalar joint before stretching toward dorsiflexion. MAFOs can help maintain a neutral position at the ankle but will not stretch the muscle group.

Achilles tendon lengthening is the most frequent surgical intervention for equinus deformity.[115,118,142,143]

Surgeons also use the Vulpius procedure, which is a lengthening of the aponeurosis of the gastrocnemius-soleus muscle group.[143,144] Rosenthal and Simon have had success with young children as well and indicate that if the procedure is done at 6 years of age or younger, a repeat procedure can be anticipated in 6 to 7 years. In the younger patient, their recurrence rate is 14%; in children older than 6 years of age, the recurrence rate drops to 1%.[144] Strecker et al. have reported good results with a technique called heelcord advancement.[145] Overlengthening is the most common complication of surgery, and it results in a calcaneal gait or an increase in dorsiflexion during stance.[146] This gait is crouched in nature, with increased energy demands and subsequent shortening of the muscles in the hips and knees.

Postoperative care typically involves an orthotic to maintain the surgically achieved range and to provide distal stability, thereby facilitating development of proximal strength and motor control. ROM through the ankle joint and strengthening for those with some voluntary control must always be emphasized.

PES VALGUS

Pes valgus is a deformity that includes eversion, plantar-flexion, and inclination of the calcaneous with abduction of the forefoot. These positions cause a medial prominence of the talus, which is commonly accompanied by callous formation on the skin. This deformity is usually flexible and can be corrected by reducing the subtalar joint and forefoot to a neutral position with the ankle plantar-flexed. Three situations contribute to the deformity: (1) spastic peroneal muscles that change the axis of rotation of the subtalar joint to a more horizontal alignment and abduct the midfoot and forefoot; (2) gastrocnemius-soleus contracture causing plantar-flexion of the calcaneous; and (3) persistent fetal medial deviation of the neck of the talus.[51]

Crawford and associates developed a procedure called staple arthroeriesis, which involves operative limitation of joint motion. It is used in children younger than 6 years of age to correct a pes valgus deformity until they are old enough to undergo arthrodesis. The authors have reported that the procedure, which involves driving a staple into the talus and calcaneous across the subtalar joint, works so well that, in many cases, additional surgery is not needed.[147] The most common of the later procedures that are performed include (1) the Grice extra-articular subtalar arthrodesis,[115,118,142,148,149] peroneus brevis lengthening for less severe valgus,[142] (3) triple arthrodesis for rigid deformities,[115] and (4) Grice-Schede procedure.[150]

The period of postsurgical immobilization varies greatly, depending upon the specific procedure and the surgeon's preference. An orthotic will almost always be used, and motion will either be significantly limited or eliminated. Long after surgery, the therapist may note joint hypermobility at sites proximal and distal to the arthrodesis, in which case special orthotics may be required.

VARUS DEFORMITY

Varus deformity is uncommon in children with CP. It results from imbalance between weak peroneal muscles and spastic posterior or anterior tibialis muscles.[115]

A variety of surgical procedures are performed for this deformity, including lengthening or splitting and transferring of either the posterior or anterior tibialis muscle.[115,118,151–156]

Therapeutic intervention should emphasize muscle reeducation, particularly when a muscle has been transferred; ROM exercise; strengthening; and facilitation of functional activities for which foot alignment is important (e.g., standing and gait). Each child should be evaluated for an orthotic, with the recommendation discussed with the surgeon.

Lower Extremity Orthoses

The decision to use an orthosis and the choice of orthosis should be based on the physical therapist's assessment of ROM, foot alignment, voluntary control of movement in the lower extremity, and functional level of the child. Because the foot is intended to provide both stability and mobility, the effects of an orthosis on these two functions must be considered.

If the ankle and foot cannot be brought into a neutral position with the knee in extension in a non–weight-bearing position, an orthosis is contraindicated. The result of wearing an orthosis with a contracture at the ankle or foot will be that the child needs to compensate in another area of the foot to attain the ROM needed for standing and ambulating. This compensation will cause hypermobility in the joints that are compensating, and will encourage continued hypomobility in the area of contracture and limitation.

A trial of serial casting may be used in an effort to reduce Achilles tendon contracture.[95,157] Effort should be made to use nonsurgical techniques to treat tight Achilles tendons until the child is 4 years of age. Serial casting is a good option. Care must be exercised to lock the subtalar joint while applying the cast to gain dorsiflexion of the ankle, to ensure stretching of the gastrocnemius or soleus group, and to prevent hypermobility of the subtalar joint. Surgery is most likely needed if proper serial casting is unsuccessful after 2 to 4 weeks. Some of the orthoses commonly used for children with CP and their specific benefits are described.

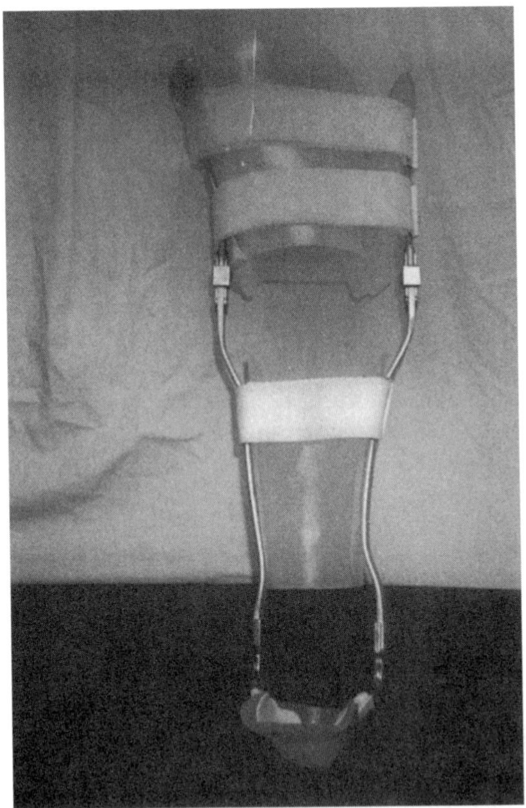

Figure 4-9 ▪ A knee-ankle-foot orthosis. (Courtesy of Carlo Cocco, Cocco Brothers, Inc., Philadelphia, PA.)

Knee-Ankle-Foot Orthosis

A knee-ankle-foot orthosis (KAFO) is rarely indicated for a child with CP because it is too heavy and cumbersome for the child (Fig. 4-9).[158] The child will typically demonstrate atypical motor patterns with the increased effort and energy required for ambulation. Below-knee orthoses will generally control the hips as well as the knees and feet, and should be considered before a KAFO is ordered.

Inhibitive Casts

The primary goal of inhibitive casts and orthoses is to reduce the influence of abnormal tonic reflexes on the foot, ankle, and leg.[159,160] Radtka et al. write that

> the inhibitive casts are purported to decrease spasticity by prolonged stretch and pressure on the tendons of the tricep surae muscle and toe flexors and to inhibit or decrease abnormal reflexes in the lower extremity by protecting the foot from tactile-induced reflexes.[161]
>
> . . . the casts are reported to prevent excessive ankle plantar flexion, improve lower-extremity muscle timing, and normalize movements of the trunk, pelvis, and lower extremity in standing and during gait. Studies have shown changes in the stretch sensitivities of the ankle plantar flexors, increased ambulation ability, improved passive ankle dorsiflexion and foot-floor contact during gait and improved stride length. . . ."[161]

Inhibitive casts have been developed over the years and come to a point of improved fabrication and aesthetic quality. There are now inhibitive ankle-foot orthoses (AFO) that are intended for the same use as the inhibitive casts. The inhibitive AFO is lightweight, flexible, and easily worn with regular shoes.[161] One type of inhibitive AFO is the dynamic ankle-foot orthosis (DAFO) with a plantar-flexion stop (Fig. 4-10).

Dynamic Ankle-Foot Orthosis

Radtka et al. described the construction of the dynamic ankle-foot orthosis (DAFO).[161] The footplate is a custom-contoured plate similar to the inhibitive cast. It has built-up areas under the toes, lateral and medial longitudinal arches, and transverse metatarsal arch with recessed areas under the metatarsal and calcaneal pad areas. These features provide support and stabilization to the arches of the foot and position the midtarsal and subtalar joints in a neutral position.[161] "The footplate is designed to reduce abnormal muscle activity and to effect biomechanical changes, including decreased excessive ankle plantar flexion and improved motions of the lower extremity, pelvis, and trunk during standing and gait."[161(p. 397)] The DAFO provides total contact to the ankle and foot when it has a plantar-flexion stop. A toe loop stabilizes the first digit while there is a forefoot strap and an ankle strap. The DAFO with a plantar flexion stop is thinner, more flexible, and shorter than the conventional MAFO (Fig. 4-11).

Molded Ankle-Foot Orthosis

A molded ankle-foot orthosis (MAFO) is indicated for control of the following:

1. A functional equinus position caused by gastrocnemius-soleus hypertonus that can be corrected with treatment
2. Genu recurvatum during stance phase that results from a functional, not structural, equinus position

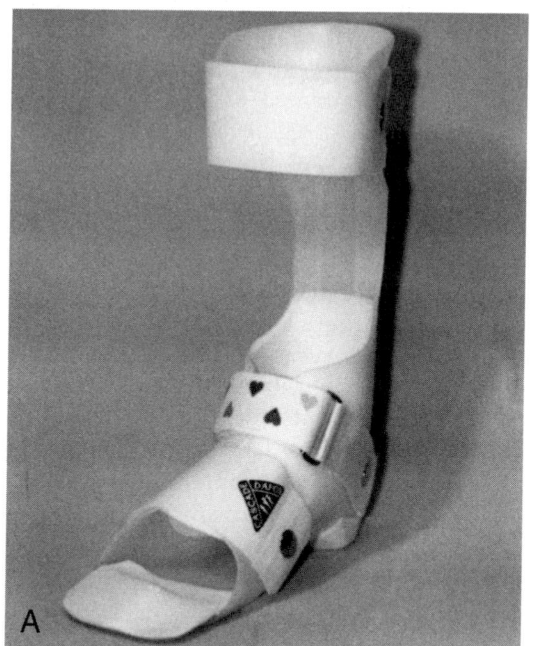

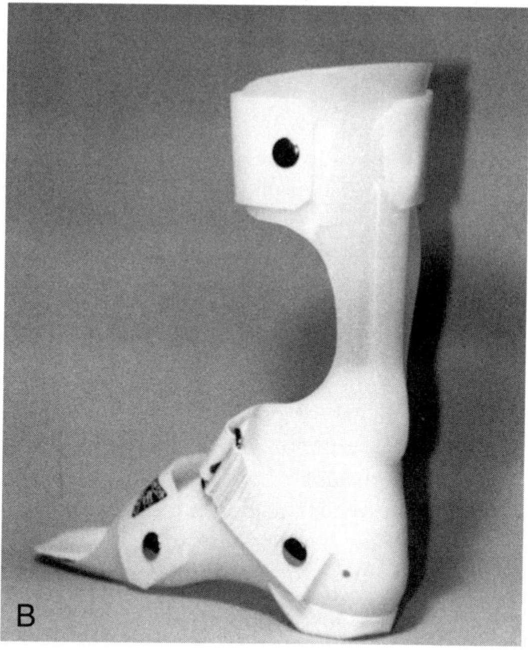

Figure 4-10 ■ Dynamic ankle-foot orthosis with a planta-flexion stop (**A**), Front view; (**B**), Rear view. (Courtesy of Cascade DAFO, Inc., Bellingham, WA.)

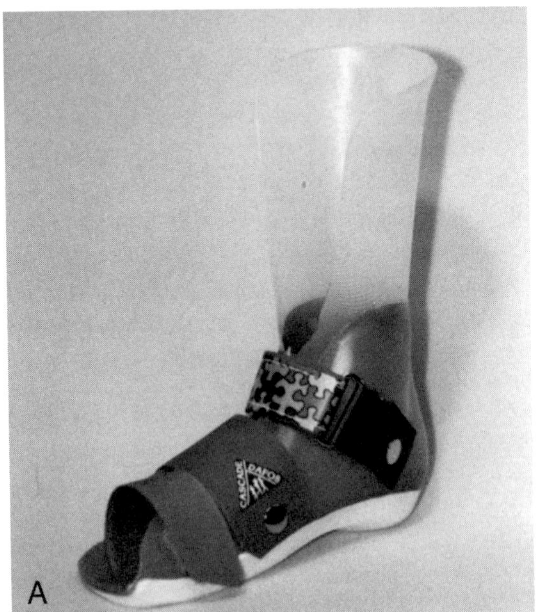

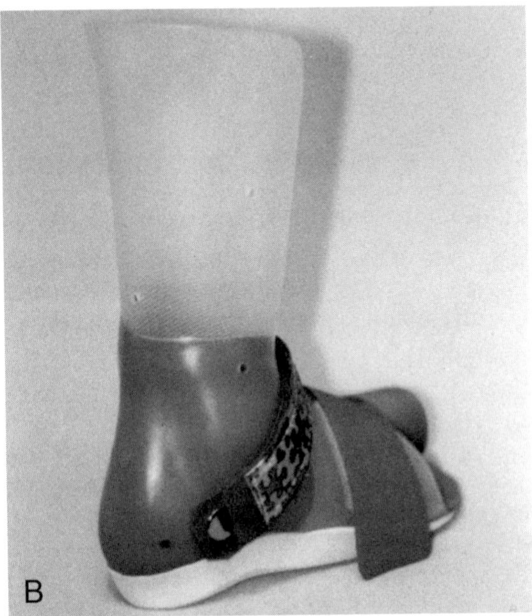

Figure 4-11 ▪ Dynamic ankle-foot orthosis with a great toe loop, forefoot strap, and ankle strap (**A**), Front view; (**B**), Rear view. (Courtesy of Cascade DAFO, Inc., Bellingham, WA.)

3. Pes valgus associated with hypertonus in the gastrocnemius-soleus group.[162]

An MAFO may also be indicated to improve gait efficiency, as its application can decrease the energy demands of gait in children with spastic diplegic CP.[69] A polypropylene solid AFO has been the most commonly prescribed brace for reducing excessive ankle plantar-flexion during stance.[161] It covers the posterior aspect of the calf with trim lines that are slightly anterior to the ankles. It has straps across the front of the ankle and the anterior upper tibia (Fig. 4-12) and controls the ankle biomechanically by using a three-force system to prevent excessive ankle plantar-flexion during stance.[161] Therapists might also make a low-temperature plastic MAFO by molding the plastic over the child's lower leg and foot once the ankles and foot have been padded properly. This is indicated when the exact orthosis is not yet known and a trial brace is warranted or when the child is quite small, is just beginning weight bearing activities and early ambulation, and the feet are likely to grow quickly in the next 6 months. These braces can be carefully modified according to the child's needs with a heat gun. The trim lines remain the same as for the polypropylene MAFOs. Continuing education courses are helpful to properly learn to fabricate this brace.

Radtka et al. studied the effects on the gait of children with CP of DAFOs with a plantar-flexion stop, MAFOs, and no AFOs.[161] Both orthoses increased stride length, decreased cadence, and reduced excessive ankle plantar-flexion when compared with no orthoses. There were no differences in the gait variables when comparing the two orthoses. However, "parents, subjects, and their physical therapists commented that the DAFO was lighter and more

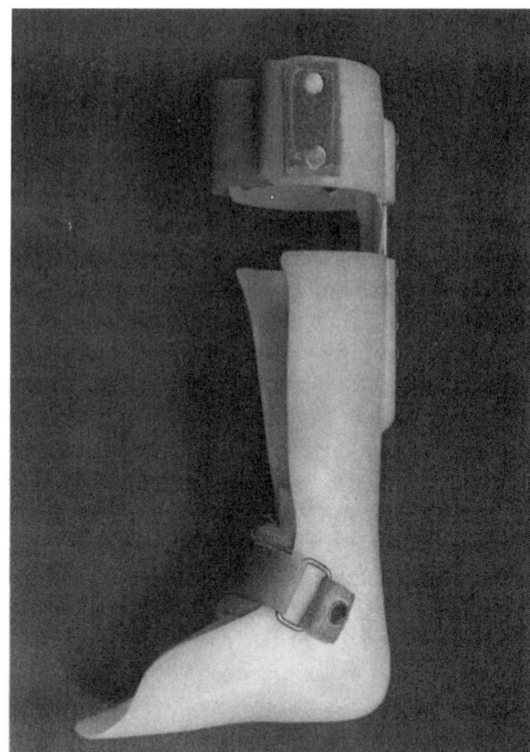

Figure 4-12 ▪ Molded ankle-foot orthosis with growth bar. (Courtesy of Carlo Cocco, Cocco Brothers. Inc., Philadelphia, PA.)

cosmetically appealing, but slightly more difficult for the children to initially learn to independently don and doff as compared with the solid AFO."[161(p. 405)] Therefore, each child should be considered on an individual basis when deciding on an orthotic intervention.

Articulating Ankle-Foot Orthosis

A hinged AFO, with an ankle articulation, is indicated when free dorsiflexion is desired but the child continues to need a plantar-flexion stop (Fig. 4-13). Significant biomechanical changes were found such as more natural ankle motion during stance and greater symmetry of segmental lower extremity motion when the ankle has freedom to move.[163,164] These orthoses inhibit plantar-flexion hypertonus while permitting free dorsiflexion, thus allowing the child increased ease in rising to stand and ambulating. They may also help strengthen the muscles crossing the ankle.

Night splinting is used to increase the length of the gastrocnemius-soleus group by maintaining a prolonged stretch into dorsiflexion (Fig. 4-14). By using an ankle articulation with an adjustable strap attached to the footplate by the toes, one can alter the degree of dorsiflexion while the child is wearing the orthosis.

Floor Reaction Orthosis

A floor reaction orthosis is indicated when knee extension cannot be maintained in stance during ambulation and excessive flexion of the

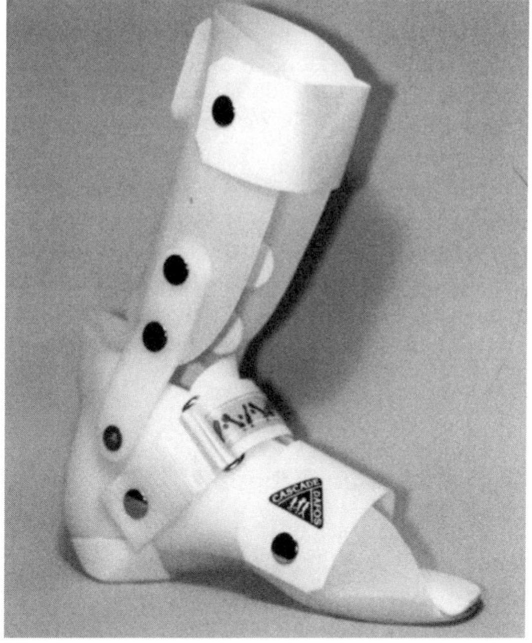

Figure 4-13 ▪ Articulating ankle-foot orthosis allows free dorsiflexion. with a plantar-flexion stop (Courtesy of Cascade DAFO, Inc., Bellingham, WA.)

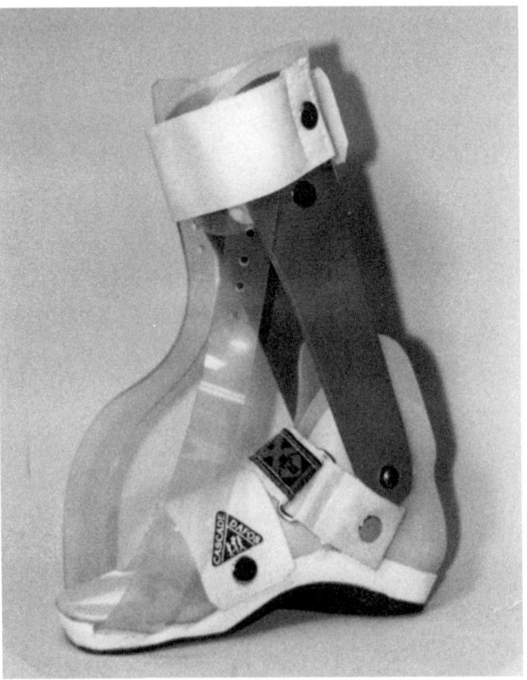

Figure 4-14 ▪ Night splint to provide prolonged stretch into dorsiflexion. Uses an adjustable strap with an ankle articulation. (Courtesy of Cascade DAFO, Inc., Bellingham, WA.)

ankle and knee is noted when the heel is in contact with the floor. Such orthoses are containdicated when full knee extension cannot be achieved passively with the child in stance and the ankle and foot in neutral alignment (Fig. 4-15).[159]

Supramalleolar Orthosis

The supramalleolar orthosis (SMO) is indicated when ankle stability is critically important but limited tibial motion is desired. This orthosis provides less support than the MAFO and allows some tibia-over-foot motion during ambulation, but provides malleolar support by having the trimlines anterior and superior to the malleoli (Fig. 4-16, *A,B*).

Shoe Inserts

A variety of shoe inserts are available, and they may be used for a number of reasons. They are indicated when there is dynamic control of the knee and ankle during gait, but assistance is required to maintain the calcaneous, subtalar, and midtarsal joints in neutral alignment. They are not helpful when the heel is held off the floor owing to hypertonus of the gastrocnemius-soleus group. The child's foot alignment, both in weight-bearing and non–weight-bearing positions, must be evaluated, as the heel cup can be designed for a specific problem. Trimlines can be anterior or inferior to either the medial or lateral malleoli, and the foot plate can be proximal or distal to the metatarsal heads (Fig. 4-17). Shoe inserts are made commercially, and they can also be made of low-temperature plastic in the clinic. They are sold under various names and are particularly popular with athletes. Some shoe companies make multiple, interchangeable inserts for their shoes, depending on the child's needs. Remember that the hindfoot must be well aligned before the forefoot can be addressed with any orthotic.

High-Top Orthopedic Shoe/Phelps Short-Leg Brace

Phelps short-leg braces with high-top shoes have limited use in the management of ankle and foot problems in children with CP. The high-top shoe, even with a stiff heel counter, does not support or maintain the calcaneous in a neutral position. The child actually reshapes the shoe so that the foot is maintained in calcaneal eversion with subtalar and midtarsal joint malalignment. Adding a medial T-strap, secured around a Phelps short-leg brace, provides pressure against the medial aspect of the foot, but does not cause the changes in alignment needed in the rear part of the foot to move the subtalar joint out of pronation.

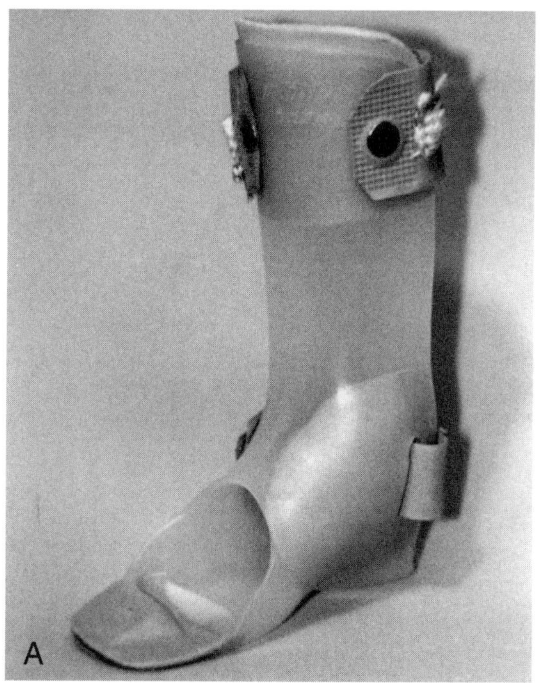

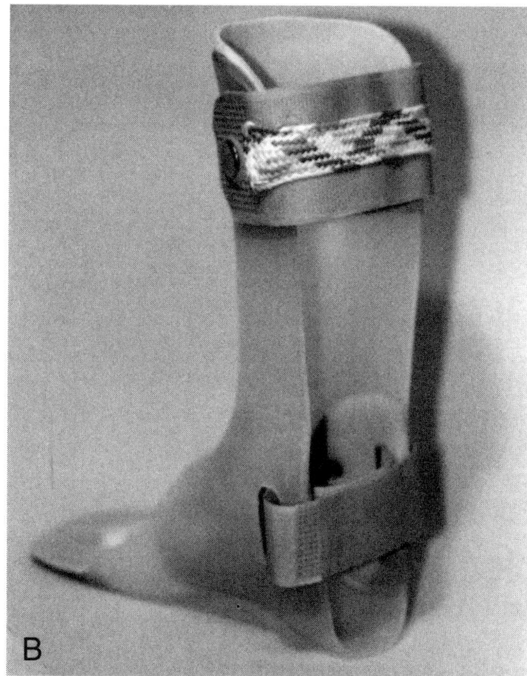

Figure 4-15 ▪ Floor reaction orthosis (**A**), Front view; (**B**), Rear view. (Courtesy of Cascade DAFO, Inc., Bellingham, WA.)

The Adolescent with Cerebral Palsy

During adolescence, children become more interested in school activities and community life opportunities. It is a time of increased peer pressure and transition into a period of growth and development when one is expected to be more self-sufficient and independent. This period may be difficult for some adolescents with CP as they become more aware of limitations and the impact of their disability on themselves, their family, and friends. Awareness of their own sexuality is developing, as well as potential interest in the opposite sex.

Growth spurts are expected during adolescence and can create difficulty for the adolescent with CP. Bones tend to grow more quickly than muscles and therefore muscle shortening, contractures, and discomfort are possibilities. As their bodies grow taller and bigger, one might find decreased endurance for aerobic activities and daily routines. Typical disabilities at this time include a lack of independent mobility and continued difficulty and slowness with self-care and hygiene skills at a time when personal privacy is increasingly important.[84] Goals for the adolescent, in response to the growth, may be to maintain or increase the level of function and work toward more independence in life skills. It is necessary to anticipate musculoskeletal changes before they occur in order to prevent the secondary impairments of contractures and decreased endurance for ambulation and other activities.

When the child encounters a larger physical space in middle school and high school, the physical therapist may need to consider alter-

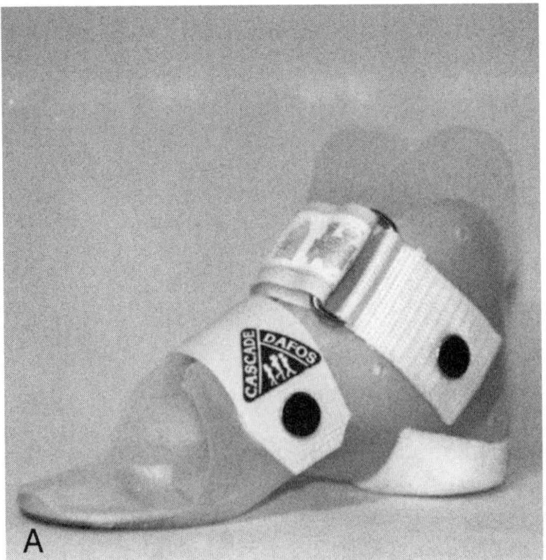

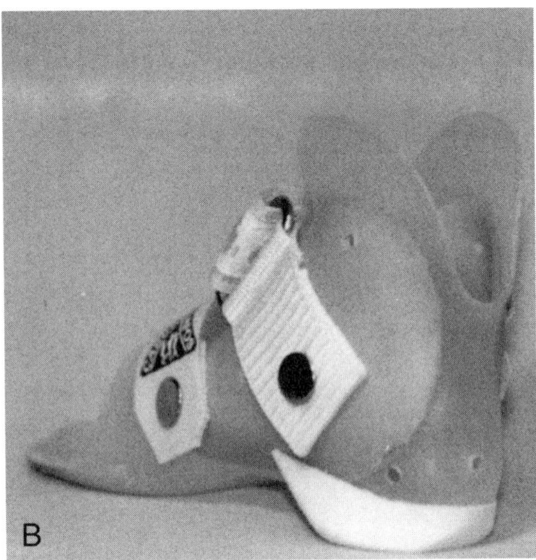

Figure 4-16 ▪ Supramalleolar orthosis. Provides medial-lateral ankle support with free dorsiflexion and plantarflexion (**A**), Front view; (**B**), Rear view. (Courtesy of Cascade DAFO, Inc., Bellingham, WA.)

nate modes for mobility. A manual or electric wheelchair may become appropriate. As the child grows, there is often more physical stress on the family members and continued family teaching is necessary, including body mechanics, lifting, performing assisted or dependent transfers, aiding mobility, and assisting in general self-care and hygiene.

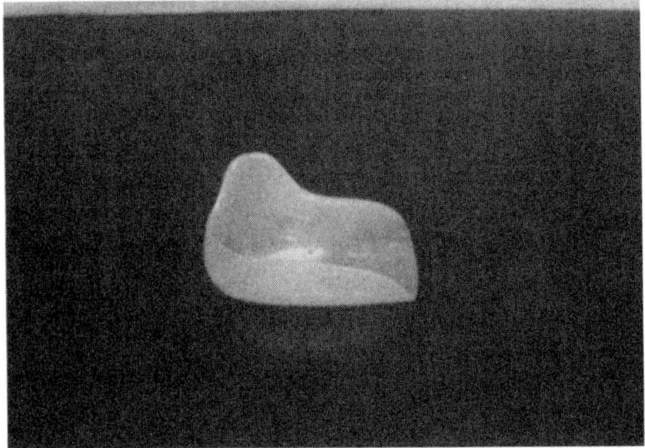

Figure 4-17 ▪ An example of a shoe insert. (Courtesy of Carlo Cocco, Cocco Brothers. Inc., Philadelphia, PA.)

The adolescent may not have the typical opportunities in the community or to socialize with peers, which may limit the social-emotional development that typically takes place at this time. "Therapists should strive to foster self-esteem and assertiveness in children and adolescents by emphasizing their abilities, finding areas in which they can excel, and helping them to acknowledge their difficulties with a view toward identifying appropriate compensations."[84]

Magill-Evans and Restall conducted a longitudinal study of self-esteem in 22 adolescents with CP and 22 nondisabled peers. They found that as adolescents, only girls with CP scored lower on physical, social, and personal self-esteem. This difference with the other groups disappeared as adults.[165] This indicates that we, as professionals, need to be diligent in our support of these children and adolescents and foster their self-esteem and independence.

Home Management

A home management program is an essential part of the treatment plan for the child with CP. The home program should be designed to reinforce positions and movements that have been practiced in the physical therapy sessions, and it should be updated frequently. The therapist must consider the daily routine of the child and family when planning a home program. Exercise that is incorporated into the activities of daily living (ADLs) and play is more likely to be carried out than a separate, formal exercise regimen lasting 30 minutes. The therapist must also consider realistically the other non–child-related demands placed on the parents. Siblings, too, can be very valuable in assisting with the child's program and incorporating activities and exercise into an established routine. "The unique, spontaneous and competitive interaction of siblings offers increased incentives for functional independence."[166]

Therapeutic exercise for the baby is easily incorporated into daily care activities. Therapeutic handling aimed at increasing movement can be done during routine activities, such as diapering, dressing, feeding, bathing, carrying, and lifting the baby from a supported position.

For the child who has an interest in other activities, a therapist might recommend taking up a musical instrument, therapeutic horseback riding, therapeutic aquatics, or any other activity that coincides with and reinforces the therapeutic goals of the child.

Consultation with the School

Communication between the therapist and the child's teacher is essential for appropriate and effective management and education of the child in the classroom. The therapist should obtain information from the teacher regarding the child's daily routine at school. With that information, joint planning for the child can result in an effective and efficient educational program.

The therapist must emphasize correct alignment while the child is sitting. Optimal height of a desk may contribute to postural control and, thus, to a greater degree of success with desktop activities. A learning position should be used, if possible, that stresses greater extension of the hip and knee. The result of keeping the child in a constantly flexed sitting position too long will likely be flexion contractures at the hip and knee. Periodic opportunity for movement, whether in physical education class or at the child's own negotiation, may also provide relief from the sitting position. There should be a sharing of the assistance and supervision required for quality of movement and safety. The physical education teacher should be informed of joint movement goals and specific types or patterns of movement that may either be deleterious or beneficial for the child. There should also be a review conducted with teachers for the purpose of and proper use of splints, braces, and other assistive or adaptive devices.

The occupational therapist and the speech-language pathologist will share information about the child's attention span, perceptual and cognitive deficits, and speech and language capabilities. This information, along with specific suggestions, should facilitate learning for the child.

Therapists should not expect teachers to handle children therapeutically for the purpose of obtaining postural control. A more realistic expectation would be maintenance of correct alignment, relief from sitting, use of adaptive or assistive devices, and attention to issues regarding safety. The therapist must recognize the teacher as an important ally in the therapeutic arena. An extensive discussion of the role of the physical therapist in the schools can be found in Chapter 15.

Case Study

Elsa is a 13-year-old girl, born with multiple cranial neuropathies. A CAT scan after birth revealed no definitive findings. A repeat CAT scan at 10 years of age revealed a migrational defect (lack of migration of some of the gray matter during the development of the brain). By 8 months of age, Elsa was diagnosed with right hemiplegia and a movement disorder. The movement disorder has been labeled myoclonus or hemiballismus at different stages in her life. Elsa had six surgeries on her eyes before 1 year of age. A trial of bilateral serial casting was completed at 3 ½ years of age for her shortened gastrocnemius-soleus groups and hamstrings. She required surgical heelcord lengthening at 5 years of age and bone graft in her left foot at 11 years of age to correct severe pronation. Elsa was initially mediated with phenobarbital for the movement disorder without any success at decreasing the hemiballistic movements. She was changed to a regimen of valproic acid, then to a dopamine agent. She is now receiving valproic acid, which has afforded the most control over the hemiballistic movements.

At 11 months of age, Elsa began therapy consisting of 1-hour sessions per week each of physical, occupational, and speech therapies. Initially in therapy, Elsa demonstrated severe hypotonia and was unable to lift her head off the surface when she was placed in a prone position. Physical therapy concentrated on increasing her function toward independent mobility on the floor, independent sitting and transitions between postures, and eventually, ambulation with assistive devices. These services remained in place until after she entered kindergarten, when physical, occupational, and speech services began twice weekly in the school system and continued to follow in the outpatient medical model for several years. Outpatient medical-based physical therapy changed to a consultative role by the time Elsa was 8 years old. At 13 years of age, she continues to receive physical and occupational therapy in school and monthly consultative medical, physical therapy services.

Academically, Elsa can read and write her work on the computer. At 13 years of age, she is changing her school placement from an academic program to a life skills program to place more emphasis on gaining independence in self-care skills. The services in the school system have focused on her ability to learn information and improve the mobility required in the school buildings and community. Services included adaptive seating in the classroom, augmentative communication in her early school experience, and using a computer for all her school work. Elsa now uses verbal communication to interact but continues to do all her school work on the computer, using her left hand on the keyboard and a trackball.

Physical therapy has emphasized independent mobility both on the floor and vertical throughout her life. Elsa started walking with a walker by the age of 3 years and progressed to a quad cane used interchangeably with a walker until 10 years of age, when Elsa required the stability of a walker full time for ambulation. She has always required orthotics and has used articulating orthotics since age 6. She has consistently required assisted ambulation to a minimum of standby supervision because of the hemiballistic movement. Elsa has great difficulty regaining her balance quickly enough to prevent a fall when she experiences the involuntary movements. At 12 years of age, Elsa changed to a posterior walker with a right forarm platform, which has afforded her more independence in the house for up to a distance of 30 feet.

For assisted mobility, Elsa began using a tricycle at 3 years of age and now uses an adult size model. She received a manual wheelchair for long distances on entering kindergarten and has remained dependent in its use because of her inability to use her right arm for propulsion. When Elsa turned 11, she was measured and fitted for an electric WC, which offers her independence in the school and the surrounding community, although supervision for safety is needed.

Elsa has had the benefit of recreational and therapeutic activities throughout her life. She has participated in hippotherapy since 4 years of age, attending dance classes for special needs children for 1 year at the same age, and attended therapeutic aquatics from ages 4 through 8. She goes to summer camp with an attendant and enjoys the pool there on a daily basis.

(continued)

Case Study (Continued)

Elsa's family has been intimately involved in all intervention decisions and has advocated for all her needs. She has benefited from a variety of interventions at home, in the medical model, in school, and in the community. Elsa has achieved a level of independence with which she is very happy and enjoys the associated interactions. She should continue to make progress toward a productive, full life with her family and friends, given the therapeutic and mechanical supports necessary for her mobility in her environment.

Other Disciplines Involved in the Care of Children with Cerebral Palsy

Because CP is a developmental disability, it affects not only the child's posture, movement, and acquisition of motor skills but also the development of perceptual skills, language, and cognition, as well as social-emotional growth. The child with CP must have a treatment program that considers the child as a "whole" person, not merely a combination of systems (see Case Study).

In addition to the child's individual needs, which may be great, the child must be seen as a member of a family unit. The impact of a disabled child on parents, siblings, and the extended family must be considered in treatment planning. Although families are often expected to carry out many of the treatment tasks at home, professionals must recognize that family members may need periodic relief or respite from the burden of care.

There must be a coordinated effort among the many disciplines involved in treating the child with CP. Medical care may include the services of a general pediatrician, neurologist, orthopedic surgeon, podiatrist, ophthalmologist, and physiatrist. There may be other health care personnel involved in the child's care, such as gastroenterologists, ear-nose-throat specialists, nutritionists, homeopaths, psychiatrists or psychologists, and neonatologists, which is dependent on the child's unique needs. Allied health professionals my include any one or all of the following: physical therapist, physical therapy assistant, occupational therapist, certified occupational therapy assistant, speech and language pathologist, and speech and language assistant. If the child is in early intervention, there will also be a teacher on the team and sometimes a teaching assistant. Nurses are included in early intervention programs when the child is termed as being medically fragile or at-risk. Communication among the team members and through the family becomes a monumental task and vital to the child's well-being and ultimate success.

The occupational therapist works with postural control and movement primarily as a prerequisite for fine motor skills as they relate to self-help activities—feeding, dressing, bathing, play, and the development of perceptual skills. During the child's adolescent years, the occupational therapist becomes more involved with prevocational testing and training.

The speech and language pathologist is also involved with the acquisition of postural control and movement against gravity. Specific attention is paid to alignment of the head, trunk, and pelvis in order to promote optimal respiration in support of speech. The coordination of breathing with oral motor skills is necessary for feeding and, on a more differentiated level, for speech. A manual or electronic communication board may be indicated if oral speech is not a possibility. Manual sign language is rarely appropriate for children with CP, who often lack the fine finger control to sign successfully. However, a system of gestures can be used appropriately in the home and classroom. In addition to the motor deficits, the child's acquisition of language concepts may be delayed.

The psychologist may be involved in formal psychological testing of the child with CP to identify cognitive strengths and deficits. The psychologist will then make recommendations for appropriate educational placement to best meet the child's needs. Psychological therapy may be indicated if behavioral or emotional problems interfere with the social and emotional growth of the child and the family.

The recreational therapist may be involved in identifying leisure interests, and may work with the child and family in the selection and pursuit of leisure activities. Identification of toys appropriate for the child's developmental level and movement capabilities may allow independent play for the child, and is among the responsibilities of the recreational therapist. Some commonly used toys may be converted so that they can be electrically operated by battery and remote control. A joystick or press plate control may be used depending on the child's level of fine motor skill. Specially adapted access switches can also be made or purchased for particular toys. Computer programs can be used for fun and academic pursuits for the child. It is important to work with an individual knowledgeable about the available hardware and software and how adaptations can be made for your child.

Community recreation centers and schools often sponsor swimming, gymnastics, horseback riding, and dance programs in which children with disabilities may participate with their able-bodied peers. An important goal for recreational programs is to develop a positive self-image and high self-esteem by emphasizing activities in which a child *can* participate successfully.

Some music schools offer instrumental lessons for children with special needs. The motivation to learn to play the piano or an instrument can be the key to progress in the fine motor arena for some children.

A social worker may assist the family in locating services for the disabled child. The social worker can also play an important role in guiding and teaching family members to be advocates for the disabled family member. The disabled child, as a member of a larger family unit, will have a significant impact on that unit. The social worker can provide counseling and support for the family to help resolve issues of concern.

Summary

Children with cerebral palsy present with a wide range of neuromuscular, sensory/perceptual, and congitive concerns. To be effective in the evaluation and treatment of the child; an interdisciplinary team must have excellent communication skills with the child, the family and/or caregiver, and one another. This chapter presents physical therapy intervention as a problem-solving approach necessary to treat each child as an individual with unique needs and goals. The ultimate goal is for the child to become a functioning member of the family unit as well as the community to the utmost capacity.

Acknowledgments

I would like to thank Judi Bierman, Barbara Cupps, and Linda Kleibhan for the sharing of information and ideas with me over the years and their encouragement for me to continue my growth. Suzanne Davis deserves thanks for sharing her knowledge and patience, for her special insight into atypical development and assessment, and for her personal friendship along the way. They are all wonderful mentors and terrific therapists.

Acknowledgments are extended to Kate Reynolds and Kate Bain for their feedback after reading portions of the manuscript and to the parents of Elsa for their support and contributions to the case history. Thanks also to Cascade DAFO, Inc. for their effort in providing pictures of their products for inclusion in this chapter.

REFERENCES

1. Nelson K. What proportion of cerebral palsy is related to birth asphyxia? *J Pediatr.* 1988;113: 572–574.
2. Nelson K. Relationship of intrapartum and delivery room events to long-term neurologic outcome. *Clin Perinatol.* 1989;16:995–1007.
3. Niswander KR, Gordon M. The Collaborative Perinatal Project. In: *The Women and Their Pregnancies.* DHEW Publication no. 73–379, 1972.
4. Ellenberg JH, Nelson KB. Cluster of perinatal events identifying infants at high risk for death or disability. *J Pediatr.* 1988;113:546–552.
5. Melone PJ, Ernest JM, O'Shea MD, et al. Appropriateness of intrapartum fetal heart rate management and risk of cerebral palsy. *Am J Obstet Gynecol.* 1991;165:272–276.
6. Boyle CA, Yeargin-Allsopp M, Doernberg NS, et al. Prevalence of selected developmental disabilities in children 3–10 years of age: the Metropolitan Atlanta Developmental Disabilities Surveillance Program, 1991. MMWR-CDC-Surveill- Summ. 1996 April 19;45(2):1–14.
7. Dias LS, Marty GR. Selective Posterior Rhizotomy In: *The Diplegic Child: Evaluation and Management.* Sussman MD, ed. Rosemont, IL: American Academy of Orthopaedic Surgeons; 1992.
8. Torfs CP, van den Berg B. Oechsli FW, Cummins S. Prenatal and perinatal factors in the etiology of cerebral palsy. *J Pediatr.* 1990;116:615–619.
9. Nelson KB, Ellenberg JH. The asymptomatic newborn and risk of cerebral palsy. *Am J Dis Child.* 1987;141:1333–1335.
10. Freeman JM, Nelson KB. Intrapartum asphyxia and cerebral palsy. *Pediatrics.* 1988;82:240–249.
11. Naeye RL, Peter EC, Bartholemew M, Landis JR. Origins of cerebral palsy. *Am J Dis Child.* 1989;143:1154–1161.
12. Skidmore MD, Rivers A, Hack M. Increased risk of cerebral palsy among very low birthweight infants with chronic lung disease. *Dev Med Child Neurol.* 1990;32:325–332.
13. Luthy DA, Shy KK, Strickland D, et al. Status of infants at birth and risk for adverse neonatal events and long-term sequelae. *Am J Obstet Gynecol.* 1987;157:676–679.
14. Graziani L, Stanley C. Intracranial hemorrhage and the preterm infant. *Intens Caring Unlim.* 1987;5:6–7.
15. Graziani L, et al. Mechanical ventilation in preterm infants: Neurosonographic and developmental studies. In press.
16. Graziani L, Mitchell DG, Kornhauser M, et al. Neurodevelopment of preterm infants. Neonatal neurosonographic and serum bilirubin studies. *Pediatrics.* 1992;89:229–234.
17. Scherzer AL, Tscharnuter I. *Early Diagnosis and Therapy in Cerebral Palsy: A Primer on Infant Developmental Problems.* New York: Marcel Dekker; 1982.
18. Blitz RK, Wechtel RC, Blackmon L, et al. Neurodevelopmental outcome of extremely low birth weight infants in Maryland. *Md Med J.* 1997 Jan;46(1):18–24.
19. Bobath B, Bobath K. *Motor Development in the Different Types of Cerebral Palsy.* London: William Heineman Medical Books; 1982.
20. Molnar GE, ed. *Pediatric Rehabilitation.* Baltimore: Williams & Wilkins; 1985.
21. Blanche EI, Botticelli TM, Hallway MK. *Combining Neurodevelopment Treatment and Sensory Integration Principles: An Approach to Pediatric Therapy.* Tucson: Therapy Skill Builders; 1995.
22. Cooper J, Majnemer, A, Rosenbaltt B, Birnbaum R. et al. The determination of sensory deficits in children with hemiplegic cerebral palsy. *J Child Neurol.* 1995 Jul;10(4):300–309.
23. Brett EM, ed. *Pediatric Neurology.* New York: Churchill and Livingstone; 1983.
24. Stanley FS, English DR. Prevalence and risk factors for cerebral palsy in a total population cohort of low birthweight (<2000 grams) infants. *Dev Med Child Neurol.* 1986;28:559–568.
25. Staheli LT, Duncan WR, Schaefer E. Growth alterations in the hemiplegic child. *Clin Orthop.* 1968;60:205–212.
26. Holt KS. *Growth Disturbances: Hemiplegic Cerebral Palsy in Children and Adults.* London: William Heinemann Medical Books; 1961. Clinics in Developmental Medicine. No 4.
27. Harada T. Erada S, Anwar MM, et al. The cervical spine in athetoid cerebral palsy. A radiological study of 180 patients. *J Bone Joint Surg Br.* 1996 Jul;78(4):613–619.
28. Kitchen WH, Doyle LW, Ford GW, et al. Cerebral palsy in very low birthweight infants surviving to 2 years with modern perinatal intensive care. *Am J Perinatol.* 1987;4:29–35.
29. Pidcock FS, Graziani LJ, Stanley C, et al. Neurosonographic features of periventricular echoden-

sities associated with cerebral palsy in preterm infants. *J Pediatr.* 1990;116:417–422.
30. Kilbride HW, Daily DK, Matriu I, et al. Neurodevelopmental follow-up of infants with birthweight less than 801 grams with intracranial hemorrhage. *J Perinatol.* 1980;9:376–381.
31. Graham M, Livens MI, Trouna JQ, et al. Prediction of cerebral palsy in very low birthweight infants: Prospective ultrasound study. *Lancet.* 1987;2:593–506.
32. Tudehope DI, Masel J, Mohay H, et al. Neonatal cranial ultrasonography as predictor of 2 year outcome of very low birthweight infants. *Aust Pediatr J.* 1989;25:66–71.
33. Allen MC, Capute AJ. Neonatal neurodevelopmental examination as a predictor of neuromotor outcome in premature infants. *Pediatrics.* 1989;83:498–506.
34. Burns YR, O'Callaghan M, Tudehope DI. Early identification of cerebral palsy in high risk infants. *Aust Pediatr J.* 1989;25:215–219.
35. Harris SR. Early neuromotor predictors of cerebral palsy in low birthweight infants. *Dev Med Child Neurol.* 1987;29:508–519.
36. Harris SR. Movement analysis—An aid to diagnosis of cerebral palsy. *Phys Ther.* 1991;71:215–221.
37. Nelson KB, Ellenberg JH. Children who "outgrew" cerebral palsy. *Pediatrics.* 1982;69: 529–535.
38. Bly L. Abnormal motor development. In: Slaton DS, ed: *Proceedings of a Conference on Development of Movement in Infancy offered by the Division of Physical Therapy, University North Carolina at Chapel Hill;* May 18–22, 1980.
39. Bobath B. *Abnormal Postural Reflex Activity Caused by Brain Lesions.* 2nd Ed. London: William Heinemann Medical Books; 1972.
40. Bobath B. The very early treatment of cerebral palsy. *Dev Med Child Neurol.* 1967;9:373–390.
41. Bobath K. *A Neurophysiological Basis for the Treatment of Cerebral Palsy.* Philadelphia: JB Lippincott; 1980.
42. Bobath B, Bobath K. An analysis of the development of standing and walking patterns in patients with cerebral palsy. *Physiotherapy.* 1962;48:3–12.
43. Cochrane CD. Joint mobilization principles: Considerations for use in the child with central nervous system dysfunction. *Phys Ther.* 1987;67: 1105–1109.
44. Fiorentino MR. *Normal and Abnormal Development—The Influence of Primitive Reflexes on Motor Development.* Springfield, IL: Charles C Thomas; 1980.
45. Illingworth RS. *The Development of the Infant and Young Child.* 8th Ed. New York: Churchill Livingstone; 1983.
46. Levitt S. *Treatment of Cerebral Palsy and Motor Delay.* 2nd Ed. Oxford, England: Blackwell Scientific publishers, 1982.
47. Magnus R. Some Results of Studies in the Physiology of Posture. Cameron Prize Lectures, University of Edinburgh; May 1926.
48. Weisz S. Studies in equilibrium reaction. *J Nerv Mental Dis.* 1938;88:150–162.
49. Bly L. The components of normal movement during the first year of life. In: Slaton DS, ed. *Proceedings of a Conference on Development of Movement in Infancy offered by the University of North Carolina at Chapel Hill,* Division of Physical Therapy, May 18–20, 1980.
50. Polgar G, Promadhat V. *Pulmonary Function Testing in Children.* Philadelphia: WB Saunders; 1971.
51. Bleck EE. *Orthopedic Management of Cerebral Palsy.* Philadelphia: WB Saunders; 1979.
52. Shands AR, Steele MK. Torsion of the femur. *J Bone Joint Surg.* 1958;40A:803–816.
53. Bly L. What is the role of sensation in motor learning? What is the Role of Feedback and Feedforward? *NDTA Network.* 1996 Sept/Oct:1–7.
54. Cupps B. Postural Control: A current view. *NDTA Network.* 1997 Jan/Feb:1–7.
55. Olney SJ, Wright MJ. Cerebral palsy. In: Suzann Campbell, ed. *Physical Therapy for Children.* Philadelphia: WB Saunders; 1994.
56. *Research Plan for the National Center for Medical Rehabilitation* Research. NIH Publication No. 93-3509, March 1993.
57. Hoppenfeld S. *Physical Examination of the Spine and Extremities.* Norwalk, CT: Appleton-Century-Crofts; 1976.
58. Michele AA. *Iliopsoas.* Springfield, IL: Charles C Thomas; 1962.
59. Beals RK. Developmental changes in the femur and acetabulum in spastic paraplegia and diplegia. *Dev Med Child Neurol.* 1969;11:303–313.
60. Jordan P. Evaluation and Treatment of Foot Disorders. Presentation at the Neurodevelopmental Treatment Association Regional Conference, New York; May, 1984.
61. Calliet R. *Foot and Ankle Pain.* Philadelphia: FA Davis, 1970.
62. Burnett CN, Johnson EQ. Development of gait in childhood. Parts 1 and 2. *Dev Med Child Neurol.* 1971;13:196–215.
63. Sutherland D, Olshen R,Cooper L, Woo SL. The development of mature gait. *J Bone Joint Surg.* 1980;62A:336–353.
64. Mylebust BM. A review of myotatic reflexes and the development of motor control and gait in infants and children: A special communication. *Phys Ther.* 1990;70:188–203.

65. Thelen E, Cooke DW. Relationship between newborn stepping and later walking: A new interpretation. *Dev Med Child Neurol.* 1987;29:380–393.
66. Saunders JB, Inman VT, Eberhart HD. The major determinants in normal and pathological gait. *J Bone Joint Surg.* 1953;35A:543–558.
67. Watt JM, Robertson CM, Grace MG. Early prognosis for ambulation of neonatal intensive care survivors with cerebral palsy. *Dev Med Child Neurol.* 1989;31:766–773.
68. Hicks R, Durinick N, Gage JR. Differentiation of idiopathic toe-walking and cerebral palsy. *J Pediatr Orthop.* 1988;8:160–163.
69. Mossberg KA, Linton KA, Fricke K. Ankle-foot orthoses: Effect on energy expenditure of gait in spastic diplegic children. *Arch Phys Med Rehab.* 1990;71:490–494.
70. Stamer M. *Functional Documentation.* Tucson, AR: Therapy Skill Builders; 1995.
71. Campbell SK. Quantifying the effects of interventions for movement disorders resulting from cerebral palsy. *J Child Neurol.* 1996 Nov;11 Suppl 1:561–570.
72. Harris SR, Atwater SW, Crowe TK. Accepted and controversial neuromotor therapies for infants at high risk for cerebral palsy. *J Perinatol.* 1988 Winter;8(1):3–13.
73. Palisano RJ, Kolobe TH, Haley SM, et al. Validity of the Peabody Developmental Gross Motor Scale as an evaluative measure of infants receiving physical therapy. *Phys Ther.* 1995 Nov; 75(11):939–948.
74. Binder H, Eng GD. Rehabilitation management of children with spastic diplegic cerebral palsy. *Arch Phys Med Rehabil.* 1989;70:482–489.
75. Molnar GE. Rehabilitation in cerebral palsy. *West J Med.* 1991;154:569–572.
76. Fetters L. Measurement and treatment in cerebral palsy: An argument for a new approach (Review). *Phys Ther.* 1991;71:244–247.
77. Kluzik J, Fetters L. Coryell J. Quantification of control: A preliminary study of effects of neurodevelopmental treatment on reaching in children with spastic cerebral palsy. *Phys Ther.* 1990;70:65–78.
78. Kamm K, Thelen E, Jensen J. A dynamical systems approach to motor development. *Phys Ther.* 1990;70:763–775.
79. Finnie NR. *Handling the Young Cerebral Palsied Child at Home.* 2nd Ed. New York: Dalton Publications, 1975.
80. Davis S. Neurodevelopmental Treatment/Bobath Eight Week Course in the treatment of children with cerebral palsy. Lecture notes. June–July 1997.
81. Birkmeier, Kristen. Curriculum and theoretical base committee update. *NDTA Network.* 1997 July/Aug;6:4;1–7.
82. Pape KE. Therapeutic Electrical Stimulation the Past, the Present, the Future. *NDTA Network.* 1996 July/Aug; 1–7.
83. Pape KE, Kirsch SE. Technology-assisted self-care in the treatment of spastic diplegia. In Sussman MD, ed. *The Diplegic Child: Evaluation and Management.* Rosemont, IL: American Academy of Orthopaedic Surgeons; 1992.
84. Olney SJ, Wright MJ. Cerebral palsy. In: Campbell SK, ed. *Physical Therapy for Children.* Philadelphia: W.B. Saunders, 1994.
85. Stuberg WA. Considerations related to weight-bearing programs in children with developmental disabilities. *Phys Ther.* 1992;72:35–40.
86. Rose J, Gamble JG, Medeiras J, et al. Energy cost of walking in normal children and in those with cerebral palsy: Comparison of heart rate and oxygen uptake. *J Pediatr Orthop.* 1989;9:276–279.
87. Logan L, Byers-Hinkley K, Ciccone CD. Anterior versus posterior walkers: A gait analysis study. *Dev Med Child Neurol.* 1990;32:1044–1048.
88. Levangie PK, Chimera M, Johnston M, et al. The effects of posterior rolling walkers on gait characteristics of children with spastic cerebral palsy. *Phys Occup Ther Pediatr.* 1989;9:1–17.
89. Canadian Medical Association. Editorial. *Can Med Assn J.* 1987;136:57.
90. Kauffman IB, Ridenour M. Influence of an infant walker on onset and quality of walking pattern of locomotion: An electromyographic investigation. *Percept Mot Skills.* 1977;45:1323–1329.
91. *Mothering* 46, Winter 1988.
92. Pronsati M. Baby walkers—Considering full price of convenience. *Adv Phys Ther.* May 18, 1992:7.
93. Black JA, Reed MD, Roberts CD. Muscle relaxant drugs for children with cerebral palsy. In Sussman MD, ed. *The Diplegic Child: Evaluation and Management.* Rosemont, IL: American Academy of Orthopaedic Surgeons; 1992.
94. Pranzatelli MR. Oral pharmacotherapy for the movement disorders of cerebral palsy. *J Child Neurol.* 1996 Nov;11 Suppl 1:S13–22.
95. Sutherland DH, et al. Injection of botulinum A toxin into the gastrocnemius muscle of patients with cerebral palsy: A 3 dimensional motion analysis study. *Gait Posture* 1996;4:269–279.
96. Koman LA, Mooney JF, Smith BP. Neuromuscular blockade in the management of cerebral palsy. *J Child Neurol.* 1996 Nov;11 Suppl 1:S23–28.
97. Koman LA, et al. Management of cerebral palsy with botulinum A toxin: Preliminary investigation. *J Pediatr Orthop.* 1993 July–Aug; 13(4):489–495.
98. Peacock WJ, Stoudt LA. Functional outcomes following selective posterior rhizotomy in children with cerebral palsy. *J Neurosurg.* 1991;74:380–385.

99. Guiliani CA. Dorsal rhizotomy for children with cerebral palsy: Support for concept of motor control. *Phys Ther.* 1991;71:248–259.
100. Abbott R, Forem SL, Johann M. Selective posterior rhizotomy for the treatment of spasticity: A review. *Child Nerv Syst.* 1989;5:337–346.
101. Oppenheim W. Selective posterior rhizotomy for spastic cerebral palsy. A review. *Clin Orthop Rel Res.* 1990;253:20–29.
102. Oppenheim WL, Staudt LA, Peacock WJ. The rationale for rhizotomy. In: Sussman MD, ed. *The Diplegic Child: Evaluation and Management.* Rosemont, IL: American Academy of Orthopaedic Surgeons; 1992.
103. Peter JC, Arens LJ. Selective posterior lumbosacral rhizotomy in teenagers and young adults with spastic cerebral palsy. *Br J Neursurg.* 1994;8(2):135–139.
104. Bloom KK, Nazar GB. Functional assessment following selective posterior rhizotomy in spastic cerebral palsy. *Childs Nerv Sys.* 1994 Mar;10(2): 84–86.
105. Thomas SS, Aiona MD, Pierce R, Piatt JH 2nd et al. Gait changes in children with spastic diplegia after selective dorsal rhizotomy. *J Pediatr Orthop.* 1996 Nov–Dec;16(6):747–752.
106. Chicoine MR, Park TS, Kaufman BA. Selective dorsal rhizotomy and rates of orthopedic surgery in children with spastic cerebral palsy. *J Neurosurg.* 1997 Jan;86(1):34–39.
107. Hendricks-Ferguson VL, Ortman MR. Selective dorsal rhizotomy to decrease spasticity in cerebral palsy. *AORN J.* 1995 Mar;61(3):514–518, 521–552, 525.
108. Heim RC, Rark TS, Vogler GP, et al. Changes in hip migration after selective dorsal rhizotomy for spastic quadriplegia in cerebral palsy. *J Neurosurg.* 1995 Apr; 82(4): 567–571.
109. Waltz JM, Andreesen WH, Hunt DP. Spinal cord stimulation and motor disorders. *Pace-Pac Clin Electrophys.* 1987;10:180–204.
110. Hugenholtz H, Humphreys P, McIntyre WM, et al. Cervical spinal cord stimulation for spasticity in cerebral palsy. *Neurosurgery.* 1988;22:707–714.
111. Albright AL, Barron WB, Fasick MP, et al. Continuous intrathecal baclofen infusion for spasticity of cerebral origin. *JAMA.* 1993 Nov 24;270(20): 2475–2477.
112. DeLuca PA. The musculoskeletal management of children with cerebral palsy. *Pediatr Clin North Am.* 1996 Oct;43(5):1135–1150.
113. Sprague JB. Surgical management of cerebral palsy. *Orthop Nurs.* 1992 July–Aug;11(4):11–9.
114. Dormans JP. Orthopedic management of children with cerebral palsy. *Pediatr Clin North Am.* 1993 Jun;40(3):645–657.
115. Green NE. The orthopedic management of the ankle, foot, and knee in patients with cerebral palsy. Neuromuscular disease and deformities. *Instructional Course Lectures.* 1987;36:253–256.
116. Gamble JG, Rinsky LA, Bleck EE. Established hip dislocations in children with cerebral palsy. *Clin Orthop Rel Res.* 1990;253:90–99.
117. Pritchett JW. Treated and untreated unstable hips in severe cerebral palsy. *Dev Med Child Neurol.* 1990; 32:3–6.
118. Jones ET, Knapp DR. Assessment and management of the lower extremity in cerebral palsy. *Orthop Clin North Am.* 1987;18:725–728.
119. Root L. Treatment of hip problems in cerebral palsy. Neuromuscular diseases and deformities. *Instructional Course Lectures.* 1987;36:237–252.
120. Osterkamp J, Caillouette JT, Hoffer MM. Chiari osteotomy in cerebral palsy. *J Pediatr Orthop.* 1988;8:274–277.
121. Smith JT. Stevens PM. Combined adductor transfer, iliopsoas release, and proximal hamstring release in cerebral palsy. *J Pediatr Orthoped.* 1989;9:1–5.
122. Patrick JH. Techniques of psoas tenotomy and rectus femoris transfer: "New" operations for cerebral palsy diplegia—a description. *J Pediatr Orthop B.* 1996 Fall;5(4):242–246.
123. Moreau M, Cook PC, Ashton B. Adductor and psoas release for subluxation of the hip in children with spastic cerebral palsy. *J Pediatr Orthop.* 1995 Sep–Oct;15(5):672–676.
124. Atar D, et al. Femoral varus derotational osteotomy in cerebral palsy. *Am J Orthop.* 1995 Apr;24(4):337–341.
125. Moens P, Lammens J, Molenaers G, Fabry G. Femoral derotation for increased hip anteversion. A new surgical technique with a modified Ilizarov frame. *J Bone Joint Surg Br.* 1995 Jan;77(1): 107–109.
126. Pope DF, Bueff HU, DeLuca PA. Pelvic osteotomies for subluxation of the hip in cerebral palsy. *J Pediatr Orthop.* 1994 Nov–Dec;14(6): 724–730.
127. Root L, Laplasa FJ, Brourman SN, Angel DH. The severely unstable hip in cerebral palsy. Treatment with open reduction, pelvic osteotomy, and femoral osteotomy with shortening. *J Bone Joint Surg Am.* 1995 May;77(5):703–712.
128. Brunner R, Baumann JU. Clinical benefit of reconstruction of dislocated or subluxated hip joints in patients with spastic cerebral palsy. *J Pediatr Orthop.* 1994 May–Jun;14(3):290–294.

129. Atar D, Grant AD, Bash J, Lehman WB. Combined hip surgery in cerebral palsy patients. *Am J Orthop.* 1995 Jan;24(1):52–55.
130. Barrie JL, Galasko CS. Surgery for unstable hips in cerebral palsy. *J Pediatr Orthop B.* 1996 Fall; 5(4):225–231.
131. McHale KA, Bagg M, Nason SS. Treatment of the chronically dislocated hip in adolescents with cerebral palsy with femoral head resection and subtrochanteric valgus osteotomy. *J Pediatr Orthop.* 1990;10:504–509.
132. Carr C, Gage JR. The fate of the non-operated hip in cerebral palsy. *J Pediatr Orthop.* 1987; 7:262–267.
133. Aronson DD, Zak PJ, Lee CL, Bollinger RO, Lamont RL. Posterior transfer of the adductors in children who have cerebral palsy. *J Bone Joint Surg.* 1991;73A:59–65.
134. Grogan DP, Lundy MS, Ogden JA. A method for early postoperative mobilization of the cerebral palsy patient using a removable abduction bar. *J Pediatr Othop.* 1987;7:338–340.
135. Harryman SE. Lower extremity surgery for children with cerebral palsy: Physical therapy management. *Phys Ther.* 1992 Jan;72(1):16–24.
136. Phillips WE, Audet M. Use of serial casting in the management of knee joint contractures in an adolescent with cerebral palsy. *Phys Ther.* 1990;70: 521–523.
137. Anderson JP, Snow B, Dorey FJ, Kabo JM. Efficacy of soft splints in reducing severe knee flexion contractures. *Dev Med Child Neurol.* 1988;30: 502–508.
138. Root L. Distal hamstring surgery in cerebral palsy. In: Sussman MD, ed. *The Diplegic Child Evaluation and Management.* Rosemont, IL: American Academy of Orthopaedic Surgeons; 1992.
139. Gage JR. Distal hamstring lengthening/release and rectus femoris transfer. In: Sussman MD, ed. *The Diplegic Child Evaluation and Management.* Rosemont, IL: American Academy of Orthopaedic Surgeons; 1992.
140. Gage JR. Surgical treatment of knee dysfunctional in cerebral palsy. *Clin Orthop Rel Res.* 1990; 253:45–54.
141. Abdennebi B, Bougatene B. Selective neurotomies for relief of spasticity focalized to the foot and to the knee flexors. Results in a series of 58 patients. Acta Neurochir Wien. 1996;138(8): 917–920.
142. Fulford GE. Surgical management of ankle and foot deformities in cerebral palsy. *Clin Orthop Rel Res.* 1990;253:55–61.
143. Yngve DA, Chambers C. Vulpius and Z-lengthening. *J Pediatr Orthop.* 1996 Nov–Dec; 16(6): 759–764.
144. Rosenthal RK, Simon SR. The Vulpius gastrocnemius-soleus lengthening. In: Sussman MD, ed. *The Diplegic Child Evaluation and Management.* Rosemont, IL: American Academy of Orthopaedic Surgeons; 1992.
145. Strecker WB, Via MW, Oliver SK, et al. Heelcord advancement for treatment of equinus deformity in cerebral palsy. *J Pediatr Orthop.* 1990;10; 105–108.
146. Segal LS, Thomas GS, Mazur JM, et al. Calcaneal gait in spastic diplegia after heel cord lengthening: A study with gait analysis. *J Pediatr Orthop.* 1989;9:697–701.
147. Crawford AH, Kucharzyk D, Roy DR, et al. Subtalar stabilization of the planovalgus foot by staple arthroereisis in young children who have neuromuscular problems. *J Bone Joint Surg.* 1990;72A: 840–845.
148. Drvaric DM, Schmitt EW, Nahams JM. The Grice extra-articular subtalar arthrodesis in the treatment of spastic hindfoot valgus deformity. *Dev Med Child Neurol.* 1989;31:665–669.
149. Guttman GG. Subtalar arthrodesis in children with cerebral palsy: Results using iliac bone plug. *Foot Ankle.* 1990;10:206–210.
150. Hamel J, et al. A combined bony and soft-tissue tarsal stabilization procedure (Grice-Schede) for hindfoot valgus in children with cerebral palsy. *Arch Orthop Trauma Surg.* 1994;113(5): 237–243.
151. Johnson WL, Lester EL. Transposition of the posterior tibial tendon. *Clin Orthop Rel Res.* 1989;245:223–227.
152. Medina PA, Karpman RR, Yeung AT. Split posterior tibial tendon transfer for spastic equinovarus foot deformity. *Foot Ankle.* 1989;10:65–67.
153. Barnes MJ, Herring JA. Combined split anterior tibial tendon transfer and intramuscular lengthening of the posterior tibial tendon. *J Bone Joint Surg.* 1991;73A:734–738.
154. Kagaya H, et al. Split posterior tibial tendon transfer for varus deformity of hindfoot. *Clin Orthop.* 1996 Feb;(323):254–260.
155. Roehr B, Lyne ED. Split anterior tibial tendon transfer. In: Sussman MD, ed. *The Diplegic Child: Evaluation and Management.* Rosemont, IL: American Academy of Orthopaedic Surgeons; 1992.
156. Green NE. Split posterior tibial tendon transfer: The universal procedure. In: Sussman MD, ed. *The Diplegic Child: Evaluation and Management.* Rosemont, IL: American Academy of Orthopaedic Surgeons; 1992.
157. Mazur JM, Shanks DE. Nonsurgical treatment of tight achilles tendon. In: Sussman MD, ed. *The Diplegic Child: Evaluation and Management.*

Rosemont, IL: American Academy of Orthopaedic Surgeons; 1992.

158. Jones ET, Knapp DR. Assessment and management of the lower extremity in cerebral palsy. *Orthop Clin North Am.* 1987;18:725–738.
159. Sussman MD, Cusick B. Preliminary report: The role of short-leg, tone reducing cases as an adjunct to physical therapy of patients with cerebral palsy. *Johns Hopkins Med J.* 1979;145:112–114.
160. Hanson CJ, Jones LJ. Gait abnormalities and inhibitive casts in cerebral; palsy: Literature review. *J Am Podiatr Med Assoc.* 1989;79:53–59.
161. Radtka SA. A comparison of gait with solid, dynamic, and no ankle-foot orthoses in children with spastic cerebral palsy. *Phys Ther.* 1997; 77(4):395–409.
162. Cusick B. Tone-reducing casts as an adjunct to the treatment of cerebral palsy. Lecture notes, Philadelphia; May 19, 1981.
163. Middleton EA, Hurley GR, McIlwain JS. The role of rigid and hinged polypropylene ankle-foot orthoses in the management of cerebral palsy: A case study. *Prosthet Orthot Int.* 1988;12:129–135.
164. Carmick J. Managing equinus in a child with cerebral palsy: Merits of hinged ankle-foot orthoses. *Dev Med Child Neurol.* 1995 Nov;37(11): 1006–1010.
165. Magill-Evans JE, Restall G. Self-esteem of persons with cerebral palsy: From adolescence to adulthood. *Am S Occup Ther.* 1991 Sept;45(9): 819–825.
166. Craft MJ, Lakin JA, Oppliger RA, Clancy GM, Vanderlinden DW. Siblings as change agents for promoting the functional status of children with cerebral palsy. *Dev Med Child Neurol.* 1990;32: 1049,1057.

Spina Bifida

Elena Tappit-Emas

Incidence and Etiology

Spina bifida is a disability causing locomotor dysfunction in children that is second only to cerebral palsy in incidence. With an incidence in the United States that approaches 1 in every 1000 live births, spina bifida is the second most common birth defect after Down syndrome. Studies examining the possible causes of spina bifida have evaluated genetic, environmental, and dietary factors that might affect its occurrence. No definitive cause, including chromosomal abnormalities, has yet been identified.[1,2]

Many factors may lead to spina bifida, and a genetic predisposition may be enhanced by the existence of numerous environmental factors. Low levels of maternal folic acid prior to conception has been implicated by several studies.

One study by Duff, Nutr, and Cooper found a significant though temporary increase of children born with neural tube defects on the island of Jamaica who were conceived during the several months immediately following hurricane Gilbert in September of 1988. The normal diet of the island is rich in folic acid from fresh fruit and vegetables. The hurricane destroyed much of the island's crops, and for a temporary period, fresh produce was scarce.[3] This study as well as an annotation by Seller proposes a need to fortify commonly eaten foods with folic acid such as orange juice, cereals, flour, rice, and salt.[4]

Maternal use of valproic acid, an anticonvulsant, is also known to induce this defect in offspring. Recently, maternal hyperthemia caused by saunas, hot tub and electric blanket use, and maternal fevers during the first trimester of pregnancy were studied.[5] Only hot tubs showed any tendency to increase the risk of spina bifida.

A high occurrence (4.5 per 1000 births) is seen in families of Irish and Celtic heritage, but Japanese families show a low occurrence of only 0.3 per 1000 births. A changing pattern of occurrence has appeared in the United States. An increase in spina bifida has been seen in children born to Hispanic and African-American families, perhaps owing to environmental factors and pollution as populations have shifted to industrialized urban areas.[6] Families in which spina bifida is present have a 2% to 5% greater chance than the general population of having a second child with the disorder.

Prognosis

In previous decades, long-term survival of children with spina bifida was reported to range from as low as 1% without treatment to 50% with treatment. A survival rate of more than 90% is expected today with aggressive treatment of the spinal defect and associated problems. This chapter presents the primary problems and concerns for this population, including hydrocephalus, motor and sensory deficits in the lower extremities, and related issues of clinical significance.

The use of antibiotics to limit infection, starting in 1947, and the surgical insertion of ventricular shunts in 1960 to limit hydrocephalus were major advances in treatment. Recently, early and consistent use of intermittent clean catheterization to empty the bladder completely has dramatically improved the survival rate by controlling urinary tract infection and renal deterioration, both of which have been major causes of mortality. These measures, along with the practice of early back closure, continue to improve the survival of children with spina bifida. With this improved survival rate has come an increase in the number of severely affected children. However, there is also an increased number of less severely involved patients who would likely have not survived with earlier treatment protocols. Therefore, the full spectrum and complexity of this disability can now be appreciated. Clinicians now have the opportunity, unavailable in previous eras, to work with and learn a great deal from this heterogeneous group.[7,8]

Definitions

The terms myelomeningocele, meningomyelocele, spina bifida, spina bifida aperta, spina bifida cystica, spinal dysraphism, and myelodysplasia are synonymous. Spina bifida is a spinal defect usually diagnosed at birth by noting the presence of an external sac on the infant's back (Fig. 5-1). The sac contains meninges and spinal cord protruding through a dorsal defect in the vertebrae. This defect may occur at any point along the spine but is most commonly located in the lumbar region. The sac may be covered by a transparent membrane that may have

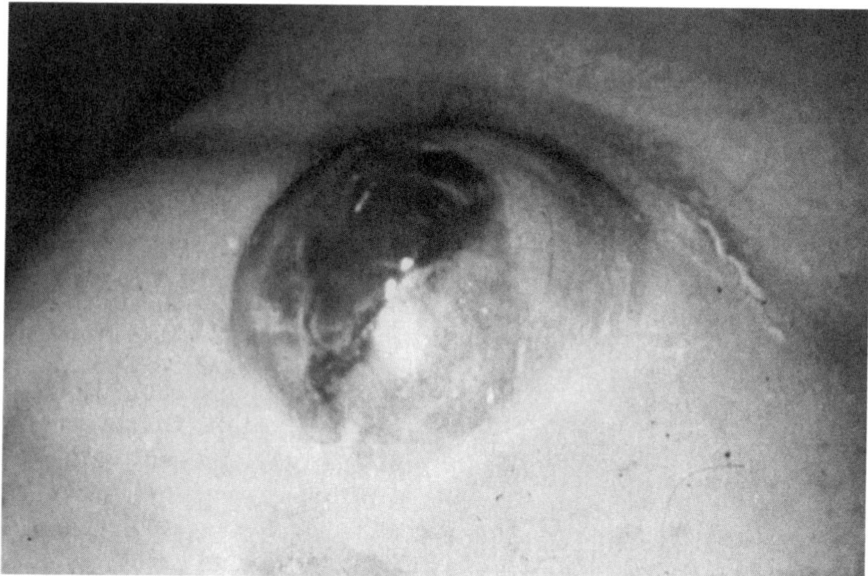

Figure 5-1 ▪ Spina bifida defect in a newborn infant before surgical repair.

neural tissue attached to its inner surface, or the sac may be open with the neural tissue exposed. The lateral borders of the sac have bony protrusions formed by the unfused neural arches of the vertebrae. The defect may be large, with many vertebrae involved, or it may be small, involving only one or two segments. The size of the lesion is not necessarily predictive of the child's functional deficit.[6,8,9]

Spina bifida occulta and myelocele are less severe anomalies associated with spina bifida. *Spina bifida occulta* is a condition involving nonfusion of the halves of the vertebral arches, but without disturbance of the underlying neural tissue. This lesion is most commonly located in the lumbar or sacral spine and is often an incidental finding when roentgenograms are taken for unrelated reasons. Spina bifida occulta may be distinguished externally by a midline tuft of hair, with or without an area of pigmentation on the overlying skin. Between 21% and 26% of parents of children with spina bifida cystica have been found to have the occulta defect. Otherwise, spina bifida occulta has only a 4.5% to 8% incidence in the general population.[6,8,10] Neurologic and muscular dysfunction were previously thought to be absent in individuals with spina bifida occulta. However, recent work by Fidas et al. has revealed a high association of mild urinary tract disorders in these individuals.[11]

A *myelocele* is a protruding sac containing meninges and cerebrospinal fluid (CSF), but in this condition, the nerve roots and spinal cord remain intact and in their normal positions. Motor and sensory deficits, hydrocephalus, and other central nervous system (CNS) problems are not associated with a myelocele.[9]

Lipomeningocele, a superficial fatty mass in the low lumbar or sacral level, is another defect of the vertebrae that is usually included in this group of diagnoses. Neurologic deficits and hydrocephalus are not expected in patients with a lipomeningocele. However, there is a high incidence bowel and bladder dysfunction resulting from a tethered spinal cord in this population.[12,13] Refer to additional information regarding tethered cord later in this chapter.

Embryology

Spina bifida cystica, one of several neural tube defects, occurs early in the embryologic development of the CNS. Cells of the neural plate, which forms by day 18 of gestation, differentiate to create the neural tube and neural crest. The neural crest becomes the peripheral nervous system, including the cranial nerves, spinal nerves, autonomic nerves, and ganglia. The neural tube, which becomes the CNS, the brain, and the spinal cord, is open at both the cranial and caudal ends. The cranial end closes on approximately the 24th day of gestation. Failure to close results in a fatal condition called anencephaly. The caudal end of the neural tube closes on day 26 of gestation. Failure of closure or fusion at any point along the caudal border initiates spina bifida cystica or myelomeningocele. Common clinical signs of spina bifida cystica include absence of motor and sensory function (usually bilateral) below the level of the spinal defect and loss of neural control of bowel and bladder function. Unilateral motor and sensory loss has been reported. The pattern of loss may also be asymmetric. The functional deficits may be partial or complete, but they are almost always permanent.[8,14,15]

Hydrocephalus and the Chiari II Malformation

Hydrocephalus and the Arnold-Chiari malformation are CNS abnormalities that are commonly associated with spina bifida. *Hydrocephalus* is an abnormal accumulation of CSF in the cranial vault. In individuals without spina bifida, hydrocephalus may be caused by overproduction of CSF, a failure in absorption of the fluid, or an obstruction in the normal flow of CSF through the brain structures and spinal cord. Obstruction by the Arnold-Chiari malformation is considered to be the cause of hydrocephalus in most children with spina bifida. This malformation, also known as the *Chiari II malformation,* is a deformity of the cerebellum, medulla, and cervical spinal cord. The posterior cerebellum herniates downward through the foramen magnum, and brain stem structures are also displaced in a caudal direction. The CSF released from the fourth ventricle may face an obstruction by these abnormally situated structures, and its flow through the foramen magnum may be disrupted. Traction on the lower cranial nerves may also occur with this malformation. Studies using magnetic resonance imaging (MRI) have shown that most children with spina bifida have the Chiari II malformation. Among those with this malformation, the likelihood of hydrocephalus developing is greater than 90%.[16–19]

Theories related to the development of the Chiari II malformation are of interest. Previously, it was thought that the primary spinal defect acted as an anchor on the spinal cord, preventing it from sliding proximally within the spinal canal as the fetus grew. It was believed that this traction on the cord pulled down the attached brain-stem structures into an abnormally low position. Hydrocephalus was thought to result solely from the hydrodynamic consequence of this blockage.[20] In 1989, a study by McLone and Knepper linked the occurrence of spina bifida, the Chiari II malformation, and hydrocephalus.[21] These researchers postulated that a series of interrelated, time-dependent defects occur during the embryologic development of the primitive ventricular system, causing the Chiari II malformation and hydrocephalus. Their findings indicate that most affected children also have small posterior fossae that are unable to accommodate the hind brain and brain-stem structures. Therefore, neither downward traction nor downward pressure from hydrocephalus causes the malformation. Significantly, McLone and Knepper found that more than 25% of the neonates with spina bifida had head circumferences measuring below the 5th percentile.[21] These researchers have postulated that spina bifida results from mistimed steps in the development of the ventricular system initiated by failure of closure of the neural tube. This explanation has received widespread acceptance among both neuroanatomists and neurosurgeons. The explanation is of great interest to physical therapists who have speculated about the cause of CNS dysfunction in children with spina bifida. These children differ greatly from those with only hydrocephalus, with whom they are often compared. The McLone and Knepper theory begins to offer an anatomic rationale for the CNS abnormalities seen in many patients, and offers a viable basis for future investigation.[21]

Approximately 2% to 3% of children with spina bifida show significant effects of the Chiari II malformation on brain-stem and cranial nerve function Display 5-1. Tracheostomy and gastrostomy may be life-saving measures for these symptoms, which are reported to resolve as the child grows and the brain matures. In severe cases of Chiari II malformation, significant upper extremity weakness and opisthotonic postures may be seen. Posterior fossa decompression and cervical laminectomy to relieve pressure on the brain stem and cervical spinal structures are accepted courses of treatment but are associated with varying degrees of success. It is of interest that no correlation has been found between the severity of a child's symptoms and the degree of hydrocephalus. In fact, no correlation has yet been found between the child's motor level and any other finding. Therefore, attempts to predict which children will have significant difficulties have been unsuccessful. Examination by MRI has revealed severe abnormalities in some children who are asymptomatic. There is speculation that brainstem auditory evoked potentials may provide some diagnostic assistance in the future. Physicians believe that there is much to learn at the microscopic level about this abnormality.[6,8,22–25]

DISPLAY 5-1

Symptoms Associated with Chiari II Malformation

Stridor—especially with inspiration
Apnea—when crying, or at night
Gastroesophageal reflux
Paralysis of vocal cords
Swallowing difficulty
Bronchial aspiration

Prenatal Testing and Diagnosis

Increasingly sophisticated prenatal testing has allowed the early diagnosis of spina bifida. Such testing provides information that allows families to make informed decisions about a pregnancy. For the family that chooses to bring their baby to term, appropriate and well-coordinated medical care can be arranged in anticipation of the birth.

Alpha-fetoprotein (AFP) is normally present in the developing fetus and is found in the amniotic fluid. AFP reaches its peak levels in the fetal serum and, subsequently, in the amniotic fluid from the 6th to the 14th week of gestation. After the 14th week, however, AFP continues to leak into the amniotic fluid through the exposed vascularity of the spina bifida defect. Abnormally high levels of AFP in the amniotic fluid provides strong evidence for a neural tube defect. Testing for AFP by amniocentesis and, more recently, in maternal blood samples, has been responsible for detection of approximately 89% of neural tube defects. Unfortunately, the tests used have the potential for both false-positive and false-negative results. Therefore, AFP results are routinely compared clinically with the results of ultrasonographic imaging.[8,16]

Improved ultrasound equipment and experienced technicians have enabled obstetricians to observe and document several cranial abnormalities that have a high correlation with the presence of spina bifida. Because a small back lesion on a neonate can be difficult or impossible to detect, clinicians are now using cranial signs as an indication of the abnormality. These clinical findings are then followed by ultrasonographic studies performed for the purpose of locating the back lesion.[26,27]

There has been speculation regarding the best method of obstetric delivery when spina bifida is detected. A cesarean section may have a protective effect on the neural tissue of the back, thus improving the functional status of the child. Cesarean section reduces the trauma to the exposed nerves of the back that would occur during vaginal delivery. Moreover, a cesarean delivery avoids the bacterial contamination of the neonate's open lesion associated with passage through the vaginal canal, thereby reducing the risk of meningitis. A cesarean section also avoids trauma to the back from a breech presentation, which could affect the infant's neurologic function. Finally, back closure can be accomplished more rapidly following a scheduled cesarean section than after an unscheduled vaginal delivery.[28–32]

Management of the Neonate

General Philosophy of Treatment

Philosophies of treatment for the neonate with spina bifida vary throughout the world and among institutions within the United States. Because the back lesion was not universally thought to be life-threatening, institutions were free to develop their own protocols for the timing and intensity of treatment for these infants. However, the results of studies comparing various treatment regimens support the efficacy of early intervention. Immediate sterile care of the lesion to prevent infection is essential, and surgical closure of the back within 72 hours of birth is now the goal for most institutions.[6,8,33]

The objective of back surgery is to place the neural tissue into the vertebral canal, cover the spinal defect, and achieve a flat and watertight closure of the sac (Fig. 5-2). The open spine provides direct access to the spinal cord and brain. By preventing infection and its associated brain damage, the child's level of function, both physical and cognitive, will be preserved. McLone and associates have shown that babies who suffer gram-negative ventriculitis are less adept intellectually than uninfected babies.[35] These findings are significant in that intellectual function was not significantly affected by either hydrocephalus or the level of paralysis.[6,33–35]

Although in many institutions children with spina bifida are treated aggressively with imme-

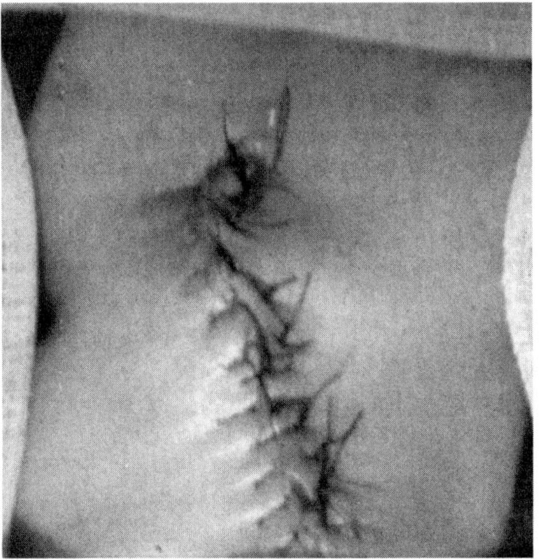

Figure 5-2 ▪ The same defect as shown in Figure 5-1, after surgical repair.

diate back closure and rapid management of hydrocephalus, some institutions practice selective treatment. That is, there will be more aggressive management for those children who appear to be less involved. In these institutions, the care for the neonate with spina bifida will vary depending on the level of lower extremity paralysis. Other factors influencing treatment decisions include the presence of accompanying abnormalities, such as hydrocephalus, kyphoscoliosis, and renal problems. Other institutions attempt to educate parents about their child's status and the implications of spina bifida on their lives. The parents may then act in a thoughtful manner in combination with the medical staff to choose a mutually acceptable course of action. During this period of education, which may last several hours or several weeks, the infant will usually be treated to maintain a stable condition and prevent infection.

This early period also provides time for the medical staff to gather information about the child's condition. This information is shared with the family so that discussion about hydrocephalus or orthopedic deformities, which require more involved early care, can begin. It is important to note that an accurate prediction of the child's potential is difficult in the early days. A vast number of variables will influence the child's condition and function in the coming years, so clinicians must be wary about presenting information about the child's future. An exception, of course, may be in the case of a severely impaired child with multiple congenital anomalies as well as spina bifida whose outcome is apparently bleak.[36–38]

Preoperative Assessment

In many centers, the preoperative assessment is done by one physician experienced in the overall care of children with spina bifida. Consults are then requested for specific services necessary for each baby. More commonly, however, a team of experts will evaluate the baby and continue to monitor the child throughout the course of hospitalization. These professionals comprise the treatment team that will be involved in long-term care of the child.

The neurosurgeon is concerned initially with the location and extent of the infant's back lesion. Kyphoscoliosis presents a complication to back surgery and may lead to impaired wound healing because of excessive pressure over the suture site. Skin grafting is occasionally necessary to gain adequate skin coverage of a large lesion. Congenital scoliosis with accompanying fused ribs at the level of the back lesion usually predicts rapid progression of the scoliosis during the growth periods of childhood. The resultant effect of progressive scoliosis on pulmonary function may be life-threatening, even with bracing and surgical intervention.

A neonatologist or pediatrician may be consulted to assess the general health of the baby and to identify other congenital defects or cardiopulmonary dysfunction that may be present but that are unrelated to the spinal lesion.

The urologist will request urodynamic testing during the early neonatal period. However, immediate postnatal attention may not be indicated.

A comprehensive orthopedic evaluation may not be imperative, but the surgeon can offer insight into orthopedic problems that are present at birth. Difficulties that may be anticipated may also be discussed. Valuable information and education for the family and medical team can be provided as a result of early orthopedic intervention. Evaluation of the lower extremities and spinal alignment will help establish a plan of orthopedic care for the baby's first weeks of life. This plan of care can incorporate other appropriate staff for coordinated intervention.[6,8,38–39]

Management of Hydrocephalus

After back closure, 10% of affected infants recover, have the sutures removed, and leave the hospital without further complication. The remaining 90% will begin to develop hydrocephalus during the next several days or weeks. After back closure, the natural drain for CSF is unavailable and CSF pressure begins to rise in the cranium. Of the 90% who will develop hydrocephalus, approximately 25% are born with evidence of hydrocephalus and need immediate shunt insertion. Studies show that an additional 55% will develop hydrocephalus within several days of birth. The remaining babies will need shunting within 6 months. The neurosurgeon carefully monitors changes in the baby's head circumference, and studies such as ultrasonography, computed tomography, or MRI, provide baseline information about the size of the lateral ventricles. Later comparisons can assist in determining the appropriate time for insertion of a shunt.

Changes in the baby's state often indicate increased intracranial pressure. As the enlarged ventricles cause the brain to expand within the flexible cranial vault of the infant, many symptoms are seen singularly or in combination. The two most common symptoms include *"sunsetting,"* a downward deviation of the eyes, and separation of the cranial sutures with a bulging anterior fontanelle.

The increasing fluid pressure may stabilize without surgery in some individuals, but it is impossible to predict when this will occur, how great the pressure will become, or how large the head will grow. Vital signs become depressed and respiratory arrest can occur when pressure on the brain stem structures becomes too great. Some individuals will survive without treatment for the hydrocephalus and become severely impaired.[6,7,38]

Surgical insertion of a shunt will relieve the signs and symptoms associated with increased intracranial pressure. The shunt is a thin, flexible tube that diverts CSF away from the lateral ventricles. It is secured at the proximal and distal ends and is radiopaque for easy location by radiographic studies. The ventriculoatrial (VA) shunt moves excess CSF from one lateral ventricle to the right atrium of the heart. Because infections of the system can lead to septicemia, ventriculitis, superior vena cava occlusion, and pulmonary emboli, this type of shunt is not used as commonly as in past years. The ventriculoperitoneal (VP) shunt is currently the preferred treatment for hydrocephalus. Although occlusion of this type of shunt may occur more easily than with the VA shunt, complications associated with the VP shunt are far less severe. As it exits the lateral ventricle, the shunt can be palpated distally along the neck, under the clavicle, and down the chest wall, just below the superficial fascia. The shunt inserts into the peritoneum, where CSF is reabsorbed and the excess excreted[39,40] (Fig. 5-3).

Although shunt insertion is a common operation for most neurosurgical teams, it is yet another event for the infant who has already had at least one major procedure to close the back lesion. In order to spare the infant a second anesthesia, several centers have begun to perform simultaneous back closure and shunt insertion. Advocates of this approach also believe

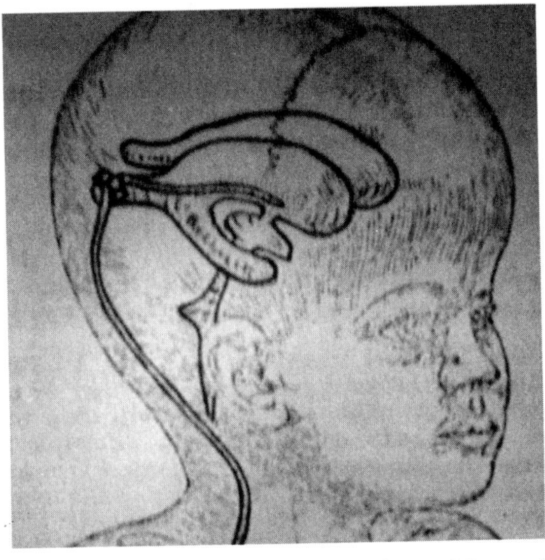

Figure 5-3 ■ Location of the lateral ventricles and placement of ventriculoperitoneal shunt.

that healing of the back wound from the inside is compromised when the CSF pressure builds internally. With the double surgery, more rapid healing of the back wound is expected. Neither negative sequelae nor increased postoperative complications have been reported for the double procedure.[41,42]

After surgery, a plan for physical therapy, based on the infant's condition, can be developed. The priority is for rapid healing, an uneventful recovery, and a speedy discharge to home. It is appropriate to wait at least 24 to 48 hours postoperatively before initiating physical therapy. In many cases, the extent of hydrocephalus prior to surgery will affect the decision about the baby's return to oral feeding, position changes, range of motion exercises, and normal handling in the upright position. Premature aggressive handling after surgery is not safe, particularly for the baby with a very large head circumference. Intracranial pressure can drop dramatically after shunt insertion, and vascular insult can occur if the baby is held upright prematurely.[38]

Physical Therapy for the Infant with Spina Bifida

Overview

Physical therapy can begin in the early preoperative period before back closure. Ideally, the therapist who provides the preoperative evaluation will continue treating the baby throughout the hospitalization. This same therapist can then provide long-term monitoring and education as the baby progresses to the outpatient department or specialty clinic. This staffing approach provides consistent support for parents during these early, difficult times. Also, the importance of staff continuity becomes increasingly important as the child grows and changes in function occur. The therapist with a good baseline of observations and documentation about the baby can be a valuable resource for the medical team. When a therapist has monitored the baby through the early period of care, the ability to detect subtle changes later is enhanced.[38]

Manual Muscle Testing

A manual muscle test by the physical therapist can provide objective information regarding the presence of active movement and the quantity of muscle power present in the baby's lower extremities (Display 5-2). Manual muscle testing should be performed before back surgery whenever possible. Testing is repeated approximately 10 days after surgery, then at 6 months, and yearly thereafter. The goal of these early testing sessions is to assist the medical staff in identifying the level of the back lesion by assessing the lower extremity movement or lack thereof.[38]

Consideration must be given to positioning of the baby for the muscle test during the early stage of care. Depending on the status of the back lesion or surgical site and to protect the involved area, the infant's position may be limited to prone or side-lying. Although these positions make it difficult to test the hip rotators accurately, careful observation and palpation should allow for identification of most other muscle groups (Figs. 5-4 and 5-5).

DISPLAY 5-2

Information Provided by Manual Muscle Testing for Children with Spina Bifida

Baseline analysis for use in long-term comparisons
Assessment of remaining muscle function
Evaluation of muscular imbalance at each joint
Prediction of the degree and character of existing deformity
Prediction of potential for future deformity
Assistance in determining the need for surgery and bracing

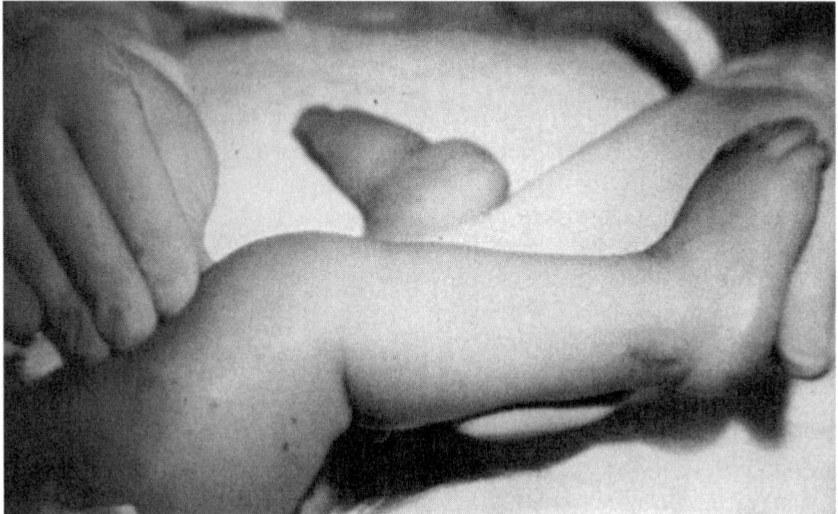

Figure 5-4 ▪ Palpation and observation of the quadriceps muscle during a preoperative assessment of the function of the lower extremities.

A motor level is assigned according to the last intact nerve root found. Identification of this motor level allows consistency of communication among professionals involved with the baby. However, children assigned to the same motor level will vary widely in their muscle function, so it is very important to locate and grade each individual muscle as it becomes feasible.[43]

Extraneous factors may influence movement ability during the infant's first hours of life. The

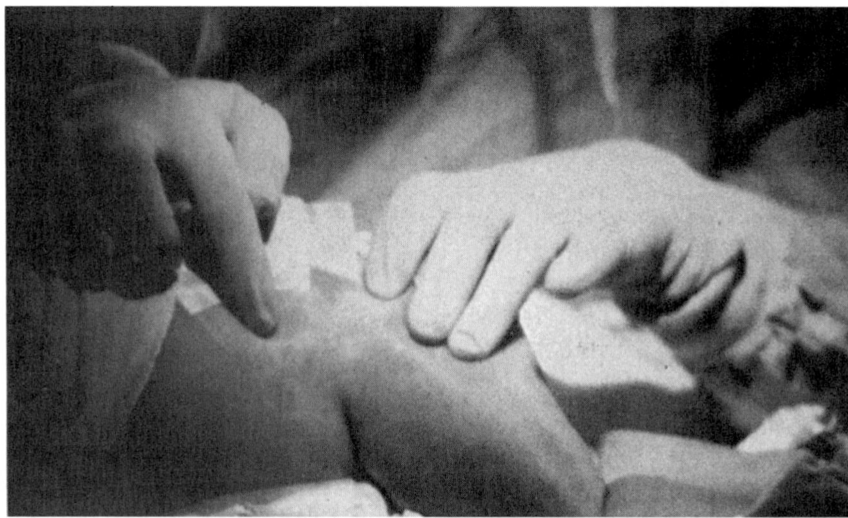

Figure 5-5 ▪ Stimulation of the infant as a means of eliciting movement for testing the gluteus maximus and medius muscles.

effects of maternal anesthesia, increased cerebral pressure from hydrocephalus, and general lethargy and fatigue from a difficult or long labor may depress spontaneous movements. Conversely, these same factors may render the baby hyperirritable when stimulated. Tickling the baby above the level of the lesion or around the neck and face is a stimulus to keep the baby moving. Movements of the extremities can be observed and contractions palpated by stabilizing the limb proximally. Proper limb stabilization is necessary to avoid misinterpreting the origin of a movement. The principles for muscle testing in this population are much the same as those for older patients. Gentle resistance to movement at one part of the leg may help increase the strength of a movement at a distal part of the limb. Allowing movement to occur at only one joint at a time will allow a more accurate interpretation. For example, holding the hip and knee firmly in either partial flexion or extension and preventing movement at those joints will enable the therapist to detect weak ankle motion that might otherwise have gone unnoticed. After locating each area of movement, the therapist must then assess the strength of the muscle responsible for the observed movement. Above all, patience and ingenuity will improve the accuracy of this measure of the baby's motor ability.[38,44]

The therapist should note whether or not muscles are functioning, which muscles are strong and can move a joint through its entire range, and which are weak and can move the joint only partially. This distinction will make determination of the motor level more precise. The ability to distinguish between active and reflexive movement, although sometimes difficult during the early period, can facilitate identification of the lesion level.[44]

Reflex movement is common in infants with thoracic paralysis. In these patients, there is no activity at the hip joint, but movement is noted distally at the knee or ankle. This movement, which looks like fasciculations of the muscle belly with a weak, continuous movement at the joint, may be seen when the baby is sleeping or when the other joints in that limb are not moving. The movement is usually observed in a flexor muscle and may be seen at the Achilles tendon in the form of plantar flexion. Reflex movements represent sparing of local reflex arcs. However, cortical control of the movement has been interrupted by the spinal defect. This reflex movement is of concern because of its involuntary nature and because it is unopposed by an active antagonist at the same joint. Therefore, this unchecked reflex activity can become a deforming force that often requires surgical intervention. The movement is often misleading to staff and family who may interpret the movement as a useful, functional motion. However, because the motion is not cortically initiated, it seldom has any functional value.[38]

Manual muscle testing grades can be modified until the child can be positioned appropriately for gravity and gravity-eliminated responses. Modification of testing procedures is also suggested until the child can follow verbal cues and be tested with resistance so as to increase the consistency and reliability of results. One successful method developed at Children's Memorial Hospital in Chicago uses an X to indicate the presence of strong movement, or O for an absent response, T for trace movement (when contraction is palpated but movement cannot be seen), and an R to indicate reflex movement. This scheme of grading, when combined with the existing scale of 0 through 5, or "absent" to "normal" classifications, provides significant information about the lower extremities.

This evaluation can help predict muscle imbalance and the consequential potential for deformity. If a deformity is present, early muscle testing can identify whether the cause of the limitation is passive, as a result of malpositioning in utero, or active, resulting from muscle imbalance around the joint. Distinguishing the cause of joint limitation is important for the orthopedic surgeon who may wish to operate early on the lower extremities. The surgeon will want to spare potentially useful muscle function and eliminate movement that will only be deforming in nature. If the stimulus for movement is questionable, the surgeon may choose to wait until the child is older and a more accurate evaluation is possible before deciding on the type of surgery.[43]

Some centers have attempted to use electromyographic (EMG) studies to evaluate lower extremity innervation. EMG studies are interesting from an academic standpoint but offer little functional information about the baby and are not widely regarded as valuable.

It is also of interest that poor correlation exists between early manual muscle testing and the child's future level of function. Future function depends upon strength of the lower extremity musculature, the child's total CNS function, motivation, intellectual capacity, and the family's capacity for long-term support and interest. These variables are only a few factors that can influence the functional potential of the growing child with spina bifida. They affect the child's success at using the movements present in the lower extremities. These concerns are addressed in greater detail in subsequent sections of this chapter.[46]

Results of early manual muscle tests can be compared with later tests in order to monitor the child's neuromuscular stability. It is a pleasant surprise to find increased movement or strength after back closure, but any decrease in movement must immediately be brought to the attention of the neurosurgeon. Deterioration of lower extremity motor function may indicate a surgical error, the development of hydromyelia, or a tethered spinal cord, each of which requires neurosurgical intervention.[47]

Range of Motion Assessment

Preliminary assessment of range of motion (ROM) can be performed prior to back closure. Normal neonates have flexion contractures of up to 30 degrees at the hips, 10 to 20 degrees at the knees, and ankle dorsiflexion of up to 40 or 50 degrees. Limitations in ROM in the baby with spina bifida should not be considered an indication for immediate and aggressive stretching. Early limitations of range require a safe plan of management for several weeks. When it becomes apparent that limitations will be both severe and long-lasting, a long-term plan can be developed that will likely include surgical correction.[48,49]

Several common limitations are seen in the neonate with spina bifida. Extreme tightness of the hip flexors is common in the child with motor level involvement at L-2 to L-3 or L-3 to L-4 owing to the presence of a strong iliopsoas with no opposing force offered from weak or absent hip extensors. Hamstrings, which exert a secondary hip extension force, are also lacking. Adductor tightness is also likely as a result of adductor innervation and the absence of the antagonist gluteus medius. If the baby has an insufficient range of hip flexion to tolerate prone positioning, the neurosurgeon and nursing staff must be informed in an effort to prevent possible fractures of the femur. Adapted prone positioning, with legs draped over a raised platform in the operating room, may be indicated during back closure. A modified prone or side-lying position postoperatively is safest. The physical therapist is often the first to note the need for special positioning following the preoperative assessment of range of motion.[50]

Dorsiflexion or a calcaneous deformity at the ankle is a common contracture seen at birth. The child with L-5 innervation has strong dorsiflexion, provided by the anterior tibialis and toe extensors, but weak or absent toe flexors and lack of plantar-flexion from the gastrocnemius/soleus group. Plans may call for splinting the ankle at 90 degrees for optimal alignment during the early days in the hospital. In addition to splinting, gentle passive exercise often helps reduce this deformity.

Provided that the baby is medically stable and the physician agrees, daily ROM exercise for the lower extremities can begin at bedside as early as the day after back closure. Although options are limited after surgery, prone and side-lying positions are adequate to perform all motions needed in the lower extremities at this time.[8,38,50]

Postoperative Physical Therapy

In order for the physical therapist to develop a complete and appropriate program for the infant who has undergone back closure and shunting, the results of both the neurologic and orthopedic evaluations must be considered. To be most effective, the therapist should also be sensitive to the state of the family members, who will have begun to visit their baby more regularly.

COMMUNICATION

In most cases, parents of infants with spina bifida experience a very different and more difficult postpartum period than had been anticipated. Their baby was probably transferred to a tertiary care facility shortly after birth. Often, the needs of the recovering mother are superseded by the needs of the father and other family members to attend to the infant. Inaccurate information about spina bifida, in general, and their child, in particular, may further compromise family coping skills during this physically and emotionally difficult time. It has been reported that parents are often told by staff members that their child will be mentally retarded, will never walk, and will require institutionalization. These professionals, although well-intentioned, are not experienced in current methods of evaluation and treatment of children with spina bifida and may only recall information from a previous era in which a bleak outlook for these babies was the norm rather than the exception. This misinformation causes many parents to become confused and frustrated, especially when the specialty team in the hospital presents apparently conflicting information. Communication between the therapist and other team members is important. All persons working with the infant must know and understand each other's findings. Information given to the family must be appropriate and consistent and should always be presented in a sensitive manner.[6]

Reflecting a positive and caring attitude during treatment sessions is an important objective for the physical therapist, as this approach may help normalize the family's involvement with the infant. A home program can be taught to the family immediately. This is a constructive way for the therapist to begin interacting with family members and to facilitate their interaction with the infant. The therapist should encourage the family to observe and participate in the infant's care during hospitalization in order to prepare them for providing care at home. Waiting to educate the family until the last few days of hospitalization places increased stress on the family members, who must learn much from many people in a short time. An unexpectedly quick discharge may also leave no time for family education, which should be spread over the entire period of hospitalization, with follow-up sessions scheduled during outpatient or clinic visits.

EXERCISE

Passive ROM exercises should be brief and should be performed only two or three times each day. The therapist can combine individual leg movements into patterns of movement so that the family need only learn three or four patterns for the home program. An example would be to combine flexion of the hip and knee of one leg, while holding the opposite leg in full extension. With the baby supine, both hips can be abducted at the same time, leaving only the foot and ankle to be done individually[36] (Figs. 5-6 and 5-7).

These ROM exercises are performed gently with the hands placed close to the joint being

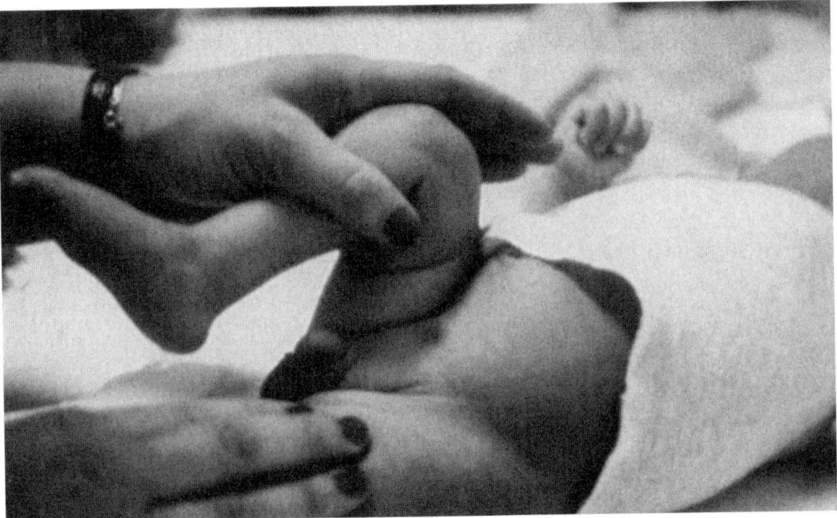

Figure 5-6 ▪ Exercises for range of motion of the lower extremities. Full flexion of one hip and knee is combined with an extension of the opposite extremity.

moved in order to use a short lever arm, thereby preventing unnecessary stress to soft tissue and joint structures. Several repetitions of each pattern, holding the joint briefly at the end of the range, should maintain and may increase ROM in joints with mild or moderate limitations. If severe limitations exist, exercise of the area affected may require additional time and repetitions. Aggressive stretching should be avoided, regardless of the severity of the joint limitation.

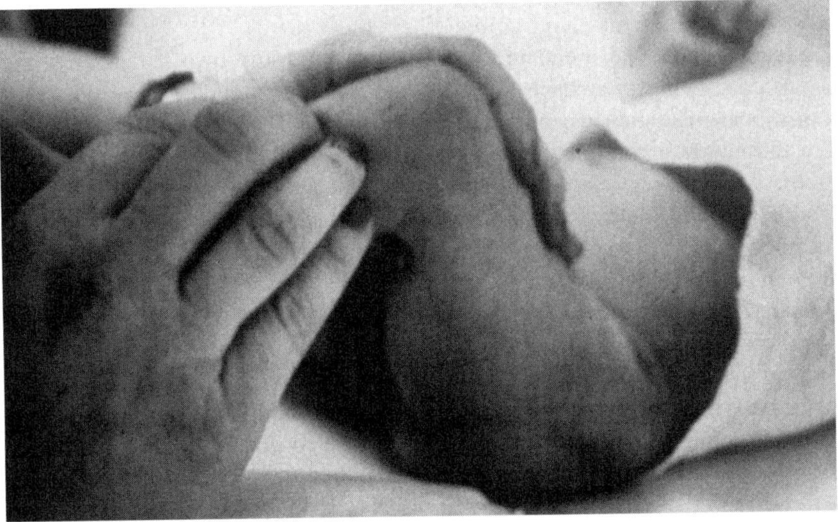

Figure 5-7 ▪ Placement of the hand for a range of motion exercise of the knee. Note the use of a short lever arm.

By participating in the educational process and exercise program during this early time, parents are encouraged to touch and move their baby's legs while being observed by the therapist. Opportunities to handle their baby with supervision can help alleviate concern that many families express about further injuring the infant. With the therapist's comforting and supportive words, the exercise program offers a valuable opportunity for positive parent–child interaction.

Passive ROM exercises must continue throughout the child's life. The goal is that the child will ultimately learn to perform the exercises independently. Passive exercise is often forgotten by therapists and parents as the child becomes more active, starts crawling, and therapy shifts to concentrate on gait training. Although many therapists consider the latter activities to be adequate to maintain range, regardless of the level of motor activity, only the innervated portions of the limb are being actively moved. If ROM exercises are discontinued, contractures will develop. For many children, contractures may develop over years, but for others, range is lost within a short time. With loss of range, function will also diminish.[8,16,38]

POSITIONING AND HANDLING

The physical therapist often assumes responsibility for developing a program of positioning for the hospitalized baby. Although many positioning options are available as discharge nears, options during the first few postoperative days may be limited to prone or side-lying positions. As the child's medical status stabilizes and tolerance to movement improves, it is advisable to avoid leaving the child immobile for long periods. Handling and carrying strategies can be practiced by the therapist and then recommended to the parents. Finding a comfortable chair is most important, and once seated, the therapist or family member can hold the child prone over the lap, rocking or swaying slowly side to side. This position is restful for the parent and provides novel movement for the infant. The baby may also enjoy a slow walk around the hospital floor while being held up and slightly over one of the parent's shoulders. This position gives the infant an opportunity to attempt to raise its head and look around. If a supine position is contraindicated, parents may gently cradle the infant prone across their forearms as they walk or sit. These positions will provide the family with a repertoire of acceptable handling methods when they come to visit their baby. Parents may feel less awkward if they do not need a nurse or therapist to hand them the baby on each visit. These positions are also nonthreatening for the infant, who needs time to recover and who will not respond well to aggressive handling of the trunk, head, or extremities. One must remember that the primary postoperative goals for such infants are uncomplicated healing of the back wound, speedy recovery from shunt insertion, and discharge from the hospital.[38]

Short periods of supine and supported upright sitting in the therapist's arms should not affect the course of back wound healing. A variety of positions helps normalize the baby's experiences during waking hours, while eating, or quietly observing the surroundings. These short periods are also useful for the therapist, who can note the baby's responses to gravity in these positions, feel for changes in muscle tone, and observe any significant asymmetries, particularly through the shoulders and neck. Documenting this information will provide a useful baseline against which to compare later developmental findings.[6,8,38]

Families should first watch, then try to duplicate, the activities recommended for their baby. If a parent does not show some hesitation or anxiety on first handling the baby, it may indicate a poor understanding of the baby's condition and may contribute to subsequent poor judgment in other areas of care. Even for families with experience raising other children, some level of fear or anxiety at first is a healthy sign.

The therapist can begin to "role release" as the hospitalization proceeds, delegating to the parents some ROM and handling activities. As this change in roles occurs, the therapist can begin to concentrate on other areas of the child's plan of care. At many hospitals, the therapist is asked to repeat the lower extremity manual muscle test prior to the infant's discharge.

The therapist can also observe the baby's state, noting changes secondary to hydrocephalus and shunt insertion, so as to provide additional baseline information that may help identify a later shunt malfunction. When a malfunction occurs, in addition to the signs and symptoms presented in Table 5-1; a change in the baby's tone and responsiveness to movement may also be noted.

The family should be encouraged to be active in gathering information about their infant. They should be encouraged to play with and observe the baby, not only to foster positive interaction but also to aid the medical staff in assessing the infant's function. Interaction with the medical team becomes less frequent as the child grows and becomes increasingly medically stable. Observations by parents can help identify problems at an early stage so that appropriate medical care can be sought.

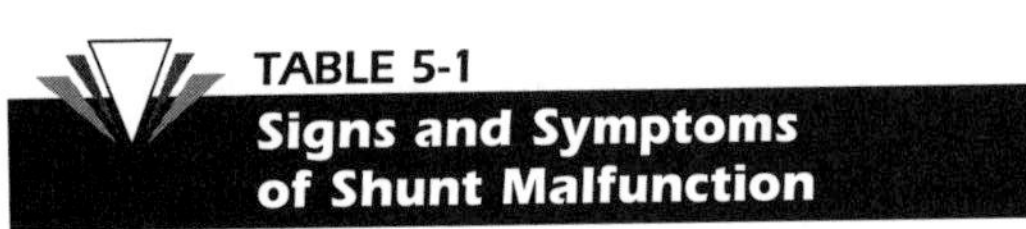
TABLE 5-1
Signs and Symptoms of Shunt Malfunction

Infants

Bulging fontanelle	High-pitched cry
Vomiting	Irritability
Change in appetite	Lethargy
"Sunset" sign of eyes	Seizures
Edema, redness along shunt tract	Exclusive rate of growth of head circumference
	Thinning of skin over scalp

Toddlers

Vomiting	Lethargy
Irritability	Seizures
Headaches	New nystagmus
Edema, reddness along shunt tract	New squint

School-Aged Children

Headaches	Vomiting
Lethargy	Seizures
Irritability	Decreased school performance
Edema, redness along shunt tract	Personality changes
Handwriting changes	Memory changes

SENSORY ASSESSMENT

The physical therapist should perform a sensory assessment of the neonate with spina bifida. To gather information about possible sensory deficits, the therapist should try to ascertain areas of the infant's lower extremities that are sensitive or insensitive to touch. This sensory information, along with the results of muscle testing, can be used to accurately establish the level of the spinal lesion. One reason for the early assessment is to find the level of intact sensation so that the therapist can stimulate active motion. It is the novice clinician who strokes the plantar surface of the foot, expecting to make the child move. This technique is successful only when the infant has intact sensation to the sacral nerve roots. Most infants with spina bifida have a higher level of insensitivity. The therapist may find that the level of motor function and sensation may not be similar in both legs. Early results of sensory testing may be inaccurate, depending on the state of the infant. In addition, it may be difficult to accurately assess all sensory modalities in the newborn infant (light touch, deep pressure, temperature, etc.).

As sensory findings become more stable and reproducible, the information can be shared with the family, who must become educated about their child's skin anesthesia. Educating parents about skin care for the baby is often the shared responsibility of the nursing and therapy staffs. It is sometimes difficult for parents to understand the concept that their baby has areas of the lower body and legs that are insensitive to touch. The therapist can help the family discover this information on their own. Using a gentle touch, caress, or tickle, a family member can map out areas of responsiveness when the infant is awake but quiet. The therapist should not use a pine or other sharp object to demonstrate this testing. The baby's response to a pinprick is no more valid than its response to a gentle caress, and a sharp object may increase the parent's anxiety and concern about the baby's medical care.

Insensitive areas of the lower extremities require additional protection from use and abuse because the child will be unaware of injury to denervated areas. For example, families must always test the temperature of bathwater prior to immersing the child. The infant's legs and feet should always be protected while crawling. Prior to placing the infant on the floor to play, a search for hidden objects in the carpet may prevent an accidental injury from loose carpet tacks or a small toy. Socks or booties will also help prevent problems when children begin to reach for and bite their toes, around the are of 6 to 8 months.

As the infant grows, skin insensitivity continues to be a problem. Application of new shoes or braces, for instance, requires vigilant attention to fit and avoidance of pressure areas will prevent sores or abrasions.

Normal sensation keeps the typical person from sitting immobile for long periods. Intact sensory feedback causes individuals to shift around frequently and change their weight distribution, thereby relieving pressure. Persons with areas of insensitivity, however, tend to develop skin problems secondary to sitting because they do not shift their weight, change their position, or relieve pressure. Similarly, typical persons are able to adjust their gait to avoid abrasion when there is pressure from an ill-fitting shoe. Such readjustment does not occur with the child who has spina bifida, as areas of pressure are not perceived by the child with abnormal sensation. It is important, therefore, to introduce any new orthosis gradually. The orthotic should be worn for only a few hours each time, and the skin should be inspected to determine whether any pressure areas are present. When areas of redness consistently last for longer than 30 minutes, an adjustment of the orthosis is indicated. This plan for skin accommodation is best implemented over a weekend or in the evening, when the child has more time at home. It is best not to send the child for a full day of school with a new orthosis until proper fit is ensured. Time spent addressing these issues initially may save the child from losing valuable time later as a result of immobility, serious infections, or additional hospitalizations.[8,16,38]

Care for the Young Child

Ongoing Concerns and Issues

After the initial medical care for the child with spina bifida, a plan of long-term care should be developed. Various approaches to continued care are seen throughout the United States, with many children seen by specialists located in one institution. Conversely, a primary care pediatrician may choose to refer the child to professionals in several locations as specific needs are identified. Professionals in the community who are affiliated with early intervention programs or private offices may provide care, but when care is divided among several sites, a new role may emerge for the parents. They may be forced to become case managers for their child to facilitate continuity of care and communication among the professionals. This added responsibility may present a large burden for many families and may result in less-than-optimal care for their children. It appears that, because of the multiple specialty areas needed to provide comprehensive care for children with spina bifida, care may be delivered best by experienced professionals who work together as a coordinated team. That is why many pediatric facilities attempt to organize an interdisciplinary clinic for children with spina bifida, where several primary specialists can see the child on the same day. Families are encouraged to continue their child's care at a spina bifida specialty clinic if at all possible. With a team of specialists working together to complement one another, both the child and parents can benefit. Communication is facilitated and expedited with professionals in one location. Information can be shared to increase learning and maintain a current outlook. If problems are detected, the necessary personnel are present to address the concern without the need for another appointment. With consistency and coordination, trust in the professional staff can develop more easily, thereby enabling the family to be less stressed and potentially better able to cope with their child's needs.[6,8,38,51]

The child will need to return frequently to the clinic during the first year of care for evaluation by various specialists. The neurosurgeon will monitor the status of the back closure, hydrocephalus, and shunt (Display 5-3).[6,8] The orthopedist will evaluate limb flexibility, strength, and joint integrity. Splints and surgery are planned to prepare the child for standing (Display 5-4).[8,38] The urologist will monitor bowel and bladder function, assess renal status at regular intervals, and plan a course of care that includes intermitting catheterization and pharmacologic management (Display 5-5).[52–54] A bowel program that may involve periodic toileting, diet, medication, and biofeedback and behavior modification may be implemented to attain fecal continence.

As the child stabilizes in each of the specialty areas, visits to the clinic will become less frequent. It is not unusual for the child to be seen at 6-month intervals over several years and then yearly if there are no ongoing problems or major concerns. However, more frequent visits are necessary when a chronic problem requires close monitoring or treatment.

DISPLAY 5-3

Goals of Neurosurgical Care for Patients with Spina Bifida

Assess the location and size of the back defect
Perform closure of the back defect
Assess the extent of lower extremity paralysis
Assess and treat hydrocephalus
Monitor the function of the ventricular shunt
Monitor the patient for acute and chronic CNS abnormalities
Monitor the patient for CNS deterioration, tethered cord, and hydromyelia

DISPLAY 5-4

Goals of Orthopedic Surgical Care for Patients with Spina Bifida

Prevent joint contracture
Correct musculoskeletal deformities
Prevent skin breakdown from structural malalignment
Provide resources to achieve best mobility
Monitor the patient for CNS deterioration, tethered cord, and hydromyelia

Developmental Difficulties

It has become apparent that CNS deficits exist in a number of children with spina bifida. In many cases, the effects of the deficits will have a

DISPLAY 5-5

Goals of Urologic Care in Patients with Spina Bifida

Preserve renal function
Provide for adequate bladder emptying
Provide for urinary continence
Monitor the patient for CNS deterioration, tethered cord, and hydromyelia

negative impact on gross motor, fine motor, perceptual motor, and cognitive function. The effects of these deficits can be more detrimental than the lower extremity paralysis or hydrocephalus that initially accompanies the condition. The Chiari II malformation has been identified and studied for several decades but only in recent years has there been mention of this malformation as it relates to CNS dysfunction. Using MRI, a more sophisticated imaging system than previously available, structural abnormalities have been identified visually.[21] The specific extent of anatomic abnormalities and severity of the Chiari II can be determined by MRI. However, as previously noted, the clinical effects of the malformation in a particular child still cannot be predicted.

Up to 85% of children with spina bifida have low tone, with minimal to moderate developmental delay. Delayed and abnormal head and trunk control, righting, and equilibrium responses are the most common difficulties. Eventually, these delays may be attributed to the Chiari II malformation, as children with only hydrocephalus do not exhibit movement problems with the same frequency or severity as those with both spina bifida and hydrocephalus.[8,38,55–58]

CNS problems are apparent early in the baby's life. Prolonged instability of the head and upper body is noted in the baby with spina bifida. When parents carry, lift, or move their young infant, the child with poor neck stability may retain the startle response longer than the normal infant. Often, parents compensate for this by supporting the baby's head in a manner that is more protective than usual so as not to elicit the startle response. This additional support begins a cycle in which the added support further limits the experiences and opportunities for motor behavior the baby receives. This limitation reduces the chances for the child to practice independent head control and may prolong the deficit.

The typical baby spends time in various positions from the beginning of life and experiences the effects of gravity on the head and body. Typical infants will begin to stabilize their head over the shoulders in the supported upright position. This response is seen before the baby can lift its head from a prone or supine position. As the infant gains control of the head in space, a feedback mechanism develops between the baby and parent in which the baby communicates the need for support. Progressively less support is given, and new ways to carry the infant are attempted as the baby's head becomes more stable. The development is most apparent when the baby is held upright in the parent's arms while being carried. At first, the parent's hand is placed behind the baby's head to prevent it from falling backward. Several weeks later, we see this supporting hand only when parents raise or lower the baby. In just a few additional months, no guarding of the head is required when the baby is upright.

In the infant with normal tone, there is physiologic stability of the head that is not present in the infant with hypotonus. Joint proprioception through the cervical spine and the normal stretch reflexes of the soft tissue structures of the neck permit the baby's head to fall slowly into gravity, with movement or position change, but only to a small degree. The infant can hold the head reasonably steady without much active participation.

The head of an infant with low tone as a result of spina bifida will fall further forward or sideways before these stabilizing responses occur. The responses to gravity may be slow and weak. A mechanical disadvantage is added as the baby grows and the head becomes larger and heavier, and the task of head righting is made more difficult by the additional weight and weak musculature.

When the infant with spina bifida is placed in various positions and attempts to stabilize the head, compensatory patterns of movement may develop to provide some degree of success. Elevation of the shoulders is considered to be developmentally immature alignment for the infant who should have head stability by 4 months of age. This less mature method of head stabilization also interferes with the development of righting skills owing to inappropriate use of the neck musculature. Also, the upper arms are held stiffly at a time when the infant should be experimenting with and enjoying increased movement and abilities of the upper extremities.

Several months later, the child with insufficient trunk strength and stability to maintain the body upright against gravity may use the upper extremities as a prop while sitting. The shoulders remain elevated to provide stability for the head. The arms are held in internal rotation with scapular protraction. The forearms are pronated with wrist and hand flexion. Weight bearing on the hands is limited to the radial aspect. Without development of further head and trunk control, the child may remain stuck, unable to move into or out of sitting. To assist with positional changes, the motivated child may develop abnormal strategies to move. These strategies are usually passive, involving little muscle activity from the neck and trunk, and thus do not help to improve the strength and coordination of the body. The child may throw the head to one side and collapse, or may lean forward over the legs to crawl out of the sitting position.

This pattern of propping is also seen when the baby attempts to lift the head and look around while in a prone position. Side-to-side weight shifting over the hands and arms will not occur. When the child lifts an arm to reach for a toy, the prop is removed, stability is lost, and the head drops. Even with experience, this pattern does not improve. The child may tilt the head to one side to perform a weight shift and to free one arm to reach, but the head cannot be maintained upright against gravity.

When a typical baby lifts an arm to reach for an object, a weight shift to one side occurs. The head and chest remain elevated, and the trunk, neck, and lower extremity musculature actively stabilize the baby's position. The baby does not depend on upper extremity support to lift the head. With weight shifting and movement in a prone position, the arms become more externally rotated while the forearms increase in supination with pressure across the ulnar surface of the hands. Increasing tactile stimulation across the hands helps reduce the sensitivity of the grasp response. The normal upper extremity weight-bearing progression aids in the opening of the baby's flexed fingers and hands. Experiences in the prone position also provide considerable proprioception through the joints of the upper extremities. The child with spina bifida needs coordination and strength in the upper extremities to use assistive devices for ambulation and to perform paper and pencil tasks in school. But using the upper extremities in lieu of head and trunk support will limit the motor experiences of the arms and hands and may also contribute to acquisition of abnormal truncal skills.

Paralysis of the lower extremities decreases the sensorimotor stimulation that the legs provide to the remainder of the body. Tactile, proprioceptive, and vestibular input is reduced secondary to the motor and sensory limitations of the legs. The degree to which this loss affects the individual depends on the movement and sensation available in the legs and the child's CNS status. If a child is able to explore the environment actively and independently, he or she will gain knowledge about his or her body in relation to the environment. A typical baby has a vast number of experiences, and learning is gleaned from many modalities. When movement and exploration are limited, learning is affected. Lower extremity paralysis, in combination with low tone and poor head control, makes movement difficult for many children with spina bifida, thereby decreasing the child's motivation to move. With negative reinforcements for movement, more sophisticated sensorimotor skills and learning can be hampered.

Therapists must appreciate the impact of these impediments on learning in children with spina bifida. This information can be used to facilitate and encourage handling strategies that enhance more normal development and movement skills.[59–65]

Handling Strategies for Parents

Instructions for parents should begin before the child is discharged from the hospital and should continue until adequate and acceptable function is observed. Parents should be aggressive in their approach but tempered by the medical status and age of their child. Teaching sessions should include verbal instruction as well as many opportunities for the parents to observe the therapist handling their baby.

Although parents and staff often focus on the most conspicuous deficit—lower extremity paralysis—the physical therapist has the responsibility of also incorporating into the instructional program information that will promote the family's understanding of and development of gross, fine, and perceptual motor abilities above the waist. Gradual instruction can be offered based on the status of the infant and the capacity of the family. Frequent gentle reminders can be given in early treatment sessions about the spinal defect and the CNS problems seen in some children. The family should be warned of potential problems, especially the child's difficulty in developing control of the head, neck, and trunk. The therapist may describe means of lessening or preventing such problems.

It is initially useful to teach the family to look for signs suggesting these additional difficulties. Hypotonus in the child may cause a delay in acquisition of antigravity head control in all directions.[55] Parents should not permit the baby to be held or positioned with the head at severe angles to the body. These positions will allow muscles and other soft tissues to overstretch. The infant who lacks active neck flexion will be asymmetric in a supine position and will have difficulty turning the head from side to side. Abnormal compensatory patterns of movement will be seen when the baby tries to move its head. The prone position, too, may lead to frustration if neck extensor strength is poor. As the infant tires of keeping the head turned to one side, it may begin to cry. In response, the parent may lift the baby or roll it into a different position. By responding in this manner, the parent unknowingly assumes responsibility for a motor skill that the child must master. Parents should be educated that their behavior can interfere with appropriate neck and trunk muscle development that is needed to lift the head correctly.

Literature on normal development indicates that infants acquire head stability in supported upright postures before they can lift their heads from prone or maintain midline control in supine. Gaining the ability to stabilize the head while upright facilitates strengthening of all the musculature needed to lift and control the head while prone or supine (Figs. 5-8 and 5-9). With these thoughts in mind, the therapist can recommend that parents offer their baby with spina bifida experience in all positions, with a strong emphasis on upright postures.[39,43,62]

Parents can be taught to carry their awake, alert child with the head unsupported to facilitate development of head control, but without allowing the head to fall suddenly in an uncontrolled manner, thereby eliciting a startle response. Holding the baby high on the shoulder rather than at the chest level also facilitates development of head control (Fig. 5-10). Another useful strategy is for the parents to sit at a table while holding the baby in a supported sitting position on the table at eye level. In this position, the parent can encourage visual play and can provide experiences for independent head control. The infant could be held around the shoulders at first and then at chest level, depending on its balance ability.

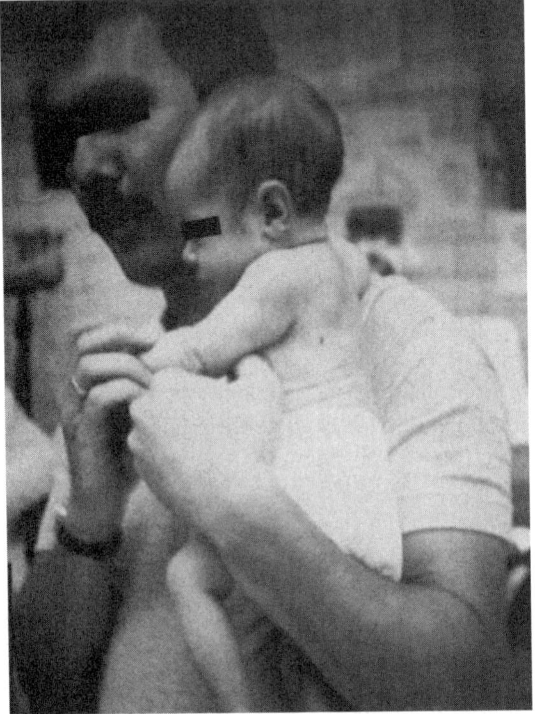

Figure 5-8 ■ Typical infant at 6 weeks of age. The infant is stabilizing the head while in an upright position. Note the erect alignment of the thoracic spine in an infant with normal muscle tone.

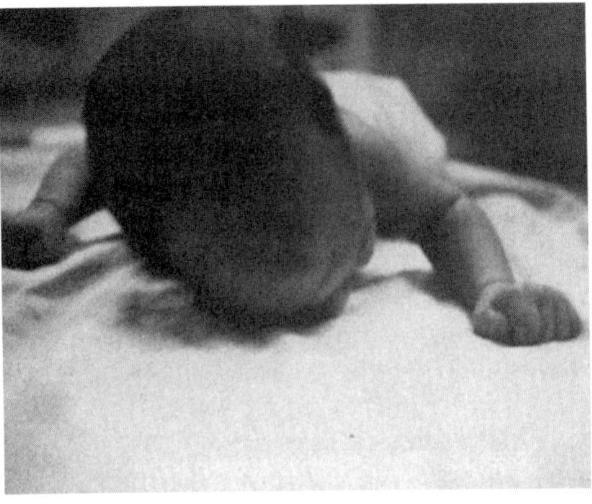

Figure 5-9 ■ The same infant as shown in Figure 5-8 is barely able to elevate the head to turn it from side to side in a prone position.

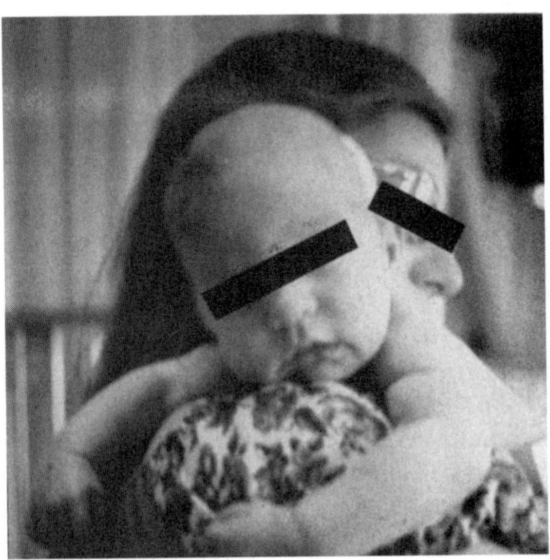

Figure 5-10 ■ Infant is being carried high on the adult's shoulder to stimulate independent movement of the head and an improved position of the upper extremities.

Parents should be instructed to observe the infant for prolonged asymmetries or sensitivity to certain movements. The therapist should demonstrate good, symmetric alignment of the baby in various positions (Fig. 5-11).

Because of CNS deficits, children with spina bifida often require long-term therapeutic programs that may be unavailable or inconvenient to provide through the hospital. Early intervention programs in the community are recommended. Ideally, the community program should provide services for the family and child. The family often needs support and assistance once it leaves the secure environment of the hospital.

This assistance and teaching may be necessary for the family in which there are other children as well as for first-time parents. It is interesting to note that parents with older children who are accustomed to the varying rates of development of typical children may deny or minimize the developmental delays of their child with spina bifida. Time and consistent input are

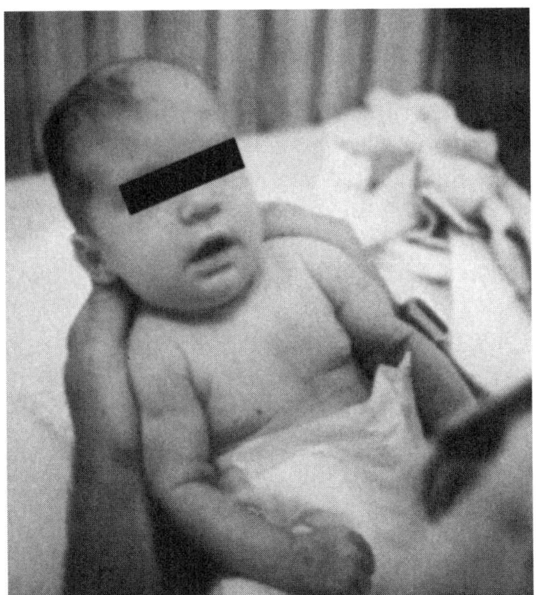

Figure 5-11 ■ This position is suggested for handling an infant in supine position. Note the attempt to provide for a symmetric posture.

required to help parents develop an effective approach to management of their child. A comprehensive program will best provide the support and services for both parents and children.

Physical Therapy for the Growing Child

Developmental Concerns

A mutually acceptable long-range plan of care should be developed cooperatively by the physical therapist, neurosurgeon, orthopedic surgeon, and family. The plan for the young child with spina bifida is based largely on objective findings from the physical therapist's evaluations. Repeated manual muscle tests and careful observation enables the therapist to identify the child's strengths and weaknesses in gross motor development and in movement of the child's lower extremities. Intervention can then be directed at specific needs within both areas of motor function (Display 5-6).

Children with spina bifida need to pursue activities that will improve righting and equilibrium responses of the head and trunk. When the therapist addresses these needs and sees improvement, there is a secondary benefit, too. While stimulating the automatic balance responses against gravity in all positions, active responses in the lower extremities are noted. These responses serve as an important part of the child's exercise program.[38]

Sitting stimulates the child's balance, improves control of the head and trunk, increases the child's visual field, and provides an opportunity for many eye-hand experiences. Head-righting and equilibrium responses can be tested by holding the child around the shoulders and slowly tilting him or her to one side. The infant should respond by returning the head toward the midline. Next, the therapist brings the infant's body to midline and repeats the activity to the other side, to diagonal directions, and straight back. If no response occurs in any direction and

DISPLAY 5-6

Goals of Physical Therapy in Patients with Spina Bifida

- Establish motor level of infant
- Perform periodic muscle testing for comparison purposes
- Instruct the patient and family in a home care program to help prevent deformity
- Provide home program instruction to facilitate motor development as close to chronologic age as is possible
- Assist in determining appropriate orthoses
- Facilitate mobility program for ambulation and wheelchair use, where indicated
- Provide information regarding the patient's neurologic function to physicians
- Monitor the patient for CNS deterioration, tethered cord, and hydromyelia

the child's head hangs, or if the child becomes upset with the activity, the movement may have been too rapid or extended too far. A slower and less challenging tilt is used until a response is noted. As the child's responses to the stimuli become more brisk and strong, the angle of tilt can be increased. As the child improves, support can be moved to the chest or waist and the same activities repeated. During this work, the oblique abdominal and lower extremity musculature will contract, in response to changes in the center of gravity, in an attempt to return the body to midline. As equilibrium responses are strengthened with this type of balance work, active hip flexion, hip adduction and abduction, knee extension, and ankle and foot movement can be elicited. It is interesting to note that children with poor upper body control and muscle strength in the lower extremities that have been graded as "trace" or "poor" by manual muscle testing often improve in leg strengths, secondary to the effects of these head and trunk activities. Therefore, it is recommended that sessions of tilting last 10 or 15 minutes and that many repetitions be provided so as to enhance strengthening of all responses (Fig. 5-12).

Neck and thoracic extensor activity and strengthening are achieved when the child can hold a position of prone extension with the head and thorax held up against gravity without use of the upper extremities. Low back extensors, gluteals, quadriceps, and plantar-flexors will also contract if they are innervated. As the child is tilted from prone slowly to the side with its head erect, strengthening of the neck musculature and head righting and equilibrium reactions in prone will occur. Trunk and lower extremity strengthening can occur by repetition of this movement pattern during routine carrying and handling activities of the infant.

Appropriate handling in the supine position can enhance the child's active head control in

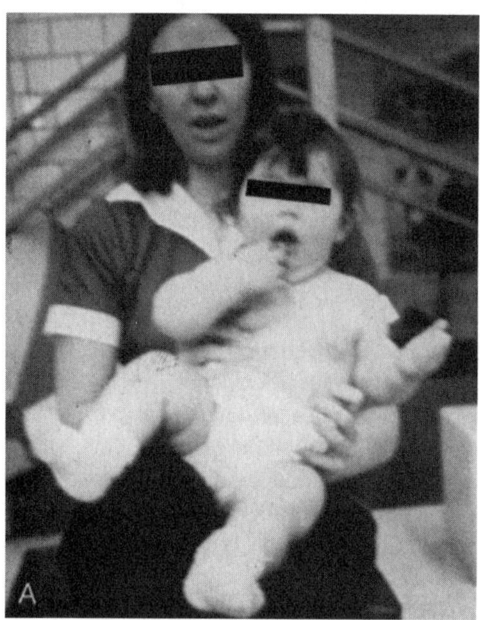

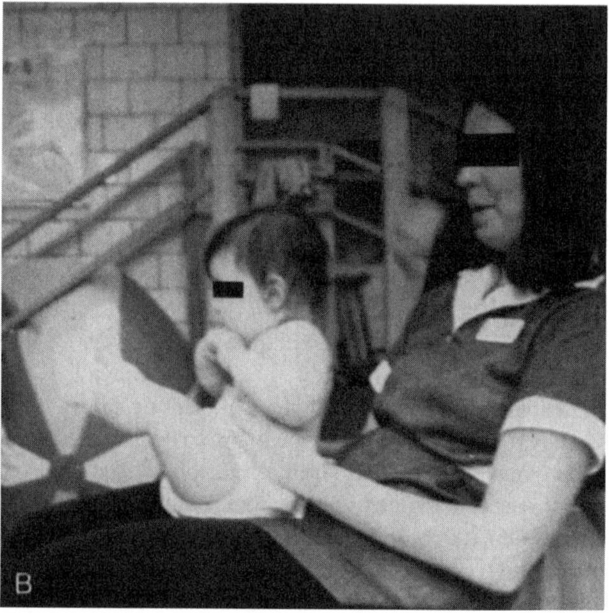

Figure 5-12 ▪ (**A**) and (**B**) Challenging the child's balance responses to elicit more sophisticated upper body abilities and strengthening of the lower extremities as they respond as well.

midline, thus decreasing the asymmetric influence of gravity on the head. The supine position also facilitates bilateral upper extremity play and disassociation of body parts through rotation of the thorax on the lumbar spine, lumbar spine on the pelvis, and lower extremities on the pelvis. When the child holds its legs up and extends them to kick and play against gravity, muscles of the lower extremities, neck, and abdomen are strengthened. Neck and trunk flexors combine with the extensors to provide for good spinal alignment in sitting.

A typical infant, as early as 2 months of age, will bear weight on the lower extremities as a result of the positive support reaction. When this response is discovered by the parents, it usually is included in the repertoire of positions used in playing with and holding the child. A great deal of proprioceptive input is provided by weight bearing. Gravity acting on the body stimulates the joint surfaces in the neck, trunk, and lower extremities. This sensory input is important for body awareness and the perception of body in space. Standing also provides a novel perception of the relationship of the body to the immediate surroundings. When the child with spina bifida bears weight, contact between the femoral head and acetabulum and muscle contractions around the hip joint may help stimulate acetabular development, thereby reducing the likelihood of hip joint dysplasia.

As the child grows, practice in standing will continue to challenge and improve body control and balance against gravity and will stimulate available muscles in the trunk and lower extremities to assist with a more independent stance. Families can be taught to assist their young child with brief periods of standing several times each day until the child can stand with less assistance, or until a standing device is provided (Fig. 5-13).[16,38]

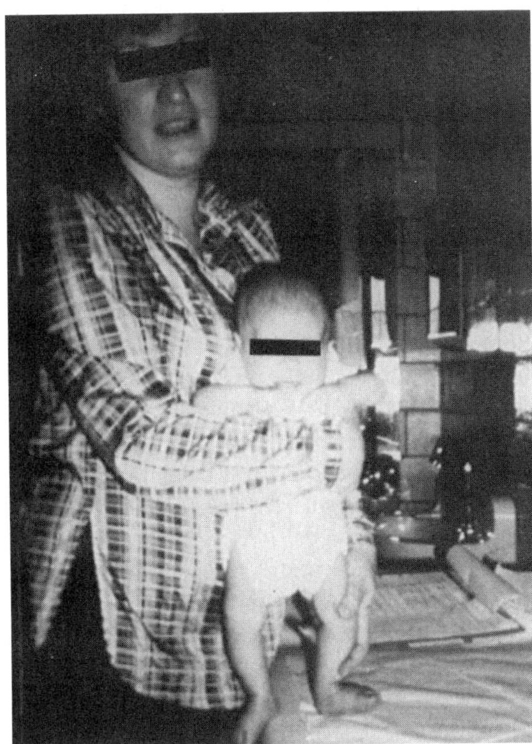

Figure 5-13 ■ Brief periods of standing throughout the day will help provide for well-aligned weight bearing in the child without fully innervated musculature of the lower extremities.

Learning to push and pull with the arms to compensate for weakness in the trunk and neck may allow the child to roll, attain the four-point position, and perhaps, to pull to a stand if lower extremity function is adequate. This progression, with its increased reliance on the arms, will ultimately lead to the child requiring a higher level of bracing than the level of lesion might indicate, as well as use of an assistive device for the unstable body during gait. This higher level of bracing will limit the child's potential despite lower extremity movement. Therefore, for the child with spina bifida, it is not sufficient merely to identify that a developmental milestone has occurred. Rather, it is important to assess the movement qualitatively, including such considerations as the child's ability to perform the movement against gravity, whether the movement is normal, and whether compensatory or abnormal patterns have developed. One can then identify patterns of movement to be enhanced or strengthened as foundations for future skills, as well as movements that should be avoided.[38]

These areas of concern can be incorporated into a safe and appropriate therapeutic regimen. The physical therapy plan should include activities performed in all positions, the use of gravity to challenge the child, and varied and changing movement stimuli to facilitate motor development. By providing these opportunities and experiences, there is an increased likelihood that the child's gross, fine, and perceptual motor abilities will be less negatively affected, and that the gross motor potential will be commensurate with the motor level of the lower extremities.

Infant Devices

The issue of seats and various baby devices should be addressed by the therapist. The available literature on development is consistent in its insistence that all infants need to be active to acquire the strength and motor control necessary to move against gravity, attain erect sitting and standing postures, and walk. The infant must receive and integrate vast amounts of sensory and motor information to build a foundation of knowledge about his or her body and to develop the ability to function effectively within the environment. Infant walkers, jumper seats, swings, bouncer chairs, and the excessive use of infant car seats can have a negative impact on motor development and sensorimotor integration. These devices may further retard the development of the infant with spina bifida who is already at risk for motor delay. (Several of these concerns are explored in greater detail in Chapter 13.)

All infants must experience the upright sitting position because of its importance for learning. This position gives the child a new visual perspective of its surroundings and provides the first sensation of the effects of gravity, the weight of the head, and the work necessary to stabilize the head over the shoulders. However, to practice and gain confidence in these early skills, the infant must be stimulated by movement—for example, while being carried in a parent's arms. The experiences of random and varied weight shifting and tilting as the parent moves and walks are physiologically important as well. Bobbing and jerking movements of the head stimulate stretch reflexes in the joint receptors of the neck, producing muscle contractions that mark the infant's beginning attempts at head control. This stimulation is essential. However, many infant seating devices offer total support. This degree of support is unwise for the infant with low tone and spina bifida who is slow to develop head control. These infants need frequent sessions with activities that challenge the head, neck, and trunk. The infant should be actively moving and turning to see its surroundings and to appreciate gravity acting on its body in different planes. To be passively entertained in seating devices allows little or no active participation in movement or in the learning process. The device passively entertains without offering any development benefits.

Consider the child who has sufficient lower extremity function to successfully move around the room in an infant walker. The child's position is often tilted to one side in the walker, with resultant poor alignment. Coordinated reciprocal movements are not necessary to gain momentum in this device, and weight bearing through the legs is often momentary and sporadic. A thrusting pattern is all that is necessary to propel the device. It is inappropriate to facilitate and strengthen these patterns because thrusting has no carryover for developing coordinated movements or providing stability to the lower extremities or trunk, both of which are vital components for ambulation and standing. Rather, infants should bear weight on their lower extremities while maintaining more normal, erect alignment of the trunk and upper body. In this way, much proprioceptive input is provided to the spine and legs. Parents who are concerned about the "weak" legs of their infant with spina bifida must be guided and encouraged to provide appropriate, active work for the child's whole body. When moving and playing, children use all parts of their body at once. A child who is excited by a bright object will move the arms and lift and kick the legs; these movements will help strengthen the innervated musculature of the legs. Holding the infant in a standing position while offering adequate support will promote control of the upper body while offering stimulation in this upright posture.

Parents often prefer that their infant be allowed to spend short periods in infant seats or walkers because of the enjoyment afforded by the devices. Because most parents strive to keep their children happy and content, the time the infant spends in these devices often increases insidiously, further reducing the time spent moving actively around the floor. In assessing the use of such devices, one must also consider the lifestyle of the family. Many parents spend much time in the car, at the market or shopping center, and other places where the infant will be placed in a supported, seated position. When the time the infant spends sleeping and eating is added to this, it may become apparent that little time is spent in more therapeutic positions. However radical an approach, the therapist may find it best to totally discourage the use of these devices except, of course, in the case of an infant car seat while traveling.[16,38,57,59–61,66]

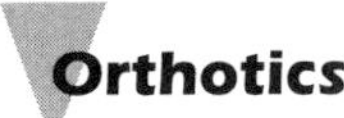

Orthotics

Introduction to Bracing

A discussion of orthotics is most logically approached by grouping the motor levels that require similar orthotic management. Thus, in this chapter, children with thoracic and L-1 to L-3 lesions are considered to have high-level paralysis, children with L-4 to L-5 lesions are considered to have low lumbar paralysis, and those with sacral lesions comprise the final group. Devices for early splinting, preambulation devices, and bracing for standing and ambulation will be discussed for each of the groups. Although the grouped motor levels have similarities, within each group are children with very different patterns of active musculature, strength, and function. Thus, one should remember that each child must be evaluated individually and, depending on the findings, a management plan developed. The information presented here may be useful for the therapist to consider and build on with future experiences.[43]

PHILOSOPHIES OF BRACING

Many clinics have a bracing philosophy that establishes a preset plateau of maximum function for children with spina bifida. In addition, several publications have supported the concept that an ultimate level of mobility exists for children at each motor level. Such a philosophy advocates establishing reasonable expectations for each child because much time, effort, and expense can be spent on orthotic management. This philosophy of bracing is thought, by some, to be an efficient method that supports the notion that functional outcome can be predicted by motor level. A clinic that follows this model would be reluctant to brace a child with a thoracic or high lumbar lesion after the early childhood years as the literature indicates that most adolescents with such lesions are mobile from a wheelchair and have discarded the possibility of ambulation. However, recent research has acknowledged that a number of variables affect the ultimate level of performance of the child, of which lower extremity function is only one. CNS function, motivation, learning capacity, and desire for movement are also very important factors that should be considered when deciding whether to proceed with or terminate an ambulation program. From an ethical standpoint, one might question whether the plateau should be set by anyone other than the patient.

The middle ground may afford a more realistic view. Adopting this approach would mean that thoughts and concerns would be shared among the medical staff, the patient, and the family when establishing goals for bracing and ambulation. Because the patient's needs and abilities could constantly be changing, the goals established would also have to be flexible. Recent changes in medical care for children with spina bifida, as well as advances in orthotics technology, seem to warrant an ongoing analysis and a creative approach to help each child attain an optimal level of performance, regardless of motor level. Achievement of a particular level of function is as important for a child with a low-level lesion as it is for one with a high-level lesion.[16,38,67]

GENERAL PRINCIPLES FOR ORTHOTICS AND GAIT TRAINING

Any discussion of bracing raises the fundamental question of whether the child should be braced high, with levels of bracing removed as motor control is mastered, or whether the child should be braced low, with sections added as the need dictates. Unfortunately, orthotic prescription is imprecise and it is a field that becomes refined with clinical experience. A brace that is applied to a moving, growing, changing child can be considered to be correct only for the period that that child remains exactly as he or she was when evaluated. This period will be shorter for the 2-year-old child than for the 10-year-old child. This means that the 5- or 6-year-old youngster who is growing rapidly and is very active may require frequent brace reevaluations, revisions, and repairs.

In order to make an appropriate brace selection, CNS function and the effects of CNS dysfunction on the child's ability to move must be considered. The orthopedic surgeon, physical therapist, and family should try to gather as much objective information about the child as possible prior to devising an orthotics program. The physical therapist should have spent time with the child and family, and should have an accurate impression of the child's motor ability. Asking parents about their perceptions of their child's motor function can provide insight into the way the family views the child. Differences between at-home and clinic performance can be identified. Parents can simply be asked to describe the ways in which the child likes to play, favorite positions, response to the upright position, degree of assistance needed to change positions, and how the child moves on the floor. (Keep in mind that it is not unusual for a parent to verbalize that the child does not seem ready to be upright.) Many changes in bracing programs are based on sound recommendations from parents, who are observing and working with the child at home.

Regardless of the brace ordered, families must be aware of whom to call and what action must be taken if the brace is inadequate or does not produce the desired result. They must also understand that the failure of, or problems with, the brace do not mean that they or their children are failures or are somehow inadequate. Families should be educated regarding both good and improper fit, when brace modification will be needed, and when it will be appropriate to add or subtract sections of the brace. With this knowledge, parents can contact the therapist or clinic with their findings so that necessary appointments can be made. Remember, changes involving increased support should not be construed as failure, regression, or lack of progress.

Decisions to change the bracing level, unlock joints, or change an assistive device should be made in a thoughtful and considered manner. The child's attitude toward and readiness for gait training plays a large part in the timeliness of these decisions. We can aim for safe and functional ambulation by 5 or 6 years of age in preparation for mobility in school, but given the numerous tasks and skills to be mastered, 5 or 6 years is not a great deal of time to prepare. Parents and therapists may feel rushed when the child is almost ready to begin school, but sufficient time must be allowed for mastery of skills at one stage before progressing to the next. Some families are forceful when expressing their desire to have their child standing and ambulating as soon as possible. The responsible method of practice is to pace the progression of skills slowly to achieve the safest, most secure, and least stressful result for the child. In keeping with this measured approach, only one change at a time should be made to the orthosis or assistive device. Otherwise, it becomes difficult to ascertain which change produced the effects observed.

A well-defined orthotic program should begin as early as the child's first day of life. After the initial evaluation of the child, the physical therapist should discuss with the orthopedic surgeon the deformities present and those likely to occur secondary to muscle imbalance around a joint. The therapist and surgeon should then develop a plan of care, including the necessary orthotics, to address current and anticipated problems. Such an early orthotics program is designed to prepare the child for upright positioning at as close to the typical age as possible. Orthopedic surgery during the first year can be coordinated to achieve the goal of upright posture.[39,68]

Thoracic Level Paralysis

The child with no motor control below the thorax has flaccid lower extremities and is at risk for developing a frog-legged deformity. This posture is common in immobile infants who remain in a supine position for long periods of time. The legs are abducted, externally rotated, and flexed at the hips and knees, with no active motion to counteract the effects of gravity. If the condition is left uncorrected, this frog-legged position will result in the muscles and other soft tissues becoming increasingly tight with time.

Prone positioning, daily ROM exercise, and gentle nighttime wrapping of the legs with elastic bandages into extension and adduction can prevent this deformity. Additional flexibility can be gained using these interventional strategies in areas where minimal to moderate tightness may already exist. As the child grows, a total body splint or total contact orthosis may be used during naps and throughout the night to prevent loss of joint range. Proper fit of the orthosis will prevent limb movement within the brace that can lead to abrasions. Because the child also needs to work on control of the head and trunk, the first orthosis, adapted with wedged rubber soles, can be used for brief periods of standing. During these sessions of standing, the child can practice and become proficient in balance activities of increasing difficulty (Fig. 5-14). Prone lying in the splint is recom-

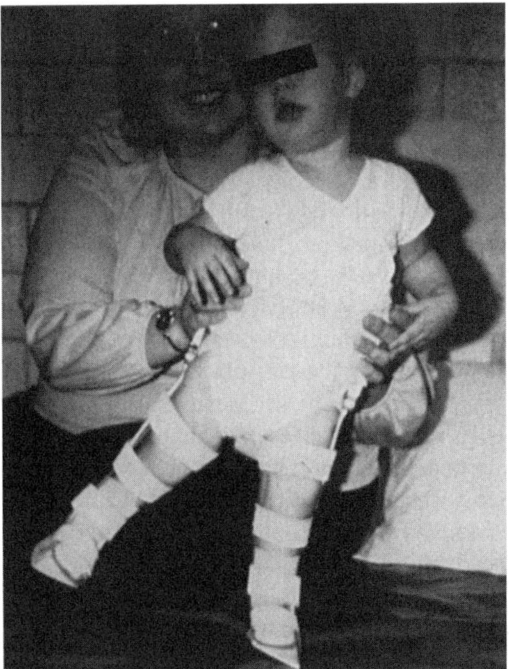

Figure 5-14 ▪ A total contact orthosis with wedged soles may be used for standing and activities involving a shift in weight.

mended to help avoid pressure over the bony prominences, such as the ischial tuberosities, sacrum, and calcaneous. Skin breakdown at these sites is common with persistent supine positioning. Inspection of the skin is essential after each session with the orthosis.

If the child has moderate to severe limitations in ROM, it is inappropriate to use the orthosis to force the limbs into better alignment. That type of problem can be managed best by surgical release of tight soft tissue structures, including the iliotibial band, hip external rotators, and knee flexors. The orthosis can be used after surgery to maintain the desired position and the newly achieved level of flexibility.

A total contact orthosis should always include a thoracolumbar section to stabilize the pelvis and lumbar spine to provide good alignment for the lower extremities. Lacking proper support of the trunk and pelvis, the child can flex the trunk laterally when in the splint, causing malalignment of the lower extremities with adduction of one hip and abduction of the other relative to the pelvis. A plantar-flexion deformity often develops in the child with total limb paralysis. Contractures involving the foot joints will make brace and shoe fit difficult; therefore, a total body orthosis should include a lower leg portion to hold the ankle in a neutral or plantigrade position for weight bearing.

For the older child with a high thoracic lesion who may spend most of the day without braces, a simple splint can be fabricated to maintain good foot position with the child seated in a wheelchair, thus allowing easy shoe fit. It might also be appropriate for such an individual to use a total body orthosis at night in order to decrease the flexion/abduction contracture that can occur in individuals who sit all day.[8,38]

High Lumbar Paralysis

Children with a motor level from L-1 to L-3 will usually exhibit strong hip flexors and adductors but no other significant strength, either poor or fair, at the hips and knees. Such children generally benefit from use of a total body splint. The splint can maintain hip and knee extension with moderate abduction (30 degrees for both legs) if used during sleep. It can also serve as the child's first standing device.

Most children with high lumbar paralysis will require bracing to stand. Bracing is indicated to support the knees and ankles and to provide medial-lateral stabilization at the hips and pelvis. A small number of children with this type of paralysis who have good balance and an intact CNS will ambulate without orthotic control at the hips and pelvis, but they will require bracing above the knees, as well as some type of assistive device. Hip subluxation and dislocation are common in children with high lumbar paralysis owing to significant muscle imbalance around the hip. There has been much discussion and debate regarding the optimal surgical approach for hip problems in such patients. The current concensus is that surgery to relocate the hip is not indicated. This approach avoids many postoperative complications, including a frozen, immobile joint, which may result from an open reduction procedure. This complication may compromise sitting and standing alignment, necessitating additional surgery. Redislocation is common owing to limited stabilization by dynamic forces around the hip. Simple surgical release of soft tissue structures may be needed if active hip flexors and adductors have tightened to the point of restricting range. With unilateral dislocation, an asymmetric pelvis will result if the involved hip becomes limited in adduction and flexion. This asymmetric posture creates an uneven foundation for sitting and standing and interferes with proper fit and alignment of braces. Evaluation for a shoe lift will also be necessary for the child with unilateral dislocation in order to equalize leg lengths with the child upright. When correction of a hip dislocation will be performed, it is appropriate for the physical therapist to be involved with the presurgical evaluation process and later with the patient and family for home program instruction.

When hip dislocation occurs, therapists and parents must continue passive ROM exercises to ensure no additional loss of flexibility. The hips will usually tighten in flexion and adduction as a result of the abnormally positioned femur. There is often fear that additional damage will occur with ROM exercises, but this is seldom, if ever, the case. Rather, more harm is done by discontinuing the exercise.[8,38,68,69]

Orthotics for Children with High Paralysis

When children with T-12 to L-3 motor levels are almost 12 months old and exhibit adequate head control, they should be considered for upright positioning in the A frame (or the Toronto standing frame). This frame can be used for short standing sessions during the day in an attempt to duplicate the activities of typical children who pull to a stand for short periods but are predominantly mobile on the floor (Fig. 5-15). A schedule of upright positioning for 20 to 30 minutes four or five times each day seems manageable for most parents. Because the devices are freestanding, this represents the child's first opportunity to be upright for play without having hands-on assistance from a parent or using the upper extremities for support. Self-feeding and fine motor activities are ideal during this standing time. Parents should be instructed to challenge their child during the standing period by working on head-righting and balance skills. A recommended activity is to slowly tilt the frame in one direction, watching for the child's righting response in the head and trunk, then repeating the tilt in another direction for the first 5 to 10 minutes of each stand-

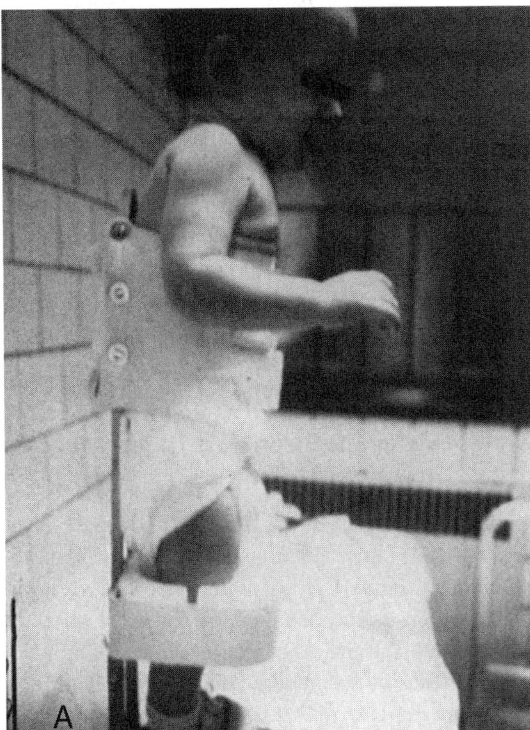

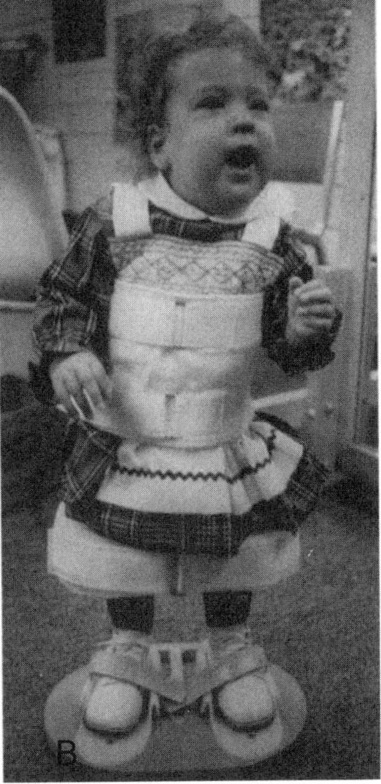

Figure 5-15 ▪ Toronto A frame showing good alignment for standing. (**A**) Side view. (**B**) Front view.

ing session. The frame should be tilted slowly and at a small angle, and all directions should be performed. Based on the child's success, further strengthening of the responses and the musculature involved can be achieved by increasing the angle of tilting. Passive standing in front of the television is not recommended, and unsupervised standing is not advisable because the child's wiggling body may cause the frame to topple.[16,38]

As the child progresses with developmental activities, such as rolling around the floor, getting into and out of a sitting position, and attempting to crawl, the child may show an intolerance for the lack of mobility of the standing frame. This indicates that the child is ready for bracing and ambulation training. Children with moderate to severe CNS deficits and delayed head and upper extremity function may continue to use the standing frames until they are unable to properly fit into the frames (at around 4 to 5 years of age). As the child outgrows the frame, the parapodium or Orlau swivel walker are orthotic options that will provide continued and valuable time in an upright posture while providing adequate support to meet the needs of the child with significant motor delay. Regardless of the device chosen, the child must continue a program of developmental and preambulation skills to improve function in the upper body, neck, trunk, and arms. While in the device, the child can learn to weight-shift, which will cause the device to move forward. The parapodium requires a walker or crutches for progression. The Orlau swivel walker has a ball-bearing plate at its base that allows the device to move forward on a level surface without assistive devices and with only a side-to-side swivel movement by the child. As skills improve, the child can begin ambulation training in either of the devices and may progress to another, less supportive orthosis.[38]

Until recently, the standard hip-knee-ankle-foot orthosis (HKAFO) was the only option for the child with high paralysis. A thoracic corset could be added to the HKAFO for the child with limited trunk control,[70] but this resulted in an extremely immobile child with the potential for exercise ambulation only. Another option—the Louisiana State University reciprocating gait orthosis (RGO)—has since been developed. The RGO uses a system of cables with a dual-action hip joint that flexes one lower extremity while maintaining the opposite hip in locked extension for a stable stance, thereby allowing a reciprocating pattern of gait. A properly fitted RGO provides stability at all lower extremity joints and supports the trunk and pelvis over the legs. Many children who have used the RGO and an assistive device have progressed to a more energy-efficient and safer gait pattern than was possible with the HKAFO. As a child's upper trunk stability improves, the RGO can be modified without decreasing the child's abilities. By retaining the cables and dual-action hip joints but removing the chest strap and thoracic uprights, the child can use the mechanism for an assisted reciprocating gait but with less restriction to the upper body.[71–74]

The isocentric RGO is a new device that eliminates the cable system but maintains the same function as the original RGO. Clinics using the original RGO are slowly switching to the new isocentric model when patients need their first brace, or when the patient's original RGO no longer fits and a new brace is required.[75]

With hip and knee joints locked, the child ambulating with either of these reciprocating braces and an assistive device performs a lateral weight shift onto one leg and leans slightly back at the shoulders to facilitate forward flexion of the unweighted lower extremity. Repeating the weight shift and leaning to the other side produces forward flexion of the opposite lower extremity. This gait pattern requires no active motor function in the lower extremities (Figs. 5-16 to 5-18).[73]

When using the standard HKAFO with pelvic band and locked hip joints, the child can

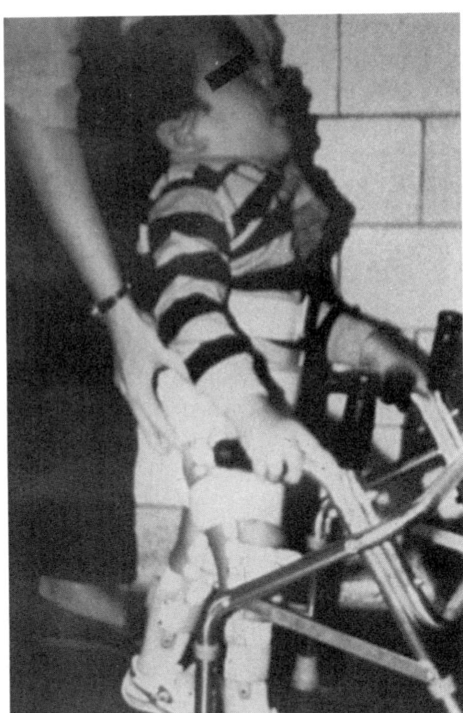

Figure 5-16 ■ Gait training with a reciprocating gait orthosis. A lateral weight shift with a slight tilt backward causes the unweighted leg to begin a swing phase.

learn a hop-to or swivel pattern of gait first, later mastering the swing-through pattern. The child with active hip flexors can attempt to walk with one or both hip joints unlocked in a reciprocating gait pattern. With both hips unlocked, the child must avoid falling forward, which is made likely by the absence of functional low back extensors or gluteals. To maintain an erect posture, the child must hyperextend the lumbar spine and shift the center of gravity posteriorly. However, this set of skills requires that the child use both upper extremities to remain erect by pushing up on the walker or crutch handles (Fig. 5-19). When using a reciprocating pattern with the hip joints unlocked on the HKAFO, the pelvic band provides control of abduction/adduction and medial/lateral rotation of the lower extremities, motion the child is unable to control actively. For some children with a high lumbar lesion and an intact CNS, the pelvic band may be removed to allow further freedom with transfers and provide a faster swing-through gait pattern. Trunk stability and hyperextension of the lumbar spine are essential for a stable stance, and these factors make these children more closely resemble patients with traumatic paraplegia than those with a congenital disability.[67,68]

Regardless of the orthosis, most young children and their therapists find the rollator walker

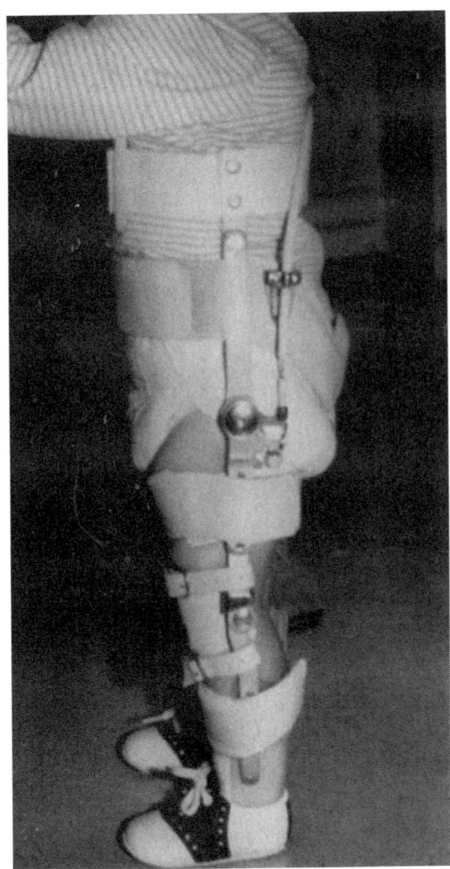

Figure 5-17 ■ Alignment and fit of an RGO with a thoracic strap and uprights, cable and dual-action hip joints.

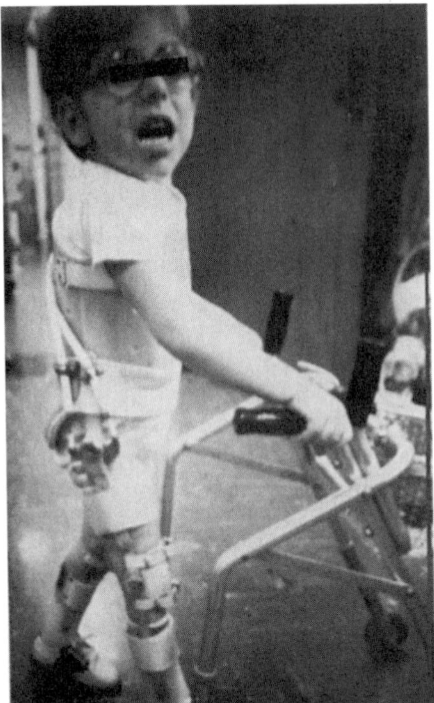

Figure 5-18 ▪ A reciprocating gait orthosis, fit over a plastic body jacket, is used to manage scoliosis. Note the erect alignment in this child with paralysis at the level of T-10.

the most effective assistive device to begin gait training. With four points of stability and two wheels on the front, the rollator provides good support and the child does not have to lift the device to advance it, as occurs when progressing a standard walker. The use of parallel bars should be avoided initially during gait training because they provide too much stability and the child may develop patterns of pulling and leaning that will be dangerous when making the transition to a walker. Exceptions may be made, however, such as in cases when a child has extreme difficulty learning to use a walker. However, in these cases, the author has found that the child who experiences great difficulty has usually been braced too low (Table 5-2).

The decision to progress the child to either axillary or forearm crutches will depend on the child's ability. The normal progression cannot be easily predicted or plotted, and a degree of experimentation is always necessary. A child wearing a body jacket to control scoliosis will often find axillary crutches difficult to use. Although axillary crutches encourage an upright position, they are best used for reciprocating or hop-to gait patterns. The swing-to and swing-through patterns are most safely and efficiently accomplished with forearm crutches. Over the years, however, the child may develop a tendency to lean forward onto the forearm crutches in an habitual posture, and this weight-bearing pattern may lead to an upper thoracic kyphosis

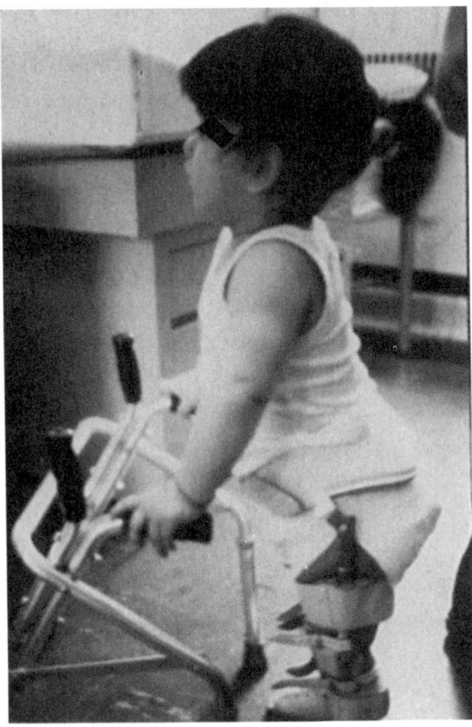

Figure 5-19 ▪ Hip-knee-ankle-foot orthosis with hips unlocked. The child maintains balance with a hyperextended lumbar spine and support from a walker.

TABLE 5-2
Ambulation Sequence: T-12 to L-3 Motor Level

	CNS Status		
	Typical→ Mild Deficit	**Mild → Moderate**	**Moderate → Severe**
Preambulation orthosis	Toronto A Frame	Toronto A Frame	Toronto A Frame
Assess	Ambulation bracing at 15–24 months	Ambulation bracing at 15–24 months	Continue with A Frame
Ambulation orthosis	HKAFO, locked hips; rollator walker	RGO; thoracic uprights; rollator walker	Orlau swivel walker; no assistive device
Progress	As above, hips unlocked	RGO; remove uprights; rollator walker	RGO; thoracic uprights; rollator walker
Progress	As above, crutches	As above, crutches	
Progress	KAFO, pelvic band removed; crutches	Assess for further changes; consider standard HKAFO or KAFO	Assess for further changes

HKAFO, hip-knee-ankle-foot orthosis; KAFO, knee-ankle-foot orthosis; RGO, reciprocating gait orthosis.

with elevated and protracted scapulae. If kyphosis begins to develop, the therapist and family must work together with the child to maintain a flexible, erect thoracic spine and well-aligned shoulders. Prone lifts and shoulder external rotation with depression exercises, in both the prone and supine position, will help strengthen the lower trapezius muscles, which may reduce the severity of the kyphosis.

As children with a high-level paralysis approach adolescence, many choose wheelchairs for mobility to achieve more competitive function with their peers. As transition to a wheelchair occurs, children who discard bracing usually spend little or no time standing. They will also experience the growth spurts and weight gains that are normal for all adolescents. Spending a full day in the wheelchair increases the likelihood of flexion contractures, which are very common in nonambulatory adolescents and which can restrict proper wheelchair skills and activities. Therefore, children who choose wheelchair mobility should also maintain a regimen of positioning and physical activity aimed at avoiding joint contractures and musculoskeletal deterioration. Prone positioning, standers, parapodiums, or braces can be used during prescribed therapy sessions at home or school. Swimming, wheelchair sports, wheelchair aerobics, and other activities that help control weight and improve cardiovascular function may also be included in the activity regimen.

As with infants, consideration of upper extremity and trunk strength, coordination, and mobility is appropriate with the older children and young adults with spina bifida. Significant changes in size and weight can result in loss of strength, immobility, and ultimately, diminished abilities.[8,38,67,68,70,76,77]

Low Lumbar Paralysis

Children with L-4 or L-5 motor function usually have strong hip flexors and adductors. Gluteus medius and tensor fascia lata may contribute to hip abduction, although the strength of these muscles may vary from "poor" to "good." Hip extension from the gluteus maximus is usually absent. These children are at risk for early hip dislocation or later progressive subluxation, depending on the relative strengths of the muscles surrounding the hip joint. Inherent ligamentous laxity in the child with low tone also contributes to hip joint instability.

Manual muscle testing of the muscles around the knee usually shows strong quadriceps and medial hamstrings (semitendinosus and semimembranosus) but absent lateral hamstring function. Kicking and crawling during early childhood can produce an internal tibial torsion deformity owing to the unopposed pull on the tibia by the medial hamstrings. This imbalance in forces can cause a toeing-in posture during standing and gait, which is first seen as the child pulls to a stand and begins to cruise.

Careful manual muscle testing is crucial in children with these lower lesions because there is often great variation of motor ability at the ankle and foot (Display 5-7). Anterior and posterior tibialis muscles, long and short toe extensors, peroneus longus and brevis muscles, and toe flexors may be functional, but the strength in these muscles may vary from "poor" to "normal." If significant imbalances in strength are found, patients may need to be splinted at night to prevent a progressive loss of flexibility.

When dorsiflexors are stronger than plantarflexors, a calcaneous deformity may have been present at birth, or it may develop through early childhood. An exceptionally high arch—a pes cavus deformity—may be caused by the unopposed action of the anterior tibialis, which results in a foot with a reduced weight-bearing surface. The distribution of body weight is limited to the heel and ball of the foot. Bracing and shoe fit can be difficult, and surgery is often indicated to weaken or eliminate deforming forces, realign the bones, and provide a greater weight-bearing surface over the entire sole of the foot.

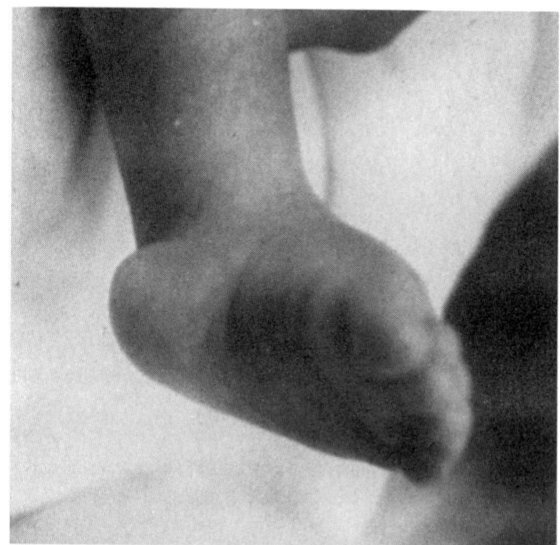

Figure 5-20 ▪ *Talipes equinovarus (clubfoot deformity) in a neonate.*

DISPLAY 5-7

Common Foot Deformities in Patients with Spina Bifida

Pes calcaneous—calcaneovarus, calcaneovalgus
Talipes equinovarus—clubfoot
Pes equinus—flatfoot
Convex pes valgus—rocker-bottom foot, vertical talus
Pes cavus—high arch with toe clawing
Ankle valgus

A calcaneovarus or calcaneovalgus foot may occur in children with low-level paralysis when there is an absence of the gastrocnemius/soleus muscle group. Various combinations of strengths and weaknesses in the musculature of the foot and ankle can produce abnormal foot alignment and abnormality of the weight-bearing surfaces of the foot. The orthopedic surgeon may consider muscle lengthening procedures and tendon transfers in an attempt to balance the dynamic forces around the joints.

Clubfoot (talipes equinovarus) is the most common foot deformity in children with spina bifidia who have an L-4 or L-5 motor level (Fig. 5-20). Diagnosis and management of clubfoot has prompted extensive discussion by orthopedic surgeons. Many now suggest early taping and gentle manipulation, followed by application of a well-padded splint, rather than serial casting, which had been used extensively in recent years. This change is approach is a response to the problem of pressure over the bony prominences resulting from casting and the associated problems of irritation and skin breakdown. Clubfoot is often very resistant to conservative treatment, however, and surgical correction often provides improved distribution of weight-bearing and easier orthotic fit. Recurrence of clubfoot secondary to incomplete surgical correction is not uncommon, and may lead to irritation and skin breakdown from a brace or shoe. Gentle stretching exercises to maintain flexibility and well-padded, properly fitting brace are important, although additional surgery to correct the deformity is common. When tendon lengthening is used in lieu of total excision of tendons to correct clubfoot, the deformity is more likely to recur. Since children with this level of motor paralysis will always need bracing to stabilize the ankle, tendon excision has no real negative impact on the child's brace level or ambulation potential. Initial surgical correction should be planned to correct the deformity completely in order to prevent additional procedures. Consistent stretching of the skin and soft tissue of the medial foot prior to clubfoot repair has been found to prevent wound dehiscence, a common complication resulting from the skin being stretched thin and taut to cover the longer, corrected foot following surgery.[8,38,77,78]

Debate continues regarding surgery for the child with unilateral or bilateral hip dislocation and an L-4 or L-5 motor level. When deciding on a course of management, the surgeon must consider the child's total function, including lower extremity strength and developmental skills. Surgical correction may be avoided if high bracing and assistive devices are indicated by the pattern of lower extremity weakness. Surgery may also be avoided for the child with poor lower extremity strength and significant CNS involvement. Surgery may be indicated for the child with good motor control of the trunk and strong quadriceps.

This child may eventually be able to walk with AFO or unlocked KAFO level bracing and an assistive device. Active gluteus medius muscles may indicate the child's potential for ambulation with low bracing and no assistive device. Therefore, some surgeons may choose to relocate the child's hips to prevent or correct significant gait deviations that would hamper the child's unassisted walking.

Surgery might also prevent later degenerative changes in the unstable hip that could cause pain around the hip joint in the child with normal sensation. However, other surgeons contend that bilateral dislocations should never be repaired surgically for fear that postoperative complications may diminish the child's potential for gait. Unilateral dislocation should be corrected only in the child with intact CNS function who has the potential for ambulation with short bracing, and who is unlikely to have gait deviations that require an assistive device.[39,77,79,80]

It is apparent from this section as it is from the literature that the management of hip dislocations in spina bifida is a confusing and controversial subject. The therapist can play a role in assisting the physician to identify any influences a hip dislocation may have on the child's muscle strengths and weaknesses, skill in the upright position, and trunk and pelvic alignment. This information may then enable the physician to evaluate the treatment options better and choose accordingly.

Children with L-4 to L-5 paralysis and significant CNS deficits are often unable to control their trunk in an upright position. This inability often conveys to the therapist the impression (often false) that a higher level of paralysis exists. The therapist and the family should continue their attempts to remediate the effects of the CNS deficit, including low tone and poor motor control, by improving coordination of the head, shoulders, and trunk. At around

3 years of age, the child may be working from a Toronto standing frame and, later, may use an RGO for gait training. Both devices offer a psychological and motivational boost for a child who has been slow to develop. If gait training is patient and thoughtful, there could be relatively easy success. Before the advent of the RGO, many children with poor trunk stability and low lumbar paralysis were fit with low bracing. These inappropriate orthotics and the ineffective attempts at gait training they caused resulted in frustration for children, parents, and therapists alike. The RGO seems to provide significant benefits to this group of children.[39,73]

The child with a lesion at L-4 to L-5 without any apparent CNS deficit can be provided with braces according to their lower extremity function (Table 5-3). Many of these children are able to pull to a stand or are attempting to stand by 10 to 12 months of age, and will not require a standing frame. If the child can control the knees while upright, use of an ankle-foot orthosis (AFO) can be initiated (Fig. 5-21). "Twister" cables, which provide a rotatory force, may be added later if rotation needs correction. Internal rotation, emanating from unequal forces behind the knee, is most common (Fig. 5-22). However, external rotation of both legs, or a combination of internal rotation of one leg and external rotation of the other leg, may occur. Twister cables can be adjusted to control any of these combinations, and are

TABLE 5-3
Orthotic Management for L-4 to L-5 and Sacral Motor Lesions

	L-4 to L-5	Sacral
Muscles present	Hip flexors and adductors Quadriceps Medical hamstrings Anterior tibialis Some gluteus medius Some foot intrinsics	All, with possible exception of gluteus maximus, gastrocnemius-soleus group, and foot intrinsics
Preambulation orthotics	Toronto standing frame (some children may pull to stand, bypassing the frame, and begin with bracing*)	Usually none needed*
Ambulation bracing	RGO; KAFO with weak quadriceps AFO with or without "twisters" if torsion is present*	AFO with weak gastrocnemius-soleus or crouched gait. Some need no bracing, but shoe insert may help maintain proper foot alignment
Assistive devices	Rollator walker or crutches. An independent gait is possible for some, usually with a gluteus medius lurch and lumbar lordosis.	Possibly a walker early on; most progress to an independent gait*
Expected functional level	Ambulatory in life unless increased body weight; flexion contractures; poor CNS status; further complications may reduce ambulatory status	Independent gait with moderate to minimal deviations based on patterns of weakness

*Control of upper body and CNS status may modify these levels.

RGO, reciprocating gait orthosis; KAFO, knee-ankle-foot orthosis; AFO, ankle-foot orthosis.

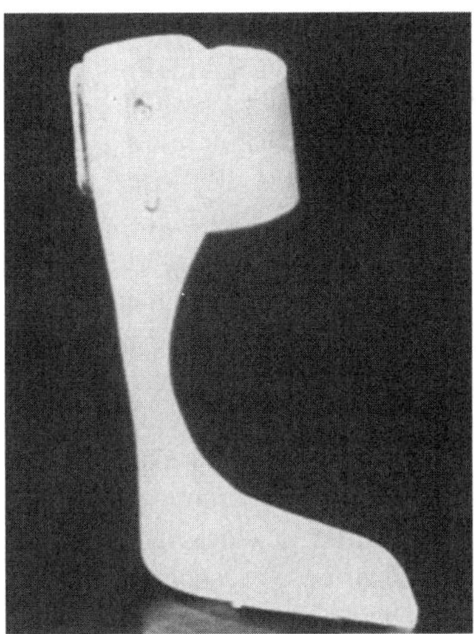

Figure 5-21 ■ A plastic ankle-foot orthosis is aligned at 90 degrees or at a neutral position.

valuable in aligning the lower extremities during gait. The child may learn to control minimal rotational deviation and avoid later surgical correction. Twister cables may also assist in allowing the loose ligamentous structures at the knee to tighten, thereby correcting the source of some of the deviation. For children who retain the rotational deformity, surgery is usually recommended around the age of 6 years. The procedure should correct the bony malalignment and transfer the active medial hamstrings to a more midline orientation so that the deformity does not recur.

A knee-ankle-foot orthosis (KAFO) may be used for a child with weak quadriceps and difficulty maintaining either unilateral or bilateral knee extension when upright. A patellar pad will help maintain knee extension while reduc-

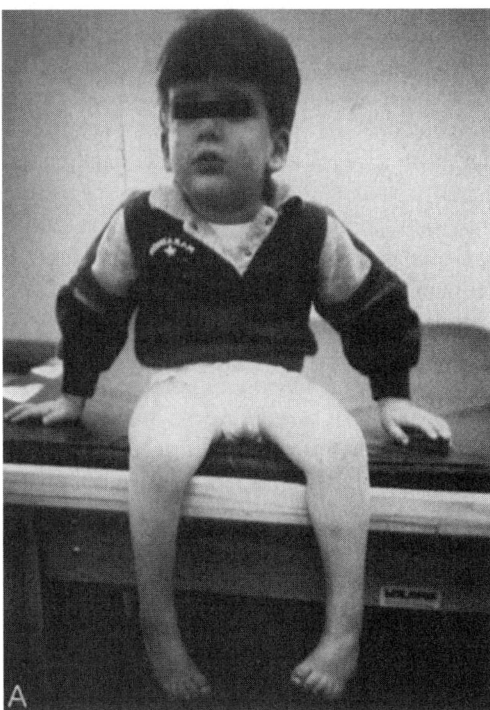

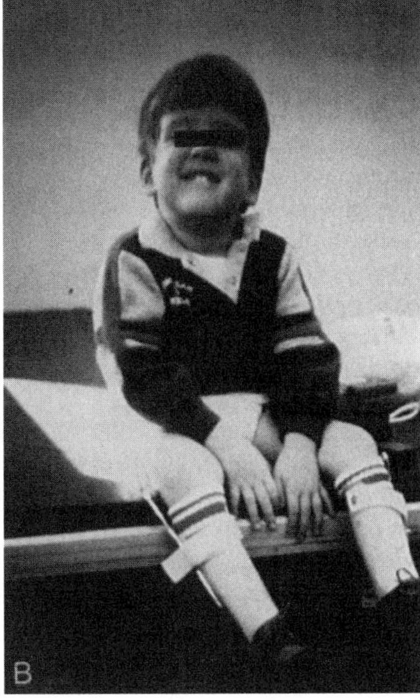

Figure 5-22 ■ (**A**) and (**B**) A child with an L-4 to L-5 motor level and significant in-toeing is portrayed. Twister cables are attached to an ankle-foot orthosis to control rotation or torsion until surgery is indicated.

ing the pressure exerted across the thigh and tibial straps of the KAFO. This reduction in pressure decreases the probability of the skin breakdown at those sites. Although a pad at the knee adds to the time spent donning and doffing the brace, it appears to be a valuable component that ensures a level of knee extension that the more proximal and distal straps alone will not offer. If unilateral knee flexion is noted, the child should be examined prior to considering a KAFO in order to eliminate the possibility of a leg length discrepancy causing flexion of the longer limb during stance.[8,38]

Some clinics use a "floor reaction" or "anti-crouch" orthosis for children who have difficulty attaining knee extension. This orthosis is an AFO with an anterior shell that facilitates knee extension at heel strike. The orthosis is theoretically sound and successful with other disabilities. But problems of pressure across the anterior tibia have caused some centers to avoid this device.

A recent study presented by Hunt et al. explored the use of a hinged AFO that limited range of motion at the ankle from 5 degrees of dorsiflexion to 10 degrees of plantar-flexion. It demonstrated a positive influence on walking velocity; therefore, this brace may warrant further investigation.[81]

Regardless of the orthosis chosen, a careful assessment of the resulting gait pattern will indicate the likelihood of success or failure of a particular device.

The child with an L-4 or L-5 motor level is often able to begin ambulation after one or two sessions of gait training with a rollator walker. The family can continue working with the child at home after only a brief demonstration in the clinic. Crutch training for the young child is often more involved and lengthy, and clinicians believe that crutches may be ill-advised until the child reaches 4 or 5 years of age and has a good level of skill and self-confidence in the upright position. The child must also have a sufficient attention span to benefit, without stress, from the crutch training sessions. Some children with L-4 to L-5 paralysis will attempt independent, unassisted ambulation. The gait pattern usually includes a hyperlordotic lumbar spine and a side-to-side gluteus medius lurch. The degree of these deviations depends on the strength of the hip extensors and abductors relative to the flexors and adductors. Gait will appear more normal when good back and abdominal strength can assist with alignment of the lumbar spine and pelvis.

Despite the high degree of activity demonstrated by these children, ROM exercise remains important. A prone program is useful to counteract the hyperlordotic posture of the spine that occurs secondary to the anterior pelvic tilt with flexed hips during ambulation. Lying prone for prescribed periods during the day and through the night can minimize development of hip flexion contractures. Moderate to severe hip flexion contractures are the single most influential factor leading to the deterioration of ambulation skill in these children. Hip flexion contractures of 20 degrees or more in the child using AFOs and crutches will diminish gait velocity to 44% of normal. A 10-degree contracture reduces gait velocity to 65% of normal. Activity to maintain spinal mobility, to prevent a fixed lordotic spine, and supine and sitting activities to address abdominal muscle strength are also recommended for the long-term program at school and in the home.[39,77,79,82]

Sacral Level Paralysis

The child with sacral paralysis will have a greater degree of muscle function throughout the lower extremities than a child with spina bifida at any other motor level. In the child with sacral paralysis, muscular forces around the hips and knees are in better balance, with full or partial innervation of the hip extensors and lateral hamstrings. Strong function of the gluteus medius, medial hamstrings, and quadriceps is expected in this population. The incidence of hip subluxation and dislocation is lower than at other motor levels. Significant hip flexion contractures should not develop, and abnormal torsions of the femur and tibia are not as prevalent as with lesions at other levels. Because of the additional musculature available at the proximal joints, the gait pattern of the child with sacral innervation more closely resembles a normal gait.

Manual muscle testing demonstrates considerable variation in muscle function among children with lesions at this motor level. Variation is greatest at the foot and ankle, with the gastrocnemius/soleus being the major group that may still be weak. The toe flexors may be present and may provide some secondary ankle plantar flexion, but they are usually not strong enough to stabilize the ankle and totally replace a weak gastrocnemius/soleus. As a result, AFOs will be indicated for most of these children.

The child with sacral innervation may not need external support at the ankle if strong plantar-flexors are present. Close observation, however, is necessary during childhood when there is rapid growth and changes in weight. The gastrocnemius/soleus group that is rated as having "poor" or "fair" function may adequately stabilize the tibia of a small child for proper standing and walking for short distances. As the child grows, the lever arm of the muscle will lengthen, often resulting in changes in muscle efficiency and alignment. The loss of mechanical advantage means that additional strength is needed for stabilization, but this may not be available. The gastrocnemius/soleus group controls the forward movement of the tibia over the foot as the stance phase of gait progresses from heel-strike. When strength is inadequate, a crouched gait may develop. Because the tibia is permitted to roll forward too far and too rapidly into excessive dorsiflexion, hip and knee flexion will result. The child should be observed walking during the physical therapy assessment. With strong gluteus medius and quadriceps muscles, the child may be able to stand erect, but without adequate gastrocnemius/soleus muscle function, excessive dorsiflexion and knee flexion will be noted during gait. Flexion contractures can develop if this posture is not remediated. Surgical lengthening of tight hamstrings will be necessary as a result of the changes noted above, and a once-independent ambulator may need assistive devices for support. The child may develop limited ambulation capacity owing to the added energy needed for this type of gait. The crouched gait and its associated problems can be prevented simply by using an AFO when the child begins to walk. The child whose posture is maintained by an orthosis may choose to go for short periods without bracing (to a party or special event) without compromising future potential.[38]

The information now available from podiatric specialists indicates that this group of children may benefit from having molded shoe orthoses placed within the typically prescribed AFO. This arrangement may prevent many of the hindfoot and midfoot malalignments that can arise as the children grow older. Articulating ankle joints that permit limited dorsiflexion may be indicated for some children who are likely to benefit from the opportunity to use active musculature in the ankle and foot.[81,82]

The child with sacral innervation will commonly have some mild gait deviations. Compared with the child with a higher motor level, the child with sacral paralysis may appear not to need therapeutic intervention. However, benefits will likely be accrued from a program that will "fine tune" the gait. Thoracic and abdominal strengthening is recommended to address the oblique abdominals as well as the rectus abdominus. The child should also practice correct alignment of the shoulders, trunk, pelvis, and limbs during standing and ambulation. Tactile, verbal, and visual reinforcement can all be used to help the child learn and maintain proper posture for long periods of time. Children involved in a long-term program like this may still have an abnormal gait pattern but when they choose, can assume a more correct alignment.

The child with a sacral innervation usually exhibits some mild gait deviations. Compared with the child with a higher motor paralysis, the child with a sacral paralysis may not appear to need therapeutic intervention. Actually, an intense, short-term program may not be indicated. However, benefits can be noted from a therapeutic program to "fine tune" the child's gait that continues over a long period of time, with short periods of direct intervention by the therapist, especially at times of increased growth. Thoracic and abdominal strengthening for the oblique abdominals as well as the rectus abdominus and strengthening to all extensors of the trunk and limbs is recommended. The child should practice correct alignment of the shoulders, trunk, pelvis, and limbs during standing and ambulation. Tactile, verbal, and visual reinforcement can all be used to help the child learn and maintain proper posture for progressively longer periods of time. Children involved in a long-term program like this may still exhibit an abnormal gait pattern most of the time, but they may assume a more correct alignment for short periods of time. As the child ages, the desire may develop to replicate this alignment and the child will then have the skill to do so. It is a pleasure to work with children who can reach high levels of motor function. The process of working with a child like this is also an educational opportunity for the clinician. The therapist must learn to observe closely and analyze subtle gait deviations and to deduce the areas of trunk and limb weakness that contribute to the deviation so an appropriate intervention plan can be made. The development of careful and critical observational skills will ultimately benefit all patients (Fig. 5-23).

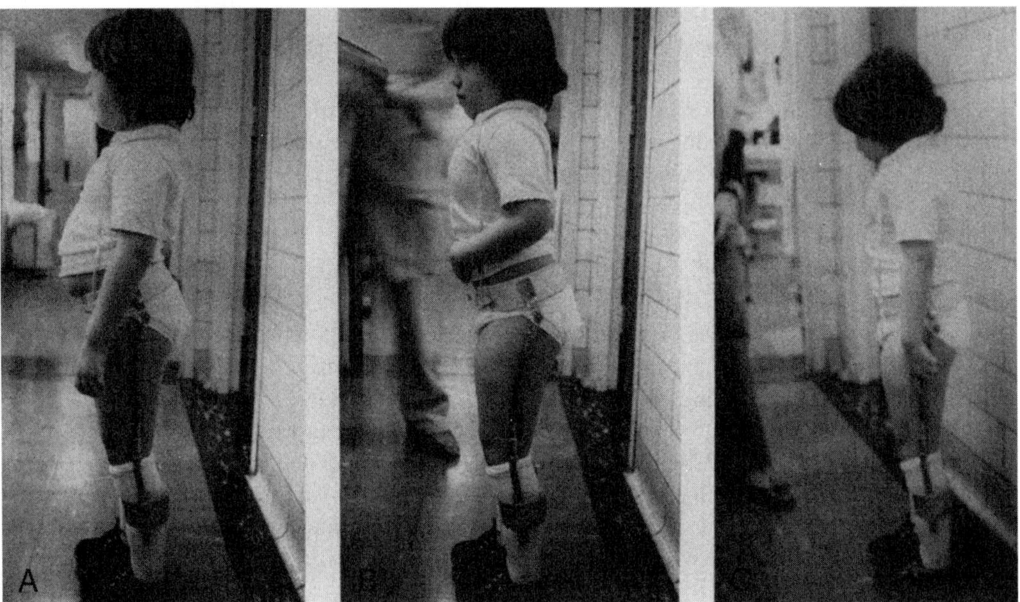

Figure 5-23 ▪ Nine-year-old girl with an S-1 motor level. (**A**) An independent gait has been achieved with ankle-foot orthoses and twisters. Note the poor alignment and low tone of the trunk, as well as the anterior pelvic tilt with hip flexion. (**B**) Following a long-term program of active exercises for problem areas, she works hard to align the thorax and lumbar spine cortically and improve pelvic alignment. (**C**) Increasing success with more correct posture.

Compared with children with involvement at other motor levels, fewer children with sacral paralysis have hydrocephalus and require a shunt, and fewer exhibit pathologically low tone. Therefore, many of the CNS and biomechanical factors that negatively influence the child with spina bifida are not prevalent in children with low-level lesions. As a result, children with sacral paralysis who present with hip instability are treated aggressively if they appear to have the potential for unassisted gait.[6,38]

The use of preambulation devices may be unnecessary if the child acquires strong balance responses in the trunk and is developing a normal quality of movement. At between 10 and 15 months of age, the child may be pulling to stand independently, just as would a typical child of that age. A foot splint, commonly worn at night to maintain alignment, may also be used during the day to stabilize a weak ankle for standing while awaiting definitive bracing.

For the child with CNS difficulties, it is important to follow the same course of therapy that would be prescribed for a child with a higher level lesion. The program can include activities that address flexion and extension strength against gravity through the head and trunk, and balance and equilibrium skills in all positions. The program should also include passive and active exercises for the lower extremities to prevent joint contractures.[38]

Three-Dimensional Gait Analysis

The development of increasingly sophisticated gait technology is providing objective information that enables therapists, orthotists, and orthopedic surgeons to study and understand more accurately the gait and gait parameters of patients with spina bifida. Widely held beliefs and treatment protocols that were developed using subjective or anecdotal evidence may now be validitated or discarded by utilizing the three-dimensional information. Orthotic prescriptions can be better tailored to the needs of the child when the effects of the orthosis can be understood, especially on the sagittal plane kinematics, walking speed, progression of ground reaction forces across the foot, and the three plane motions of the pelvis, hips, and knees. Dias, Sarwark, and Vankoski at the gait lab of Children's Memorial Hospital in Chicago have found that the comparison of children with spina bifida to normal gait parameters has not provided the most meaningful information to guide and evaluate treatment plans.[83,84] They state that children with spina bifida at a given lesion level demonstrate characteristic gait patterns that are reasonably homogenous. These identifiable patterns then become a baseline from which comparisons can be drawn, enabling the clinician to focus on realistic goals for that patient and to evaluate more fairly the result of interventions, either conservative or surgical. In a recent publication it was found that in the absence of the gluteus medius, gluteus maximus, and ankle plantar-flexors, certain compensatory movements at the pelvis and hip were consistently noted to enable the children to maintain independent ambulation. This gait pattern of the child with a lumbosacral level lesion is characterized by exaggerated movement at the pelvis and pelvic obliquity, increased stance phase hip abduction, increased stance phase knee flexion, knee valgus, and increased ankle dorsiflexion.[84] In another study, Williams et al. reported a 24% incidence of late knee pain these ambulatory patients with lumbosacral level lesions. The apparent knee valgus was found to be a result of a combination of internal pelvic and hip rotation and stance phase knee flexion. The use of gait analysis for early detection of these abnormal knee moments can direct the clinician toward the most appropriate treatment, either tibial derotation osteotomy or the use of KAFOs, to assist the patient to avoid pain and deterioration of gait. The continued use of crutches was also found to be an important deterrent to later arthritic joint changes and pain with this population of children. Even though the children were able to walk unaided at any early age, crutches reduced the exaggerated range of movements through the lumbar spine, pelvis, hips, and knees. Finally, it is interesting to note that many gait labs include the results of manual muscle testing and gross motor assessments provided by the physical therapist when evaluating the child's total movement skills and developing a treatment plan for intervention.[83–87]

Casting After Orthopedic Surgery

Earlier in this chapter, various deformities commonly associated with different motor levels were mentioned, as were surgical procedures to correct these deformities. Following many procedures, the child is usually in some type of cast for a temporary period of immobilization to allow the surgical site to heal undisturbed. Casts should never be considered to be a benign treatment method for the child with spina bifida. Pressure and irritation of insensate skin are always risks. Fractures, loss of joint flexibility, and loss of gross motor skills are commonly noted on removal of the cast. Children with minimal CNS deficits may lose postural security and antigravity muscle strength during immobilization. It is troublesome to see children lose skills that they have worked long and hard to gain.

Most surgeons agree that children should be casted for the shortest possible time needed for adequate healing. Because of problems related to immobility, and to minimize hospitalizations, multiple anesthesias, and periods of immobility, surgeons try to plan several procedures that can be performed at one operative session. One should remember that periods of immobility are, nonetheless, necessary. Casting is an important part of the orthopedic program to reduce deformity and ultimately gain function. With some forethought and planning for the child and family, therapists can assist in making this period less of a problem.[38,88–90] Returning children as quickly as possible to their preoperative status, or to an improved status, is a postoperative objective for the therapist. Recommendations for treatment and management of the child can be discussed with the family before surgery in order to ensure that the child's needs are understood and adequate preparation is made. Most families experience a great deal of stress at this time, and the therapist may have to be available for several short sessions to accomplish all the necessary teaching.

Many children will be in hip spica casts following hip surgery. If surgery is performed for a unilateral problem, the full hip spica may still be used to stabilize the pelvis and opposite limb, thereby preventing movement and malalignment at the surgical site. With the surgeon's approval, prone positioning will help prevent pressure sores on the calcaneous, sacrum, and ischial tuberosity, and will challenge the child to lift and extend the head to watch television, read, or play. Prone positioning in a reclining wheelchair or scooter board can provide mobility if the child can use the upper extremities for propulsion; this also reduces the need for the child to be carried or moved around the house. Similar prone positioning on a wagon for long walks outdoors may help the family survive this period with less anxiety because the child is occupied and happy. Some clever families have adapted hand trucks or dollies to safely stand and move their older, heavier child (Fig. 5-24). After several days, physicians may permit the child to stand, a position that can be maintained for long periods, especially during meals and for play. If the cast is asymmetric, towels propped under the feet will help to level the child. To ensure safety, it is necessary to lean the child on a chair, table, or sofa that will not move. In addition, it may be necessary for a family member to remain with the child to prevent falling. Families living in multilevel homes may have to prepare a temporary bedroom for the child on the first floor. An old mattress or a few thick blankets on the floor are usually comfortable. Instruction in strategies for safely lifting and

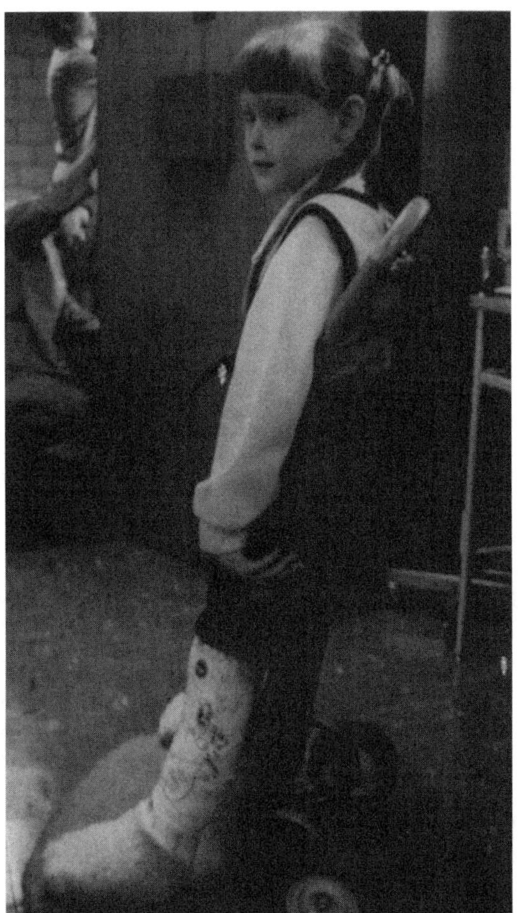

Figure 5-24 ■ A parent finds an imaginative and safe way of standing and moving their older child in a hip spica by adapting a commercially available hand truck.

turning the child while using good body mechanics will be appreciated by the family and the child, and are the responsibility of the physical therapist.

Regardless of the age of the child in a spina cast, daily exercise periods are important to prevent loss of neck and trunk strength and to maintain the automatic balance responses. Prone lifts, supine head lifts, standing, and tilting for 15 to 20 minutes in all directions should be instituted several times each day. As the child attempts to maintain balance, muscles are working above and within the cast. This activity places stress on the bones of the lower extremities, thereby reducing demineralization and, possibly, the risk of a fracture when the cast is removed. Postural insecurity will also be reduced as vestibular and proprioceptive stimulation are provided by these challenging antigravity activities (Fig. 5-25).

In many clinics, the child is admitted for a period of intensive therapy aimed at ensuring the child's return to function following cast removal. Lower extremity ROM and strength are the immediate concerns, along with improvement in balance and the equilibrium responses

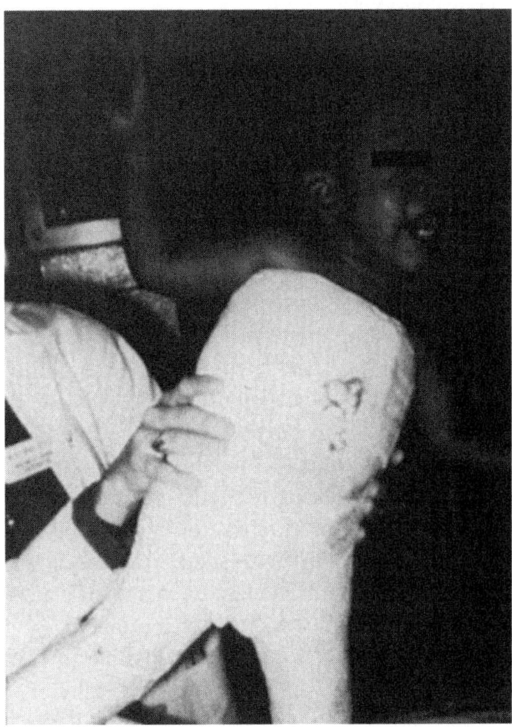

Figure 5-25 ■ Child with a hip spica cast after hip reduction surgery. Note how the child is both standing and being tilted. Standing, when the surgeon approves, about 10 days after surgery, is one aspect of the home care program.

of the neck and upper body, and a return to the child's former level of physical function. An increase in function can be achieved in a short period of time if the therapist properly targets all of the child's needs and does not address only lower extremity flexibility.

If the child has a high-level lesion, surgery was likely performed to gain passive flexibility for good limb alignment and brace fit. For such a child, a review of ROM exercises with the parents, an orthotic evaluation, and a review of activities to further improve upper body control may be all that is needed after cast removal. The child may then be monitored, until adequate function is achieved, through an outpatient clinic, community facility, or school physical therapy program.[38]

The child with a high-level lesion who demonstrates a significant loss of motion at the hip or knee is at risk for fracture. A brief hospitalization may be indicated to regain the lost mobility. The child might also be sent home in a bivalved cast, with a program of frequent ROM exercise and sedentary activities if the family is able to comply.[89,90]

Procedures to relocate or stabilize the hip joint in children with L-4 to L-5 lesions include simple tendon lengthening, femoral or pelvic osteotomy, or the more complex Lindseth procedure, which involves transfer of the external obliques. Candidates for the Lindseth procedure are those children with the potential for unassisted gait and an intact CNS. Admission to the hospital after cast removal following a Lindseth procedure may be necessary to ensure that joint mobility and balance skills are again safe and acceptable, and that the child is working toward ambulation without an assistive device.

A period of 6 to 12 weeks in a hip spica cast can reduce mobility in the lumbar spine and the lower extremities. Usually, it is difficult for the child to achieve a 90-degree angle at the hips when sitting because of tightness in the hamstrings and hip extensors after being in extension in the cast. Hip and low back tightness frequently causes abnormal alignment in sitting, with the child's pelvis rocked posteriorly, and a secondary thoracic spine kyphosis that requires remediation. Gentle activities are indicated to increase pelvic and hip mobility and strength. Active thoracic extension with active hip flexion and use of abdominal muscles will help in attaining and holding a 90-degree sitting alignment. Care should be taken to avoid placing the child in a sitting position for extended periods of time until mobility is regained at the hips and spine.

Parents should be warned to prohibit their child from crawling after removal of a spica cast, because crawling requires hip and knee flexion exceeding 90 degrees. Hip rotation is also required as the child moves into and out of sitting and the four-point position. If the necessary flexibility and range is not present in these motions when the cast is removed, fractures may occur.[38]

Following surgery of the knees or ankles, children will have either long- or short-leg casts and the family will require instructions to avoid excessive supine positioning and sitting. These positions place pressure on the heels and will lead to skin breakdown. Flexion contractures and their associated deformities are a major concern. Sitting, crawling, and knee-walking with short leg casts will foster increased tightness of the hip and knee flexors. Information regarding alternative positions should be offered to avoid positions that encourage flexion. Prone-lying is the preferred position, and standing and ambulation are preferred activities, when feasible. Ambulation is achieved quickly when walkers, rather than crutches, are used as assistive devices during this temporary period. Lack of good balance through the trunk, poor prioception, and possibly malaligned casts makes crutch-training difficult. By comparison, instruction with a walker is usually a faster and safer choice. Strengthening exercises can be used for back, hip, and knee extensors, along with exercises for the trunk to help keep the child mobile during the period of casting. With such a program the child will also be likely to demonstrate a greater degree of readiness for returning to the previous, or an improved, level of function once the cast is removed.

Central Nervous System Deterioration

Throughout life, the individual with spina bifida, clinicians, and family members should be vigilant regarding any change in function that could indicate hydromyelia or a tethered spinal cord. These neurologic conditions can affect the patient's mobility, urologic function, activities of daily living (ADLs), and educational capacity. If diagnosed and treated in a timely fashion, the effects can be temporary. If left untreated, the symptoms can worsen and become permanent. Clinicians must be knowledgeable about these problems because their effects can be discovered by the physical therapist during routing evaluations or reevaluations, manual muscle testing, or parent interview.[79]

Hydromyelia

Hall, Lindseth, and associates conducted a study of rapidly progressive scoliosis occurring in patients with spina bifida and found some children with excessive CSF migrating into the spinal cord.[91] Pockets of excess CSF indicated that normal CSF circulation was impaired. This collection of fluid down the spinal cord caused areas of pressure and necrosis of peripheral nerves, which resulted in the weakness that produced the rapidly progressive scoliosis. Other symptoms that have been found to be associated with hydromyelia include progressive upper extremity weakness and hypertonus. If the problem was caused by a shunt malfunction, one might expect enlarged ventricles, but computerized tomography (CT) scans have shown no such increase in the size of lateral ventricles. Nonetheless, revision of the VP shunt has produced improvement in the symptoms. In some centers, a percentage of affected children have required spinal shunting at the level of the fluid pockets to ensure that the excess fluid would be completely eliminated. Lindseth, an orthopedic surgeon, has become a strong advocate for further investigation of all cases of rapidly progressive scoliosis. He believes it is important to detect any CNS complication and not treat the scoliosis as a purely skeletal abnormality. Left untreated, the hydromyelia can cause continuing deterioration in upper and lower extremity function as the fluid collects along the spinal cord.[8,16,38,91,92]

Tethered Spinal Cord

At approximately 10 weeks' gestation, the vertebral column and spinal cord of the fetus are the same length. Spinal nerves exit horizontally at their corresponding vertebrae. By 5 months' gestation, the vertebral column has grown more rapidly than the spinal cord, which at that time ends at S-1. At birth, the cord is at L-3, and by adulthood, the cord is at the L-1 to L-2 vertebral level.

A tethered spinal cord occurs when adhesions anchor the spinal cord at the site of the back lesion. The child is growing rapidly, but the cord is not free to slide upward as normally occurs, instead remaining bound at the level of the back defect. Excessive stretch to the spinal cord causes metabolic changes and ischemia of the neural tissue, with associated degeneration in muscle function. Rapidly progressive scoliosis, hypertonus in the lower extremities, and changes in urologic function may be attributed to tethering of the cord. Changes in gait pattern may be seen in older children. Occurrences of increased tone on passive ROM, asymmetric changes in manual muscle testing results, areas of decreasing strength, or discomfort in the back or buttocks should alert the therapist to this possible problem. Close examination by professionals and vigilance by parents can usually identify early functional changes associated with a tethered cord (Display 5-8). Peterson suggests that based on his study population, those children with repaired lesions at levels above L-3 begin to exhibit symptoms of tethered cord before age 6 and those with lesion levels below L-4 tend to become symptomatic after age 6. He also found that children with unrepaired back defects exhibit symptoms much earlier than age 6, regardless of where the lesion level is located.[93] When tethering is suspected, myelography may be utilized to confirm the diagnosis. Subsequent neurosurgical release can free the cord. It may not migrate to its appropriate position when freed, but further growth of the child may proceed without incident. If the release is performed in a timely manner, irreversible neurologic damage can usually be prevented. However it is becoming more clear that total correction of all the symptoms should not be assumed.[38,93–95,97–100] McClone et al. found in their study of 30 children who received surgical intervention for tethered cord that the greater number of children who exhibited improvement of their scoliosis were those who had curves of less than 50 degrees. During a 2- to 7-year follow-up, although 38% of the children began to show progression of their curves owing to retethering, the remaining children showed a stabilized or improved spinal alignment.[94]

DISPLAY 5-8

Clinical Findings that May Lead to Diagnosis of Tethered Cord

- Spasticity in muscles with saccral nerve roots
- Increased tone in legs with resistance to passive ROM
- Sudden increase in lumbar lordosis
- Back or buttock pain
- Development of scoliosis at a young age
- Rapidly progressing scoliosis
- Scoliosis above level of paralysis
- Change in urologic function
- Change in gait pattern
- Progressive weakening in leg musculature

Scoliosis

Hydromyelia and tethered cord should always be suspected if scoliosis develops in a child with a motor lesion below T-12. The child with thoracic paralysis does not have active trunk musculature to provide antigravity strength and is always at risk for scoliosis. However, a child with a lumbar or sacral lesion with full trunk muscle innervation should be evaluated when any curvature develops over a short time period. Clinics that provide surgical treatment for hydromyelia and tethered cord report a reduction in the overall occurrence of scoliosis requiring spinal fusion. Following untethering of the spine, there is a significant reduction, but no reports of total correction, of curvature.[92–96,100]

A group of children with spina bifida may develop scoliosis without evidence of a CNS problem. When scoliosis occurs and trunk alignment is poor, children will require additional upper extremity support to remain erect in sitting and standing. In sitting, the uneven pelvis causes pressure at areas of increased weight-bearing. Braces become ill-fitting, which can lead to deterioration of mobility, and changes in balance cause the gait to become more difficult. Propelling a wheelchair may become more strenuous because the child must work both to maintain an upright posture and to use the upper extremities effectively.

Spinal braces are useful for the child without trunk support, but surgical fusion is inevitable for most of these children. There are numerous methods for and preferred approaches to spinal fusion, and the periods of immobility and restrictions on daily activity vary with each. The type of instrumentation employed and the area and extent of the fusion will also influence these parameters.

If the fusion extends to the sacrum, pelvic mobility will diminish, and ambulatory ability will be affected. Gait analysis has shown greater excursion of movement at the pelvis in ambulatory children with spina bifida than in typical children. Given this information, surgeons have been reluctant to fuse the sacral area of ambulatory children if this can be avoided. The upper extremity and trunk movement necessary for successful wheelchair propulsion are also limited if flexibility of the distal spine is diminished or absent.

The physical therapist must be concerned with the patient's postoperative activity level and resumption of mobility. Maintaining flexibility and strength in all extremities and preventing skin problems during this period of immobility must be a priority. When full activities are permitted, it is important to reassess the patient to determine whether function has been lost. Spinal fusion will influence the performance of many ADLs, and new skills and adaptive strategies will need to be developed.[8,38]

Latex Allergy

Allergic reactions to latex in the population of individuals with spina bifida has become a relatively recent (1989) but serious concern. Latex is a natural rubber used in a wide variety of products that come into contact with human skin and other body surfaces. In the health field, a vast number of commonly used items contain or are made exclusively from latex. Latex has been depended on for its impermeable qualities and strength while still providing sensitivity to touch. This makes it an excellent material for use in sterile gloves, where it has provided dependable protection to the medical community to prevent the spread of illness. It is durable as well as elastic, which accounts for its popularity and wide usage for various types of flexible tubing and in the toy industry (Display 5-9).

Although it is believed that only 1% of the general population is allergic to latex, the results of various studies agree that 18% to 37% of patients with spina bifida exhibit a significant

DISPLAY 5-9

Partial List of Commonly used Products Containing Latex

Balloons
Pacifiers
Chewing gum
Dental dam
Rubber bands
Elastic in clothing
Beach toys
Koosh balls
Some types of disposable diapers
Glue
Paints
Erasers
Some brands of band-aids
Bulb syringes
Ready-to-use enemas
Ostomy pouches
Oxygen masks
Pulse oximeters
Reflex hammers
Stethoscope tubing
Suction tubing
Vascular stockings
Crutch axillary pads, tips, and hand grips
Kitchen cleaning gloves
Swim goggles
Wheelchair tires
Some wheelchair cushions
Zippered food storage bags

sensitivity to latex. It was also found that 7% to 10% of health care workers exhibit a latex sensitivity. Allergic reactions may appear as watery and itchy eyes, sneezing, coughing, hives, and a rash in the area of contact. More serious reactions may produce swelling of the trachea, and changes in blood pressure and circulation, resulting in anaphylactic shock. Diagnosis of latex sensitivity is based on a clinical history, observation of the reaction, and immunologic findings following the use of a skin prick allergy test. The cause, to date, is not known but it is theorized that early, intense, and consistent exposure to latex products results in the development of the sensitivity. Some of the more severe symptoms were believed to be a result of inhalation of the powder contained in most sterile latex gloves. The powder makes the gloves easy to don and doff, and it can become airborne upon removal of the gloves. However, further investigation found this was not a consistent irritant.

The Food and Drug Administration and the Centers for Disease Control and Prevention are investigating the problem and supporting efforts to find the components of latex that are responsible for the allergy, developing methods of producing safe nonallergenic rubber, and labeling products with a latex content. A blood test has been developed which is being used during preemployment testing for health care workers and for patients with spina bifida. There has been evidence that the latex allergy is also related to a sensitivity to bananas, chestnuts, avocados, and kiwi fruit in some patients, and this relationship is also being investigated.

Some valuable information regarding patient safety and education was obtained from E.L.A.S.T.I.C. = Education for Latex Allergy/ Support Team Information Coalition. They recommend that parents, older patients or their caregivers carry an auto-injectible type epinephrine in case of a serious allergic reaction. They recommend having a supply of sterile nonlatex gloves on hand for emergency use. All sensitive individuals should wear a Medic Alert bracelet, necklace, or dog tags. Neighborhood paramedic teams, the fire department, and local Emergency Medical Services who might respond to an emergency call should be alerted to the patient's sensitivities. Keeping a set of nonlatex gloves near the front door in case of such an emergency is also encouraged. Families and patients are encouraged to also become familiar with products that must be avoided. A complete list of latex products and alternative nonlatex products is available from the Spina Bifida Association of America. Refer to the end of this chapter for other sources for latex information and latex-free products, and resources.[101–110]

Perceptual Motor and Cognitive Performance

The population of children with spina bifida represents a diverse and varied group. The children vary considerably in the problems that are present and their abilities, and therapists must be aware of possible difficulties that may affect the learning potential of their patients. This section provides a brief overview of the vast amount of information that is available on this topic (see the resources cited at the end of this chapter).

Great interest and concern have been expressed regarding the cognitive, sensory, and perceptual motor function of children with spina bifida. Studies have shown that the intelligence of this population is unrelated to motor level, severity of hydrocephalus prior to shunt insertion, or number of shunt revisions. Those complications that do influence intellect in this population include untimely treatment of hydrocephalus, cerebral infection, and other CNS problems.[6,34]

Intelligence testing for children with spina bifida places them within the normal range for most tests but below the population mean. Willis and associates found test scores in this population to be particularly low in performance IQ, arithmetic achievement, and visual motor integration.[111] When the children were retested at an older age, the arithmetic achievement and visual motor integration scores declined even further, but the reading and spelling abilities did not decline. These problems are thought to be attributable to a visual-perceptual-organizational deficit that influences the child's ability to solve mathematic and visual-spatial problems.[111]

Other studies have noted a high degree of attention deficit or distractibility in some children with spina bifida, these problems were especially profound in those who showed poor language development. These children had poor development of auditory figure-ground, which allows a child to recognize and to attend to relevant features in the auditory environment. A child with difficulty in this area may not be able to identify relevant auditory input and discard the irrelevant. Therefore, in a rich auditory environment, extraneous sounds distract the child from the assigned task. These children often do better in a quiet, secluded testing situation, but classroom performance for similar tasks can be poor. Horn et al. found limited development of language comprehension in many of the children tested.[112] Individual vocabulary comprehension was normal, but comprehension of a story was poor. The children had difficulty identifying and retaining relevant features of the story and discarding the unimportant ones. Difficulty learning and memorizing lists of unrelated words has also been noted. However, memory for related facts was better, such as when answering questions about a short story.[112]

In the studies just mentioned, little information was available regarding early medical treatment of the child. Methods of treatment for hydrocephalus and ventricular infections were not delineated. Other factors that influence sensorimotor learning and testing outcome, including level of mobility and sensation in the trunk and lower extremity, were not mentioned. Therefore, it is difficult to determine precisely which factors may be responsible for the problems that influence learning. Decreased opportunity to develop manual skills has been thought to be a factor, as have the mobility limitations that affect the child's experiences with moving the body relative to stationary objects and manipulation and movement of those objects. Theoretical rationales for dysfunction include potential cerebellar damage from the Chiari II malformation. CNS damage affects the range, direction, force, and rate of voluntary movements and the manner in which movement is interpreted.

Any discussion of perceptual development should include problems of ocular function. Compared with the normal population, strabismus occurs six to eight times more frequently in those children with spina bifida. Visual-spatial problems during manipulation activities have also been noted in some children with spina bifida. The lack of conjugate gaze influences spatial relationships, constancy of size, and development of normal visual perception. Other, more frequent ocular problems in children with spina bifida include nystagmus, poor ocular motility, and other convergence defects. These abnormalities have been attributed to brainstem dysfunction, although there has been no correlation by MRI studies of the severity of the Chiari II malformation and these ocular defects.

The consensus is that children with spina bifida need a broad range of movement and learning experiences during the early years. Increased experiences in many areas may decrease the impact of any specific limitations. Testing with age-appropriate materials is critically important, and eliminating test items that include a motor component affords a more accurate and valid result[113–119] (Fig. 5-26).

Wheelchair Mobility

Much of this chapter has been devoted to bracing and ambulation issues, but some type of seated mobility must also be considered for the

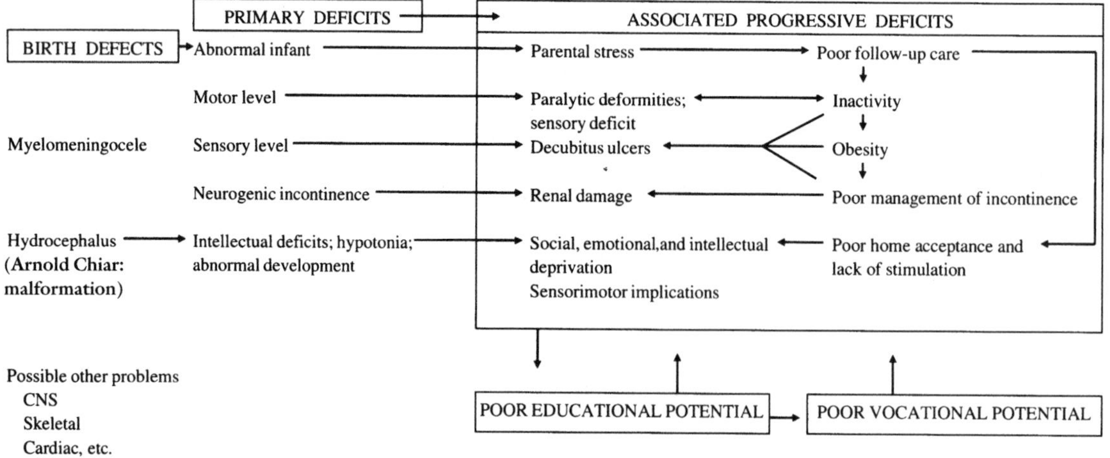

Figure 5-26 ▪ Primary and progressive deficits in children with spina bifida. (Adapted from Syllabus of Instructional Courses, American Academy for Cerebral Palsy, 1974.)

many children for whom this is appropriate and necessary. Any decision to use one of the many devices should include the patient, family, and professional staff involved with the child. It is appropriate first to determine the need for and proposed uses of seated mobility. Is it for recreation and peer group interaction, indoor or outdoor use, or for use at school or preschool? A first device might be a hand-propelled caster cart or star car ordered through a medical supply company. Many commercially available electric cars or motorcycles can be modified with a hand switch rather than the usual foot pedal. These devices are inexpensive and low to the ground, facilitating transfer to the floor or to a standing position. They are cosmetically appealing and are acceptable to both disabled and typical children alike. They can be fast and safe when used in the proper environment, and provide beneficial stimulation and opportunities for socialization. The child's upper extremity ability and the presence of abnormal tone can guide the therapist in selecting the correct device, whether manual or electric. Excessive upper extremity work to propel and maneuver a device may frustrate the child and produce unacceptable changes in tone. One study examined young children with otherwise poor mobility who used motorized chairs. Benefits that were noted included increased curiosity, initiative, motivation, communication, exploration, and interaction with objects in the environment. There were also significant decreases in dependency and in demanding and hostile behaviors.[120]

The family that needs a wheelchair so that their child can be included on trips out-of-doors can use a stroller until the child is 5 to 6 years of age. Strollers are available in larger sizes, and can be used in combination with ambulation. It is not unusual for a typical child to ride in a stroller for periods of time during a family outing either.

A traditional wheelchair can be obtained prior to the child starting school. Safe transportation on the school bus is an issue. The therapist may have to research the method of transportation to be used. The smallest child can be carried onto the bus and secured in a regular seat. The child would then ambulate at school. Knowing which wheelchairs can be safely secured on the bus in a particular community will be helpful for the child who is not ready to ambulate (Fig. 5–27).

Other indications for a wheelchair include lack of efficient community mobility, resulting in limited cognitive and psychosocial experiences; marginally functional or unsafe ambulation; speed in ambulation that is inadequate to maintain a level consistent with peers and/or family; and increasing recreational activities.

The therapist should remember the increased risks for the child in a wheelchair. Scheduling time to use the chair and time out of the chair should be considered. The chance of abandonment of a gait program by a child who may have the potential of reaching a high level of efficient ambulation is always a risk of wheelchair use. Flexion contractures of the hips and knees, pressure problems, and spinal deformity are other issues for the seated child. Therefore, the child should spend time both out of the chair and out of the seated position every day. Prone positioning, standing in a prone or a supine stander, and ambulation are options available for the child.

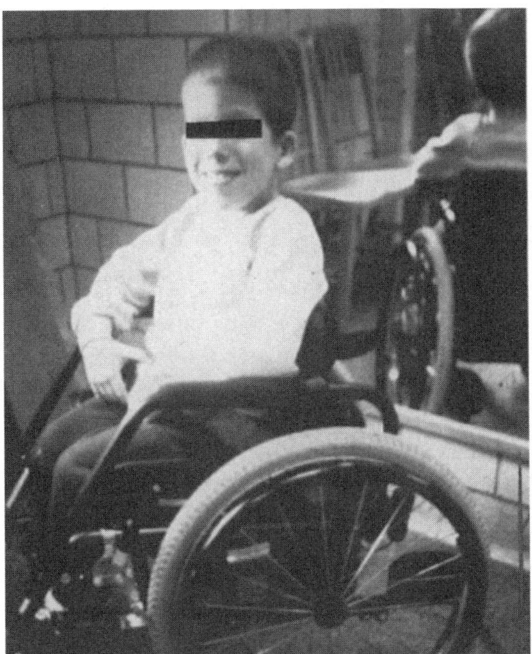

Figure 5-27 ▪ A light-weight wheelchair is selected for long-distance use in the school and community. This child also uses a reciprocating gait orthosis for shorter distances in the home and school.

As the child matures and mobility needs change, an electric wheelchair or cart can provide added speed and efficiency. A motorized device, which will conserve energy, may be very important for the individual facing a full and hectic day at school or work.

Various wheelchair cushions may prevent or reduce the development of pressure sores. Several materials are available, including high-density foam, which can be modified for even weight distribution. Regardless of the cushion chosen, activities for pressure relief are the best means of preventing skin breakdown on the posterior thighs and buttocks and should be performed, without fail, throughout the day. Frequent wheelchair push-ups and out-of-chair time should be incorporated into the daily schedule to provide for regular pressure relief.[8,16,38,120–122]

Recreation and Leisure Activities: Aquatics

As the child with spina bifida gets older and enters school, the time available for free periods of play and movement on the floor may be greatly reduced. Generally speaking, a full-time academic curriculum in an integrated or regular education setting provides little chance in which recreation can be pursued. Gym class with an instructor who is imaginative and motivated to collaborate with a physical therapist on ways to include the student with spina bifida into the regular array of activities will help the child along the route of finding activities in which he or she is able to participate and those that he or she might also enjoy. The child enrolled in a special education curriculum may have additional sessions scheduled into the school day for the development of recreation and leisure skills as part of their curriculum. But, as is true with the population of typical children who are school age, the child with spina bifida is often dependent on the knowledge and resources of family and friends to provide them with exposure to new, novel, and consistent recreational pursuits after the school day ends. Identifying activities that can be learned and pursued throughout one's life should be considered an important part of the total care plan for the individual with spina bifida. The physical therapist has a valuable role in assisting the patient and his or her family to find appropriate programs that offer wheelchair games and sports or adaptive programs for the child who is ambulatory. Being asked to give an opinion or a recommendation for adapted bicycles and other home exercise or recreation equipment is not uncommon. Helping to keep the child active with this advice is an important contribution. The child with spina bifida should be encouraged to regularly participate in activities that provide an appropriate cardiovascular challenge, muscle strengthening, improved eye-hand coordination, wheelchair maneuvering skills, and sportsmanship from which all children can benefit.

The inclusion and expansion of aquatics within the physical therapy profession has resulted in a significant increase in the body of research and information available for the therapist who has the opportunity to add aquatics to his or her clinical repertoire. The interest in health and fitness within the general population has resulted in many more accessible pool facilities available for both recreation and therapeutic purposes. Providing opportunities to explore and enjoy the benefits of moving in water may assist the child with spina bifida to enjoy this recreational activity that can be fun. Learning water safety and basic swimming skills can be taught to the young child and utilized throughout his or her lifetime. Water competency with or without the use of flotation devices can enable the person with spina bifida to experience a level of independent freedom of movement unavailable on land. More advanced aquatic skills can also be incorporated into a multifaceted therapeutic program that can be designed for the individual, taught, and monitored by the physical therapist who has access to a pool facility. By utilizing the natural properties of resistance and buoyancy of the water, strengthening of the body, increasing cardiovascular efficiency, and fun can result. This therapist has found that providing physical therapy sessions in the pool can be a useful tool in the rehabilitation program of the child following orthopedic surgery. Children who are already comfortable in the water are easily motivated to work hard on an exercise program when the excitement and novelty of the water environment is added. Brief free swim periods can be the rest time in between working or they can be the rewards for a child who did a good job. Taking a break on that mat usually results in the patient not moving, whereas the child usually continues to move in the water. Lap swims, races, and in-pool team games such as search and retrieve, basketball, volleyball, or tag are just a few of the many possibilities. (Display 5-10).

The Adult with Spina Bifida

Care of the patient with spina bifida does not end with the move to an adult facility for medical care. Being aware of the abilities, problems, and concerns of the adult with spina bifida is helpful for the clinician specializing in pediatric care. By analyzing the aging process and its effect on the patient, the therapist may develop a perspective that will influence younger patients. Seeing the long-term effects of many surgical and other therapeutic interventions can provide insight into areas of weakness and can improve the approach to care by modifying existing management protocols.[123]

DISPLAY 5-10

Examples of Therapeutic Strategies That Can Be Used in a Pool Setting

Provides strengthening to innervated lower extremity musculature, upper extremities, and trunk:

1. Movement of legs in all directions, all planes, with combination patterns of movement not feasible on a two-dimensional gym mat. Can be passive range of motion, active, active assistive, and resistive, depending on need.
2. Use of flotation device in deep water with legs down in the water, kicking in place against water's resistance.
3. Pushing off from pool side or therapist's hands while prone or supine on water surface to strengthen extension musculature and enjoy the sudden propulsion through the water.
4. Swimming laps with only leg motions while holding kick board or in an inner tube if necessary.
5. Lap swims using webbed gloves for added propulsion and resistance and a variety of strokes to address all muscles of shoulders. Flotation cuffs can be used around ankles if necessary to prevent legs from dragging on pool floor and provide extension if active gluteal musculature is not present.
6. Resistive swimming with therapist holding legs and preventing forward movement prone or supine.
7. Supine, within flotation ring, lifting legs out of water and twisting them side to side for work on all abdominals.
8. Ball toss and catch, basketball, newcomb, or volleyball in various water depths depending on children's ages and abilities.

In a study of patients with spina bifida, Dias et al. found that 80% lived with parents or other relatives.[124] Half of those individuals were older than 30 years of age. Eighty-two percent had achieved some level of independence, whereas 6% were totally dependent. Seventeen patients had married and were living away from family members. The degree of independence was not related to the lesion level or degree of ambulation achieved.[124] Dunne and Shurtleff identified some common complaints of adults with spina bifida, including obesity, social incontinence, recurrent urinary tract infections, chronic decubiti, joint pain, hypertension, neurologic deterioration, and depression.[125] McClone and colleagues cited other problem areas affecting the adult with spina bifida, including job training, employment, and achieving psychological and physical independence from family.[126] These studies indicate that the adult population has multiple and varied needs that may best be met by a multidisciplinary team approach.

Summary

There are many approaches to treating children with spina bifida. The disability is a complex one that requires an understanding of the many systems that are affected by its presence. The information presented in this chapter provides a background for a better understanding of this birth defect. Depending upon the setting in which the physical therapist is employed, certain sections of the chapter may be more or less relevant. Concerns and strategies for intervention suggested throughout this chapter reflect a general philosophy that physical therapists must be knowledgeable and aware of all facets of the disability. The therapist should also be sensitive to the protocols and concerns of the other professionals treating the child. The true challenge to the physical therapist is to integrate these various perspectives into a creative treatment plan that produces the best result for each child.

Combining experimentation and exploration, the therapist will discover new ideas for treatment that will help the child progress to his or her most productive and functional ability.

REFERENCES

1. Morrisey RT. Spina bifida: A new rehabilitation problem. *Orthop Clin North Am.* 1978;9:379–389.
2. Myers GJ. Myelomeningocele: The medical aspects. *Pediatr Clin North Am.* 1984;31:165–175.
3. Duff WE, Nutr M, Cooper ES. Neural tube defects in Jamaica following Hurricane Gilbert. *Am J Public Health.* 1994;Mar 84(3):473–476.
4. Seller M. Risks in spina bifida: Annotation. *DMCN.* 1994;36:1021–1025.
5. Lunsky AM, Ulcicus M, Rothman KJ, et al. Maternal heat exposure and neural tube defects. *J Am Med Assoc.* 1992;268:882–885.
6. McClone D. Neurosurgical management and operative closure for myelomeningocele. Presented at the Annual Myelomeningocele Seminar; 1982; Chicago.
7. Scarff TB, Fronczak S. Myelomeningocele: A review and update. *Rehab Lit.* 1981;42:143–147.
8. Tachdjian MO. *Pediatric Orthopedics.* 2nd ed. Vol 3. Philadelphia: WB Saunders; 1990; 1773–1880.
9. Behrman RC, Vaughn VC, eds. *Nelson's Textbook of Pediatrics.* 11th Ed. Philadelphia: WB Saunders; 1979.
10. Wolraich M. The association of spina bifida occulta and myelomeningocele. Presented at the 2nd Symposium on Spina Bifida; 1984; Cincinnati, Ohio.
11. Fidas A, MacDonald HL, Elton RA, et al. Prevalence of spina bifida occulta in patients with functional disorders of the lower urinary tract and its relation to urodynamics and neurophysiological measurements. *Br Med J.* 1989;298:357–359.
12. D'Agasta SD, Banta JV, Gahm N. The fate of patients with lipomeningocele. Presented at the American Academy of Cerebral Palsy and Developmental Medicine (ACPDM); 1987; Boston.
13. Kanev PM, Lemire RJ, Loeser JD, et al. Management and long-term follow-up review of children with lipomyelomeningocele. *J Neurosurg.* 1990; 73:48–52.
14. Moore KL. *The Developing Human: Clinically Oriented Embryology.* Philadelphia: WB Saunders; 1974.
15. Robbins SL. *Pathologic Basis of Disease.* Philadelphia: WB Saunders; 1974.
16. Umphred DA. *Neurological Rehabilitation.* St. Louis: CV Mosby; 1985.
17. Sharrard WJ. Neuromotor evaluation of the newborn. In: *Symposium on Myelomeningocele.* St. Louis: CV Mosby; 1972.
18. Peach B. The Arnold-Chiari malformation. *Arch Neurol.* 1965;12:165.
19. Peach B. The Arnold-Chiari malformation. *Arch Neurol.* 1965;12:109.
20. McCullough DC. Arnold-Chiari malformation—theories of development. Presented at the 2nd Symposium on Myelomeningocele; 1984; Cincinnati, OH.
21. McLone DG, Knepper PA. The cause of Chiari II malformation: A unified theory. *Pediatr Neurosci.* 1989;15:1–12.
22. Lutschg J, Meyer E, Jeanneret-Iseli C, et al. Brainstem auditory evoked potential in myelomeningocele. *Neuropediatrics.* 1985;16:202–204.
23. Hesz N, Wolraich M. Vocal cord paralysis and brainstem dysfunction in children with spina bifida. *Dev Med Child Neurol.* 1985;27:528–531.
24. Hoffman HJ, Hendrick EB, Humphreys RP, et al. Manifestations and management of Arnold-Chiari malformation in patients with myelomeningocele. *Child's Brain.* 1975;1:255–259.
25. Staal MJ, Melhuizen-de Regt MJ, Hess J. Sudden death in hydrocephalic spina bifida aperta patients. *Pediatr Neurosci.* 1987;13:13–18.
26. Pilu G, Romero R, Reece A, et al. Subnormal cerebellum in fetuses with spina bifida. *Am J Obstet Gynecol.* 1988;158:1052–1056.
27. Benacerraf BR, Stryker J, Frigotto FD. Abnormal ultrasound appearance of the cerebellum (banana sign): Indirect sign of spina bifida. *Pediatr Radiol.* 1989;171:151–153.
28. Thiagarajah S, Henke J, Hogge WA, et al. Early diagnosis of spina bifida: The value of cranial ultrasound markers. *Obstet Gynecol.* 1990;76: 54–57.
29. Bensen J, Dillard RG, Burton BK. Open spina bifida: Does cesarean section delivery improve prognosis? *Obstet Gynecol.* 1988;71:532–534.
30. Luthy DA, Wardinsky T, Shurtleff DB, et al. Cesarean section before the onset of labor and subsequent motor function in infants with myelomeningocele diagnosed antenatally. *N Engl J Med.* 1991;324:662–666.
31. Shurtleff DB, Luthy DA, Benedetti TJ, et al. Perinatal management, cesarean section and outcome in fetal spina bifida. Presented at the American

Academy of Cerebral Palsy and Developmental Medicine; 1987; Boston.
32. Hogge WA, Dungan JS, Brooks MP, et al. Diagnosis and management of prenatally detected myelomeningocele: A preliminary report. *Am J Obstet Gynecol.* 1990;163:1061–1064.
33. Raimondi AJ, Soare P. Intellectual development in shunted hydrocephalic children. *Am J Dis Child.* 1974;127:664–671.
34. McLone DG, Czyzewski D, Raimondi AJ, et al. Central nervous system infections as a limiting factor in the intelligence of children with myelomeningocele. *Pediatrics.* 1982;70:338–342.
35. Ellenbogen RG, Goldmann DA, Winston KW. Group B streptococcal infections of the central nervous system in infants with myelomeningocele. *Surg Neurol.* 1988;29:237–242.
36. Banta J. Long-term ambulation in spina bifida. Presented at the American Academy of Cerebral Palsy and Developmental Medicine; Chicago; 1983.
37. Murdoch A. How valuable is muscle charting? *Physiotherapy.* 1980;66:221–223.
38. Schafer M, Dias L. *Myelomeningocele: Orthopedic Treatment.* Baltimore: Williams & Wilkins; 1983.
39. *An Introduction to Hydrocephalus.* Children's Memorial Hospital; Chicago, IL; 1982.
40. Raimondi AJ. Complications of ventriculoperitoneal shunting and a critical comparison of the 3-piece and 1-piece systems. *Child's Brain.* 1977;3:321–342.
41. Bell WO, Sumner TE, Volberg FM. The significance of ventriculomegaly in the newborn with myelodysplasia. *Childs Nervous System.* 1987; 3:239–241.
42. Bell WO, Arbit E, Fraser R. One-stage myelomeningocele closure and ventriculo-peritoneal shunt placement. *Surg Neurol.* 1987;27: 233–236.
43. Manning J. Facilitation of movement—the Bobath approach. *Physiotherapy.* 1972;58:403–408.
44. Daniels L, Williams M, Worthingham C. *Muscle Testing: Techniques of Manual Examination.* Philadelphia: WB Saunders; 1956.
45. Strach EH. Orthopedic care of children with myelomeningocele: A modern program of rehabilitation. *Br Med J.* 1967;3:791–794.
46. Asher M, Olson J. Factors affecting the ambulatory status of patients with spina bifida cystica. *J Bone Joint Surg.* 1983;65A:350–356.
47. Bunch W. Progressive neurological loss in myelomeningocele patients. Presented at the American Academy of Cerebral Palsy and Developmental Medicine Conference; San Diego; 1982.
48. Coon V, Donato G, Houser C, et al. Normal ranges of hip motion in infants. *Clin Orthop.* 1975;110:256–260.
49. Haas S. Normal ranges of hip motion in the newborn. *Clin Orthop Related Res.* 1973;91:114–118.
50. Dias L. Hip contractures in the child with spina bifida. Presented at the 2nd Symposium on Spina Bifida; 1984; Cincinnati, OH.
51. Banta JV, Lin R, Peterson M, et al. The team approach in the care of the child with myelomeningocele. *J Prosthet Orthot.* 1989;2:263–273.
52. Lie HR, Lagergren Rasmussen F, et al. Bowel and bladder control of children with myelomeningocele: A Nordic study. *Dev Med Child Neurol.* 1991;33:1053–1061.
53. Brem AS, Martin D, Callaghan J, et al. Long-term renal risk factors in children with myelomeningocele. *J Pediatr.* 1987;110:51–55.
54. Anagnostopoulos D, Joannides E, Kotsianos K. The urological management of patients with myelodysplasia. *Pediatr Surg Int.* 1988;3: 347–350.
55. Wolf LS. Early motor development in children with myelomeningocele. Presented at the American Academy of Cerebral Palsy and Developmental Medicine; Washington, DC; 1984.
56. Mazur JM. Hand function in patients with spina bifida cystica. *J Pediatr Orthop.* 1986;6:442–447.
57. Anderson P. Impairment of a motor skill in children with spina bifida cystica and hydrocephalus: An exploratory study. *Br J Psychol.* 1977;68:61–70.
58. Dahl M, Ahlsten G, Carlson H, et al. Neurological dysfunction above cele level in children with spina bifida cystica: A prospective study to 3 years. *DMCN.* 1995;37:30–40.
59. Bobath B. Motor development, its effect on general development and application to the treatment of cerebral palsy. *Physiotherapy.* 1971;57: 526–532.
60. Bobath B. The treatment of neuromuscular disorders by improving patterns of coordination. *Physiotherapy.* 1969;55:18–22.
61. Bobath B. The very early treatment of cerebral palsy. *Dev Med Child Neurol.* 1967;9:373–390.
62. Caplan F. *The First Twelve Months of Life.* New York: Grosset and Dunlap; 1973.
63. Turner A. Upper-limb function in children with myelomeningocele. *Dev Med Child Neurol.* 1986; 28:790–798.
64. Turner A. Hand function in children with myelomeningocele. *J Bone Joint Surg (Br).* 1985; 67:268–272.
65. Agness PJ. Learning disabilities and the person with spina bifida. Presented at the Spina Bifida Association of America Meeting; 1980; Chicago.

66. Cronchman M. The effects of babywalkers on early locomotor development. *Dev Med Child Neurol.* 1986;28:757–761.
67. Charney EB, Melchionni JB, Smith DR. Community ambulation by children with myelomeningocele and high level paralysis. Presented at the American Academy of Cerebral Palsy and Developmental Medicine; San Francisco; 1989.
68. Beaty JH, Canale ST. Current concepts review. Orthopedic aspects of myelomeningocele. *J Bone Joint Surg (Am).* 1990;72:626–630.
69. Menelaus M. Hip dislocation: Concepts of treatment. Presented at the 2nd Symposium on Spina Bifida; 1984; Cincinnati, Ohio.
70. Stauffer ES, Hoffer M. Ambulation in thoracic paraplegia. *J Bone Joint Surg.* 1972; 54A:1336. Abstract.
71. Hoffer MM, Feiwell EE, Perry R, et al. Functional ambulation in patients with myelomeningocele. *J Bone Joint Surg.* 1973;55A:137–148.
72. Yngve D, Douglas R, Roberts JM. The reciprocating gait orthosis in myelomeningocele. *J Pediatr Orthop.* 1984;4:304–310.
73. Dias L, Tappit-Emas E. Boot E. The reciprocating gait orthosis: The Children's Memorial experience. Presented at the American Academy of Developmental Medicine and Child Neurology; 1984; Washington, DC.
74. Douglas R, Larson PF, D'Ambrosia R, et al. The LSU reciprocating gait orthosis. *Orthopedics.* 1983;6:834–839.
75. Center for Orthotics Design, Inc.
76. Williams L. Energy cost of walking and of wheelchair propulsion by children with myelodysplasia. *Dev Med Child Neurol.* 1983;25:617–624.
77. McDonald CM, Jaffe KM, Mosca VS, et al. Ambulatory outcome of children with myelomeningocele: Effect of lower extremity muscle strength. *Dev Med Child Neurol.* 1991;33: 482–490.
78. Neto J, Dias L, Gabriel A. Congenital talipes equinovarus in spina bifida: Treatment and results. *J Pediatr Orthop.* 1996;16:782–785.
79. Schopler SA, Menelaus MB. Significance of the strength of the quadriceps muscles in children with myelomeningocele. *J Pediatr Orthop.* 1987; 7:507–512.
80. Sherk HH, Uppal GS, Lane G, et al. Treatment versus nontreatment of hip dislocations in ambulatory patients with myelomeningocele. *Dev Med Child Neurol.* 1991;33:491–494.
81. Hunt, et al. The effects of fixed and hinged ankle-foot orthoses on gait myoelectric activity in children with myelomeningocele. Meeting Highlights of AACPDM. *J Pediatr Orthop.* 1994;14:2:269.
82. Knutson LM, Clark DE. Orthotic devices for ambulation in children with cerebral palsy and myelomeningocele. *Phys Ther.* 1991;71:947–960.
83. Vankoski S, Dias L. Children with spina bifida benefit from gait analysis. *Vicon Motion Systems. The Standard.* 1997;1:4–5.
84. Vankoski S, Sarwark J, Moore C, et al. Characteristic pelvis, hip and knee kinematic patterns in children with lumbosacral myelomeningocele. *Gait Posture.* 1995;3:1:51–57.
85. Ounpuu S, Davis R, Bell K, et al. Gait analysis in the treatment decision making process in patients with myelomeningocele. 8th Annual East Coast Gait Laboratories Conference.
86. Duffy C, Hill A, Cosgrove A, et al. Three-dimensional gait analysis in spina bifida. *J Pediatr Orthop.* 1996;16:786–791.
87. Williams J, Graham G, Dunne K, et al. Late knee problems in myelomeningocele. *J Pediatr Orthop.* 1993;13:701–703.
88. Drummond D. Post-operative fractures in patients with myelomeningocele. *Dev Med Child Neurol.* 1981;23:147–150.
89. Rosenstein BD, Greene WB, Herrington RT, et al. Bone density in myelomeningocele: The effects of ambulatory status and other factors. *Dev Med Child Neurol.* 1987;29:486–494.
90. Lock TR, Aronson DD. Fractures in patients who have myelomeningocele. *J Bone Joint Surg (Am).* 1989;71:1153–1157.
91. Hall P, Lindseth R, Campbell R, et al. Scoliosis and hydrocephalus in myelomeningocele patients: The effect of ventricular shunting. *J Neurosurg.* 1979;50:174–178.
92. Mazur JM, Menelaus MB. Neurologic status of spina bifida patients and the orthopedic surgeon. *Clin Orthop Rel Res.* 1991;264:54–64.
93. Petersen M. Tethered cord syndrome in myelodysplasia: Correlation between level of lesion and height at time of presentation. *DMCN.* 1992; 34:604–610.
94. McClone D, Herman J, Gabriele A, et al. Tethered cord as a cause of scoliosis in children with a myelomeningocele. *Pediatr Neurosurg.* 1990;91: 16:8–13.
95. Banta J. The tethered cord in myelomeningocele: Should it be untethered? *Dev Med Child Neurol.* 1991;33:167–176.
96. McLaughlin TP, Banta JV, Gahn NH, et al. Intraspinal rhizotomy and distal cordectomy in pa-

tients with myelomeningocele. *J Bone Joint Surg (Am)*. 1986;68:88–94.

97. Mazur J, Stillwell A, Menelaus M. The significance of spasticity n the upper and lower limbs in myelomeningocele. *J Bone Joint Surg (Br)*. 1986; 68:213–217.
98. Flanagan RC, Russell DP, Walsh JW. Urologic aspects of tethered cord. *Urology*. 1989;33:80–82.
99. Kaplan WE, McLone DG, Richards I. The urological manifestation of the tethered spinal cord. *J Urol*. 1988;140:1285–1288.
100. Grief L, Stalmasek V. Tethered cord syndrome: A pediatric case study. *J Neurosci Nurs*. 1989;21: 86–91.
101. Centers for Disease Control. Anaphylactic reaction during general anesthesia among pediatric patients, United States. Jan 1990–Jan 1991. *MMWR*. 1991;40:437–443.
102. Allergic Reactions to Latex-Containing Medical Devices: FDA Medical Alert. Food and Drug Administration. March 29, 1991.
103. Meeropol E, Frost J, Pugh L, et al. Latex allergy in children with myelomeningocele. *J Pediatr Orthop*. 1993;13:1–4.
104. D'Astous J, Drouin M, Rhine E. Intraoperative anaphylaxis secondary to allergy to latex in children who have spina bifida. *JBJS*. 1992;74-A: 1084–1086.
105. Meehan P, Galina M, Daftari T. Intraoperative anaphylaxis due to allergy to latex. *JBJS*. 1992; 74-A:1103–1109.
106. Lu L, Kurup V, Hoffman D, et al. Characterization of a major latex allergen associated with hypersensitivity in spina bifida patients. *J Immunol*. 1995;155:2721–2728.
107. Medical Sciences Bulletin. Jan. 13, 1997. http://pharminfo.com/pub/msb/latex.html.
108. Spina Bifida Association of America. http://www: infohiway.com/spinabifida/latex.html.
109. Good Latex Allergy Survival Skills. Jan. 3, 1997. http//www.netcom.com/~ecbdmd/Glass.html.
110. Latex Allergy. Jan. 13, 1997. http://www. Waisman.Wisc.Edu/~rowley/sbkids/Sb_latex. html.
111. Willis KE, Holmbeck GN, Dillon K, et al. Intelligence and achievement in children with myelomeningocele. *J Pediatr Psychol*. 1990;15:161–176.
112. Horn DG, Pugzles Lorch E, Lorch RF, et al. Distractibility and vocabulary deficits in children with spina bifida and hydrocephalus. *Dev Med Child Neurol*. 1985;27:713–720.
113. Wolfe GA, Kennedy D, Brewer K, et al. Visual perception and upper extremity function in children with spina bifida. Presented at the American Academy of Cerebral Palsy and Developmental Medicine; San Francisco; 1989.
114. Cull C, Wyke MA. Memory function of children with spina bifida and shunted hydrocephalus. *Dev Med Child Neurol*. 1984;26:177–183.
115. Mauk JE, Charney EB, Nambiar R, et al. Strabismus and spina bifida. Presented at the American Academy of Cerebral Palsy and Developmental Medicine; 1987.
116. Lennerstrand G, Gallo JE. Neuro-ophthalmological evaluation of patients with myelomeningocele and Chiari malformations. *Dev Med Child Neurol*. 1990;32:415–422.
117. Rothstein TB, Romano PE, Shoch D. Meningomyelocele. *Am J Ophthalmol*. 1974;77:690–693.
118. Horn DG, Lorch EP, Lorch RF, et al. Distractibility and vocabulary deficits in children with spina bifida and hydrocephalus. *Dev Med Child Neurol*. 1985;27:713–720.
119. Ruff HA. The development of perception and recognition of objects. *Child Dev*. 1980;51:981–992.
120. Butler C. Effects of powered mobility on self-initiated behaviors of very young children with locomotor disability. *Dev Med Child Neurol*. 1986; 28:325–332.
121. DeLateur B, Berni R, Hangladarom T, et al. Wheelchair cushions designed to prevent pressure sores. *Arch Phys Med Rehabil*. 1976;57:129–135.
122. Fiewell E. Seating and cushions for spina bifida. Presented at the 2nd Symposium on Spina Bifida; 1984; Cincinnati, OH.
123. Borjeson MC, Lagergren JL. Life conditions of adolescents with myelomeningocele. *Dev Med Child Neurol*. 1990;32:698–706.
124. Dias LS, Fernandez AC, Swank M. Adults with spina bifida: A review of seventy-one patients. Presented at the American Academy of Cerebral Palsy and Developmental Medicine; Boston; 1987.
125. Dunne KB, Shurtleff DB. The medical status of adults with spina bifida. Presented at the American Academy of Cerebral Palsy and Developmental Medicine; 1987.
126. McClone DG. Spina bifida today: Problems adult face. *Semin Neurol*. 1989;9:169–175.

BIBLIOGRAPHY

Williamson GG. *Children with Spina Bifida: Early Intervention and Pre-School Programming*. Baltimore: Brooks Publishers; 1987 (Family concerns and PT/OT interventional strategies).

Scherzer A, Tscharnuter I. *Early Diagnosis and Therapy in Cerebral Palsy*. New York: Marcel Dekker; 1982 (Handling strategies for young children).

OTHER SOURCES FOR LATEX INFORMATION

Spina Bifida Association of America, Tel. 800-621-3141.
FDA Latex Hotline, Tel. 301-594-3060.

LATEX FREE PRODUCTS CAN BE ORDERED FROM THE FOLLOWING

Alternative Resource Catalog, Tel. 708-503-8298.
NO LATEX Industries, Tel. 800-296-9185.
Relia Care Express, Tel. 888-225-1941.

Neuromuscular Disorders in Childhood and Physical Therapy Intervention

Julaine M. Florence

Children with neuromuscular disorders have a lifelong challenge to maintain function. That challenge can be met with the help of a knowledgeable physical therapist. In this chapter, the term *neuromuscular disease* refers to disorders whose primary pathology affects any part of the motor unit from the anterior horn cell out to the muscle itself. Common to all of these disorders is muscle weakness, which may be produced by pathology at any part of the motor unit. When characterizing neuromuscular disorders and their pathology, it is convenient to consider the various anatomic divisions of this motor unit: the anterior horn cell, peripheral nerve, neuromuscular junction, and the muscle.

Neuromuscular diseases may be either hereditary or acquired and are variously classified as myopathies, in which the cause of the muscle weakness is attributable to pathology confined to the muscle itself, or neuropathies, in which the muscle weakness is secondary to an abnormality of either the anterior horn cell or peripheral nerve. Further characterization is based on a particular disorder's characteristic pattern of presentation.

The term *muscular dystrophy* describes a group of myopathies that are genetically determined and have a steadily progressive degenerative course. Further classification of the muscular dystrophies is based on their clinical presentation, including the distribution of weakness and mode of inheritance.

The terms *spinal muscular atrophy* and *motor neuropathy* refer to neurogenic disorders whose underlying pathology affects the anterior horn cell or the peripheral nerve. Further classification is based on clinical presentation and mode of inheritance.

The neuromuscular disorders vary significantly in their presentation, pathology, and progression but are linked with regard to physical therapy intervention by their common characteristic of muscle weakness leading to loss of function and physical deformity. A physical therapist with an understanding of these disorders can help identify, predict, intervene, and possibly prevent unnecessary complications throughout the course of each disorder. The purpose of this chapter is to provide an overview of select neuromuscular diseases, including clinical presentation, pathology, diagnosis, disease progression, medical treatment, and physical therapy intervention.

Because Duchenne muscular dystrophy (DMD) is one of the most common myopathies and best known of the dystrophies affecting children, much of this chapter is devoted to a discussion of this disorder. Physical therapy interventions and principles that apply to the management of weakness and deformity in patients with DMD are also applicable to other neuromuscular diseases that present with similar symptoms and complications. Knowledge of the various disorders will allow appropriate decisions to be made about the suitability and timing of various physical therapy interventions. Other neuromuscular diseases that are reviewed in this chapter include myotonic and fasioscapulohumeral dystrophy and the spinal muscular atrophies.

Duchenne Muscular Dystrophy

Duchenne muscular dystrophy, also known as pseudohypertrophic muscular dystrophy or progressive muscular dystrophy, is one of the most prevalent and severely disabling of the childhood myopathies.

DMD is among the most severely disabling of all childhood disorders. Unlike disorders such as cerebral palsy or poliomyelitis, DMD represents a progressive disease in which the child becomes weaker and usually dies of a respiratory infection or cardiorespiratory insufficiency in the late teens or early 20s. Estimates of DMD's incidence vary between 13 and 33 patients per 100,000 live male births.[1] There is an X-linked inheritance pattern to DMD whereby male offspring inherit the disease from their mothers, who are most often asymptomatic. Advances in molecular biology have shown the defect to be a mutation at XP21 in the gene coding for the protein, dystrophin.[2,3]

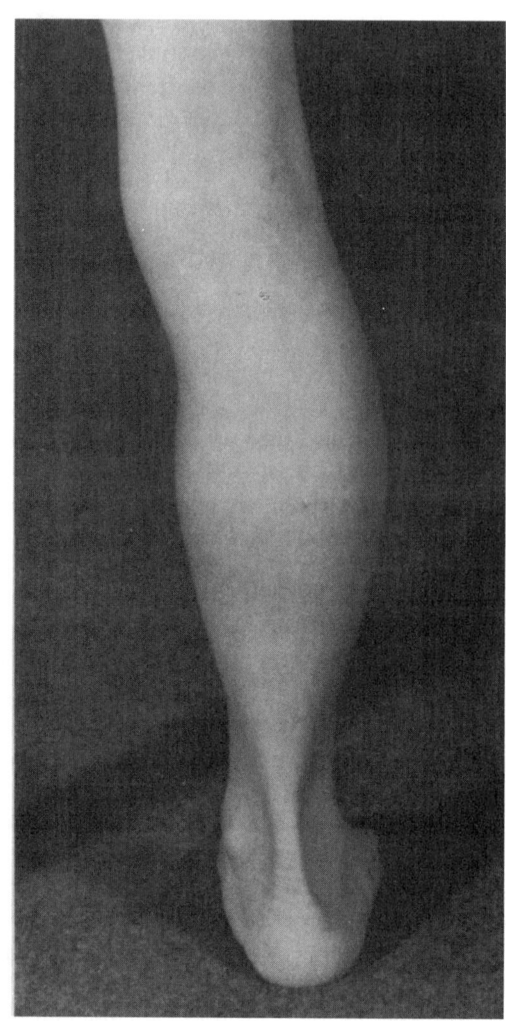

Figure 6-1 ▪ Duchenne dystrophy. Pseudohypertrophy of the calf. (From Lovell WW, Winter RB, eds. *Pediatric Orthopaedics.* 2nd Ed. Philadelphia: JB Lippincott; 1986:264.)

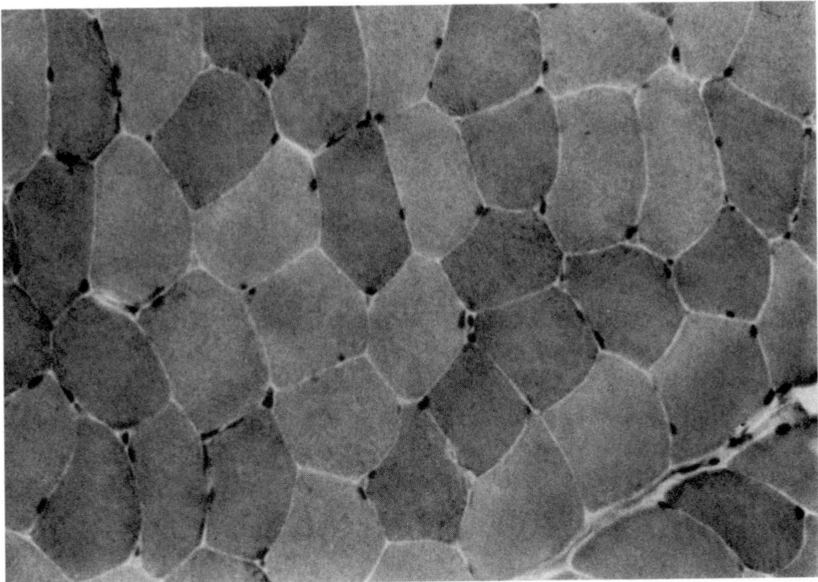

Figure 6-2 ▪ Normal adult muscle. Muscle fibers are cut in a plane transverse to their long axis and appear to have round, oval, or slightly irregular profiles. One or more darkly stained nuclei are seen at the edge of most fibers. (Trichrome, x300) (From Maloney, Burks, Ringel, eds. *Interdisciplinary Rehabilitation of Multiple Sclerosis and Neuromuscular Disorders.* Philadelphia: JB Lippincott; 1984:202.)

Clinical Presentation and Progression

The onset of the disorder is insidious, usually resulting in symptoms before 3 years of age; however, symptoms may not be noticed for months or years, and the disease may be misdiagnosed for years.[4]

Earliest symptoms may include a reluctance to walk or run at appropriate ages, falling, difficulty getting up off the floor, toe walking, clumsiness, and an increase in size of several groups of muscles. The gastrocnemius is the most notable muscle that commonly shows this "pseudohypertrophy," but the infraspinatus and deltoid muscles are also commonly enlarged (Fig. 6-1). These pseudohypertrophic muscles have a firm consistency when palpated. Histologic examination of muscle shows degeneration of muscle fibers with increased connective tissue and adipose cells (Figs. 6-2 and 6-3). Motor and sensory neurons are undamaged, and there is no significant change in either the central nervous system (CNS) or in the vascular system.[5] A high rate of intellectual impairment and emotional disturbance has been associated with DMD.[6]

The clinical presentation gives the first clues to the diagnosis, which is confirmed by the results of laboratory studies. Laboratory findings include an abnormally high serum creatinine kinase level, myopathic electromyogram (EMG), and abnormal muscle biopsy results (see Fig. 6-3)[5] or characteristic deletion on genetic analysis.[2,3] With the availability of genetic analysis, all male family members may be screened for the disorder and all female family members may be screened for their carrier status.

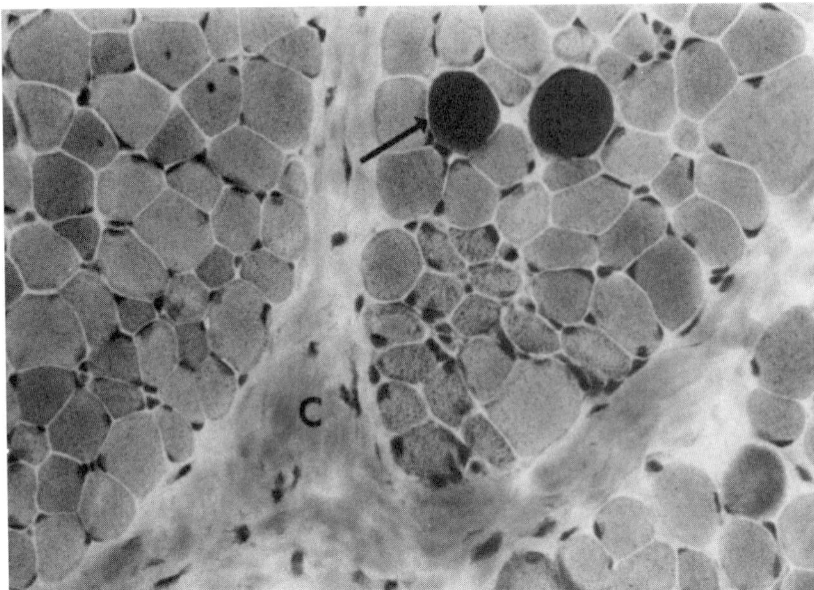

Figure 6-3 ■ Duchenne dystrophy. Compare these fibers with those of normal muscle in Figure 6-2. Dystrophic changes include a marked variability in fiber size; dark, "opaque" fibers (*arrow*); and abnormal quantities of fibrous connective tissue (*C*). (Trichrome, × 300) (From Maloney, Burks, Ringel, eds. *Interdisciplinary Rehabilitation of Muscular Dystrophy and Neuromuscular Disorders.* Philadelphia: JB Lippincott; 1984:203.)

The weakness is steadily progressive with the boys losing strength at 0.322 units per year (SD = 0.318) on a 10-point scale (see Fig. 6-4). This average muscle score represents the sum score of 34 muscles graded using the Medical Research Council Scale[7] for manual muscle testing, converted to a 10 point scale.[8] This slope of decline associated with the increasing age of the child was documented by following 378 boys, 6 to 18 years of age with the diagnosis of DMD, for a mean of 2.7 years (SD = 3.1, maximum = 10.7 years). This natural history study[9] of DMD was conducted by the Collaborative Investigation of Duchenne Dystrophy (CIDD) group. These natural history data have been reanalyzed with the inclusion of 95 new cases for presentation in this chapter (Figs. 6-4, 6-5, and 6-7). Although the overall decline in strength is 0.3 units per year, different muscles decline at varying rates (Fig. 6-5), with proximal muscles tending to be weaker earlier in the course of the illness and to progress faster.

Early weakness of the hip and knee extensors often results in an exaggerated lumbar lordosis that is characteristic of the early stages of disease. The lordosis occurs in response to the attempt to align the center of gravity anterior to the fulcrum of the knee joint and posterior to the falcrum of the hip joint. This realignment gives maximum stability at both joints. The child attempts to broaden the base of support during walking and thus develops a gait that resembles waddling. The child may develop iliotibial band contractures, which are made worse by this wide-based stance. As the weakness progresses, the child rises from the floor by "climbing up the legs." This maneuver, known as Gower's sign, is indicative of proximal muscle weakness (Fig. 6-6).

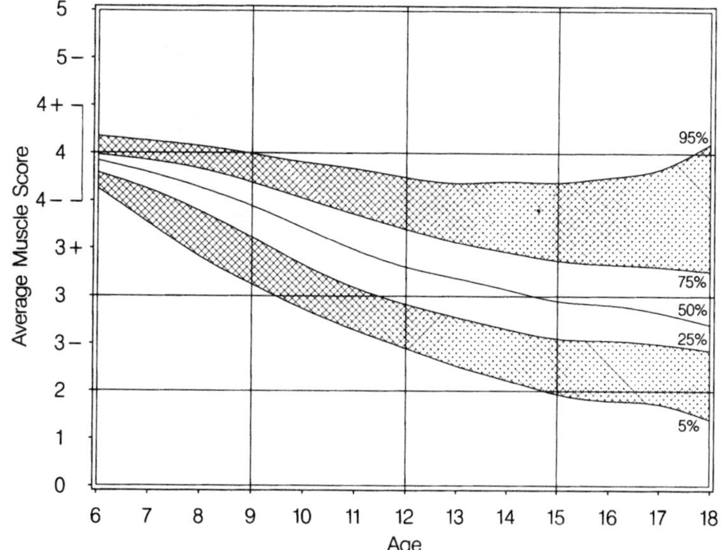

Figure 6-4 ▪ Average muscle scores plotted as percentiles of the population. The center line represents the 50th percentile. The shaded areas span the 5th to the 25th and the 75th to the 95th percentile. (Courtesy of the Collaborative Investigation of Duchenne Dystrophy [CIDD] Group).

As the disease progresses, there is a tendency to develop contractures. These contractures typically result in plantar-flexion at the ankle, with inversion of the foot and flexion at both the hips and knees.

This early loss of range of motion (ROM), noted in the hip flexors, iliotibial bands, and heel cords, limits stance and ambulation in that patients find it difficult to achieve the mechanical alignment necessary to hold themselves in an

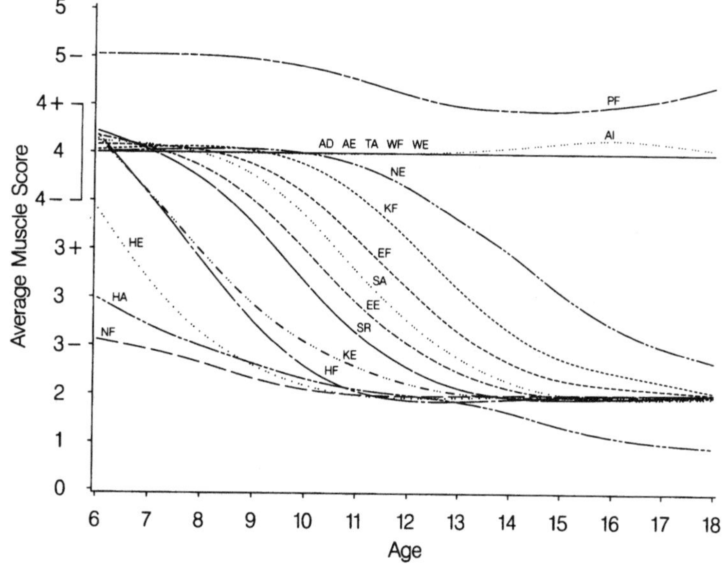

Figure 6-5 ▪ The lines represent the 50th percentiles for the strength of individual muscles plotted against age. PF, plantar-flexor; AI, ankle invertor; AD, ankle dorsiflexor; AE, ankle invertor; TA, thumb abductor; WF, wrist flexor; WE, wrist extensor; NE, neck extensor; KF, knee flexor; EF, elbow flexor; HE, hip extensor; SA, shoulder abductor; EE, elbow extensor; HA, hip abductor; SR, shoulder external rotator; KE, knee extensor; HF, hip flexor; NF, neck flexor. (Courtesy of the Collaborative Investigation of Duchenne Dystrophy [CIDD] Group).

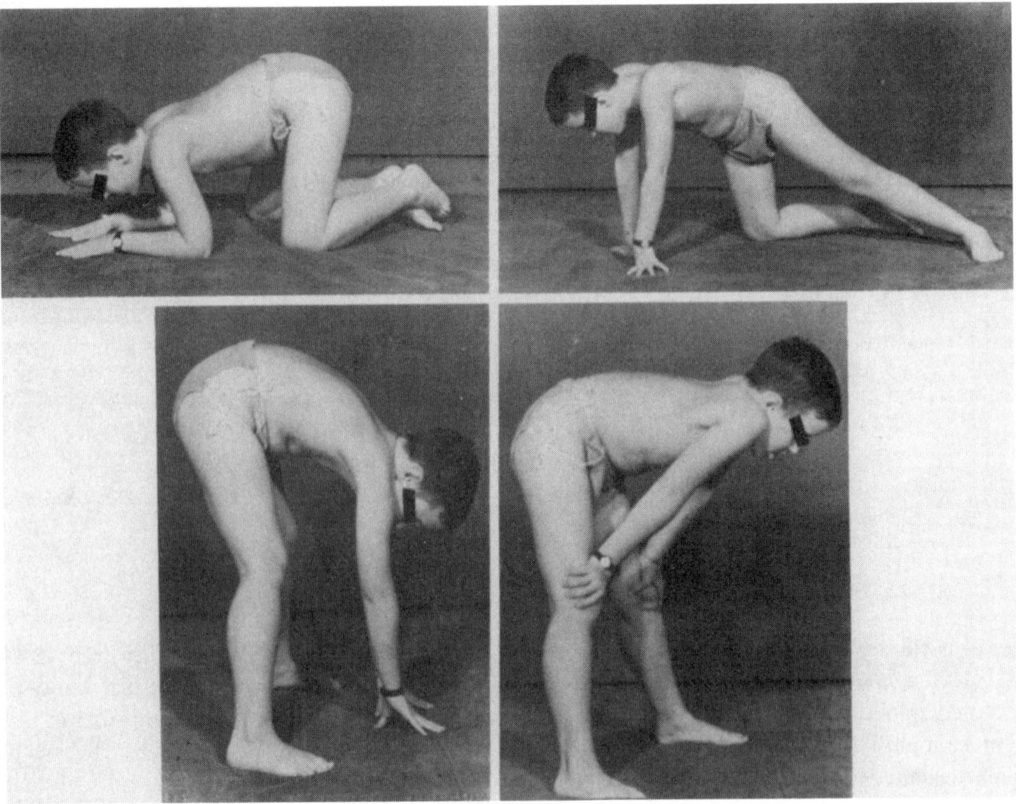

Figure 6-6 ▪ Gower's sign. This series of maneuvers is necessary to achieve an upright posture, and it occurs with all types of pelvic and trunk weakness. The child "climbs up the legs" when rising from the floor. (From Lovell WW, Winter RB, eds. *Pediatric Orthopaedics.* 2nd ed. Philadelphia: JB Lippincott 1986:265.)

upright posture using their weak musculature. As these boys spend more time sitting, an increasing degree of contracture is seen at the hips, knees, and elbows.

Functional activities may be performed more slowly by children with DMD than by normal children, but most of those affected are able to walk, climb stairs, and stand up from the floor without too much difficulty until 6 or 7 years of age. At this time, a relatively rapid decline in function has been documented, which generally results in a loss of unassisted ambulation at 9 to 10 years of age and loss of ambulation, even in long-leg braces, at 12 to 13 years of age.[9] A graphic representation of the ages at which the children have increasing difficulty with various functional activities is presented in Figure 6-7. These functional activities are considered to be "milestones" and represent significant points in disease progression. The arm grades awarded were developed by Brooke and associates[9] (Table 6-1), whereas the leg grades are based on a scale proposed by Vignos (Table 6-2).[10]

As is demonstrated by the range and distribution of percentiles in Figures 6-4 and 6-7, the clinical course of disease progression in individual children is not homogeneous. The mildest of the X-linked progressive dystrophies has been

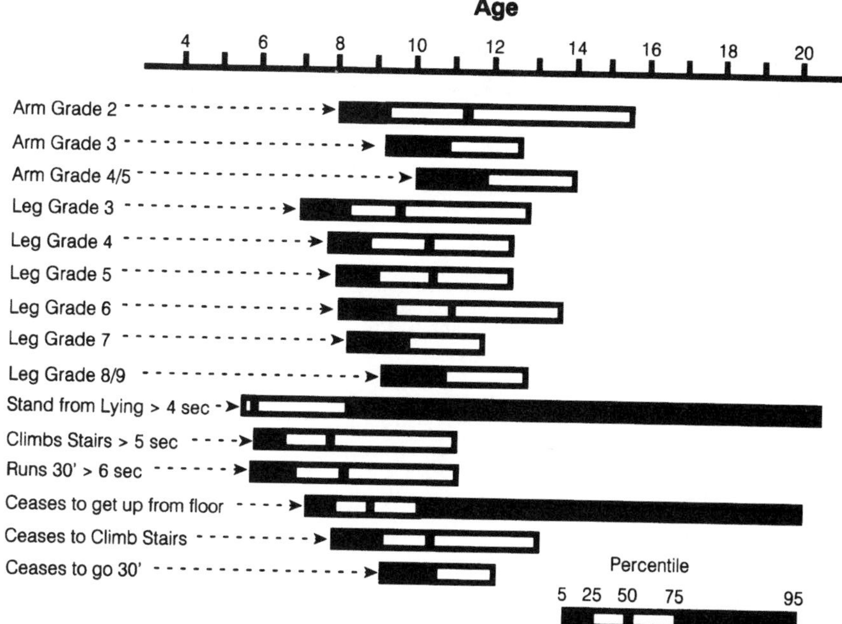

Figure 6-7 ▪ Graphic representation of the ages (expressed as percentiles) at which children with Duchenne muscular dystrophy have increasing difficulty with functional tasks. (Courtesy of the Collaborative Investigation of Duchenne Dystrophy [CIDD] Group.)

termed Becker muscular dystrophy. This classification applies to individuals who maintain independent ambulation until after the age of 15 years. Brooke and colleagues have coined the term "outliers"[9] to describe a population of boys who fulfill the diagnostic criteria for DMD but who, when compared to the DMD population's usual pattern of disease progression, fall outside the usual limits. Investigators are studying genetic heterogeneity with regard to DNA mutations and resulting dystrophin expression in an attempt to explain the varying levels of clinical severity associated with DMD.[11]

Scoliosis develops as the age of the child with DMD increases; significant curves are generally not noticed until after the age of 11 years.[12] This scoliosis tends to progress as the back muscles become weaker and as the child spends less time standing and more time sitting, resulting in a positional scoliosis (Fig. 6-8) which, over time, becomes fixed.

In addition to the voluntary muscles, DMD affects other organs. As the respiratory musculature atrophies, coughing becomes ineffective and pulmonary infections become more frequent, often leading to the patient's early death. Dystrophic cardiomyopathy is common and often contributes to death.[13] Although intelligence may be reduced among children with DMD, this deficit is not progressive and is not related to the severity of disease.[14] Although not progressive, this intellectual deficit may hinder the child's development and may make a physical evaluation of the child difficult. Fortunately, children with DMD seldom lose bowel or bladder control, and other neurologic signs do not appear.

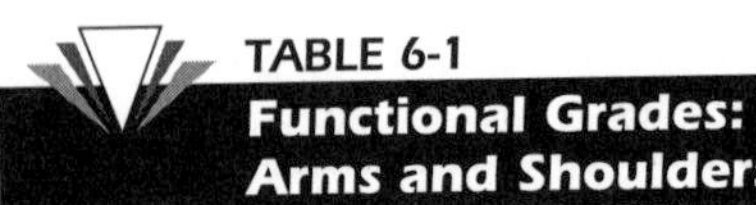

TABLE 6-1
Functional Grades: Arms and Shoulders

Grades	Functional Ability
1	Standing with arms at the sides, the patient can abduct the arms in a full circle until they touch above the head.
2	The patient can raise the arms above the head only by flexing the elbow (i.e., by shortening the circumference of the movement) or by using accessory muscles).
3	The patient cannot raise hands above the head, but can raise an 8-oz glass of water to the mouth (using both hands if necessary).
4	The patient can raise hands to the mouth, but cannot raise an 8-oz glass of water to the mouth.
5	The patient cannot raise hands to the mouth, but can use the hands to hold a pen or to pick up pennies from a table.
6	The patient cannot raise hands to the mouth and has no useful function of the hands.

Treatment

Although definitive treatment is lacking, proper management, as outlined by Ziter and Allsop, can prolong the maximum functional ability of the child.[15] This program of management begins once the diagnosis is established, and it is initiated concurrently with parental counseling in an attempt to reduce the guilt, hostility, fear, depression, hopelessness, and numerous other emotions commonly experienced by the parents.

> The clinician faced with this situation can propose a positive approach based on the following: 1) some of the complications which magnify the functional disability of DMD are predictable and preventable; 2) an active program of physical therapy and the timely application of braces can prolong ambulation and more closely approximate the normal independence of later childhood; and 3) if a specific treatment ever becomes available, those in optimal physical condition are most apt to benefit.[15]

There is no pharmaceutical treatment that will cure DMD, but several studies[16,17] have confirmed an initial report that prednisone increases strength in patients with DMD.[18] Further investigation has shown that prednisone, despite its many side effects, keeps those affected by DMD "stronger for longer."[19,20] Other pharmaceutical interventions that have been studied in hope of finding a treatment as effective as prednisone, without the side effects, include deflazacort (a corticosteroid)[21] and oxandrolone (an anabolic steroid).[22]

Myoblast transplant has been proposed as a treatment for DMD with the aim of replacing

TABLE 6-2
Functional Grades: Hips and Legs

Grades	Functional Ability
1	Walks and climbs stairs without assistance
2	Walks and climbs stairs with the aid of a railing
3	Walks and climbs stairs slowly (elapsed time of more than 12 seconds for four standard stairs) with the aid of a railing
4	Walks unassisted and rises from a chair, but cannot climb stairs
5	Walks unassisted but cannot rise from a chair or climb stairs
6	Walks only with assistance or walks independently with long-leg braces
7	Walks in long-leg braces, but requires assistance for balance
8	Stands in long-leg braces, but is unable to walk even with assistance
9	Is in wheelchair
10	Is confined to bed

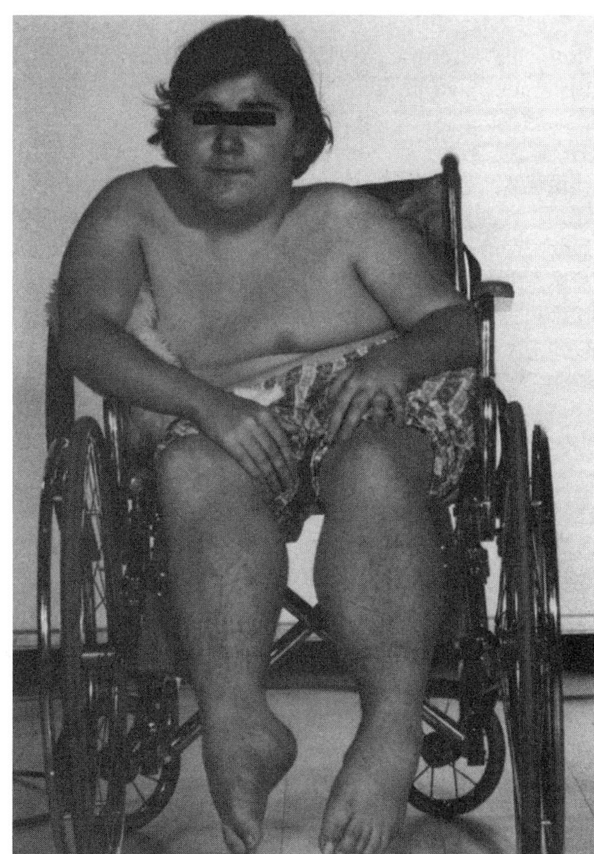

Figure 6-8 ▪ Obesity with fixed equinocavovarus and scoliosis in a child with advanced Duchenne muscular dystrophy. (From Maloney, Burks, Ringel, eds. *Interdisciplinary Rehabilitation of Muscular Dystrophy and Neuromuscular Disorders.* Philadelphia: JB Lippincott; 1984:290.)

the missing protein dystrophin.[23] However, at present, this procedure is still being investigated. Various other strategies for replacing the defective gene and missing protein are under study, but currently none are available for clinical use.[24]

Physical Therapy Evaluation

Each child with DMD should undergo a physical therapy evaluation. Such an evaluation involves the gathering of information that contributes to the development of a plan of care.[25] That care plan will be based largely on the functional significance of the therapist's findings.

FUNCTIONAL ABILITY

Systematic and serial recording of standard tasks shows that the child with DMD is in one of two general phases: stable performance or declining performance. During the stable phase, which may continue for several years, the child may demonstrate normal performance of various tasks during the serial evaluations, despite a continuing decline in strength. A discrepancy exists in the age at which the aforementioned tasks are failed, as illustrated in Figure 6-7.

Ziter and associates[26] and Allsop and Ziter[27] have demonstrated that, although functional ability appears to remain at a constant stage in many children with DMD, actual muscle strength continues to decline insidiously. These findings suggest that, although timed functional tests are useful in determining the patient's current status, they have limited value in monitoring the progressive loss of strength in DMD. As a result of these studies, Allsop believes that, when timed trials are used as dependent variables in drug trials, they may overestimate therapeutic efficacy. A patient who appears to be stable in a series of timed trials may actually be experiencing a continual decline in strength, in which case the drug has had no effect on the progression of the myopathy.

Brooke and coworkers[28] and Florence and associates[8] have presented a clinical evaluation protocol for DMD—assessing strength, pulmonary function, and functional tasks in combination—that has been demonstrated to be reliable in documenting disease course in patients with DMD.[9] In addition, the protocol is able to detect not only the therapeutic effect of pharmaceutical intervention but the time course and differences in various dose levels of such intervention.[23]

MUSCLE TESTING

Measurement of muscle strength by way of manual muscle testing (MMT) remains a valid approach to assessing the progression of disease in children with DMD.[8] MMT has been shown to be both reliable[24] and sensitive to changes in strength in patients with DMD.[29]

Because muscle weakness is characteristic of all myopathies, MMT must be a routine part of the physical therapy evaluation of the child with myopathy. Serial use of MMT provides data against which the efficacy of management can be monitored. The longitudinal results of MMT in children with DMD show a linearity in the decline of muscle strength. Although some authors describe an apparent stabilization of strength between 5 and 8 years of age, Allsop and Ziter,[27] Ziter and associates,[26] and Brooke et al.[9] have found neither plateaus nor accelerated periods of the disease process. Bracing does not slow down the deterioration, and use of a wheelchair does not increase the rate of decline.

By the time the child reaches 7 years of age, or with serial strength scores recorded for 1 year, it is possible to estimate the rate of progression as either rapid (>10% deterioration per year), average (5% to 10% deterioration per year), or slow (<5% deterioration per year). There is a variation in the rapidity of progression, and MMT, along with performance of functional tasks, helps determine when bracing or wheelchairs will be needed.

The following muscles are routinely graded:

Upper trapezius	Rhomboids
Lower trapezius	Iliopsoas
Deltoid	Quadriceps
Serratus anterior	Gluteus maximus
Pectorals	Gluteus medius
Latissimus dorsi	Anterior tibialis
Triceps	Abdominals

Although this list of muscles may be useful for monitoring the child's status in the clinical setting, the only muscle groups in which reliability of testing has been documented are those graphed in Figure 6-5. It has been demonstrated that, although MMT is a reliable means of assessment in DMD when performed by the same examiner, the interrater reliability of MMT varies among individual muscles and grades.[8,30] It is apparent that one's purpose for performing MMT—whether it is to answer clinical questions or to serve as a research measurement tool—determines the vigor with which one approaches strength testing.

Because of the difficulty in testing the serratus anterior, a supplementary position may be used. The child holds both hands at eye level with arms horizontally abducted and elbows extended. The amount of scapular winging is noted and a subjective grade is given. The traditional testing position is then attempted in order to achieve a more refined and specific grade.

Although the iliopsoas muscle is tested in the standard position, its ability to generate force decreases at an early stage in the disease. Most of the hip flexion strength is generated by the long head of the rectus femoris and by the sartorius. No attempt is made to differentiate between the often nonexistent sternal head and the clavicular portion of the pectoralis major.

In the later stages of the disease, differentiation between the fair and fair–poor range of muscle strength becomes difficult to ascertain for the abdominal muscles. Weakened neck flexors provide additional resistance to the abdominal muscles. This resistance is caused by the head not being able to flex onto the thorax during abdominal contraction, thereby resulting in a longer lever arm for the abdominal muscles.

Hand-held myometry and various fixed tensiometer systems have been used in attempts to better quantify muscle strength in boys with DMD.[31,32]

RANGE OF MOTION

Standard assessment of joint motion with goniometry should be done periodically. Pandya and associates studied the intratester and intertester reliability of goniometry for children with DMD.[33] They found high intratester values, but intertester values varied. As a result, they have recommended that serial goniometric evaluations be done by the same examiner.[33] Early loss of ambulation is more frequently caused by loss of motion and contracture than by weakness in specific muscle groups. Loss of full ankle dorsiflexion, knee extension, and hip extension, with resultant contractures, occurs commonly in patients with DMD. Measurement of ankle dorsiflexion, knee extension, hip extension, and iliotibial band (ITB) tightness are probably the most important aspects of goniometric testing.

Physical Therapy Intervention

We believe that physical therapists manage patients and their problems, not diseases. The primary problems encountered by children with DMD include the following:

1. Weakness
2. Decreased active and passive ROM
3. Loss of ambulation
4. Decreased functional ability
5. Decreased pulmonary function
6. Emotional trauma—individual and family
7. Progressive scoliosis

When physical therapy management has been appropriate, physical pain should not be a problem for the child. After a physical examination of the patient, the physical therapist can identify current problems and, based on a thorough understanding of the disease process, should be able to predict the next major difficulties to be encountered. Based on the specific areas of concern for each family, it is possible to identify four major goals of management common to all children with DMD.

1. Prevent deformity.
2. Prolong functional capacity.
3. Facilitate the development and assistance of family support and support of others.
4. Control pain, if necessary.

As the preceding four goals are accomplished, we fulfill our general goal for all individuals with neuromuscular disease, that of helping them be as independent and comfortable as possible within the limits of their disability.

To address the preceding goals, one must think about the specifics of preventing deformity through the prescription of ROM exercises and stretching, splinting, and appropriate positioning. Prolonging functional capacity of ensuring safety while functioning may require the prescription of specific orthotics or adaptive equipment.

Support for the family may be aided by good rapport with the medical personnel; family education in regard to the disease process and its implications; referral to the Muscular Dystrophy Association (MDA), where they would have access to other families facing similar problems; and the educational, social, financial, and medical care opportunities offered by the MDA. The child and family may be aided by appropriate timing of referral to other associated medical personnel, including orthotist, occupational therapist, adaptive equipment supplier, social service worker, dietician, or medical specialists including orthopedic surgeon, pulmonologist, or cardiologist.

Pain control may or may not be necessary and is often dependent on how successful stretching and bracing strategies were in the child's earlier years. Appropriate stretching, fit and positioning in wheelchairs, cushions, alternating pressure pads, or specialized mattresses and hospital beds can go a long way in assisting the control of discomfort in these children.

HOME PROGRAM

Because much of the responsibility for daily treatment must be assumed by the family or friends of the patient with DMD, an effective program of care at home is essential. Although sustaining enthusiasm and adherence with the home program may be difficult, the likelihood of success can be improved by giving simple instructions, requesting a limited number of exercises and repetitions each day, and offering extensive feedback and positive reinforcement to people in the support system. By reducing the anxiety associated with non-adherence and outlining both short- and long-term goals for the family, adherance and rapport can be improved. In the case of a single-parent family, we suggest extra support from older siblings, clergy, social groups, neighbors, and schools. The home program is convenient and inexpensive. Professional physical therapy once or twice each week is probably neither necessary nor cost-effective, unless it is provided within the school setting. Periodic reevaluation, retraining, and motivation sessions for parents are mandatory.

PREVENTING DEFORMITY

The tendency for development of plantar-flexion contractures is usually the earliest problem. Daily stretching of the Achilles tendons should slow down the development of this deformity. The use of night splints in combination with heelcord stretching has been shown to play a significant role in preventing the often relentless equinovarus deformity associated with DMD.[12] No studies are available on which to base a passive stretching prescription, but the regimen often prescribed is between 10 and 30 repetitions, held for 5 to 10 seconds each, performed at least once, and preferably twice, daily.

As soon as the physical therapist sees any change in length of the hamstring muscles during a periodic evaluation, hamstring stretching is added to the home program. As with the Achilles tendon, hamstrings are stretched daily by performing ten repetitions of 10 seconds each. The ITB, hip flexors, and foot evertors are other structures that must be monitored carefully for loss of ROM, which usually occurs in all these structures as a result of either weakness or static position.

If plantar-flexion contractures and the resultant knee, ITB, and hip flexion contractures are allowed to continue unchecked, the child will progress much sooner than necessary to the late ambulation stage and will lose the ability to ambulate at an earlier age than with intervention.

ACTIVITY LEVEL/ACTIVE EXERCISE

Normal activities for a young boy are stressed when possible, and active resistive exercise is not encouraged. There should be no concern about the level of activity causing undue fatigue unless fatigue is present after a full night's sleep. There is no evidence that a home program of specific active exercise changes the course of progressive weakness in the boys with DMD.

Several studies have indicated that submaximal exercise has limited value in increasing strength or changing function in DMD.[34,35] At the same time, however, these studies have demonstrated no negative effects of exercise. Others have documented an increased level of metabolic stress associated with increased activity in boys with DMD[36] and with endurance exercise in individuals with other neuromuscular diseases.[37] This increased metabolic stress may be an indicator of muscle damage, although neither study documented a negative effect on muscle strength or function.

Scott et al. have suggested a possible beneficial effect of chronic low-frequency electrical stimulation in DMD. They demonstrated an increase in maximum voluntary strength of the tibialis anterior muscle of boys who were so stimulated for 6 weeks.[38] The effects of prolonged low-frequency stimulation are being investigated in other muscle groups. This finding is very interesting but, once again, such stimulation targets the strength of only one muscle group. With appropriate selection of muscles, this treatment may promote prolonged maintenance of function, but it does not address the systemic nature of the disorder.

PROLONGING AMBULATION

As patients with DMD become weaker, their gait pattern is altered in an attempt to improve stability during walking. Stride length decreases, and the width of the base of support increases to provide a more stable base. The ITB accommodates to the new, shortened position associated with the wider base of support. Weakness in the gluteus medius becomes more pronounced, and the child assumes the typical waddling gait.

The lordotic curve increases with progressive weakness of the gluteus maximus. As that muscle weakens, the child attempts to increase stability, moving the center of gravity posterior to the fulcrum of the hip joint by pulling the arms back and by exaggerating the lordosis. Stability at the hip joint during standing is now provided passively by structures anterior to the hip joint, primarily the iliofemoral ligament. Even a mild knee flexion contracture would make ambulation difficult or impossible with the child in this position.

Treatment programs combining passive stretching and lower extremity bracing have demonstrated a reduction in the rate of progression of lower extremity contractures and have prolonged ambulation.[39,40] Various surgical interventions—including Achilles tendon lengthening and Yount fasciotomies,[41] tibialis posterior transpositions,[42] and percutaneous tenotomies[43,44]—in combination with vigorous physical therapy and orthotic intervention, have been reported to improve and prolong ambulation.[45–47] However, there is a paucity of prospective studies that statistically substantiate which type of intervention is appropriate during what time period, and whether the patient and/or family was satisfied with such intervention. A recent prospective study has demonstrated "that a comprehensive program of single early surgical intervention followed by a definite course of rehabilitation can significantly stabilize and possibly prolong ambulation without resorting to long leg braces."[48]

Whatever the surgical methods, a vigorous postoperative physical therapy program should aim to get the patient up and standing and walking as soon as possible. Active joint stretching will help maintain, and may even increase, ROM at those joints that have been percutaneously released; this is because with release of the superficial layers, there is improved access to the deeper structures that may be shortened. The goal of the postoperative physical therapy program is independent ambulation with a minimum of 3 to 5 hours per day of standing and/or walking. Even when no steps are possible, the child is asked to stand at least 1 hour a day (in a standing table if necessary). Optimal stance is with the back in extension so that the center of gravity falls behind the hip joint. Some have proposed that this extension promotes a straight spine, as it keeps the facets locked in extension, thereby prohibiting side-bending.

WHEELCHAIR USE

The decision to buy a wheelchair should be delayed until all other means of ambulation have been exhausted. However, use of a wheelchair or "buggy" strictly for long-distance transport may be most helpful for the child and family.

Only when a family is adamant in its opposition to bracing, or if braced independent ambulation is no longer possible, should a wheelchair be considered for the primary means of mobility. In many cases, efforts aimed at prolonging ambulation will cease when the child sees the improved independence, increased comfort, convenience, reduced fatigue, and peer attention afforded by wheelchair use. Deformities, particularly hip, knee, and ankle flexion contractures and scoliosis, will often increase when the child uses a wheelchair. Even when ambulation is not possible, use of a standing table of some type helps postpone these deformities and may reduce the risk of early pulmonary complications.

Because the wheelchair is a personal piece of equipment for the child, he or she should be involved in decisions regarding its design, and color. The therapist and the child should discuss the following wheelchair options.

1. Wrap-around, removable adjustable-height desk arms
2. Swing-away, elevating, detachable leg rests with heel loops. Elevation can be done periodically during the day to help maintain knee extension and prevent ankle edema.
3. Solid seat to maintain the pelvis in a horizontally aligned position that may help postpone the development of scoliosis
4. Lateral trunk supports for thoracic positioning (Fig. 6-9)

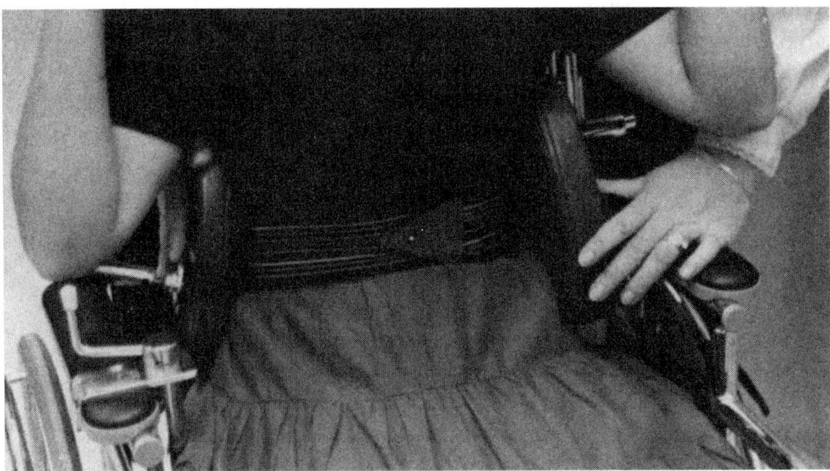

Figure 6-9 ■ Adjustable scoliosis pads fitted on a wheelchair facilitate trunk positioning. (From Maloney, Burks, Ringel, eds. *Interdisciplinary Rehabilitation of Muscular Dystrophy and Neuromuscular Disorders.* Philadelphia: JB Lippincott; 1984:275.)

5. Appropriate width—it is best to select a chair that is too narrow rather than one that is too wide.
6. Reclining back—may be useful in the later stages of disease when the upright posture is not tolerated; may promote spinal extension
7. Seat cushion to provide comfort and prevent decubiti
8. Headrest
9. Molded seat or back insert
10. Seat belt

During the later stages of the disease, if it is financially feasible, a powered wheelchair will provide for continued independent mobility. A proportional drive will make it both easier and safer for the child to manipulate the powered wheelchair and should be considered along with the previously mentioned items.

WEIGHT CONTROL

The need to guard against obesity is as important for the child who is limited to a wheelchair as for the ambulatory child. Despite good use of transfer techniques and proper body mechanics by others, excessive weight gain can reduce the child's transfers and may restrict both mobility and social activity. Moreover, excessive weight gain in the child with neuromuscular disease may not only reduce mobility but may also have a deleterious effect on self-esteem, posture, and respiratory function.

Edwards and associates have demonstrated that controlled weight reduction in obese children with DMD is a safe and practical way to improve mobility and self-esteem.[49] However, it is probably easier to prevent excessive weight gain in the young, ambulatory child than to initiate severe dietary restriction in an obese, seated adolescent. It has been proposed that this philosophy of weight control be promoted early for children with neuromuscular disease (taking into account the need for fat intake in early development). Normal growth charts make no allowance for the progressive loss of muscle in DMD, so if the child continues to gain weight according to normal standards, accumulation of fat tissue may occur as, at this stage, there is muscle wasting in DMD. Griffiths and Edwards studied the relationships between body composition and breakdown products of muscle.[50] They developed a chart, based on their research, which gives ideal weight guidelines for weight control in boys with DMD.[50] The physical therapist can play a major role in promoting this weight control philosophy with the child and family. When weight control is not effective, use of a hydraulic lift becomes important. One or more family members must be trained in the safe and proper use of such a lift.

MINIMIZING SPINAL DEFORMITY

As the child's sitting time increases, so does kyphoscoliosis. Previous clinical observations have documented that he convexity will likely be toward the dominant extremity.[51] Because of this relationship, we recommend that the child with adequate bilateral manual skills have the wheelchair drive moved from side to side every 6 months in order to prevent the scoliosis from becoming structural.

Various pads fitted onto wheelchairs, or custom-molded backs and seats fitted into wheelchairs, have been used in an attempt to provide appropriate hip and spinal positioning while the patient is seated in the wheelchair, but no studies are available to prove their clinical efficacy. A light plastic body jacket extending from the pelvis to under the armpits has been used by some in an attempt to slow down or maintain the position of the spine, but again there are no studies to confirm its effectiveness. For this type of spinal orthosis to be effective, it must be worn the entire time the child is out of bed, which may be both impractical and uncomfortable. Moreover, such an orthosis does not work well on an obese individual, and it may reduce a child's ability to take a deep breath.[25]

The increasing sophistication of spinal instrumentation within the field of orthopedics has made spinal fixation an option for children with DMD. Previously, the amount of "down time" following surgery precluded these children from choosing this option, both because of the muscle weakness and the risk of respiratory complications. Currently, physical therapy plays an important role in getting these children "up and moving" within days to a week after surgery, depending on their medical status. Any child with a thoracolumbar curve that has progressed past 30 degrees should be considered for spinal fixation, taking into consideration the child's functional level and cardiac and respiratory status. Initially, referrals for spinal stabilization were attempts on our part to improve or stabilize our patients' respiratory function, as we were concerned about the mechanical disadvantage the kyphoscoliosis placed on the already weak respiratory muscles, as well as the potentially deleterious effect of this scoliosis on respiratory function. Recent studies have demonstrated no salutary effect of segmental spinal stabilization on respiratory function based on either short- or long-term follow-up, but all studies have documented improved sitting comfort, appearance, and stabilization, or improvement of kyphoscoliosis.[52–54]

FACILITATING SLEEP

Air mattresses or commercial flotation pads often improve sleeping comfort for children with advanced deterioration who have difficulty positioning themselves or changing position at night. These devices also provide relief for family members who might otherwise be up three to five times per night to turn the patient. A hospital bed may be useful in the later stages of disease to assist with positioning and transfers, as well as to elevate the head of the bed in an attempt to ease the respiratory distress that can occur during sleep as the contents of the abdominal cavity push against the diaphragm, increasing the effort required in taking a deep breath.

RESPIRATORY CONSIDERATIONS

The major cause of respiratory complications in DMD is the progressive weakness of the muscles of respiration. This weakness may or may not be exacerbated by the mechanical disadvantages associated with kyphoscoliosis. The signs and symptoms of respiratory insufficiency include excessive fatigue and daytime sleepiness, headaches on awakening (secondary to increased carbon dioxide levels that may accompany decreased respiratory efficacy while supine), sleep disturbances (nightmares), or feeling the need to strain to "gulp for air."

A good history and periodic pulmonary function testing with the child in both the seated and supine positions are the most effective means of monitoring respiratory insufficiency. In addition, family members should be trained in the techniques of bronchial drainage, chest percussion, and assisted coughing. One study demonstrated improved pulmonary function after performance of breathing exercises, but this effect was not sustained.[55]

If the history and pulmonary function test results suggest that the lungs are not being adequately ventilated, the child should be referred to a pulmonologist for further testing and discussion of options for assisted ventilation. Nasal positive pressure ventilation may be used at night to assist breathing and to provide a rest for overworked respiratory muscles.[56] An adjustment period is often necessary when this type of ventilation is used, but after a period of time the patient often derives the benefits of improved sleep and increased energy and alertness in the daytime. Ventilatory assistance might be required both day and night for children with advanced respiratory failure. Thanks to modern technology, this is a feasible option.[57] Technology has provided advances so that speech and eating are not severely affected by a tracheostomy, and ventilators are compact, battery-driven devices that can be attached to an appropriately modified wheelchair. The physical therapist may play a major role in positioning and adapting wheelchairs for individuals requiring assisted ventilation. This type of multidisciplinary program can optimize function and prolong life. Not all individuals choose these options, and some do not have the resources to pursue them, but those who have the means generally report a very satisfying life, including higher education and gainful employment.[58]

ACTIVITIES OF DAILY LIVING

The physical therapist should routinely assess the child's ability to perform activities of daily living (ADLs). The patient's ability to feed himself, turn pages in a book, and do necessary personal hygiene tasks must all be assessed periodically. The physical therapist may choose to request an occupational therapy consultation. A home visit is most helpful in assessing adaptive equipment needs.

FACILITATING FAMILY SUPPORT

The physical therapist plays an important role in providing support, motivation, and training of the patient with DMD and his family members. Successful family support depends on the early involvement of the physical therapist and the ability of the therapist to have the family comply with a home program that is monitored and adapted appropriately. Assessment of the social situation of the family should be part of each visit.

The mild to moderate intellectual impairment in these young boys often imposes both educational and emotional handicaps, in addition to the obvious physical changes accompanying DMD. The child learns that the disease will continuously erode the quality and quantity of his existence, and the resultant reliance and dependence on others frequently gives rise to stress within the family. Although he or she is not a psychotherapist, the physical therapist must be aware of the emotional factors involved with the illness and must provide strong emotional support, as well as help in reinforcing and attaining goals and preventing conflicts. A healthy emotional environment for the family and the child with DMD is at least as important to the child as the prevention of contractures.

MANAGEMENT OF PAIN

Most of the pain that occurs in these disorders is mechanical in nature and caused by limited ability to move in the bed or wheelchair either because of their muscle weakness or joint contracture. If the aforementioned goals are achieved, management of pain should be minimal. Pain occurs at the limits of ROM in all joints, and because contractures reduce the ROM, they also increase the opportunity for the development of pain. If pain becomes a problem, routine methods of treatment and appropriate positioning techniques should help minimize the discomfort.

SUMMARY

A successful treatment program should result in several additional years of independent ambulation, improved self-sufficiency, substantial postponement of the restrictions imposed by a wheelchair, and the maintenance of the maximal functional independence allowed by the child's level of strength. See Case Study (A.M., 10-year-old Caucasian with Duchenne Muscular Dystrophy).

Case Study—A.M., 10-Year-Old Caucasian with Duchenne Muscular Dystrophy

A.M. is a 10-year-old Caucasian boy with a diagnosis of Duchenne muscular dystrophy. He was diagnosed at 4 years of age when it was noted that he was slow getting up off the floor after story time at preschool and appeared unable to keep up with his school mates. He has been followed periodically by physical therapy since that time for family education in range of motion and active stretching exercises and for monitoring the status of his muscle strength, function, and joint contractures.

At 4 years of age, the family had been instructed in stretching of the heelcords to be performed on a daily basis and A.M. had been fitted with night splints to maintain a neutral position at his ankles during sleep. (He was encouraged to wear his "moon boots" throughout the night, but if it was only 2 to 3 hours at neutral before he took them off, this shorter period was considered beneficial.) At 5 to 6 years of age, the stretching of hip flexors and iliotibial bands had been added to the daily stretching regimen.

At this time, A.M. comes to physical therapy with the chief complaint of an increased number of falls (~4/day), and increased difficulty rising from a chair, ascending and descending stairs, and he can no longer get off the floor without the use of "furniture" along with his Gower's maneuver.

Strength in the UE graded in the "good" range, with the LE grading "fair" to "poor," in the proximal muscle groups. Measurements of joint contractures revealed hip flexors that measured −30 degrees bilaterally, iliotibial bands at −35 degrees bilaterally, knees at neutral and −20 degrees at the right ankle and −25 degrees on the left. In the UE, ROM was within normal limits bilaterally and functionally still independent.

Stretching exercises were reviewed and emphasized with the family. In conference with the orthotist and neuromuscular physician, it was decided that A.M. would be fit and trained to stand and walk with long leg braces. A.M. and his family would be instructed to use them for "practice" an hour a day, so he would be ready to graduate to full-time use as walking became more difficult.

Contracture releases were also discussed with the family as an option if use of the long leg braces was difficult, and a future referral to the orthopedic surgeon was discussed. A.M. and family were instructed to return to physical therapy in conjunction with being fitted by the orthotist with the long leg braces. The need for a wheelchair, only to be used for long-distance transport, was addressed, but neither family nor child were ready for that major step. They had a "buggy" that they used for long distances, and A.M. did not feel a stigma attached to using a "buggy." The topic of a wheelchair was dropped and noted in the chart to be picked up at a later date.

Contact was made with the treating physical therapist in the school district for her/his suggestions or comments.

Other Related Disorders

Although the neuromuscular disorders have varying etiologies and lack a cure, these disorders result in similar physical problems that can be managed by applying similar principles. As previously presented for DMD, the major physical therapy goals include preventing deformity, prolonging functional capacity, facilitating family knowledge and involvement through education and counseling, and helping in the management of pain, if necessary.

For each disorder, treatment should help prevent complications. None of the habilitative approaches used can alter the underlying neuromuscular destruction. Prevention should serve as the focus of our efforts. The basic tenets of treatment should ensure that a carefully planned home program is carried out and appropriately monitored. In addition to these tenets, weight control is important. Caloric intake and physical activity level must be considered, and the family must be educated about the secondary complications associated with obesity.

Myotonic Dystrophy

Myotonic dystrophy (MTD) is an autosomal dominant disorder whose location is on chromosome 19.[59] In the most typical form of MTD, the symptoms are first noticed during adolescence and are characterized by myotonia, a delay in muscle relaxation time, and muscle weakness. As the weakness progresses, the myotonia often decreases. The individual will present to the clinic with complaints of weakness and stiffness. Stiffness, which is often the major complaint, is characteristic of the myotonia. Patients often have a characteristic physical appearance that includes a long, thin face with temporal and masseter muscle wasting; frontal balding; and weakness and wasting of the sternocleidomastoids. The pattern of weakness in MTD presents first with distal wasting and weakness, manifested by a foot drop and difficulty opening jars. Proximal muscle weakness occurs in the later stage of the disease. The most severe form of MTD is congenital and is associated with generalized muscular hypoplasia, mental retardation, and a high incidence of neonatal mortality. Children with congenital MTD are born to mothers afflicted with the disorder. Because MTD is inherited in an autosomal dominant pattern, an individual with the disease has a 50/50 chance of each offspring having the disease. The severe congenital form of MTD is characterized by maternal transmission only. The latter group is often plagued with severe mental retardation, speech disturbances, delayed motor milestones, distal weakness, and spinal deformities. With survival to adulthood, these individuals follow the pattern of the classic course of the disease, in which cataracts are common. There is involvement not only of skeletal muscle, but smooth muscle and cardiac conduction defects are often seen, particularly first-degree heart block. There may be associated infertility, decreased respiratory drive, and numerous endocrine problems. Currently, there is no treatment for the disorder, and the etiology of the genetic defect is unknown. There is no curative pharmacologic treatment, although some medications may be used to ameliorate the symptoms of myotonia. The objectives of current therapeutic intervention are to reduce the distal wasting and weakness and control the spinal deformities.

Death in these individuals is usually caused by heart block or problems secondary to decreased respiratory drive. The respiratory complications may be severe and, when mechanically ventilated, these patients are very difficult to wean. The congenital forms of MTD may be accompanied by severe developmental delays, in which case intervention that employs various motor development approaches may be beneficial.

Facioscapulohumeral Dystrophy

Facioscapulohumeral dystrophy (FSH) can arise at any time from childhood until adult life. There is an autosomal dominant pattern of inheritance.[59] The gene defect appears to be located on chromosome 4. Initial muscular involvement includes the face and shoulder girdle, but subsequent progression may include the pelvic girdle and trunk musculature. Progression of the disease is usually insidious, with long periods of apparent arrest of the process. Some cases occur in which there is a rapid progression and disability, but most patients survive and are active throughout adulthood and do not die prematurely. The disease commonly begins during childhood, but because of its wide variance, it may show up as late as the third or fourth decade. Therefore, a child at risk for inheritance of FSH should not be pronounced free of the disease just because no signs or symptoms occurred during childhood.

Although the progression of weakness in FSH proceeds proximal to distal, as in DMD, the pattern of muscle weakness is different. The lower trapezius and facial musculature in patients with FSH show weakness the earliest, but unlike DMD, the latissimus dorsi is seldom involved. During the early stages of the disease, a physical therapist with good muscle testing skills may be the person best qualified to identify or diagnose the muscle disease. A good test of facial weakness involves having the child blow air into the cheeks to cause them to bulge but not to let air escape through the lips. The therapist can then exert manual pressure on the cheeks to see the point at which the orbicularis oris muscle allows air to escape. The major problem for the physical therapist is to determine the difference between normal and reduced strength in the facial muscles. The brachioradialis is another characteristically weak muscle in children with FSH. However, because a strong biceps brachii confounds testing of the brachioradialis, palpation and observation are the main tools for identifying weakness in this muscle.

The main problem caused by FSH early in the course of the child's life is pain in the upper thoracic region that results from lack of stability secondary to weakness of the trapezius, rhomboids, and other scapular musculature (Fig. 6-10). In severe cases, some recommend a modified Taylor brace to support the midthoracic region and to retract the scapulae (when properly fitted and stabilized at the pelvis). In those cases when the deltoid is preserved but scapular stabilization is absent, a scapulothoracic fusion may be helpful.[60,61]

Spinal Muscular Atrophy

Three categories of spinal muscular atrophy (SMA) occur in childhood:

1. Infantile SMA, or Werdnig-Hoffman disease
2. Intermediate SMA (type II muscular atrophy or chronic Werdnig-Hoffman disease)
3. Juvenile SMA (Kugelberg-Welander disease)

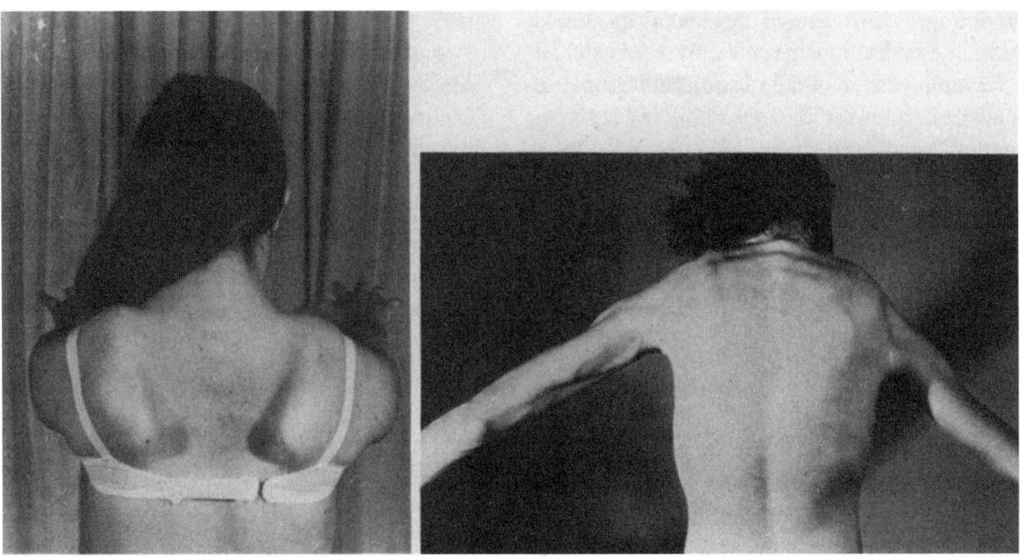

Figure 6-10 ■ Facioscapulohumeral dystrophy. Bilateral scapular winging and elevation are indicative of diffuse shoulder girdle involvement. (From Lovell WW, Winter RB, eds. *Pediatric Orthopaedics*. 2nd Ed. Philadelphia: JB Lippincott; 1986:268.)

All of these conditions are inherited as autosomal recessive disorders located on chromosome 5.[62,63] All three have pathology affecting the anterior horn cell, and, although all are located in chromosome 5, there are primary differences in their clinical presentation. Diseases of the anterior horn cell (motor neurons) are associated with wasting and weakness of the muscles. Sensory changes are absent. In the childhood and juvenile forms, the lower motor neurons are chiefly affected and the diseases are often similar. This similarity is in contrast to amyotrophic lateral sclerosis, an adult form of motor neuron disease, which is less often inherited and more commonly associated with upper motor neuron involvement.

INFANTILE SPINAL MUSCULAR ATROPHY

Infantile SMA is almost always noted within the first 3 months of life. The mother often complains of decreased fetal movement. At birth, the affected child is hypotonic, has difficulty feeding, commonly has respiratory distress, and may present with "failure to thrive." Muscle wasting is often severe, and spontaneous movements are few. The pattern of breathing is abnormal, with the abdominal muscles playing a greater role than the thoracic muscles (i.e., these children are "belly breathers"). The child may continue to have difficulty feeding and swallowing. On close inspection, the tongue may be atrophic, and when the child cries, one may see fasciculations or "jumping" of the tongue. Deep tendon reflexes are usually decreased or absent, and plantar responses are usually flexor or absent. No sensory abnormalities are noted. During the first several years of life, hospitalizations for pulmonary infections are common. These children do not achieve motor milestones at a normal rate, if at all. Most children with infantile SMA do not survive beyond 3 years of age, with respiratory failure being responsible for their death.[5]

INTERMEDIATE SPINAL MUSCULAR ATROPHY

Intermediate SMA (or type II SMA) also affects infants but is more benign than the acute or infantile (Werdnig-Hoffman) form. This form of SMA refers to a group of "floppy" children with lower motor neuron disease who are slow to attain motor milestones. Prior to differentiation between infantile SMA and intermediate SMA, it was noted that a group of children with SMA never walked but did not die at an early age. These children are presumed to have had intermediate or type II SMA. Today, these children are usually involved in habilitative intervention, including physical therapy and orthotic training, to provide for early standing or ambulation. Type II SMA usually presents after 3 to 6 months of age when the children are noted to be slow in reaching their motor milestones. These children are characterized by weakness and wasting of the extremities and trunk musculature. Feeding and swallowing difficulties are seldom a problem. There is often a fine tremor when the child attempts to use the limbs. This is not a true intention tremor, but has been referred to as a mini-polymyoclonus.[5] These children may or may not learn to walk. Most will require orthotic intervention to ambulate, but often, the ambulation is not functional. Nonetheless, it is important in these children to encourage stance, to maintain joint mobility, to prevent problems associated with long-term wheelchair sitting, and to attempt to keep the patient's back as straight as possible for as long as possible. These children often survive into adulthood but are vulnerable to pulmonary infection at any point. Children with intermediate SMA are predisposed to the complications, such as joint contractures and kyphoscoliosis, that affect other children with neuromuscular weakness. Although respiratory insufficiency is a problem in both the infantile and intermediate forms of SMA, there is not the same cardiac involvement as is seen in Duchenne muscular dystrophy because the children with SMA appear to have normal cardiac tissue. In both forms of SMA, the diagnosis is made on the basis of the clinical presentation and laboratory tests, including electromyography, which will show denervation with fibrillations and a paucity of motor units. Nerve conduction velocity tests are usually normal for the child's age. Muscle biopsy helps confirm the diagnosis by demonstrating a characteristic pattern of denervation. However, a muscle biopsy does not often differentiate between infantile and intermediate SMA. There is no diagnostic test available that can differentiate accurately between infantile and intermediate SMA; therefore, initial prognosis is often based on the clinical acumen of the physician and recommendations by other professionals. Most often, the prognosis is left for time to tell and is dependent primarily on the number of respiratory infections suffered each year.[5]

Both diseases have been located on chromosome number 5,[59] but no other etiology is apparent. Studies of anterior horn cell metabolism have not been helpful, and current treatment is primarily symptomatic. The treatment approach includes physical therapy, orthotics, spinal management, wheelchair seating, and appropriate treatment of respiratory distress.

Administration of neurotrophic factors as a pharmacologic treatment has been proposed for individuals with anterior horn cell disease. There studies are presently under way in adult motor neuron disease syndromes.

JUVENILLE SPINAL MUSCULAR ATROPHY (KUGELBERG-WELANDER DISEASE)

Juvenile SMA is characterized by symptoms of progressive weakness, wasting, and fasciculations that are noted between the ages of 5 and 15 years. Proximal muscles are usually involved first, and because of the age of presentation, this disease may be confused with the muscular dystrophies. Deep tendon reflexes are decreased, but contractures are unusual, and progressive spinal deformities are uncommon. A mild, progressive weakness is common. Diagnosis is established on the basis of the clinical picture and the results of diagnostic laboratory studies, including an electromyogram and muscle biopsy, which show denervation. As with other forms of SMA, treatment is supportive in the hope of gaining time until a neurotrophic factor may become available to either cure or retard the progression of this disease.

Summary

The disorders discussed in this chapter are all characterized by weakness and wasting of the skeletal musculature, progressive deformity, and increasing disability. The physical therapist plays an important role as counselor, motivator, facilitator, and provider of emotional support for the affected child and family. These expanded roles may be as important as the actual physical assistance and training that physical therapists traditionally provide.

REFERENCES

1. Dubowitz V. *Muscle Disorders in Childhood.* London: WB Saunders; 1978:22.
2. Koenig N, Hoffman EP, Bertelson CJ, et al. Complete cloning of the Duchenne muscular dystrophy (DMD) cDNA and preliminary genomic organization of the DMD gene in normal and affected individuals. *Cell.* 1987;50:509–517.
3. Hoffman EP, Brown RH, Kunkel LM. Dystrophin: The protein product of the Duchenne muscular dystrophy locus. *Cell.* 1987;51:919.
4. Crisp DE, Ziter FA, Bray PF. Diagnostic delay in Duchenne muscular dystrophy. *JAMA.* 1982;247: 478–480.
5. Brooke MH. *Clinicians' View of Neuromuscular Disease.* 2nd Ed. Baltimore: Williams & Wilkins; 1986:117–159.
6. Leibowitz D, Dubowitz V. Intellect and behavior in Duchenne muscular dystrophy. *Dev Med Child Neurol.* 1981;23:577–590.
7. Medical Research Council of the United Kingdom. *Aids to Examination of the Peripheral Nervous Sys-*

tem: Memorandum No. 45. Palo Alto, CA: Pedragon House; 1978.

8. Florence JM, Pandya S, King W, et al. Clinical trials in Duchenne dystrophy. Standardization and reliability of evaluation procedures. *Phys Ther*. 64: 41–45.
9. Brooke MH, Fenichel G, Griggs R, et al. Clinical investigations in Duchenne dystrophy. Part 2. Determination of the "power" of therapeutic trials based on the natural history. *Muscle Nerve*. 1983;6:91–103.
10. Vignos PJ, Spencer GE, Archibald KC. Management of progressive muscular dystrophy of childhood. *JAMA*. 1963;184:89–96.
11. Koenig M, Biggs AH, Moyer M, et al. The molecular basis for Duchenne vs Becker muscular dystrophy: Correlation of severity with type of deletion. *Am J Hum Genet*. 1989;45:498.
12. Brooke MH, Fenichel G, Griggs R, et al. Duchenne muscular dystrophy: Patterns of clinical progression and effects of supportive therapy. *Neurology*. 1989;39:475–481.
13. Griggs RC, Reeves W, Moxley RT. The heart in Duchenne dystrophy. In: Rowland LP, ed. *Pathogenesis of Human Muscular Dystrophies*. Amsterdam: Excerpta Medica; 1977:661–671.
14. Prosser JE. Intelligence and the gene for Duchenne muscular dystrophy. *Arch Dis Child*. 1969;44: 221–230.
15. Ziter FA, Allsop K. The diagnosis and management of childhood muscular dystrophy. *Clin Pediatr*. 1976;15(6):540–548.
16. Brooke MH, Fenichel G, Griggs R, et al. Clinical investigation of Duchenne muscular dystrophy. Interesting results in a trial of prednisone. *Arch Neurol*. 1987;44:812–817.
17. Mendell JR. Randomized, double-blind six-month trial of prednisone in Duchenne's muscular dystrophy. *N Engl J Med*. 1989;320:1592–1597.
18. Drachman DB, Tokya RV, Meyer E. Prednisone in Duchenne muscular dystrophy. *Lancet*. 1974;2: 1409–1412.
19. DeSilva S, Drachman D, Mellits D, et al. Prednisone treatment in Duchenne muscular dystrophy. Long-term benefit. *Arch Neurol*. 1987;44:818–822.
20. Fenichel G, Florence J, Pestronk A, et al. Long-term benefit from prednisone therapy in Duchenne muscular dystrophy. *Neurology*. 1991;41: 1874–1877.
21. Florence J, Burden N, Brunham S, et al. A Canadian/U.S. multi-center study of deflazacort versus prednisone in maintaining muscle strength in Duchenne/Becker Muscular Dystrophy. *Phys Ther*. 1994;74:5.
22. Fenichel G, Pestronk A, Florence J, et al. A beneficial effect of oxandrolone in the treatment of Duchenne muscular dystrophy: A pilot study. *Neurology*, 1997;48:1225–1226.
23. Mendell J, Kissel J, Amato A, et al. Myoblast transfer in the treatment of Duchenne muscular dystrophy. *N Engl J Med*. 1995;333(13):832–838.
24. Wolff J, Malone R, Williams P, et al. Direct gene transfer into mouse muscle in vivo. *Science* 1990; 247:1465.
25. Florence J, Brooke M, Carroll J. Evaluation of the child with muscular weakness. *Orthoped Clin North Am*. 1978;9(2):421–422.
26. Ziter FA, Allsop KG, Tyler FH. Assessment of muscle strength in Duchenne muscular dystrophy. *Neurology*. 1977;27:981–984.
27. Allsop KG, Ziter FA. Loss of strength and functional decline in Duchenne dystrophy. *Arch Neurol*. 1981;38:406–411.
28. Brooke MH, Griggs R, Mendell J, et al. Clinical trial in Duchenne dystrophy. The design of the protocol. *Muscle Nerve*. 1981;4:186–197.
29. Griggs R, Moxley R, Mendell J, et al. Prednisone in Duchenne dystrophy. A randomized, controlled trial defining the time course and dose response. *Arch Neurol*. 1991;48:383–388.
30. Florence J, Pandya S, King W, et al. Intrarater reliability of manual muscle test (Medical Research Council Scale) grades in Duchenne muscular dystrophy. *Phys Ther*. 1992;72:115–126.
31. Stuberg W, Metcalf W. Reliability of quantitative muscle testing in healthy children and in children with Duchenne muscular dystrophy using hand held dynamometers. *Phys Ther*. 1988;68(6):977–982.
32. Brussock C, Haley S, Munsat T, et al. Measurement of isometric force in children with and without Duchenne muscular dystrophy. *Phys Ther*. 1992;72(2):105–114.
33. Pandya S, Florence JM, King W, et al. Reliability of goniometric measurements in patients with Duchenne muscular dystrophy. *Phys Ther*. 1985;65: 1339–1342.
34. Vignos P, Watkins M. The effect of exercise in muscular dystrophy. *JAMA*. 1966;197:121–126.
35. de Lateur B, Giaconi R. Effect on maximal strength of submaximal exercise in Duchenne muscular dystrophy. *Am J Phys Med*. 1979;58:26–36.
36. Florence JM, Fox P, Planer J, et al. Activity, creatine kinase, and myoglobin in Duchenne muscular dystrophy: A clue to etiology? *Neurology* 1985; 35:758–761.
37. Florence JM, Hagberg J. Effect of training on the exercise responses of neuromuscular disease patients. *Med Sci Sports Exer*. 1984;16:460–465.

38. Scott O, Vrbová S, Hyde S, et al. Chronic electrical stimulation: Muscle function studies in children with neuromuscular disease. In: Rose FC, Jones R, Vrbova G. *Comprehensive Neurologic Rehabilitation.* Vol. 3. New York: Demos; 1989:307–313.
39. Harris SE, Cherry DB. Childhood progressive muscular dystrophy and the role of physical therapy. *Phys Ther.* 1974;54:4–12.
40. Scott OM, Hyde SA, Goddard C, et al. Prevention of deformity in Duchenne muscular dystrophy. A prospective study of passive stretching and splintage. *Physiotherapy.* 1981;67:177–180.
41. Archibald DC, Vignos PJ Jr. A study of contractures in muscular dystrophy. *Arch Phys Med Rehabil.* 1959;40:150–157.
42. Spencer GE. Orthopaedic care of progressive muscular dystrophy. *J Bone Joint Surg (Am).* 1967;49: 1201–1204.
43. Roy L, Gibson DA. Pseudohypertrophic muscular dystrophy and its surgical management: Review of 30 patients. *Can J Surg.* 1970;13:13–20.
44. Siegel IM. Management of musculoskeletal complications in neuromuscular disease. Enhancing mobility and the role of bracing and surgery. In: Fowler WM Jr, ed. *Advances in the Rehabilitation of Neuromuscular Diseases: State of the Art Reviews.* Vol. 4. Philadelphia: Hanley & Belfus; 1988;553–575.
45. Ziter FA, Allsop KG. The value of orthoses for patients with Duchenne muscular dystrophy. *Phys Ther.* 1979;59:1361–1365.
46. Heckmatt JZ, Dubowitz V, Hyde SA, et al. Prolongation of walking in Duchenne muscular dystrophy with lightweight orthoses. Review of 57 cases. *Dev Med Child Neurol.* 1985;27:149–154.
47. Vignos PJ. Management of musculoskeletal complications in neuromuscular disease: Limb contractures and the role of stretching, braces and surgery. In: Fowler WM Jr, ed. *Advances in the Rehabilitation of Neuromuscular Diseases: State of the Art Reviews.* Vol. 4. Philadelphia: Hanley & Belfus; 1988:509–536.
48. Bach JR. Orthopedic surgery and rehabilitation for the prolongation of brace-free ambulation of patients with Duchenne muscular dystrophy. *Am J Phys Med Rehabil.* 1991;20:323–331.
49. Edwards RHT. Weight reduction in boys with muscular dystrophy. *Dev Med Child Neurol.* 1984;26:384–390.
50. Giffiths R, Edwards R. A new chart for weight control in Duchenne muscular dystrophy. *Arch Dis Child.* 1988;63:1256–1258.
51. Johnson E, Yarnell S. Hand dominance and scoliosis in Duchenne muscular dystrophy. *Arch Phys Med Rehabil.* 1976;57:462–464.
52. Miller F, Moseley C, Koreska J, et al. Pulmonary function and scoliosis in Duchenne dystrophy. *J Pediatr Orthop.* 1988;8:133–137.
53. Miller R, Chalmers A, Dao H, et al. The effect of spine fusion on respiratory function in Duchenne muscular dystrophy. *Neurology* 1991;41:37–40.
54. Shapiro F, Sethna N, Colan S, et al. Spinal fusion in Duchenne muscular dystrophy: A multidisciplinary approach. *Muscle Nerve.* 1992;15:604–614.
55. Adams M, Chandler L. Effects of physical therapy program on vital capacity of patients with muscular dystrophy. *Phys Ther.* 1974;54:494–494.
56. Leger P, Jennequin J, Gerard M, et al. Home positive pressure ventilation via nasal mask for patients with neuromuscular weakness or restrictive lung or chest-wall disease. *Respir Care.* 1989;34:73–79.
57. Bach J, O'Brien J, Krotenberg R, et al. Management of end-stage respiratory failure in Duchenne muscular dystrophy. *Muscle Nerve.* 1987;10:177–182.
58. Bach JR, Campagnolo DI, Hoeman S. Life satisfaction of individuals with Duchenne muscular dystrophy using long-term mechanical ventilatory support. *Am J Phys Rehabil.* 1991;70:129–135.
59. Griggs R, Mendell J, Miller R. *Evaluation and Treatment of Myopathies.* Philadelphia: FA Davis; 1995:114–128.
60. Bunch WH. Scapulo-thoracic fusion for shoulder stabilization in muscular dystrophy. *Minn Med.* 1973;56:391–394.
61. Copeland SA, Howard RC. Thoracoscapular fusion for facioscapulohumeral dystrophy. *J Bone Joint Surg.* 1978;60B:547–551.
62. Guillian T, Brzustowicz L, Castilla L, et al. Genetic hemogeneity between acute and chronic forms of spinal muscular atrophy. *Nature* 1990;345: 823–825.
63. Brzustowicz L, Lehner T, Castilla L, et al. Genetic mapping of chronic childhood-onset spinal muscular atrophy to chromosome 5q 11.2–13.3. *Nature* 1990;344:540–541.

Traumatic Brain Injury in Childhood

Amy Both

Definition

Traumatic brain injury (TBI),[1] a frequent cause of morbidity and mortality in the pediatric population, occurs when an external, mechanical force either accidentally or intentionally impacts the head. TBI is characterized by a period of diminished or altered consciousness that ranges from brief lethargy to prolonged unconsciousness or even brain death.[2] Symptoms vary greatly depending on the location of the lesion and the extent of underlying brain injury. TBI is not associated with congenital injury or degenerative insult. It is also referred to as brain injury, head injury, or closed head injury. Many children with TBI recover uneventfully. Others, however, are left with partial or total functional disability and/or psychosocial impairment.

Incidence

Each year 1 million children sustain TBI,[3] and between 100,000 and 200,000 require hospitalization.[4,5] Of those hospitalized, over 25,000 children die[6] and 15,000 to 30,000 experience significant long-term physical, intellectual, communication, psychosocial, and behavioral deficits.[7] Brain injury is the leading cause of trauma death in children between 1 and 19 years of age and is responsible for 43% of the accidental deaths in children 5 to 9 years of age in the United States.[6,8,9]

The incidence of TBI is two times greater in boys than girls, with an overall risk of 4% in boys and 2.5% in girls.[10,11] Premorbid personality and behavior have been found to predispose children to brain injury.[12] Children who are aggressive, fearless, and have difficulty with discipline are at an increased risk of injury.[13] In addition, there is evidence that once a child sustains a TBI, the likelihood of injury again increases.[14]

Brain injury and death rates vary considerably by race and socioeconomic status.[15] Among children in the United States under 15 years of age, death rates from accidental injury are highest for Native Americans, followed by African Americans, Hispanics, and Caucasians.[15] Asians have the lowest overall death rates from TBI. For all races, death rates are inversely related to socioeconomic status.[15] Thus, children of families with low incomes have higher death rates than children of families with upper and middle incomes.

Causes of Injury

Falls

Falls account for 35% of all pediatric TBIs that require hospitalization or result in death.[15] Two-thirds of the trauma injuries in infants are caused by falls from heights or stairs, but of these, only 8% result in severe injury.[17] However, because of the high center of gravity in younger children and the tendency to fall head first, infants and preschool age children are more susceptible to severe injury from falls of less than 4 feet than older children.[15,16] Among preschoolers, 51% of the trauma injuries occur from falls, including falls from playground equipment, of which only 6% are serious.[15] Older children usually escape severe injury in falls from heights of less than 10 feet.[15,16] Although many falls occur accidentally, falls of less than 10 feet bear investigation for potential child abuse.[15,16]

Motor Vehicle Accidents

Motor vehicle accidents (MVAs) account for approximately 25% of all pediatric TBIs and account for the vast majority of serious injuries with multiple trauma.[2] Approximately 70% of the children injured in an MVA will be in a coma for some period of time.[6,9] The incidence of MVAs contributing to TBI progressively increases between 4 and 14 years of age, with the majority of injuries occurring when the child is a bicyclist or pedestrian.[18] MVAs are the most common cause of trauma death in children 5 to 9 years old.[15]

In contrast, the majority of motor vehicle injuries sustained during adolescence occur when the adolescent is an unprotected occupant in the automobile. The shift in cause of TBI is associated with obtaining a driving license and driving and drinking among teenagers.[15] A number of studies indicate that up to 40% of adolescents are intoxicated at the time of a motor vehicle crash.[19,20]

Gunshot Wounds

Firearm injuries occur from accidental gun discharges, homicides, and suicides and rank second only to MVAs as the leading cause of trauma death in school-age children and adolescents.[19,21] The incidence of gunshot wounds among male inner city youth is extremely alarming as the children are often both the victims and the perpetrators.[21–23] More than twice as many children survive their injuries as die, with approximately 25% having permanent sequelae.[21]

Abuse/Assault

Physical abuse in infants and young children is prevalent, accounting for approximately 24% of the children who are abused requiring hospital admission[24] and 80% or more of the head trauma deaths in children under 2 years of age.[24–26] Abuse frequently results in head injury owing to the vulnerability of the immature brain and the weak supporting neck musculature. Abuse resulting in TBI is characterized by a marked discrepancy between the explanation of how the injury occurred and the nature and severity of the injury. Early identification of abuse is critical to prevent repeated or progressive injury.

Sports/Recreational Activities

Sports and recreational causes account for approximately 21% of the brain injuries to school-age children and adolescents.[15] High-risk contact sports, such as football and boxing, result in up to half of the injuries.[15] TBI is also seen in other recreation activities when head protection is either not used or forgotten, including diving, baseball, cycling, horseback riding, and rugby.

Mechanisms of Injury

Impression Injuries

Impression injuries occur when a stationary head is impacted by a solid object, such as a rock or a blunt object. Impression injuries produce skull fracture and focal lesion at the site of the impact. The presence of skull fracture is associated with an increased risk of intracranial injury; however, the absence of skull fracture does not reliably exclude a significant intracranial injury.[27,28]

Acceleration-Deceleration Injuries

Acceleration-deceleration injuries are caused when a moving head hits a relatively fixed object, such as the ground or a windshield. The young infant is particularly susceptible to acceleration-deceleration injuries as there is less restraint of motion in the neck.[29] Therefore, acceleration-deceleration injury in infancy may result in greater differential displacement of the skull and cranial contents.[29] The direction of acceleration injuries may be translational (linear) or rotational (angular). Most TBIs are a result of a combination of both translational and rotational injuries.

TRANSLATIONAL INJURY

In translational injury, the head in motion strikes a stationary object and responds with lateral displacement of both the skull and the brain. The injury that results from the initial impact of the skull on the brain is known as *coup*. The lesion that occurs in the direction opposite of the initial force is termed *contrecoup*. Contrecoup occurs as the brain decelerates against the bony structures of the skull.

ROTATIONAL INJURY

Rotational injury occurs when the skull rotates as the brain remains stationary. The effect is angular forces on the brain, surface contusions, lacerations, and shearing trauma.[30] Rotational injury can result in either focal or diffuse brain damage.

Primary Brain Damage from Trauma

Primary brain damage (Table 7-1)[29–32] from trauma is a direct result of the forces that occur to the head at the time of initial impact.

Concussion

Concussion is a clinical state characterized by altered awareness and loss of memory immediately following trauma. Impaired consciousness can last a few seconds to several hours and is related to the transmission of stretching forces to the brainstem as the brain is thrown back and forth in the cranial vault.[33] Concussion can be seen without obvious pathologic changes to the brain; however, it may also cause by mild diffuse white matter lesions or neurochemical injury.[34] Following concussion, a child may exhibit clinging behavior, disturbances in sleep, irritability, or more distractibility than usual. These behavior changes can last a few days to a few months.[34]

Contusion

A contusion is a bruising or hemorrhage of the crests or gyri in the cerebral hemispheres. Contusion can be seen following a crush injury, blunt trauma, or during an inertial load injury, such as acceleration-deceleration of the brain within the skull.[29] Contusions occur most commonly in the frontal and temporal lobes of the brain because of bony irregularities in the cranial vault.[34]

Skull Fractures

Skull fractures are seen in both closed head injuries and open, compound head injuries. Brain injury can occur both with and without the presence of skull fracture.[27,28,35] Linear communited fractures result from impact with low-velocity objects and depressed fractures generally result from impact with higher velocity objects. Linear fractures can produce contusions, hemorrhage, and cranial nerve damage.[29] Depressed skull fractures of greater than 5 mm are considered significant.[29] Depressed fractures can pro-

TABLE 7-1
Damage from Head Trauma[29–32]

Primary Head Injury	Secondary Head Injury	Other Consequences
Immediate impact/concussion	Cerebral edema	Hydrocephalus
Skull fracture	Increased intracranial pressure	Seizures
Cerebral contusion	Herniation syndromes	Infection
Intracranial hemorrhage: epidural, subdural	Ischemic/hypoxic damage	Endocrine disorders
Diffuse axonal injury	Neurochemical events	

duce herniation syndromes, contusions, lacerations, and cranial nerve damage.[29]

Intracranial Hemorrhages

Intracranial injury can occur with or without immediate loss of consciousness or skull fracture.[27,28] Two types of intracranial hemorrhage frequently seen following pediatric TBI are extradural and intradural hematomas. The rate of blood collection and the location of the hematoma are related to severity and outcome.[36] Hematomas that accumulate rapidly carry grave prognoses and require immediate surgical evacuation.[30,37]

EXTRADURAL HEMATOMAS

Extradural or epidural hematomas develop because of the tearing of an artery in the brain, primarily the middle meningeal artery and its branches. In children, epidural hematomas usually follow skull fracture or bending of the skull into the brain.[36] With unilateral epidural hematoma, there is often herniation of the temporal lobe.[37] Coma may ensue and cardiorespiratory arrest is possible.

INTRADURAL HEMATOMAS

Intradural hematomas include subdural and intracerebral hematomas. Acute subdural hematomas occur secondary to injury to veins in the subdural space. Subsequent recovery depends on both the time before hemorrhage evacuation and the extent of damage to underlying brain tissue.[36] Subdural hematomas are frequently seen with inertial injuries and occur commonly in the temporal and frontal lobes.[34] Subdural hematomas are associated with higher mortality rates and poorer functional outcomes. Intracranial hematomas can result from trauma or rupture of a congenital vascular abnormality.[38] Very severe injuries may cause large intracerebral hematomas that can rupture into the ventricles, causing intraventricular hemorrhage.[34]

Diffuse Axonal Injury

Diffuse axonal injury (DAI) is a microscopic phenomenon not commonly visible on CT scan. DAI is seen following rotational injury within the cranial vault.[29] The shearing trauma results in diffuse disturbance of cellular structures following TBI. DAI is associated with much of the significant brain damage seen in TBI, including sudden loss of consciousness, extensor rigidity of bilateral extremities, and autonomic dysfunction.[34]

Secondary Brain Damage from Trauma

Secondary brain damage from trauma (see Table 7-1)[29] evolves as a result of the pathophysiological changes initiated by the primary trauma. Research suggests that secondary brain damage from trauma develops over a period of several hours or days.[34] Secondary injuries account for a significant amount of the overall damage that occurs in TBI and prevention of secondary brain damage is a major goal of the acute management of the child with TBI.[36]

Cerebral Edema

Perhaps the most frequently occurring cause of secondary injuries is cerebral edema. Unchecked cerebral edema accompanied by an increase in intracranial pressure can lead to multiple cerebral infarctions, brain herniation, brain-stem necrosis, and irreversible coma.[30,37] Control of brain swelling is often difficult and may require the use of a combination of the following techniques: narcotic sedation, diuretics, barbiturates, systemic neuromuscular paralysis, or hyerventilation.[36,37]

Intracranial Pressure

When a mass, such as a hematoma or cerebral edema, is present following TBI, intracranial pressure (ICP) increases in response to the pressure exerted on the brain. Initial increases in ICP are accommodated by the mechanisms of the ventricular system.[39] However, when the compensatory mechanisms are no longer effective, ICP rises.

In infancy, increases in ICP will cause bulging of the fontanels and separation of the sutures. This may continue to be seen until the child is 4 or 5 years of age and fusion of the sutures is complete.[37] In older children, as ICP rises, the contents of the cranial vault are forced downward through the foramen magnum. This causes brain-stem compression and may lead to difficulty breathing and even cardiorespiratory arrest.[29,37] Prolonged increased ICP may lead to the development of post- traumatic hydrocephalus.[29,37]

Herniation Syndromes

Herniation syndromes result from displacement of the brain by an expanding lesion and cerebral edema. Depending on the location of the lesion, herniation can cause obstructive hydocephalus, brain shift past midline, or brain-stem compression.[34] Herniation can lead to neurologic deterioration of a grave nature, with resultant decreasing levels of consciousness, altered respiration, hypertonicity, hemiparesis, and decorticate posturing.[34,37]

Hypoxic-Ischemic Injury

The supply of oxygen and nutrients to the brain is dependent on adequate cerebral perfusion. Alterations of cerebral perfusion, raised ICP, or lack of oxygen to the brain may result in hypoxic-ischemic brain damage.[34] Ischemia frequently occurs in the tissue surrounding cerebral contusions or hematomas and ultimately leads to further brain damage. Severe hypoxic injury and diffuse axonal injuries are most likely to cause severe disabilities, including prolonged post-coma unawareness.[34,40]

Neurochemical Events

When trauma occurs to the brain, there is a disruption of the blood–brain barrier and a release of excitatory neurotransmitters and oxygen-free radicals into the blood system.[34] Oxygen-free radicals have an extremely toxic effect on the brain and are damaging to cell membranes and vessel walls.[41,42] The damage from oxygen-free radicals causes internal disruption of neuronal functioning and further brain damage.[41,42]

Other Consequences from Brain Damage

Hydrocephalus

Hydrocephalus can be differentiated as either communicating or noncommunicating types. In communicating hydrocephalus, all components of the ventricular system are enlarged and ICP may only be intermittently elevated. Communicating hydrocephalus is seen in the vast majority of posttraumatic cases.[43] Noncommunicating hydrocephalus refers to enlargement of the ventricles of the brain owing to an obstruction of the flow and impaired absorption of cerebrospinal fluid. Children with hydrocephalus may present with changes in mental status, lethargy, nausea/vomiting, headache, gait ataxia, and urinary incontinence.[43] Neurosurgical ventriculoperitoneal shunting procedures are performed in children with hydrocephalus to improve the flow and absorption of cerebrospinal fluid.[43]

Seizures

The occurrence of early posttraumatic seizures is more common in children than adults, with an incidence of approximately 10%.[44,45] Early posttraumatic seizures in children are frequently of a generalized onset type, such as grand mal and tonic-clonic seizures.[45,46] Partial or focal seizures and seizures of late onset are uncommon in children.[45,46] The development of early seizures has been found to be associated with more severe injury, diffuse cerebral edema, acute subdural hematoma, and open, depressed skull fractures with damage to the brain.[47] The frequency of seizure activity within the first year after TBI may be predictive of further recurrence.[48] Thus, children who do not experience seizure within the first year following injury are unlikely to develop seizures at a later time.

Infections

Penetrating injuries, such as gunshot wounds and depressed skull fractures, carry inherent risk of brain infection. In addition, neurosurgical procedures to insert ICP monitors and shunts for increased cerebrospinal fluid also carry risk of brain infection. Two common infections following penetrating wounds are meningitis and brain abscess.[43] The physical therapist can assist the medical team by monitoring for signs of infection, such as fever, headache, confusion, neck stiffness and increased ICP.

Endocrine Disorders

Although rare, hypopituitarism and precocious puberty are both reported in children following TBI.[49,50] Linear growth and weight are closely followed so that the need for medical intervention may be determined. The physical therapist should report any concerns of increased weight gain or the development of secondary sexual characteristics to the child's physician.

Clinical Rating Scales

Clinical rating scales are used to standardize the description of patients with TBI, monitor progress, determine a general plan for appropriate medical intervention, predict outcome, and assist with clinical outcomes research.

Coma Scales

Coma is defined as a complete state of unconsciousness in which the child does not open his eyes, follow commands, speak, or react to painful stimuli.[51] To assist with determining the level of unconsciousness, Glasgow neurosurgeons, Teasdale and Jennett, developed a coma assessment scale known as the Glasgow Coma Scale (GCS).[51] It is a standardized tool for assessing the neurologic status of a trauma victim and is based on the patient's best response to three categories: motor activity, verbal responses, and eye opening.

Two variations of the GCS, the Children's Coma Scale (CCS)[52] and the Pediatric Coma Scale (PCS)[53] have been found useful in assessment of outcome in children (Table 7-2). The

TABLE 7-2
Comparison of Glasgow Coma Scale and Adelaide Pediatric Coma Scale[29]

Glasgow Coma Scale (Adults)		Adelaide Pediatric Coma Scale	
Eyes Open			
Spontaneously	4		
To speech	3	As in adults	
To pain	2		
None	1		
Best Motor Response			
Obeys commands	6		
Localizes pain	5	Obeys commands	5
Withdraws	4	Localizes to pain	4
Flexion to pain	3	Flexion to pain	3
Extension to pain	2	Extension to pain	2
None	1	None	1
Best Verbal Response			
Oriented	5	Oriented	5
Confused	4	Words	4
Words	3	Vocal sounds	3
Sounds	2	Cries	2
None	1	None	1

CCS is commonly used in children under 36 months of age, whereas the PCS is used in children 9 to 72 months of age.[54] In addition, the PCS developed interpretive norms for several age groups between birth and 5 years (Table 7-3). Children whose coma scores were below the norm for age tended to have poorer outcomes.

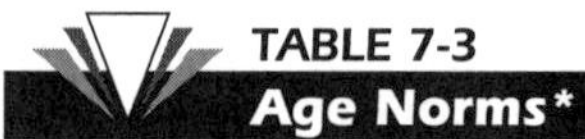

TABLE 7-3
Age Norms*

0–6 months	=	9
6–12 months	=	11
12–24 months	=	12
2–5 years	=	13
>5 years	=	14

*For the Adelaide Pediatric Coma Scale Score[29]

Orientation and Amnesia Assessment

Posttraumatic amnesia (PTA) is defined as the interval between injury and the moment at which an individual can recall a continuous memory of what is happening around him or her.[55] Evaluation of PTA in children is challenging, as traditional assessment methods rely on the subject's verbal response. Because standard orientation questions are inappropriate for children owing to their limited cognitive and language skills, the Children's Orientation and Amnesia Test (COAT)[56] was developed. The COAT is reliable for children between the ages of 4 and 15.[56] Although the COAT is useful in the age range established, a reliable method of assessing PTA in children under 4 years of age has not been established.[57]

Rancho Los Amigos Level of Cognitive Functioning

The Rancho Los Amigos Levels of Cognitive Function Scale (Rancho Scale)[58] is a descriptive scale of cognitive and behavioral functioning. It is used primarily during inpatient rehabilitation. The Rancho Scale summarizes neurobehavioral function and serves to enhance communication between staff. The Rancho Scale is also useful as a framework for the physical therapist to identify probable treatment issues and to develop treatment strategies based on the current level of cognitive function. The main limitation of the Rancho Scale is that there are poor correlations between the "phases of recovery" and prediction of discharge functional ratings.[59] In addition, cognitive function and behavior may fluctuate depending on the environment as well as fatigue or stress (see Box).

Pediatric Rancho Scale

The Pediatric Rancho[60] is an adapted version of the Rancho Los Amigos Scale that can be used to evaluate young children between the ages of infancy through 7 years of age. Like the Rancho Scale, the Pediatric Rancho Scale serves to enhance communication of recovery among staff and to assist with developing a framework for treatment management based on cognitive level (see Box).

Rancho Los Amigos Levels of Cognitive Functioning

I. *No Response:* Patient appears to be in a deep sleep and is completely unresponsive to any stimuli.
II. *Generalized Response:* Patient reacts inconsistently and nonpurposefully to stimuli in a nonspecific manner regardless of stimulus presented. Responses may be physiologic changes, gross body movements, and/or vocalization and are often limited and delayed. Often, the earliest response is to deep pain.

(continued)

Rancho Los Amigos Levels of Cognitive Functioning (Continued)

III. *Localized Response:* Patient reacts specifically but inconsistently to stimuli. Responses are directly related to type of stimulus presented. May withdraw an extremity and/or vocalize when presented with a painful stimulus. May follow simple commands such as closing eyes or squeezing hand in an inconsistent, delayed manner. May also show vague awareness of self-discomfort by pulling at nasogastric tube, catheter, or resisting restraints. May show a bias responding to familiar persons. Once external stimuli are removed, may lie quietly.

IV. *Confused-Agitated:* Patient is in a heightened state of activity, and agitation is generally in response to own internal confusion. Behavior is bizarre and nonpurposeful relative to immediate environment. Verbalizations frequently are incoherent and/or inappropriate to the environment. May cry or scream out of proportion to stimuli and even after removal, show aggressive behavior, attempt to remove restraints or tubes, or crawl out of bed. Gross attention to environment is very brief; selective attention is often nonexistent. Patient lacks any recall. Severely decreased ability to process information and does not discriminate among persons or objects; is unable to cooperate directly with treatment efforts. Unable to perform self-care without maximal assistance. May have difficulty performing motor activities such as sitting, reaching, and ambulating on request.

V. *Confused-Inappropriate:* Patient is able to respond to simple commands fairly consistently. However, with increased complexity of commands or lack of any external structure, responses are nonpurposeful, random, or fragmented. Demonstrates gross attention to the environment but is highly distractible and lacks ability to focus attention on a specific task. With structure, may be able to converse on an automatic level for short periods of time. Verbalization is often inappropriate and confabulatory. Memory is severely impaired; often shows inappropriate use of objects; and may perform previously learned tasks with structure but is unable to learn new information. Responds best to self, body, comfort, and family members. May show agitated behavior in response to discomfort or unpleasant stimuli. Can usually perform self-care activities with assistance. May wander off, either randomly or with vague intentions of "going home."

VI. *Confused-Appropriate:* Patient shows goal-directed behavior but is dependent on external input or direction. Response to discomfort is appropriate and is able to tolerate unpleasant stimuli when need is explained. Follows simple directions consistently and shows carryover for relearned/newly learned tasks such as self-care. Responses may be incorrect owing to memory problems, but they are appropriate to the situation. Past memories show more depth and detail than recent memory. No longer wanders and is inconsistently oriented to time and place. Selective attention to tasks may be impaired. May have vague recognition of staff, has increased awareness of self, family, and basic needs.

VII. *Automatic-Appropriate:* Patient appears appropriate and oriented within the hospital and home settings; goes through daily routine automatically but frequently robot like. Patient shows minimal to no confusion and has shallow recall of activities. Shows increased awareness of self, body, family, food, people, and interaction in the environment. Has superficial awareness of, but lacks insight into condition; decreased judgment and problem solving. Lacks realistic ideas/plans for the future. Shows carryover for new learning but at a decreased rate. Requires supervision for learning and safety purposes. WIth structure is able to initiate social or recreational activities.

VIII. *Purposeful-Appropriate:* Patient is able to recall and integrate past and recent events and is aware of and responsive to environment. Shows carryover for new learning and needs no supervision once activities are learned. May continue to show a decreased ability relative to premorbid activities, abstract reasoning, tolerance for stress, and judgment in emergencies or unusually circumstances. Social, emotional, and intellectual capacities may continue to be at a decreased level but functional in society.

Hagen C, Makmus D, Durham P, et al. Levels of cognitive functioning. In: *Rehabilitation of the Head-Injured Adult: Comprehensive Physical Management.* Downey, CA: Professional Staff of Rancho Los Amigos Hospital; 1979:87–90.

Predictors of Injury Severity and Outcome

The outcome of a child following TBI is affected by a number of factors, including location and morphologic characteristics of the injury, complications that occur during the initial stabilization of the injury, the age of the child at the time of injury, the length of coma, the duration of PTA, the severity of the injury, premorbid psychological and cognitive adjustment, and the family response to the injury.[55,61,62] Of all the factors listed, the duration of coma appears to be the single most consistent predictor of outcome.[55,61] The rate of recovery following TBI is most rapid in the first few months and continues throughout the first year after the accident.[63] In children with severe injury, some improvement is noted in the second year following TBI.

Duration of Coma

Duration of coma is directly related to a trend seen in outcome.[64,65] The longer the coma, the worse the outcome. For children with mild TBI and loss of consciousness for one night, the results on long-term outcome measures of cognition, achievement, and behavior are in-distinguishable from those of uninjured children.[62,63] In contrast, children with moderate to severe TBI and coma lasting more than a few days

Pediatric Rancho Scale

V. *No Response to Stimuli:* Complete absence or observable change in behavior to visual, auditory, or painful stimuli.

IV. *Generalized Response to Sensory Stimulation:* Reacts to stimuli in a nonspecific manner, reactions are inconsistent, limited in nature, and often the same regardless of stimulus present. Responses may be delayed. Responses noted include physiologic changes, gross body movement, or vocalizations. First responses are often to pain. Gives generalized startle to loud sounds. Responds to repeated auditory stimulation with increased or decreased activity. Gives generalized reflex response to painful stimuli.

III. *Localized Response to Sensory Stimuli:* Reacts specifically to stimulus. Responses are directly related to type of stimuli presented. Responses include blinks when strong light crosses field of vision, follows moving object passed within visual field, and turns toward or away from loud sound or withdraws from painful stimuli. Reactions can be inconsistent and delayed. May inconsistently follow simple commands such as close eyes, move an arm. May show vague awareness of self by pulling at tubes or restraints. May show a bias by responding to family and not others.

II. *Responsive to Environment:* Appears alert and responds to name. Recognizes parents or other family members. Imitates examiner's gestures or facial expressions. Participates in simple age-appropriate vocal play/vocalizations. Gross attention but highly distractible. Needs frequent redirection to focus on task. Follows commands in an age-appropriate manner and is able to perform previously learned tasks with structure. Without external structure, responses may be random or nonpurposeful. May be agitated by external stimuli. Increased awareness of self, family, and basic needs.

I. *Patient Is Oriented to Self and Surroundings:* Shows active interest in environment and initiates social contact. Can provide accurate information about self, surroundings, orientation, and present situation as age-appropriate.

Staff from Denver Child's Hospital. Notes from Pediatric Rehab: Traumatic Brain Injury. Denver CO; 1989.

experience a variety of physical, cognitive, language, and psychological sequelae that may improve following the injury or remain permanent.

When examining functional outcome at 1 year after TBI, 73% of the children who were in a coma the median duration of 5 to 6 weeks were independent in ambulation and self-care.[66] Better outcomes occurred in the group with less than 6 weeks of coma and worse outcomes occurred in the group with more than 12 weeks of coma. In the latter group, less than one third had a normal intelligence quotient, nearly half had significant behavior problems, and three fourths needed special education placement at school.[66]

Depth of Coma

In addition to the duration of coma, the depth of coma, as measured by the GCS, is easy to assess and correlates well with prognosis and functional outcome.[55] Using the GCS scores, mild injuries are those described as having a GCS score of 13 to 15, moderate injuries have a GCS score of 9 to 12, and severe injuries have a GCS score of 8 or less.[18,67]

Most children who sustain mild brain injury, as determined by the GCS, are expected to experience a full recovery within several weeks.[68] However, for children moderately and severely injured, the degree of initial impairment on the GCS is related to both the degree of recovery and residual deficit.[62] Strong correlations in severity on the GCS and outcome have been noted especially in the areas of intelligence, academic performance, and motor performance.[62]

Duration of Posttraumatic Amnesia

The length of PTA has been used to classify the severity of TBI. Severity of injury is mild if PTA lasts less than 1 hour, moderate if PTA lasts between 1 and 24 hours, and severe if PTA lasts longer than 1 day.[69] As a further refinement, severity is very mild if PTA lasts 5 minutes or less, very se vere if PTA lasted over 7 days, and extremely severe if PTA lasts longer than 4 weeks.[69] In children, the duration of PTA has been found to be more predictive of future memory function than the GCS.[56]

Age

The capacity of the brain to guard against and respond to trauma changes with age.[18] Although at one time young children were thought to be spared greater dysfunction following TBI, newer research has demonstrated an increased vulnerability of the young child to the effects of TBI.[29,70] In infants, the skull is thin and easily deformable, thus increasing the susceptibility to injury from trauma.[29,67] In addition, immature myelination in the cerebral hemispheres places the child at risk for injury, as the younger child's brain is soft and compressible.[67]

The age of the child at the time of injury also appears to correlate with increased risk for specific impairments. Young children are more vulnerable to the effects of diffuse injury on memory than older children. Children that experience TBI before the age of 5 years exhibit more profound language deficits than when injury occurs in later childhood.[71] In addition, children who are severely injured between the ages of 15 and 21 years are at higher risk than older adult patients for late behavioral and emotional sequelae.[72]

Although the plasticity of the developing brain can allow for dramatic recovery of function, the effects of a diffuse insult produced by TBI may ultimately result in greater cognitive impairment in the developing brain than in the mature brain.[70] Moreover, deficits may remain hidden until a time in which the child needs to participate in higher level academic activities. Clearly, the young child is vulnerable to brain injury.

Other Factors

It has been difficult to use early physiologic markers as predictors of outcome in children with TBI, as they are generally unreliable.[61,66] Large percentages of children with hypertension, seizures, fixed and dilated pupils, flaccidity, or prolonged forceful posturing have been reported to have good long-term outcomes.[73]

Physical Therapy Assessment Evaluation of the Child with TBI

When a child with TBI is referred for treatment, a thorough physical therapy evaluation is necessary to ensure appropriate treatment planning and implementation. The evaluation (Display 7-1) should contain, but may not be limited to, inclusion of information on past medical history, psychosocial status, cognitive/behavioral status, basic sensorimotor status, and functional status. While performing the evaluation, consideration should be given to the child's tolerance level and attention span, as deficits in either area may limit the physical therapist's ability to complete the evaluation in one session. The physical therapist may also need to incorporate play into the assessment in an effort to enhance cooperation and obtain a more accurate picture of the child with TBI.

Subjective Evaluation

MEDICAL HISTORY

The therapist must thoroughly review the child's medical and surgical history prior to initiating the physical examination. Information should be gathered regarding the mechanism of the injury, severity of damage, and significant changes in the clinical picture over time. Particular attention should be given to reports from CT scans, x-rays, and other diagnostic tests.

PSYCHOSOCIAL INFORMATION

Interviewing the parents, siblings, and/or caregivers of the child with TBI is imperative, as successful therapeutic intervention should be family- and child-centered.[74] The family is the expert in knowing their child and often can give helpful advice to the therapist regarding the best way to motivate the child in therapy. Families should be encouraged to collaborate with the rehabilitation team in the development of appropriate treatment goals and a discharge plan. Family or psychosocial information may also be gained by talking to the social worker.

Objective Evaluation

Children who sustain TBI may experience a complex array of impairments and functional limitations in physical abilities, emotional development, and cognitive/behavioral functioning (Display 7-2).[75]

COGNITIVE/BEHAVIORAL STATUS

A comprehensive cognitive evaluation is beyond the scope of practice of the physical therapist. However, cognition should be grossly assessed by the physical therapist to assist in determining realistic treatment goals and appropriate therapeutic intervention. Physical therapy evaluation of cognition should include the following areas: arousal/orientation, attention span and focus, behavior/affect, memory, language mental flexibility, problem solving, judgment, and insight.

LEVEL OF AROUSAL/ORIENTATION. Trauma that damages the frontal lobe and brain-stem may result in impairment of arousal and orientation of the child with TBI. In addition, medications used to diminish spasticity, seizures, or pain may decrease arousal.[36] Impairment in arousal may be expressed as lethargy, drowsiness, or even coma. Decreased levels of arousal will interfere with the child's ability to attend to

DISPLAY 7-1

Physical Therapy Evaluation/Assessment Format

Medical History

Onset and mechanism of injury
Diagnostic test results (CAT scan, MRI, x-rays)
Medical precautions
Vital signs
Autonomic nervous system function
Skin Integrity
Respiratory status
Bowel and bladder status
Dysphagia status
Medications

Psychosocial Information

Family and support system
Educational/prevocational status
Cultural issues
Discharge environment

Cognitive/Behavioral Status

Level of arousal
Orientation
Attention
Behavior/affect
Memory
Language/communication
Executive functions
Neuropsychological or psychological assessments

Basic Sensorimotor Status

Hearing/Auditory Processing
Vision, perception, and visuospatial ability
Sensation
Range of motion
Strength
Muscle tone
Abnormal movement patterns, posture, and reflexes
Balance and balance strategies
Praxis and coordination
Speed of movement
Endurance

Functional Status

Bed/floor mobility
Transfers/transitions
Sitting and standing skills
Ambulation on level surfaces
Stair ascension/descension
Ambulation outside/rough terrain
Advanced gross motor skills/sports
Generalization of functional abilities

DISPLAY 7-2

Common Clinical Impairments and Functional Limitations

Physical	Emotional	Cognitive/Behavioral	Functional
Headaches	Mood swings	Decreased arousal	Limited bed mobility
Dizziness	Denial	Disorientation	Limited transfers
Visual disturbance	Anxiety	Distractibility	Poor sitting control
Visuospatial impairment	Depression	Inattention	Poor standing control
Hearing loss	Irritability	Impaired concentration	Gait impairment
Sensory loss	Guilt/self-blame	Confusion	Impaired hygiene skills
Cranial nerve injury	Emotional lability	Agitation	Impaired dressing skills
Spasticity	Low self-esteem	Memory deficits/amnesia	Impaired feeding skills
Ataxia/incoordination	Egocentricity	Sequencing difficulty	Fine motor impairment
Balance impairment	Lability	Slowed processing	Sexual dysfunction
Fatigue	Apathy	Impaired judgement	
Sleep disorders		Impaired problem solving	
Seizures		Speech/language problems	
		Decreased academic skills	

pertinent stimuli, follow commands, and benefit from feedback in therapy.

Attention. Trauma to the frontal lobe may impair attention in the child with TBI. Impairment in attention may affect both the ability to attend to a specific stimulus while screening out others and the ability to sustain attention over time. Impairment may be expressed as distractibility or inattention. Virtually all tasks involve attention and children with TBI who have problems with attention often have difficulty following commands and relearning motor tasks. This is especially noted when therapy is conducted in busy environments. Care must be taken to structure the environment and remove extraneous stimuli as appropriate.

Behavior/Affect. Following TBI, children may display a wide array of problems in behavior and affect (Display 7-2).[75] Two common changes in behavior noted during the time of rehabilitation are agitation and confusion. Agitation is characterized by a heightened state of activity and a severely decreased ability to process stimuli from the environment in a useful manner. The child who is agitated may be restless, irritable, and combative. Impulsivity and unsafe behavior may be observed as the child acts before thinking. Fortunately, agitation in children with TBI does not last as long as the agitated phase of recovery for adults with TBI.[57]

Confusion is characterized by general disorientation and inability to make sense out of the surrounding environment. Confusion may persist through most of the rehabilitative process. Children with TBI who are confused may interact either appropriately or inappropriately.

When problems with behavior persist and interfere with participation in therapy, it is important for the brain injury rehabilitation team to work together and implement a behavior modification program. Initially, the team must identify the unwanted behaviors and any precipitating factors, including environmental factors that contribute to the behavior problem. Agitation may be precipitated by factors such as pain, occult fractures, restraints, urinary tract infections, constipation, and overstimulation by staff, family, and friends. Precipitating factors should be addressed prior to the implementation of the behavior modification program and be removed when at all possible.

Then, rewards and reinforcements for desired behavior must be determined. The family may be very helpful in identifying rewards that are motivating and satisfying. A reward schedule must also be agreed on by the team to maximize compliance and promote the desired behavior. Once the reward schedule has been determined, the team then moves toward redirecting the child to appropriate actions by praising or rewarding approximations of desired actions. As the team works together to address the behavior problem in a consistent manner, the incidence of inappropriate actions slowly decreases. When the environment cannot be modified and behavior management is ineffective, pharmacologic management should be considered.

Memory. Memory impairment is the most common cognitive impairment in children with TBI.[76] Trauma to the temporal lobe commonly affects memory in children with TBI. Memory includes the ability to learn and recall new information as well as the ability to recall old previously learned information. The presence of memory loss, or amnesia, is an indication that a concussion has occurred. The amnesia may be retrograde, involving a period of time prior to the accident, or anterograde, extending from the incident forward in time.

Retrograde amnesia may be temporary and may cover events that occurred several months or years prior to the injury. Memory for most past events will usually return over several hours or days.[37] However, permanent retrograde amnesia may exist for the brief period of time preceding the accident.[37] Anterograde amnesia is problematic during the rehabilitation process and may interfere with new learning. Anterograde amnesia is rarely permanent.[37]

Memory deficits involve verbal recall and visual recognition. They may appear as the inability to remember the sequence of motor tasks from one treatment to another or as unsafe performance of functional skills. The omission of safety-related behaviors when performing functional motor skills, such as transfers and ambulation, may limit independence.

Memory with respect to a child's ability to learn new material is of particular interest to the physical therapist. Although retention of information learned prior to the TBI may remain unharmed, the memory for learning new information may be problematic. Problems with memory for new learning will also pose obvious problems for the child who will be returning to school. The results of a neuropsychological evaluation of a child's memory skills and capacity for new learning will be helpful in the establishment of realistic functional goals and the development of an appropriate educational and/or rehabilitation program.[36] Working jointly with the child's family and psychologist, the physical therapist may help determine the need for compensatory strategies, assistance, and environmental modification in the school setting.

Language. Language deficits in the child with TBI are addressed in depth by speech and language pathologists. Damage to the temporal lobe may result in expressive or receptive language skill deficits that will impede communication between the physical therapist and child, thus complicating therapy sessions. For example, receptive language deficits will impair a child's ability to understand verbal instructions for the performance of a gross motor task. When a receptive language impairment exists, determination of the best means of communication will decrease frustration for the child and the therapist.

Expressive language disorders impair a child's ability to communicate with others. Although the child with an expressive language disorder may be able to fully comprehend verbally communicated information and form an appropriate response mentally, a breakdown occurs between the formulation of the response and the verbal or gestural execution of what was intended. Once again, the physical therapist's knowledge of the child's most effective mode of communication may lessen the frustration related to the inability to communicate thoughts and feelings.[36]

EXECUTIVE FUNCTIONS. Trauma to the prefrontal regions of the frontal lobes results in impairment of executive functions. Executive functions refer to the ability to show initiative, plan activities, change conceptual sets, solve problems, regulate behavior in social settings, and use feedback to initiate behavioral change and monitor success.[36,75]

Deficits in executive functioning may be demonstrated by impulsive behavior, resulting in failure to observe safety precautions or the inability to recognize when behavior is socially inappropriate.[36] Mental inflexibility may be demonstrated as perseveration on a task or the inability to change activities without becoming disorganized.[36] Difficulty switching conceptual sets may also influence the ability to perform tasks with alternating patterns or reciprocal movements.

BASIC SENSORIMOTOR STATUS

ABNORMAL TONE

SPASTICITY. Because of damage to the cerebral cortex, children with TBI may present with spasticity. The degree of spasticity may range from mild to severe, with distribution that may be either unilateral or bilateral. Children who present with unilateral involvement display motor impairment and dysfunction similar to that of children with hemiplegic cerebral palsy. Children who present with bilateral involvement often have asymmetric distribution and movements dominated by primitive reflex activity.

Children with spasticity may also present with abnormal posturing of the extremities or the whole body. The upper extremities typically present with flexor synergy posturing. Flexor synergy posturing interferes with hygiene and functional use of the upper extremity for play, school work, and self-care. The lower extremities commonly present with extensor synergy posturing.

Children with TBI who are severely involved may present with whole body posturing. Whole body posturing can be decorticate (flexion of the upper extremities and extension of the lower extremities) or decerebrate (extension in all extremities) in nature and is frequently seen in the early stages of recovery. As the child improves, whole body posturing is replaced with more volitional movement, including movement utilizing synergistic patterns.

ATAXIA. Because of damage to the cerebellum and basal ganglia, children with TBI may experience ataxia and motor incoordination. The distribution of ataxia can also be unilateral or bilateral. Ataxia may initially be masked by spasticity in the early recovery period. Timing and execution of movement may be difficult, and intention may or may not be present. Gait in children with ataxia is characterized by a wide base of support and difficulty maintaining static stance. Ataxia is generally not associated with loss of range of motion unless combined with spasticity.

RANGE OF MOTION LOSS. Because of the poverty of movement and stereotypic abnormal movement patterns used, children with TBI who present with spasticity are at risk for loss of active range of motion and contracture development. Joints particularly at risk include the elbows, wrists, fingers, knees, and ankle-foot complex. Range of motion loss can occur quickly and early management is the key to effective prevention.

SENSORY DEFICITS

HEARING. Hearing loss is also common in pediatric TBI.[77] All children with moderate to severe traumatic brain injuries should have a thorough audiologic evaluation to determine the presence of hearing loss. When hearing loss is present, hearing aids, an FM transmitter, or preferential classroom seating may be indicated.[57]

VISION. Visual disturbances in children with TBI are common. These deficits may include decreased visual acuity, disturbances of visual pursuit and accommodation, field cuts, reduced depth perception, diplopia, transient cortical blindness, and retinal hemorrhages.[57] When visual problems exist, eye patching, glasses, or preferential classroom seating may help alleviate the difficulty.[57]

Transient cortical blindness lasting no longer than 30 days has been associated with nearly complete recovery of vision.[57,78] However, cortical blindness lasting more than 30 days generally carries a grave prognosis for children of school age and older. Retinal hemorrhages in young children with TBI are strongly suggestive of child abuse.[37,79,80]

VISUOSPATIAL SKILLS. Problems with vision are also associated with problems of perception and visuospatial function. Such deficits are frequently associated with lesions in the temporal or occipital lobes of the brain. Visuospatial and perceptual deficits may impair gross motor performance and functional mobility skills, thus limiting the potential for functional independence in a child. A figure-ground deficit, or the inability to distinguish a given form from the background, may make noting a change in terrain depth during gait training more difficult. Visuospatial deficits may make activities of daily living, such as donning an orthosis, more difficult. A child with deficits in visuospatial memory may demonstrate difficulty developing a mental map of his or her environment and consequently may have difficulty moving independently from place to place in home, school, or community.[36]

ORTHOPEDIC CONCERNS

HETEROTOPIC OSSIFICATION. Heterotopic ossification (HO), the formation of mature lamellar bone in soft tissue, can occur in children and adolescents following TBI.[81] The risk of incidence of HO is reported to be 14% and identified risk factors include age greater than 11 years and a longer duration of coma.[66,81] HO commonly occurs at the elbow, shoulder, hip, and knee. Early signs of HO include decreased joint range of motion and pain with testing, swelling, erythema, and increased warmth near the involved joint.

The use of physical therapy in the treatment of HO is controversial. Some studies have associated physical therapy and aggressive range of motion exercises with HO as a result of local microtrauma and hemorrhage to the tissue.[82] In general, gentle but persistent range of motion exercises and management of spasticity with medications or nerve blocks are imperative.[82] When HO results in significant functional impairment, surgical excision of the bone from the soft tissue is indicated. HO rarely results in functional impairment in younger children.[81,83]

FRACTURES. Fractures in the pelvis and lower extremities are commonly associated with the traumatic events causing pediatric TBI. Up to one third of children sustaining severe TBI have skeletal fractures in the long bones, clavicle, or spine.[84,85] Surgical repair of fractures may be delayed until the child is neurologically and medically stable. Postsurgical care may be complicated by the decreased cognitive status of the child, especially when the child is alert and confused. Therefore, the child must be closely monitored to ensure that proper alignment and weight-bearing status are maintained during functional activities.

Although x-rays identify major trauma to the extremities, care should be exercised in evaluating additional musculoskeletal complaints, as there is potential for minor trauma and occult fractures to be undetected in the acute recovery phase. Particular attention should be given to persistent complaints and activities that are poorly tolerated. In addition, children may have complaints of soft tissue injuries that would not be detected by x-ray.

FUNCTIONAL STATUS

Early evaluation of function is difficult because of the compromised cognitive status of the child. As the child is more alert and appropriate in interactions in the clinic, the use of standardized functional assessment tools may be helpful. The WeeFIM (Functional Independence Measure)[86] has been useful for evaluating functional independence in children under the age of 6 years, and the FIM can be used with older children.

The Pediatric Evaluation of Disability Inventory (PEDI)[87] has also been developed as a functional assessment tool for children. It measures both capability and performance in the domains of self-care, mobility, and social function. The PEDI can be used in children between the ages of 6 months to 7.5 years. Each of these assessment tools is more fully described in Chapter 2.

Establishing Treatment Goals

A thorough assessment leads to the development of specific long- and short-term goals. Goals should be written based on identified system impairments, qualitative movement deficits, and functional limitations. Goals should be measurable and expressed in behavioral terms. Each short-term goal should be written as a component that leads to the accomplishment of the long-term goal. Time frames in which goals will be achieved are dependent on the setting in which the child is seen as well as consideration of the child's cognitive and behavioral status.

Coordination of services through a case manager may assist with the identification of an approved range of the length of stay and the resources available to achieve the child's goals in physical therapy. When establishing goals, the physical therapist should also consider the proposed discharge environment so that the goals are correlated with where the child is going to once discharged from the rehabilitation setting.[88]

Management/Treatment

Rehabilitation of children with TBI is different from adults with TBI in that children are still completing the process of typical development. Treatment then must take into consideration both the typical developmental progression and the recovery from the neurologic insult.[89,90] Therefore, when planning treatment, the physical therapist must design programs that incorporate age-appropriate gross motor challenges at the appropriate level of cognitive function. Although the efficacy of various rehabilitation programs is not known, research is indicative of a positive trend in the benefit of rehabilitative services.[91]

Acute Medical Management

Early medical management of the child with TBI focuses on preservation of life, determination of injury severity, and prevention of secondary brain damage.[34] Once vital signs are stabilized, the child will undergo a general assessment for potential injuries and a neurologic examination. These tests may include radiographic examination of the skull and cervical spine, CT scan of the head, and the use of the GCS.

Acute medical intervention for children with TBI may include emergency surgery, the use of mechanical ventilation, and the use of pharmacologic agents. If a subdural or intracerebral hematoma is present, immediate neurosurgery is indicated.[34] A delay in performing the surgery can be life-threatening, as it helps decrease intracranial pressure and reduce pressure-related secondary brain injuries.[34]

Mechanically assisted ventilation at a rate greater than normal or hyperventilation is used to temporarily reduce intracranial pressure.[36] In addition to hyperventilation, pharmacologic agents are also used to decrease cerebral edema and minimize secondary brain damage. Drugs commonly used in the management of edema include mannitol and corticosteroids.[36] Medications may also be used to induce paralysis when the child's body movements interfere with the stability of vital signs and the administration of further medical interventions.[36]

Physical therapy in the acute stage may be deferred to a time in which the child is less medically fragile. Once the child is stable, the physical therapist may use the child's current level of cognitive functioning as a guide in planning a treatment program. It is important for the physical therapist to remember that the cognitive levels of recovery serve only as a general guideline for recovery. Not all children will experience each level of cognitive recovery nor progress through recovery in a strict hierarchical sequence. Either the Rancho Scale or the Pediatric Rancho Scale may assist with identification of current cognitive status and potential concerns for the various stages.

Acute Physical Therapy Management: Prevention

Physical therapy management for children with TBI functioning at low cognitive levels is aimed at the prevention of complications from prolonged inactivity and sensory deprivation. Common complications of prolonged inactivity may include skin breakdown, respiratory complications, and contracture development.

POSITIONING

A positioning program will assist with improving pulmonary hygiene, maintaining skin integrity, preventing contractures, and providing support for body alignment and movement. Positioning should be implemented with the assistance of the nursing staff and the family. Changes in position for the child confined in bed should be made every 2 hours. When the child is sitting, pressure relief procedures should be performed every 30 minutes. Pressure relief is accomplished by having the child recline on a mat in side-lying or by tilting the wheelchair backward to a semisupine position.

When designing a positioning program, the physical therapist should take into consideration any orthopedic and neurologic positioning precautions as well as the influence of abnormal tone and primitive reflexes on posture. Positioning in side-lying (Fig. 7-1) is helpful to decrease the influence of abnormal primitive reflexes and should be used when possible. Positioning in supine should incorporate strategies to reduce the influence of the tonic labyrinthine reflex and extensor tone. Positioning in prone, although allowable, will seldom be carried out at this phase of recovery as it interferes with accessibility for adequately monitoring the child.

Upright positioning even at an early stage of recovery may be achieved with the use of an adapted wheelchair (Fig. 7-2 and 7-3). The adapted wheelchair should incorporate either a

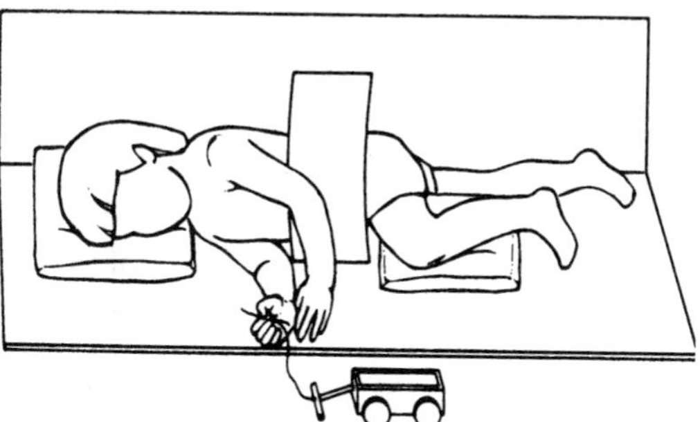

Figure 7-1 ▪ Child positioned in a side-lyer. Note that the head is maintained in line with the trunk, the upper extremities are in midline, and the lower extremities are dissociated. Gravity is eliminated, and the influence of primitive reflexes is minimized.

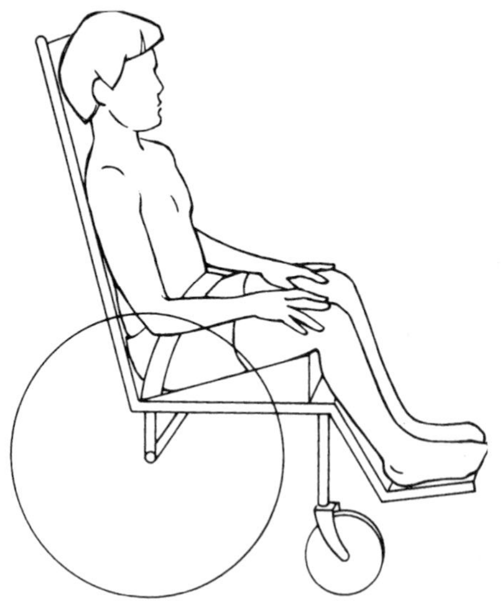

Figure 7-2 ▪ Child is supported in a wheelchair with a tall back and a seat wedge to maintain hip flexion. The back may be designed to either recline or tilt-in-space to accommodate fatigue in the child.

tilt in space or reclining seating system with postural support to assist the child in safely achieving upright while preventing overfatigue. The use of a removable headrest can be used to encourage head control when the child is more alert and can allow for rest when the child is tired.

CONTRACTURE MANAGEMENT

The importance of preventing soft tissue contractures in the acute recovery phase cannot be overemphasized. Development of contractures will delay functional independence and lead to the need for additional therapy or even surgery later in the rehabilitative phase. In addition to the use of a positioning program, range of motion and the application of splints and casts may help improve lower extremity function and prevent soft tissue contractures.[92]

Contractures in prepubertal children, who are not forcefully posturing, often may be successfully managed with positioning and splinting alone because of the child's smaller size and relative weakness.[57] Coordination of a wearing schedule is a key to enhancing the effectiveness of splinting. Wearing tolerance may be gradual, and the child must be monitored for signs of skin breakdown. In a larger child who is not forcefully posturing, serial casting followed by bivalved fiberglass cast splints may be used to manage contractures.

For children with severe extensor posturing who do not respond to a positioning program, splints or bivalved casts, serial casts are warranted (Fig. 7-4).[57] These casts must be changed initially every 3 to 5 days to prevent skin breakdown. Once it is determined that the child will tolerate the casts without skin breakdown, the casts can be worn for up to 2-week intervals until posturing diminishes and volitional control increases. Bivalved fiberglass cast splints may then be used at night to maintain range of motion. Continuous use of serial casts in a child who is alert and moving actively should not exceed 2 months.

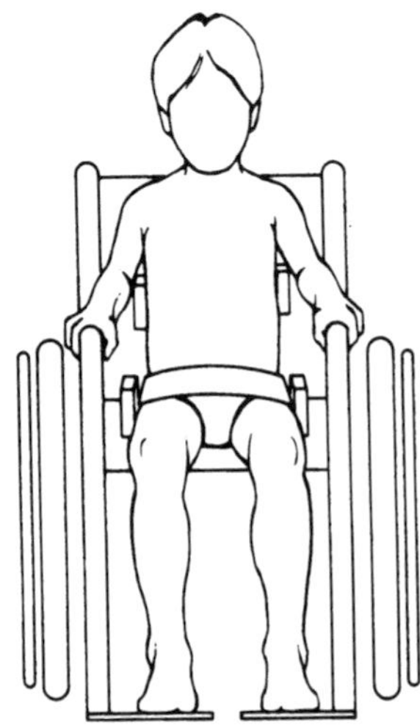

Figure 7-3 ▪ Child is sitting in a wheelchair with hip blocks and lateral trunk supports for assistance with postural control.

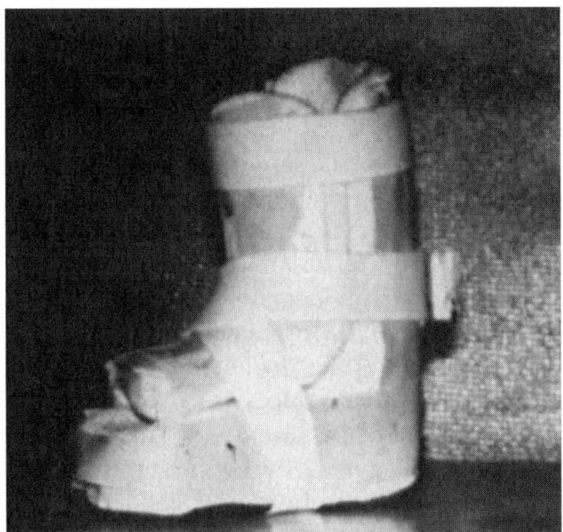

Figure 7-4 ▪ An example of a bivalved inhibitive cast.

Serial casts may be used in conjunction with oral or injectable medications to manage spasticity. Oral medications, such as dantrolene (Dantrium), although useful in decreasing spasticity, may be undesirable because of its sedating properties.[57] Diazepam (Valium) can also be used for treating spasticity but may be associated with increased agitation in children who are emerging from coma.[57] As an alternative, nerve and motor point blocks, such as phenol and Botox injections, may be more desirable in the management of spasticity in children, as there are no sedating and cognitive side effects.[57] Recent work on the use of Botox injections in children is promising. Effects of the injectable medications can last up to 3 to 6 months.[57]

Low Cognitive Level Physical Therapy Management: Stimulation

COMA STIMULATION PROGRAM

Coma stimulation programs were developed on the premise that structured stimulation could prevent sensory deprivation and accelerate recovery.[93] However, controversy exists regarding the amount of stimulation that can be safely used early in the care of a comatose child.[94] Sensory input may be provided through the vestibular, visual, tactile, auditory, and olfactory systems (Display 7-3).[95] The rehabilitation team should involve the family in selection of meaningful items to be used for stimulation. An emphasis should be placed on selecting items that reflect the child's culture, personality, likes/dislikes, hobbies, significant relationships, and pets. Items that are selected should be reevaluated periodically so that ineffective stimuli can be eliminated.

The next step in program development is to determine an appropriate schedule for stimulation. The physical therapist needs to determine the time of day at which alertness is optimal to conduct therapy and modify the child's schedule

DISPLAY 7-3

Sources of Sensory Stimulation[95]

Auditory	Visual	Olfactory	Tactile	Vestibular
Verbal orientation	Photographs	Vinegar	Hand holding	Turning
Music	Penlight	Spices	Rubbing lotion	Range of motion
Bells	Familiar objects	Perfume	Heat/cold	Sitting in chair
Familiar voice	Faces	Potpourri	Cotton balls	Tilt table
Tuning fork	Flashcards	Orange/lemon	Rough surfaces	
Clapping	Picture books		Familiar objects	

as necessary. In the event that is not possible, the physical therapist will need to modify the treatment goals within a given session and attempt to engage the child at the current level of arousal and attention.[36] Again, the family can assist by describing what a typical day for the child was like prior to injury. This information can later be used to individualize the child's program. A schedule of the coma stimulation program and the materials to be used may be kept in a box in the child's room for convenience.

Prior to implementation, the physical therapist will need to educate the family on the provision of appropriate levels of sensory stimulation, including the amount of environmental stimulation being provided. Care should be taken to create an environment that is stimulating without being overstimulating or noxious. Decreasing extraneous auditory and visual activity in the child's room or treatment area may help the child focus on commands and elicit a response related to specific treatment stimuli.

At the beginning of the coma stimulation session, the physical therapist should orient the child with TBI to his surroundings, who is interacting with him, and the current date and time. Stimulation should be brief, not lasting for more than 15 minutes, and occur frequently, eight to ten times a day in order to avoid habituation. Stimulation should be implemented in an organized fashion, orienting the child to the stimulation prior to use, using one or two sensory modalities at a time and slowly presenting meaningful items. The therapist needs to be patient and allow time for the child to respond, as processing of sensory input may be delayed. A variety of responses may occur depending on the stimulation used (Display 7-4).[95] Precautions should be taken to prevent overstimulation of the child and to ensure that the child's medical status remains stable following stimulation. Unfavorable responses to stimulation include the development of seizure activity and sustained increases in heart rate, blood pressure, and respiratory rate.[95]

For the child who is generally unresponsive or responds only to pain, the initial goal of input is to elicit any type of response to stimuli. Once again, care should be taken to monitor the child for signs of overstimulation or poor tolerance of stimulation. However, as the child becomes more alert, the therapist should focus on increasing the consistency, duration, and quality of the child's response. All team members and the family should be encouraged to document the stimuli utilized and the child's response to note progress and assist with carryover.

As the child begins to attend to therapy and follow one-step motor commands, the physical therapist can begin facilitation of movement with emphasis on head and trunk control and upper extremity movement patterns. The therapist should continue to monitor the patient for physiologic signs of sensory overload during treatment and make adjustments accordingly. As a more specific response to stimulation occurs, the physical therapist should try to improve the variety and consistency of the response and decrease delays in responding. Response should then be channeled into purposeful activity and prefunctional skills. At this

DISPLAY 7-4
Common Responses to Stimulation[95]

Auditory	Visual	Olfactory	Tactile	Vestibular
Startle reaction	Eye blink	Grimacing	Posturing	Spasticity/movement
Localization	Visual localization	Tearing	Withdrawal	Assisted ROM
Turn toward sound	Visual tracking	Head turning	Localization	Head righting
Follow commands	Visual attention	Sniffing	General response	

time, the physical therapist should also begin family education about future recovery phases and possible treatment techniques.

Mid-Cognitive Level Physical Therapy Management: Structure

When the child has emerged from coma and begins to participate in functional activities, other cognitive deficits may become evident. Selection of appropriate activities by the physical therapist should be based on cognitive as well as physical demands. However, the therapist will need to remember that the progression of cognitive and physical function can proceed at different rates.

THE AGITATED PATIENT

Initially, agitation is in response to poor regulation of stimulation and internal confusion. Factors that may contribute to agitation include overstimulation by staff, parents, and friends; restraints; occult fractures; pain; constipation and urinary tract infections. Agitation may be expressed as bizarre or aggressive behaviors. Clinicians should take care in determining what extraneous stimuli increase agitation and attempt to reduce or eliminate them when possible. Children in a confused and agitated state require the use of a highly structured environment to decrease the number of behavioral outbursts and prevent overstimulation. The physical therapist may need to give verbal reassurance to the child with TBI as some agitated behaviors can be related to fear. If precipitating factors can not be successfully reduced or eliminated, then pharmacologic management should be considered.

It is important to utilize a team approach that includes the family in the management of agitation. Common management strategies include having a quiet room with no television or telephone, limited visitors, and planned rest periods as needed. The child's family may resist suggestions to decrease visitors and stimuli, believing that talking loudly and turning on lights, television, and radio can help to increase the child's alertness and speed recovery.[56] Family education on appropriate levels of stimuli should be reinforced by staff.

It is important to protect the child who is agitated from potential injury. Restraints should be removed when possible as they may further agitation. If the unrestrained child is at risk for falling out of bed, it may be necessary to modify the room by placing the mattress on the floor or switch to an enclosed protective bed. Other protective devices include alarm devices, such as sensitized door mats and monitor bracelets used for the child or adolescent who is ambulatory and may wander away from supervision.

During the agitated phase, treatment should be modified to include activities that are familiar to the child and well liked to enhance participation and cooperation. Although the child may be able to perform familiar motor activities, the physical therapist should anticipate behavior that is essentially nonpurposeful. Appropriate tasks and activities include range of motion exercises to the child's tolerance and functional gross motor activities such as rolling, coming to sit, coming to stand, and walking. It is important for the physical therapist to work within the child's tolerance level on previously learned skills and to expect no carryover for new learning during this phase of recovery.

The child with TBI is often very unpredictable during the agitated phase, so the therapist should be prepared with numerous activity options. Choices of activities should be offered to the child when possible. When the child is uncooperative with familiar or routine activities, the physical therapist should first try to redirect the child to another therapeutic activity. If unsuccessful, the physical therapist may need to resort to involving the child in any activity in which he or she is willing to participate. Therapy of this nature is still beneficial to the child with TBI as it serves to increase attention span.

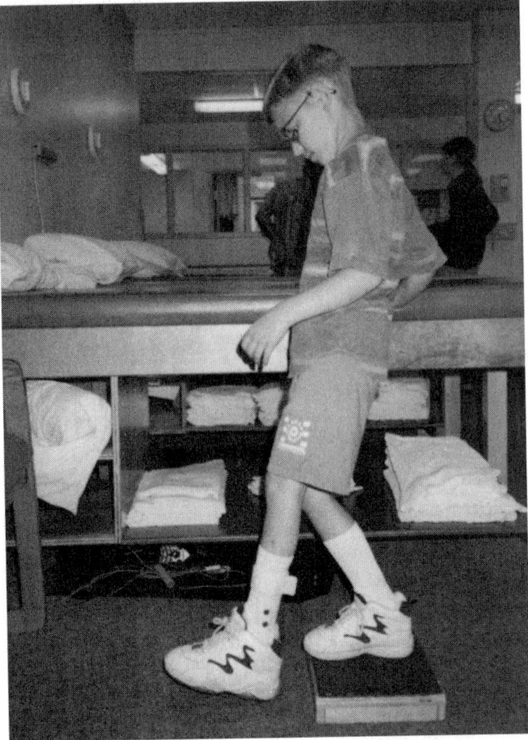

Figure 7-5 ▪ Stepping down off a small bench facilitates heelstrike with knee extension and improved eccentric control of the lower extremity. This component should later be practiced within the context of gait.

For the child who is extremely difficult to manage, cotreatment with other team members and shortened therapy sessions may be necessary for a short period of time until the child tolerates longer interactions. As attention span gradually increases, the physical therapist reinforces longer periods of attention and directs the child with TBI back to more challenging tasks.

THE CONFUSED PATIENT

Although no longer internally agitated, the child with TBI who is confused will require continued behavior management and structure during the therapy session to perform optimally. Structure may include decreasing the complexity of instructions, simplifying the environment, or breaking a motor task down into smaller components (Fig. 7-5 and 7-6). The primary goal of therapy during the confused phase of recovery is to enhance successful participation in functional tasks.

Initially, it will be necessary to keep the environment as distraction free as possible as the child may become agitated with external stimuli. In addition, the physical therapist should give the child as much structure and assistance for functional activities as necessary to allow for success. As performance improves, structure can be decreased and the child can be challenged to function in a more distracting environment.

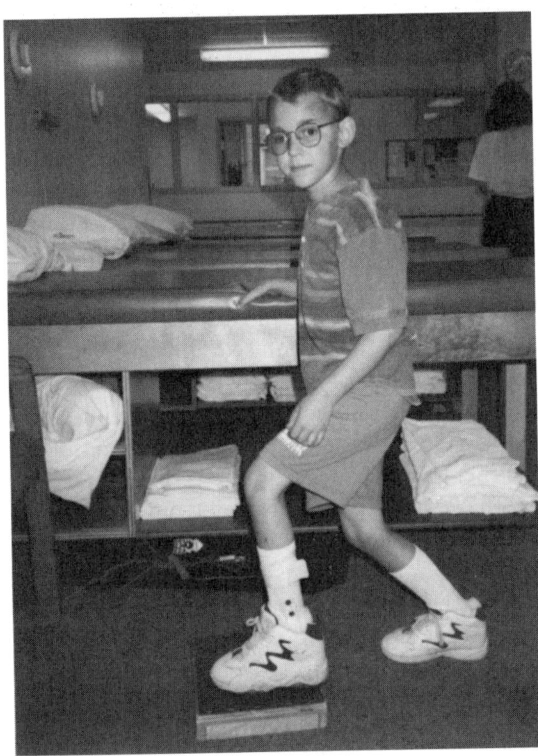

Figure 7-6 ▪ Lunges on the involved lower extremity enhance weight shifts and may help improve hip and knee control.

When the child is confused, it is helpful to work on familiar activities so that the need for verbal instruction is reduced. When giving verbal instruction, the therapist should speak slowly and keep directions simple to allow for delays in processing verbal instructions. In addition, the physical therapist may need to demonstrate new tasks instead of providing the child with verbal explanations to enhance understanding.

Orientation is very important during the confused phase of recovery. The physical therapist should remember to orient the child to his surroundings frequently and establish a familiar routine. The child's routine should allow for the same team members to see the child at the same times of the day in the same places. Thus, the child may begin to work on recall skills and begin to anticipate what is going to happen next in the day. Familiarity and routine are calming and reassuring and may assist with behavior management as well. Items such as a calendar, clock, and a schedule card may assist with orientation in an older child. In addition, the therapist may need to assist the child with topical orientation to his or her surroundings.

Encouraging the child to rely on his or her own memory for sequencing of movement or safety rules will challenge the child to become more independent. The use of a therapy journal or verbal rehearsal may help improve the child's memory. However, the therapist should be careful not to frustrate the child who has difficulty remembering. Instead of a continued open line of questioning, the therapist may offer choices and see if the child can recognize the right response. For example, a child who is learning to transfer from a wheelchair may be asked if he or she is able to scoot forward in the chair or locks the brakes first.

Although new learning is still limited, the physical therapist can begin to integrate principles of motor control and motor learning with principles of neurofacilitation to treat various focal deficits. It is the physical therapist's responsibility to select developmentally appropriate functional skills that are motivating and challenging with the correct spatial and temporal demands for the child's abilities. The physical therapist should also focus on selecting functional activities that incorporate the use of both cognitive and physical skills. For example, an activity involving maneuvering a walker through an obstacle course addresses memory for verbal commands, motor planning, and mobility skills.

An essential element in motor learning is the opportunity for practice. The child with TBI should be allowed to experience movement with assistance as necessary, make mistakes, and make corrections as his or her ability levels dictate. Practice should encourage active participation in a meaningful play activity within the current capabilities of the child. Repeated practice will be necessary for the child to learn new or previously mastered gross motor tasks. The physical therapist will have to determine a practice schedule that is related to the expectations established in the plan of care. The therapist should be aware during practice that children with TBI may display reduced endurance and increased fatigue. The therapist may need to provide rest breaks for the child both within the therapy session and in between therapies.

Determining the type of feedback to be used during therapy is another important consideration in promoting learning. The physical therapist must make choices regarding the timing, precision, and frequency of feedback. In addition, the child's cognitive and sensory function will provide a guideline for determining the appropriate feedback mode. If a child is not aware of one side of his body, kinesthetic feedback may not be helpful to enhance learning while visual and verbal feedback may be more appropriate (Fig. 7-7). Likewise if a child is aphasic, the therapist will need to facilitate learning using visual and kinesthetic information.

As the child with TBI improves, the physical therapist must modify the task and the environment in order to continue to engage the child

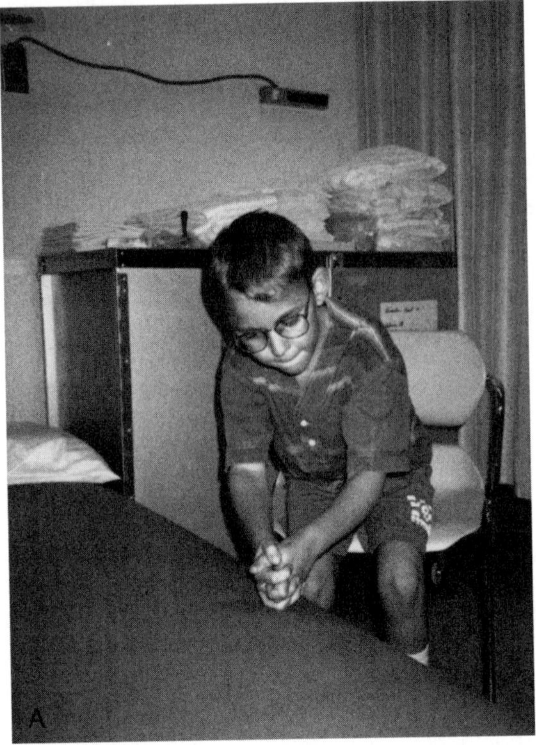

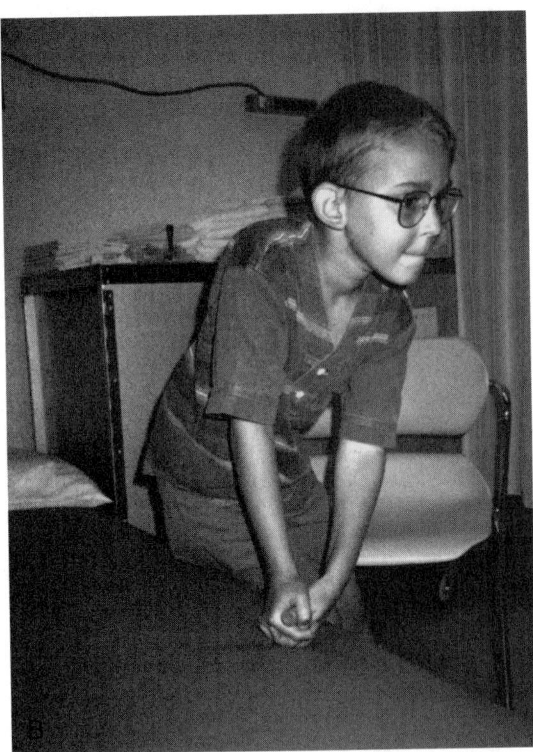

Figure 7-7 ■ (**A**) and (**B**) Verbal cues to use hands in midline during transfers may enhance the awareness of the involved side and improve safety during movement.

actively in therapy. If persistent behavioral problems exist, it may be necessary for the physical therapist to continue to use behavior modification techniques in order to increase compliance in therapy. At this stage of recovery, the child's judgment will be impaired, so it will be important to continue to protect the child from injury.

During both the agitated and the confused phases of recovery, the physical therapist should continue the use of positioning, resting splints, and casting as needed. Dynamic splints and orthotics for standing and gait activities may also assist with the management of spasticity. Tone-reducing ankle-foot orthoses (AFOs) with a footplate that supports the longitudinal as well as the transverse arches have been found to be useful in reducing lower extremity spasticity and in improving gait.[96–98] The disadvantages of braces are that they are more difficult to apply and need to be replaced more frequently than standard AFOs.[57]

Higher Cognitive Level Physical Therapy Management: School/Community Reintegration

It is important for the physical therapist to remember that not all children will reach a high level of cognitive function and have complete physical recovery. Toward the end of the rehabilitation phase, permanent losses of cognitive and physical function become more apparent and plans must be made to reintegrate the child with

TBI back into the home and/or school setting. The family, medical rehabilitation team and the school must work together and jointly plan for reentry into the school setting. The physical therapist may reevaluate the child for orthotics, assistive devices, and mobility devices necessary for function in the child's home and at school. In addition, the physical therapist may assist with recommendations regarding any environmental modifications to the child's home or school.

For the child with TBI who does reach the higher stages of cognitive recovery, the physical therapist will begin to wean the child from the cognitive cues and structure previously used in order to enhance further independence at home and/or school. Owing to the tendency of TBI to affect vision and hearing, memory, concentration, impulse control and organizational skills, the classroom environment may be particularly difficult for the child with TBI.[57] Care should be taken to not remove the structure too early as memory retention and generalization of learning to new settings occurs at slower rates.

The physical therapist should also continue to focus on treating any residual motor deficits that interfere with functional independence at home or in school. For some children, this will mean continued training with assistive devices and physical assistance for basic motor skills, such as transfers and gait (Fig. 7-8 and 7-9). For other children, who may experience only subtle problems with balance and the speed, coordination, timing, and rhythm of movement, it

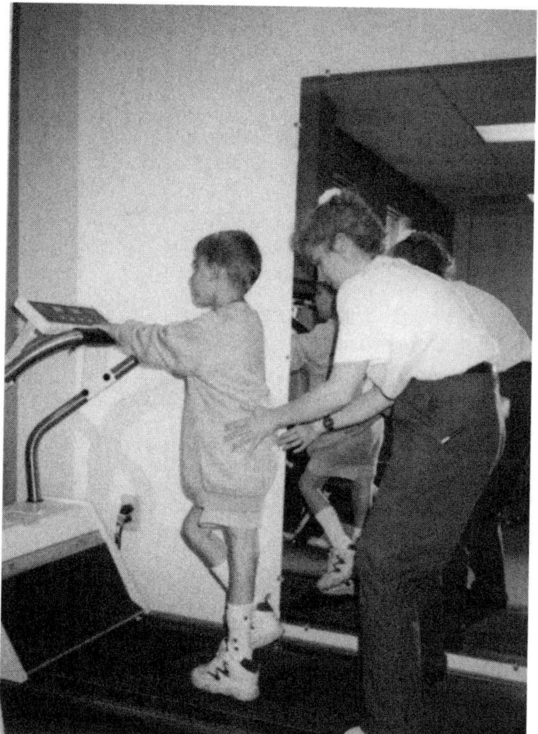

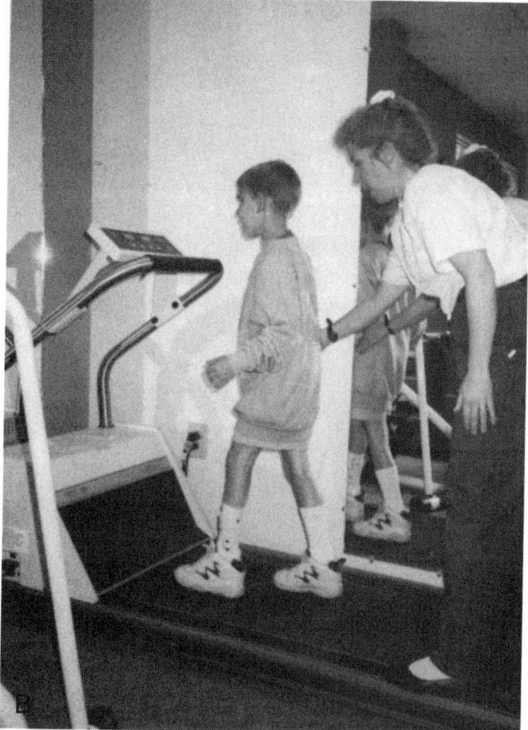

Figure 7-8 ▪ The use of a treadmill in gait training may facilitate control at various speeds. Training may be performed both with (**A**) and without (**B**) upper extremity support to challenge balance on a dynamic surface.

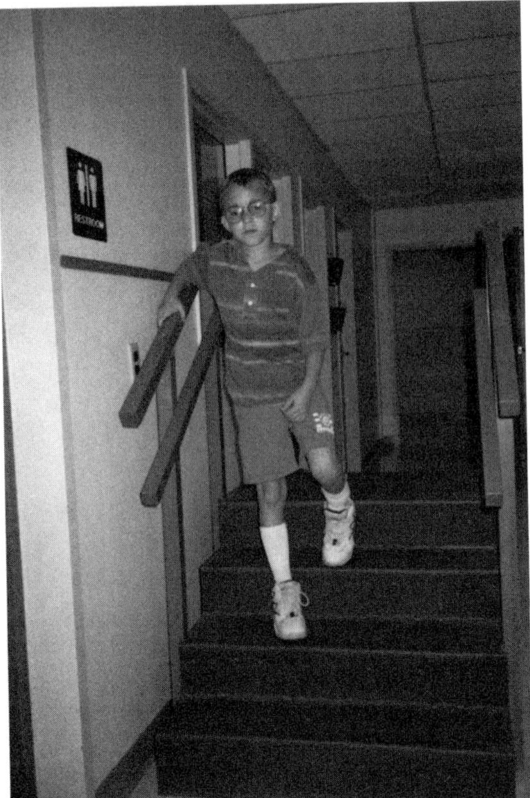

Figure 7-9 ■ In gait training on the stairs, note the increase support at the right forearm and the mild internal rotation of the right hip used to stabilize balance during descent. Verbal cues for trunk alignment and upper extremity support combined with leading with the left lower extremity may improve skill.

will mean participation in more challenging physical activities, such as walking carrying objects, running, jumping, hopping, skipping, or exercise on the (Fig. 7-10 and 7-11) balance board and therapy ball.

In addition to the problems of motor control and function, children who have experienced moderate or severe brain injury often have difficulty maintaining an appropriate level of fitness (Fig. 7-12 and 7-13). The physical therapist should design a fitness program that can be continued after contact with therapy. The physical therapist can work also with the physical education teacher in designing an adapted physical education program for the child with TBI. (Fig. 7-14).

SCHOOL ISSUES

Prior to 1990, the education system had no formal identification or tracking system for children with TBI. With the reauthorization of Public Law 94-142 in Public Law 101-476, the Individuals with Disabilities Education Act, the law now recognizes "brain injury" as a separate category of impairment in children.[57] Programs must be adapted for children with TBI. In addition to modifying the educational services the child receives, it is also reasonable to expect the

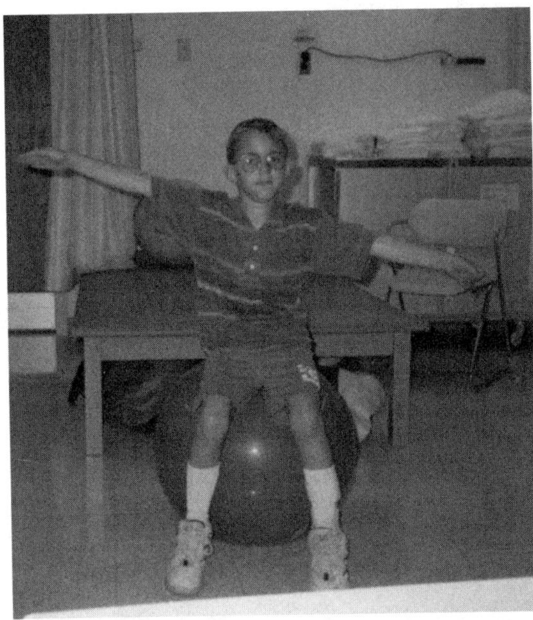

Figure 7-10 ■ The therapy ball can be used to challenge dynamic sitting balance and coordination. In addition to moving his arms to the side, the child could also practice alternating forward placement of his feet or move arms and legs in reciprocal, rhythmic patterns.

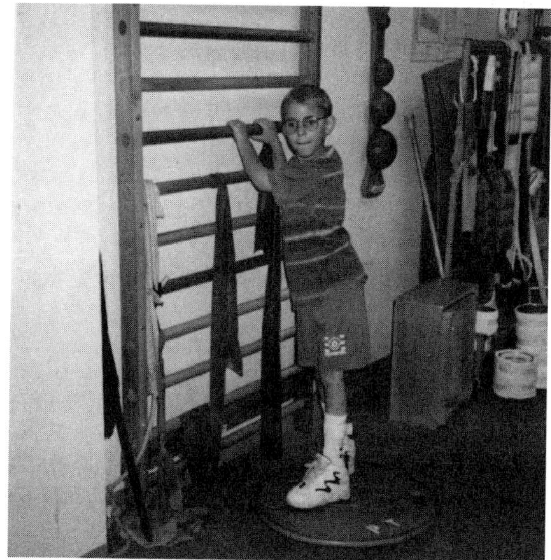

Figure 7-11 ■ A BAPS board can be used to enhance balance and coordination of the lower extremities.

school to provide physical assistance for activities of daily living, mobility, and motoric tasks, such as writing, in order to assist the child with achieving academic success. In turn, rehabilitation specialists, including physical therapists, are being called on to educate and train the existing teaching staff.[57]

Although the child with TBI may perform at a nearly age-appropriate level on achievement tests examining previously learned material, cognitive skills for future academic achievement are frequently impaired.[99] Often, the higher the preinjury IQ, the greater the IQ point loss following TBI.[100] Learning is frequently disrupted by complex information processing demands, distractions, and stress from lack of success.[62] In addition, although some children with TBI may physically appear normal, high social and academic expectations may cause the child to become frustrated and depressed. Without program modification, the child with TBI may develop significant academic and social problems during the preadolescent years.

To assist with the potential for academic success, the child with TBI will need modifications to his or her academic program. In his research, Telzrow has identified 10 educational modifications that can be used to enhance the education of moderately to severely involved children with TBI.[99] These modifications include gradual reintegration into the general classroom; behavioral programming; integration of rehabilitation therapies; low pupil-to-teacher ratios; repetition and multimodality presentation of academic material; cueing and shadowing for vocational training; emphasis on process and not volume

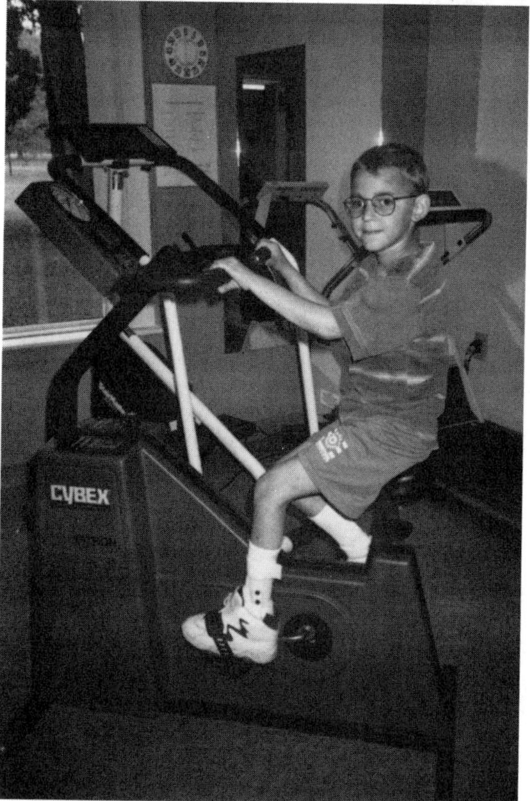

Figure 7-12 ■ Bicycling on standard exercise equipment can be used to promote aerobic exercise. It can also be done as part of training before returning to riding a standard child's bike.

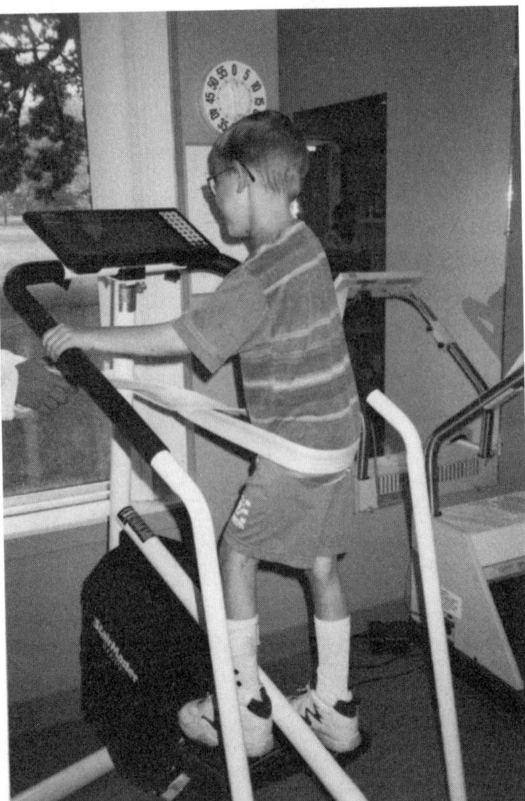

Figure 7-13 ▪ Exercise on standard exercise equipment may not only improve endurance, but it may also help improve strength. The stair stepper improves control in hip extensors and abductors, knee extensors, and ankle plantar-flexors. The strap at the hips provides a cue to maintain hip extension alignment and to increase weight bearing on the more involved side.

of material; simulations for generalization of skills to real life; readjustment counseling; and home–school liaison. In addition to these adaptations, the child with TBI may also benefit from an extended school year and additional tutoring as the prolonged summer vacation may cause some students with TBI to lose headway in academic achievement.[57] A complete discussion of physical therapy in the school system is found in Chapter 15.

Prevention

Prevention is the key to decreasing the annual incidence of TBI. Effective prevention involves decreasing the intensity of the impact to the brain, increasing options for direct prevention, and mandating protective laws.

Bicycle Helmets

The consistent use of bicycle helmets can decrease the incidence of injury as unhelmeted riders are eight times more likely to have a brain injury than helmeted bicyclists.[101] Use of helmets can also potentially prevent brain injuries from occurring in sports and recreational activities including baseball, football, horseback riding, roller blading, skateboarding, hockey, roller skating, skiing, and sledding.[2] Barriers to helmet use include the lack of awareness of recreational risks and the effectiveness of helmets, cost, and negative peer pressure. Increasing the use of helmets may be accomplished by advocating for educational programs, discount coupons, helmet subsidies, role modeling by parents, and mandatory legislative change.

Playground Equipment

Prevention can also be aimed at preventing falls from playground equipment onto unprotected surfaces. The severity of the injuries can be remarkably decreased if the height of equipment does not exceed 5 feet and materials such as sand, pea gravel, or wood chips are used under the playground equipment.[2] Surface materials must be continually maintained if they are to be effective.

Baby Walkers

Walker use in children 6 to 18 months of age is very common in the United States, and parent surveys report that 30% to 40% of children

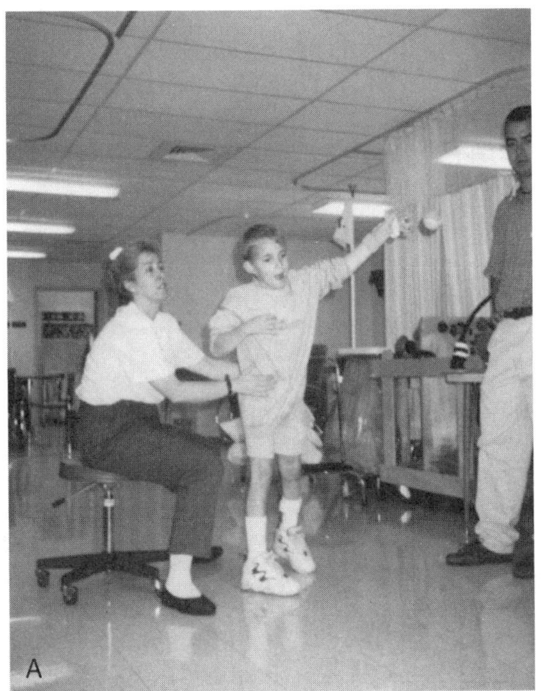

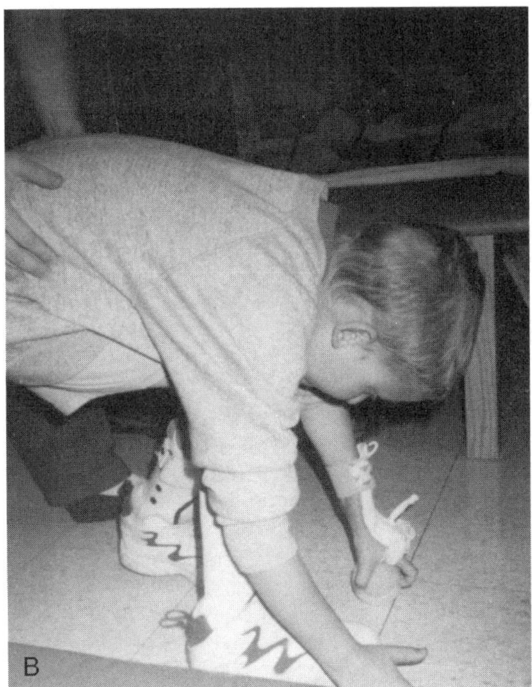

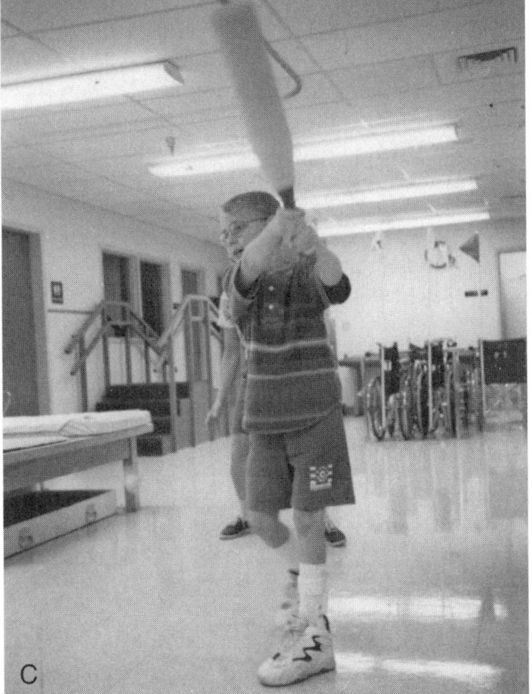

Figure 7-14 A, B, C ▪ Sports can be incorporated into therapeutic activities to enhance coordination, balance, and motor planning. A game of baseball can incorporate gross motor tasks of (**A**) throwing with the involved arm, (**B**) picking up a ground ball, and (**C**) batting.

using walkers experience some form of injury while in a baby walker.[102] It is important for parents to understand that baby walkers do not promote early walking skills. In addition, the physical therapist needs to offer some alternative, such as the use of safety gates or a play pen, that will allow the baby to move safely and freely within the home.

Traffic Behavior

The inability of children under 11 years of age to assess distances and speeds, combined with his normal impulsiveness, results in unsafe traffic behavior.[103] Even after training programs, the majority of young children still exhibit risky behavior and parents should be cautious of chil-

Case Study: Justin

Justin is a 8-year-old boy who experienced a traumatic brain injury secondary to a pedestrian-motor vehicle accident. He was unconscious at the scene of the accident and was life flighted to the nearest pediatric trauma center. On arrival to the ER, he had a Glasgow Coma Score (GCS) of 2 and his pupils were fixed and dilated. Diagnostic studies revealed diffuse right intracranial hemorrhage, a right pneumothorax, fracture of the left orbit, and multiple contusions. An ICP monitor, chest tubes, and placement of a tracheostomy tube were required for acute management.

The brain injury rehabilitation team was consulted 3 days after admission, and Justin was determined to be at a Rancho Los Amigos Scale Level II. A coma stimulation program was implemented by the brain injury team. In addition, the physical therapist initiated an inhibitory casting program to manage his left plantar-flexion posturing, which was measured at 45 degrees. A resting splint was made to maintain the right ankle in a neutral position. Justin slowly emerged from the coma over a period of 2 weeks. Subsequent treatment focused on increasing tolerance to upright on the tilt table, facilitation of head control and sitting balance, and contracture management. During the next 2 weeks Justin's medical condition stabilized and he progressed to a Rancho Los Amigos Scale Level V.

At this time, Justin's tracheostomy was removed and he was transferred to a pediatric rehabilitation center. Inhibitory casting was continued for the left plantar-flexion contracture, which was now measured at 20 degrees. Justin was given a high-back wheelchair with a custom fit modular seating system for mobility. In addition to the previous treatment strategies, Justin also began to work on transfers from supine to sit and from the wheelchair to a mat with moderate assistance. He also engaged in standing activities and gait training. Decreased motor control and hemiplegia on the left was more evident as he increased his activity level. Justin moved in synergistic patterns for both the upper and lower extremity. Strength on the right side of the body was fair. Balance and coordination in upright were poor and he required maximal assistance for standing activities.

As rehabilitation progressed, Justin's condition improved and he began to follow commands consistently and showed some recall of newly learned tasks. At the time of discharge from rehabilitation, Justin was able to propel himself in a regular wheelchair using the right extremities. He was able to transfer from the wheelchair to the mat with supervision and was able to walk short household distances with a forearm crutch on the right. He was still limited in his mobility by the left-sided spasticity. Justin had been evaluated for orthotics and was to receive a left dynamic AFO. Neuropsychological testing was completed prior to discharge and revealed deficiencies in short-term memory, attention span and focus, judgment, and agility to learn new material.

By 4 months after the injury, Justin was transitioning back into his school. His school program was modified for a half-day of inclusion in his regular classroom and a half-day of specialized classroom services. Justin would continue to receive physical therapy through the school setting. He was independent in his transfers and was ambulating with the left forearm crutch and the dynamic AFO more consistently. Justin used the wheelchair only for community mobility.

dren crossing traffic alone. More effective community approaches should focus primarily on decreasing the traffic speed, enforcing laws governing pedestrian-motor vehicle interaction, and separating the pedestrian from the traffic[2] (see Case Study).

Car Restraints

The use of occupant seat belt restraints is clearly an effective strategy for preventing injury if a crash occurs. The placement of the child in the back seat of the car and the correct use of car seats can prevent up to 90% of serious and fatal injuries to children under 5 years of age.[2] Unfortunately, misuse of child seats is still a common problem. In older children and adolescents, the use of lap and shoulder belts can prevent approximately 45% of serious and fatal injuries.[2]

REFERENCES

1. Harrison CL, Dijkers M. Traumatic brain injury registries in the United States: An overview. *Brain Injury.* 1992;6:203–212.
2. Rivara FP. Epidemiology and prevention of pediatric traumatic brain injury. *Pediatr Ann.* 1994;1: 12–17.
3. Eiben CF, Anderson TP, Lockman C, et al. Functional outcome of closed head injury in children and young adults. *Arch Phys Med Rehabil.* 1984;65: 168–170.
4. Rivara FP. Child pedestrian injuries in the United States. *Am J Dis Child.* 1990; 144:692–696.
5. Rivara FP, Mueller BA. The epidemiology and prevention of pediatric head injury. *J Head Trauma Rehabil.* 1986;1:7–15.
6. Tepas JJ, Ramenofsky ML, Barlow B, et al. Mortality in head injury: the pediatric perspective. *J Pediatr Surg.* 1990;58:236–240.
7. Kraus JF, Fife D, Cox P, et al. Incidence, severity, and external causes of pediatric brain injury. *Am J Dis Child.* 1986;140:687–693.
8. Division of Injury Control, Center for Environmental Health and Injury Control, Centers for Disease Control. Childhood injuries in the United States. *Am J Dis Child.* 1990;144:627–646.
9. Waller AE, Baker SP, Szocka A. Childhood injury deaths: National analysis and geographic variation. *Am J Publ Health.* 1989;79:310–315.
10. Rivara FP, Mueller BA. The epidemiology and prevention of pediatric head injury. *J Head Trauma Rehabil.* 1986;1:7–15.
11. Kraus JR, Fife D, Conroy C. Pediatric brain injuries: The nature, clinical course, and early outcomes in a defined United States population. *Pediatrics.* 1987;79:501–507.
12. Bijur P, Golding J, Haslum M, et al. Behavioral predictors of injury in school-age children. *Am J Dis Child.* 1988;142:1307–1312.
13. Davidson LL, Hughes SJ, O'Connor PA. Preschool behavior problems and subsequent risk of injury. 1988;82:644–651.
14. Frankowski RF. Descriptive epidemiologic studies of head injury in the United States, 1974–1984. *Adv Psychosom Med.* 1986;16:153–172.
15. Kraus JF, Rock A, Hemyari P. Brain injuries among infants, children, adolescents and young adults. *Am J Dis Child.* 1990;144:684–691.
16. Chadwick DL, Chin S, Salerno C, et al. Deaths from falls in children: How far is fatal? *J Trauma.* 1991;31:1353–1355.
17. Williams RA. Injuries in infants and small children resulting from witnessed and corroborated free falls. *J Trauma.* 1991;31:1350–1352.
18. Zimmerman RA, Bilaniuk LT. Pediatric head trauma. *Pediatr Neuroradiol.* 1994;4:349–366.
19. Center for Disease Control and Prevention. Factors potentially associated with reductions in alcohol related traffic fatalities, United States, 1990–1991. *MMWR.* 1992;41:213–215.
20. Rivara FP, Gurney JG, Ries RK, et al. A descriptive study of trauma, alcohol and alcoholism in young adults. *J Adolesc Health.* 1992;13:663–667.
21. Rivara FP. Epidemiology of violent deaths in children and adolescents in the United States. *Pediatrician.* 1983–1985;12:3–10.
22. Committee on Accident and Poison Prevention, American Academy of Pediatrics. Firearms. In: McIntire MS, ed. *Injury Control for Children and Youth.* Elk Grove Village, Il: American Academy of Pediatrics; 1987.
23. Wintemute GJ, Sloan JH. Head injury by firearm: epidemiology, clinical course, and options for prevention. *J Head Trauma Rehabil.* 1991;6:38–47.
24. Duhaime AC, Alairo AJ, Lewander J, et al. Head injury in very young children: Mechanisms, injury types, and opthalmologic findings in 100 hospitalized patients younger than 2 years of age. *Pediatrics.* 1992;90:179–185.
25. Billmire ME, Myers PA. Head injury in infants. *Pediatrics.* 1985;75:340.
26. Rivara FP, Kamitsuka MD, Quan L. Injuries to children younger than one year of age. *Pediatrics.* 1988;81:93–97.

27. Bonadio WA, Smith DS, Hillman S. Clinical indicators of intracranial lesion on computed tomographic scan in children with parietal skull fracture. *Am J Dis Child.* 1989;143:194–196.
28. Hahn YS, McLone DG. Risk factors in the outcome of children with minor head injury. *Pediatr Neurosurg.* 1993;19:134–142.
29. Kaufman BA, Dacey RG. Acute care management of closed head injury in childhood. *Pediatr Ann.* 1994;23:18–28.
30. Pang D. Pathophysiologic correlates of neurobehavioral syndromes followed closed head injury. In: Ylviasaker M, ed. *Head Injury Rehabilitation.* Austin, TX: Pro-Ed; 1985:3–70.
31. Griffith ER, Rosenthal M, Bond MR, et al., eds. *Rehabilitation of the Child and Adult with Traumatic Brain Injury.* 2nd Ed. Philadelphia: FA Davis; 1990.
32. Ylvisaker M, ed. *Head Injury Rehabilitation, Children and Adolescents.* San Diego: College Hill Press; 1985.
33. Rosman NP, Herskowitz J, Carter AP, et al. Acute head trauma in infancy and childhood. *Pediatr Clin North Am.* 1979;26:707–736.
34. Marion DW. Pathophysiology and initial neurosurgical care: Future directions. In: Horn LJ, Zasler ND, eds. *Medical Rehabilitation of Traumatic Brain Injury.* Philadelphia: Hanley & Belfus, Inc.; 1996:29–52.
35. Masters SJ. Evaluation of head trauma: Efficacy of skull films. *AJR.* 1980;135:539–547.
36. Phillips WE. Brain tumors, traumatic head injuries, and near-drowning. In: Campbell SK, ed. *Physical Therapy for Children.* Philadelphia, PA: WB Saunders Company; 1994:549–570.
37. Coffey RJ. Pediatric neurological emergencies: In: Pierog JE, Pierog LJ, eds. *Pediatric Critical Illness and Injury: Assessment and Care.* Rockville, MD: Aspen Systems Corporation; 1984:95–106.
38. Mysiw JW, Fugate LP, Clinchot DM. Assessment, early rehabilitation intervention, and tertiary prevention. In: Horn LJ, Zasler ND, eds. *Medical Rehabilitation of Traumatic Brain Injury.* Philadelphia: Hanley & Belfus, Inc.; 1996:53–76.
39. Loftgren J, Awetnow NN. Cranial and spinal components of the cerebrospinal fluid pressure–volume curve. *Acta Neurol Scandinavica.* 1973; 49:575–585.
40. Robertson CS, Contant CF, Narayan RK, et al. Cerebral blood flow, AVD02, and neurologic outcome in head-injured patients. *J Neurotrauma.* 1992;9:S349–S358.
41. Konotos HA. Oxygen radicals in central nervous system damage. *Chem Biol Int.* 1989;72:229–255.
42. Siesjo BJ, Wieloch T. Brain injury: Neurochemical aspects. In: Becker DP, Povlishock J, eds. *Central Nervous System Status Report.* Bethesda, MD: National Institute of Neurological and Communication Disorders and Stroke, National Institutes of Health. 1985;513–532.
43. Fullerton Long D. Diagnosis and management of intracranial complications in TBI rehabilitation. In: Horn LJ, Zasler ND, eds. *Medical Rehabilitation of Traumatic Brain Injury.* Philadelphia: Hanley & Belfus, Inc.; 1996:333–362.
44. Annegers JF, Grabow JD, Broover RV, et al. Seizures after head trauma: a population study. *Neurology.* 1980;30:683–689.
45. Hahn YS, Fuchs S, Flannery AM, et al. Factors influencing posttraumatic seizures in children. *Neuosurgery.* 1988:22:864–867.
46. Desai BT, Whitman S, Coonley-Hoganson R, et al. Seizures and civilian head injuries. *Epilepsia.* 1983;24:289–296.
47. Yablon SA. Posttraumatic seizures. In: Horn LJ, Zasler ND, eds. *Medical Rehabilitation of Traumatic Brain Injury.* Philadelphia: Hanley & Belfus, Inc.; 1996:363–393.
48. Salazar AM, Jabarri B, Vance SC, et al. Epilepsy after penetrating head injury: I. Clinical Correlates. *Neurology.* 1985;35:1406–1414.
49. Blendonohy PM, Philip PA. Precocious puberty in children after traumatic brain injury. *Brain Inj.* 1991;5:63–68.
50. Sockalosky ML, Kriel RL, Krach LE, et al. Precocious puberty after traumatic brain injury. *J Pediatr.* 1987;110:373–377.
51. Teasdale G, Jennett B. Assessment of coma and impaired consciousness: a practical scale. *Lancet.* 1974;2:81–84.
52. Hahn YS, Chyung C, Barthel MJ, et al. Head injuries in children under 36 months of age. *Neurosurgery.* 1988;4:34–39.
53. Reilly PL, Simpson DA, Sprod R, et al. Assessing the conscious level in infants and young children: A pediatric version of the Glasgow Coma Scale. *Childs Nerv Syst.* 1988;4:30–33.
54. Simpson DA, Cockington RA, Hanieh A, et al. Head injuries in infants and young children: The value of the Pediatric Coma Scale. Review of the literature and report on a study. *Childs Nerv Syst.* 1991;7:183–190.
55. Ruijs MB, Keyser A, Gabreels FJM. Assessment of post-traumatic amnesia in young children. *Dev Med Child Neurol.* 1992;34:885–892.
56. Ewing-Cobbs L, Levin HS, Fletcher JM, et al. The Children's Orientation and Amnesia Test: Relationship to severity of acute head injury and

to recovery of memory. *Neurosurgery.* 1990;27: 683–691.

57. Cockrell J. Pediatric brain injury rehabilitation. In: Horn LJ, Zasler ND, eds. *Medical Rehabilitation of Traumatic Brain Injury.* Philadelphia: Hanley & Belfus, Inc.; 1996:171–196.
58. Hagen C, Makmus D, Durham P, et al. Levels of cognitive functioning. In: *Rehabilitation of the Head-Injured Adult: Comprehensive Physical Management.* Downey, CA: Professional Staff of Rancho Los Amigos Hospital; 1979:87–90.
59. Johnston MV, Hall K, Carnevale G, et al. Functional assessment and outcome evaluation in traumatic brain injury rehabilitation. In: Horn LJ, Zasler ND, eds. *Medical Rehabilitation of Traumatic Brain Injury.* Philadelphia: Hanley & Belfus, Inc.; 1996:197–226.
60. Staff from Denver Child's Hospital. Notes from Pediatric Rehab: Traumatic Brain Injury. Denver, CO; 1989.
61. Kriel RL, Krach LE, Sheehan M. Pediatric closed head injury: Outcomes following prolonged unconsciousness. *Arch Phys Med Rehabil.* 1988;69: 678–681.
62. Jaffe KM, Fay GC, Polissar NL, et al. Severity of pediatric traumatic brain injury and neurobehavioral recovery at 1 year—a cohort study. *Arch Phys Med Rehabil.* 1993;74:587–595.
63. Bijur PE, Haslum M, Golding J. Cognitive and behavioral sequelae of mild head injury in children. *Pediatrics.* 1990;86:337–344.
64. MacPherson V, Sullivan SJ, Lambert J. Prediction of motor status 3 and 6 months post severe traumatic brain injury: a preliminary study. *Brain Inj.* 1992;6:489–498.
65. Wilson B, Vizor A, Bryant T. Predicting severity of cognitive impairment after severe head injury. *Brain Inj.* 1991;5:189–197.
66. Brink JD, Imbus C, Woo-Sam J. Physical recovery after severe closed head trauma in children and adolescents. *J Pediatr.* 1980;97:721–727.
67. Rivara FP. Epidemiology and prevention of pediatric traumatic brain injury. *Pediatr Ann.* 1994; 23:12–17.
68. Dikmen SS, Temkin N, Armsden G. Neuropsychological recovery: relationship to psychosocial functioning and postconcussional compliants. In: Levin HS, Eisenberg HM, Benton AL, eds. *Mild Head Injury.* New York: Oxford University Press; 1989.
69. Russell WR. *The Traumatic Amnesias.* Oxford: Oxford University Press; 1971.
70. Finger S. Brain damage, development, and behavior: Early findings. *Dev Neuropsychol.* 1991;7: 261–274.
71. Vargha-Khadem F, O'Gorman AM, Watters GV. Aphasia and handedness in relation to hemispheric side, age at injury and severity of cerebral lesion during childhood. *Brain.* 1985;108:677–696.
72. Thomen IV. Late outcome of severe blunt head trauma. A 10–15 year second follow-up. *J Neurol Neurosurg Psychiatry.* 1984;46:870–875.
73. Berger MS, Pitts LH, Lovely M, et al. Outcome of severe head injury in children and adolescents. *J Neurosurg.* 1985;62:194–199.
74. Rivara JB. Family functioning following pediatric traumatic brain injury. *Pediatr Ann.* 1994;23:38–43.
75. Koch L, Merz MA, Lynch RT. Screening for mild traumatic brain injury: A guide for rehabilitation counselors. *J Rehabil.* 1995;61:50–56.
76. Levin HS, Eisenberg HM. Neuropsychological impairment after closed head injury in children and adolescents. *Childs Brain.* 1979;5:281–292.
77. Sakai CS, Mateer C. Otological and audiological sequelae of closed head injury. *Semin Hear.* 1984; 5:157–173.
78. Griffith JT, Dodge PR. Transient blindness following head injury in children. *N Engl J Med.* 1968; 278:648–651.
79. Harwood-Nash DC. Abuse to the pediatric central nervous system. *Am J Neuroradiol.* 1992;13: 369–375.
80. Buys YM, Levin AV, Enzenauer RW, et al. Retinal findings after head trauma in infants and young children. *Opthalmology.* 1992;99:1718–1723.
81. Hurvitz EA, Mandac BR, Davidoff G, et al. Risk factors for heterotopic ossification in children and adolescents with severe traumatic brain injury. *Arch Phys Med Rehabil.*1992;73:459–462.
82. Djergaian RS. Management of musculoskeletal complications. In: Horn LJ, Zasler ND, eds. *Medical Rehabilitation of Traumatic Brain Injury.* Philadelphia: Hanley & Belfus, Inc.: 1996:459–477.
83. Sobus KML, Alexander MA, Harcke HT. Undetected musculoskeletal trauma in children with traumatic brain injury or spinal cord injury. *Arch Phys Med Rehabil.* 1993;74:902–904.
84. Molnar GE, Perrin JC. Head injury. In: Molnar GE, ed. *Pediatric Rehabilitation.* 2nd Ed. Baltimore: Williams & Wilkins; 1992:254–292.
85. Blasier D, Letts M. The orthopedic manifestations of head injury in children. *Orthop Rev.* 1989;18: 350–358.
86. Braun SL, Granger CV. A practical approach to functional assessment in pediatrics. *Occup Ther Pract.* 1991;2:46–51.
87. Feldman AB, Haley SM, Coryell J. Concurrent and construct validity of the Pediatric Evaluation of Disability Inventory. *Phys Ther.* 1990;70:602–610.

88. Maitz EA, Sachs PR. Treating families of individuals with traumatic brain injury from a family systems perspective. *J Head Trauma Rehabil.* 1995; 10:1–11.
89. Fletcher JM, Miner ME, Ewing-Cobb L. Age and recovery from head injury in children: developmental issues. In: Levin HS, Greyman J, Eisenberg HM, eds. *Neurobehavioral Recovery from Head Injury.* New York: Oxford University Press; 1987.
90. Haley SM, Cioffi MI, Lewin JE, et al. Motor dysfunction in children and adolescents after traumatic brain injury. *J Head Trauma Rehabil.* 1990; 5:77–90.
91. Hall KM, Cope DN. The benefit of rehabilitation in traumatic brain injury: A literature review. *J Head Trauma Rehabil.* 1995;10:1–13.
92. Conine TA, Sullivan T, Mackie T, et al. Effects of serial casting for the prevention of equinus in patients with acute head injury. *Arch Phys Med Rehabil.* 1990;71:310–312.
93. National Head Injury Foundation. Directory of head injury, rehabilitation services. Southborough, MA: 1990.
94. Giles GM. The status of brain injury rehabilitation. *AJOT.* 1994;48:199–205.
95. Sosnowski C, Ustik M. Early intervention: coma stimulation in the intensive care unit. *J Neurosci Nurs.* 1994;26:336–341.
96. Bronkjorst AJ, Lamb GA. An orthosis to aide in reduction of lower limb spasticity. *Orthot Prosthet.* 1987;41:23–28.
97. Hinderer KA, Harris SR, Purdy AH, et al. Effects of "tone-reducing" vs. standard plaster-casts on gait improvement of children with cerebral palsy. *Dev Med Child Neurol.* 1988;30:370–377.
98. Sankey RJ, Anderson DM, Young JA. Characteristics of ankle-foot orthoses for management of the spastic lower limb. *Dev Med Child Neurol.* 1989; 31:466–470.
99. Telzrow CF. Management of academic and educational problems in head injury. *J Learn Disabil.* 1987;20:536–545.
100. Dickerson-Mayes S, Pelco LE, Campbell CJ. Relationships among pre- and post-injury intelligence with severe closed-head injuries. *Brain Inj.* 1989; 3:301–313.
101. Thompson RS, Rivara FP, Thompson DC. A case-control study of the effectiveness of bicycle safety helmets. *N Engl J Med.* 1989:320:1361–1367.
102. Board of Trustees, AMA. Use of infant walkers. *Am J Dis Child.* 1991;145:933–934.
103. Rivara FP. Child pedestrian injuries in the United States. Current status of the problem, potential interventions and future research needs. *Am J Dis Child.* 1990;144:692–696.

Mental Retardation: Focus on Down Syndrome

Dolores B. Bertoti

The physical therapist plays a challenging and important, multifaceted role in the management of children with mental retardation. This challenge is inherent within the clinical presentation of a child with mental retardation who exhibits simultaneous and interactive impairments in the neuromotor, musculoskeletal, developmental, cognitive, and affective domains. The physical therapist must be able to not only accurately assess the child, but must also innovatively develop, implement, modify, and share with parents and other providers of service an accurate plan of care. In this chapter, an approach is offered to assist the entry-level physical therapist with assessment, treatment, and management of the child with mental retardation. The strategy presented is from a functional perspective, delineating the interactive effects of common impairments associated with mental retardation and the role of the physical therapist in managing these impairments to promote maximum best function of the child within his or her environment. Physical therapy management for the child with Down syndrome is outlined as a model strategy.

Historical Review

Society and the population of the mentally retarded have had an intriguing, interesting, and still unfolding interactional history. In the earliest of recorded interactions between the two groups, people with mental retardation were ignored, received little or no care, or were even left to die.[1] Spartan society believed in survival of only the fittest, and many people, including the physically and mentally handicapped, were left to perish.

Conversely, during the Middle Ages and in ancient Rome, it was not uncommon for wealthy people to help a "fool" or "court jester" in return for the amusement these people provided for the household and its guests.[1] Artistic work of the Middle Ages shows people serving as clowns and jesters who depict the physical characteristics of what we now identify as Down syndrome.[2] In the later Middle Ages, particularly in Europe, superstitious beliefs led to the execution of many people who were considered to be "witches and warlocks." People with mental retardation were undoubtedly included in these groups.[1] This idea that people with mental retardation were social menaces persisted throughout the 19th century, with the eventual trend away from execution but still toward punishment, imprisonment, and isolation.[3]

In the early 20th century, there was a publicly perceived need to shelter and protect people with mental retardation from the misunderstanding, abuses, and wrath of society. As a result, people with mental deficiency were isolated in asylums, shelters, and farm communities. These communities, however, rapidly became overcrowded. The goal of this public effort was clearly housing, not the provision of services.

Interest in providing services to assist people with mental retardation had a difficult beginning. In the early 1800s, Jean Marc Itard, A French physician, became intrigued with a mentally retarded youngster whom the physician had captured in the forests of Aveyron in France. Acting on his then-revolutionary premise that intellectual performance could be affected by environmental stimulation, Itard succeeded in teaching this "Wild Boy of Aveyron." Although Itard's work helped the boy improve over a 5-year period, the gains were not sufficient for acceptance of the boy into Parisian society at that time. Society frowned on the child, and Itard believed he had failed.[4]

Johann Jacob Guggenbuhl, in 1840, established a center in Switzerland for a then-innovative approach involving group teaching for children with mental retardation. His work received worldwide acclaim as a major reform. This reform influenced the work in Europe and in the United States of Edouard Sequin, who was a world leader in the development of educational and residential services for people with mental retardation. In 1876, Seguin was made president of the newly formed Association of Medical Officers of the American Institutions for Idiotic and Feeble-Minded Persons. This association later (1876) became the American Association of Mental Deficiency (AAMD),[4] currently called the American Association on Mental Retardation.[5]

In the United States, the social organization accompanying the Industrial Revolution reinforced this concept of group care of children, as well as stimulating a sense of social responsibility.[1] Throughout the 1800s, small gains fluctuated with a sense of frustration and futility, and there was a large-scale movement to house the "incurables" in large, overcrowded facilities in isolated areas.[2]

By the end of World War II, emphasis for care of people with mental retardation evolved to include "programming." This shift to a plan of activity was mainly the result of efforts by the National Association for Retarded Citizens (NARC) and other parent or professional advocacy groups.[2] A growing awareness of the negative effects of residential segregation and the limitations of existing programs led to a critical reappraisal of existing kinds of care available for people with mental retardation. Influenced by the Civil Rights Movement, the 1960s represented a time of expansion in program legislation and funds allocation for all handicapped people. Discrimination against and segregation of people with mental retardation were finally recognized as negative and undesirable.[2]

In the early 1970s, American visitors to Scandinavian countries encountered the concept of "normalization," which was defined as the principle of educating persons with handicaps to the maximum extent feasible within the "normal" environment of the nonhandicapped.[6] This process obviously required major development and use of community support systems. This era became known as the era of "deinstitutionalization." Living arrangements in the community have now become the norm for the long-term care and support of people with mental retardation.[6]

The most current approach to programming in the field of mental retardation is a functional, integrated model. Society as a whole, and therefore, the countless legislatures and service providers of today's society, view mental retardation along a changing paradigm, with a more functional definition and a focus on the interaction between the person, the environment, and the intensities and patterns of needed supports. The term readers will hear most frequently in the 1990s is "support," including needed level of support for maximum function of the individual with mental retardation in the environment.[7]

Definition

Mental retardation refers to substantial limitations in present functioning. It is characterized by significantly subaverage intellectual functioning, existing concurrently with related limitations in two or more of the following applicable adaptive skill areas: communication, self-care, home living, social skills, community use, self-direction, health and safety, functional academics, leisure, and work. Mental retardation manifests before age 18.[7]

This present definition (AAMR, 1992) reflects an important shift in thinking. Mental retardation is not a *trait,* although it is influenced by certain characteristics or capabilities of the individual. Rather, mental retardation is a *state* in which functioning is impaired. This distinction is central to understanding how the present definition broadens the concept of mental retardation and how it shifts the emphasis from measurement of traits to understanding the individual's actual functioning in daily living. For any individual with mental retardation, the description of this state of functioning requires knowledge of the individual's capabilities as well as an understanding of the structure and expectation of the individual's personal and social environment.[7]

Incidence

About 3% of the population of the United States is assumed to have mental retardation, but only 1 to 1.5 percent are actually diagnosed with this condition.[8] In 80 percent of the cases, the cause of the mental retardation is unknown. Mental retardation is four times more prevalent among males than females. Seventy-five percent of all people with mental retardation have a mild form, 20% a moderate form, and 5% have a severe or profound form.[9] One of the most prevalent forms of mental retardation is Down syndrome, with an incidence of one in 700 live births.[9]

Diagnosis

A diagnosis of mental retardation is based on the criteria embodied within the definition reflecting intellectual functioning level and adaptive skill level.

Assessment of Intellectual Functioning

The determination that a child's intellectual functioning is significantly below average is arrived at through the administration of a standardized intelligence test, usually administered by a psychologist. Fulfillment of this criterion for diagnosis of mental retardation is made on the basis of an IQ of 70 or 75 or below.[7] The instruments most commonly used for the assessment of intellectual functioning in children are the Stanford-Binet Intelligence Scale;[10] one of the Wechsler Scales, such as Wechsler Intelligence Scale for Children-III[11] or Wechsler Preschool and Primary Scale of Intelligence;[12] and the Kaufman Assessment Battery for Children.[13] These tests are usually administered by a psychologist.

Assessment of Adaptive Skill Level

Adaptive skills are those skills considered to be central to successful life functioning and are frequently related to the need for supports for persons with mental retardation. The 10 areas specifically listed in the current AAMR definition are communication, self-care, home living, social skills, community use, self-direction, health and safety, functional academics, leisure, and work. In order to fulfill the diagnostic criteria for mental retardation, deficits in two or more areas of adaptive functioning must be present, thus showing a generalized limitation in adaptive skill level.[7]

For many years, the Vineland Social Maturity Scale served as the standard measure for adaptive behavior.[14] A variety of tools are now available, including the Vineland Scale, as well as The AAMD Adaptive Behavior Scales (ABS),[15] the School Edition of the ABS,[16] the revised Vineland Adaptive Behavior Scales,[17] and the Comprehensive Test of Adaptive Behavior.[18]

Table 8-1 describes the general adaptive behavior characteristics of children and adults with different levels of mental retardation.[19]

Classification

In keeping with contemporary views of disablement,[20,21] the key elements in the 1992 AAMR definition of mental retardation are *capabilities*, *environment*, and *function*. The previously used terms of mildly, moderately, severely, or profoundly mentally retarded are no longer used. This classification language was in use until 1992 and was closely correlated with IQ scores.[22,23] Current classification carries with it an application of the new diagnostic criteria directly correlated to need for support. Needed supports will vary along a number of dimensions: First, support may be necessary in some areas of adaptive skills but not in others; second, support requirements may be time-limited or ongoing; and third, the intensities of the supports

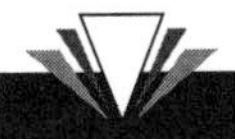

TABLE 8-1
Adaptive Behavior Characteristics of Persons with Mental Retardation

IQ	Age of the Person with Mental Retardation: Preschool	School-aged	Adult
50–55 to 70	Often appears normal; develops social and communication skill	Academic skills of 6th grade are possible; special education needs for secondary school	Can learn social and vocational skills
35–40 to 50–55	Poor social skills; can communicate; may need supervision	Can develop up to 4th grade skills with special training	Unskilled or semiskilled vocation
20–25 to 35–40	Lacks communication; poor motor skills	May learn to communicate; basic personal health habits; no academic skills	Needs complete supervision for any self-support activity
<20–25	Dependent for care; poor sensorimotor development	Some motor development; continues to be dependent for care; limited success with training	Limited motor ability and communication; continued dependency for care

Adapted from Sloan W, Birch JW. A rationale for degrees of retardation. *Am J Ment Defic.* 1955;60:262.

required, the types of support resources, and the support functions will be specific to the individual and the life cycle. There are basically four intensities of support: intermittent, limited, extensive, and pervasive. Support services may come to the child with mental retardation from four sources: the individual child (e.g., ability to make choices), other people (e.g., parent, teacher), technology (e.g., assistive devices), or habilitation services (e.g., PT, OT, Speech Therapy).[7]

Educational Classification

The original but more familiar educational classification system, first defined by Scheerenberger in 1964, is rarely used as a sole classification system.[22] Terms such as educable, trainable, and dependent are considered to be out of date but may still be seen in some educational placement descriptions. Current special education practices are shaped by both the definition of mental retardation and the need for supports. Contemporary educational placement terms follow a more functional approach, highlighting the need for support and thereby being descriptive of the child's needs for educational success. This descriptive terminology for educational support includes:

- Academic support or gifted support
- Learning support
- Life skills support
- Emotional support
- Sensory and communication support
- Visually impaired support
- Speech and language support
- Physical support
- Multiple disabilities support[23]

Physical therapy in the educational setting is detailed in Chapter 15 of this text.

Medical Classification

Medical classification, according to the Diagnostic and Statistical Manual of Mental Disorders, 4th ed. (DSM-IV),[24] uses a classification based on the degree of severity of intellectual impairment as follows:

DSM-IV Diagnoses and Codes

317	Mild Mental Retardation IQ level 50–55 to approximately 70
318.0	Moderate Mental Retardation IQ level 35–40 to 50–55
318.1	Severe Mental Retardation IQ level 20–25 to 35–40
318.2	Profound Mental Retardation IQ level below 20 or 25
319	Mental Retardation, Severity Unspecified

Etiology and Pathophysiology

Over 350 etiologies for mental retardation have been identified.[25,26] These can be broadly categorized into prenatal, perinatal, and postnatal causes. Etiologic causes with examples are depicted in Display 8-1. Movement disorders are associated with some etiologies more than others. Many children also present with a variety of associated disorders such as visual, hearing, or additional medical problems.

DISPLAY 8-1

Etiological Classification of Mental Retardation[7,25]

Prenatal Onset	Examples
1. Chromosomal disorder	Down, Turner, or Klinefelter syndrome
2. Syndrome disorders	Neurofibromatosis, myotonic muscular dystrophy, Prader-Willi, tuberous sclerosis
3. Inborn errors of metabolism	Phenylketonuria, carbohydrate disorders, mucopolysaccharide disorders (e.g., Hurler type) nucleic acid disorders (e.g., Lesch-Nyhan syndrome)
4. Developmental disorders of brain formation	Neural tube closure defects (e.g., anencephaly) hydrocephalus, porencephaly, microcephaly
5. Environmental influences	Intrauterine malnutrition, drugs, toxins, alcohol, narcotics, maternal diseases
Perinatal Causes	
6. Intrauterine disorders	Placental insufficiency, maternal sepsis, abnormal labor or delivery
7. Neonatal disorders	Intracranial hemorrhage, periventricular leukomalacia, seizures, infections, respiratory disorders, head trauma, metabolic disorders
Postnatal Causes	
8. Head injuries	Intracranial hemorrhage, contusion, concussion
9. Infections	Encephalitis, meningitis, viral infections
10. Demyelinating disorders	Postinfectious and postimmunization disorders
11. Degenerative disorders	Syndromic disorders (e.g., Rett syndrome), poliodystrophies (e.g., Friedreich ataxia), basal ganglia disorders, leukodystrophies
12. Seizure disorders	Infantile spasms, myoclonic epilepsy
13. Toxic-metabolic disorders	Reye syndrome, lead intoxication, metabolic disorders (e.g., hypoglycemia)
14. Malnutrition	Protein-calorie, prolonged IV alimentation
15. Environmental deprivation	Psychosocial disadvantage, child abuse/neglect

Primary Impairments

Neuromotor Impairments

Many types of mental retardation have associated neuromuscular, musculoskeletal, and cardiopulmonary impairments. Display 8-2 details the most common mental retardation conditions and their associated neuromotor impairments.[27–42] Most neuromuscular impairments are present as a result of primary pathology in the central nervous system (CNS). Secondary impairments then include deficits typically of concern to the physical therapist such as deficits in motor control, coordination, postural control, force production, flexibility, and balance.[43] Physical therapy assessment and treatment of these impairments for children with mental retardation are similar to those procedures used in any pediatric setting. Use of Display 8-2 can guide the pediatric physical therapist in anticipating typical management concerns associated with common mental retardation disorders. The mental retardation itself, viewed as an additional or confounding coimpairment, requires some adaptation in evaluation and treatment application because of the specific cognitive limitations presented by the child.

DISPLAY 8-2

Neuromuscular, Musculoskeletal, and Cardiopulmonary Impairments Associated with Selected Conditions of Mental Retardation

Condition	Neuromuscular	Musculoskeletal	Cardiopulmonary
Cri-du-chat syndrome[27]	Hypotonia in early childhood, sometimes later hypertonia	Minor upper extremity anomalies, scoliosis	Congenital heart disease is common
Cytomegalovirus[28] (prenatal infection)	Hypertonia, seizures microcephaly	Secondary to neuromuscular problems	Mitral stenosis, pulmonary valvular stenosis, atrial septal defect
de Lange syndrome[29,30]	Spasticity, seizures, intention tremor, microcephaly	Decreased bone age, small stature, small hands and feet, short digits, proximal thumb placement, clinodactyly 5th digit, other hand and finger defects, limited elbow extension	Neonatal respiratory problems, cardiac malformations, recurrent upper respiratory tract infections
Down syndrome[31,32]	Hypotonia, low muscle force production, slow postural reactions, slow reaction time, motor delays increase with age	Joint hyperflexibility, ligamentous laxity, foot deformities, scoliosis, atlantoaxial instability (20%)	Congenital heart disease (40%), lung hypoplasia, with pulmonary hypertension
Fetal Alcohol syndrome[30,33]	Fine motor dysfunction, visual motor deficits, weak grasp, ptosis	Joint anomalies with abnormal position or function, maxillary hypoplasia	Heart murmur—often disappears after 1st year

(*continued*)

DISPLAY 8-2

Neuromuscular, Musculoskeletal, and Cardiopulmonary Impairments Associated with Selected Conditions of Mental Retardation (Continued)

Condition	Neuromuscular	Musculoskeletal	Cardiopulmonary
Fragile X syndrome[34,35]	Hypotonia, poor coordination and motor planning, seizures	Hyperextensible finger joints, prominent jaw, scoliosis	Mitral valve prolapse
Hurler syndrome[26,30]	Hydrocephalus	Joint contractures, claw-like deformities of hands, short fingers, thoracolumbar kyphosis, shallow acetabular and glenoid fossae, irregularly shaped bones	Cardiac deformities, such as cardiac enlargement owing to right ventricular hypertension, death frequently owing to cardiac failure
Lesch-Nyhan syndrome[36]	Hypotonia followed by spasticity, chorea, and athetosis/dystonia, compulsive self-injurious behavior	Secondary to neuromuscular problems	
Prader-Willi syndrome[37,38]	Severe hypotonia and feeding problems in infancy, excessive eating and obesity in childhood, poor fine and gross motor coordination	Short stature, small hands and feet	May be associated with cor pulmonale (most common cause of death)
Rett syndrome[39–42]	Hypotonia in infancy, then gradually increasing hypertonia and lack of acquired skills, ataxia, apraxia, choreoathetosis and/or dystonia, progression from hyperkinesia to bradykinesia with age, slow reaction time, stereotypical hand movements (clapping, wringing, clenching), drooling, involuntary rhythmic tongue movement/deviation, seizures	Scoliosis, kyphosis, joint contractures, hip subluxation or dislocation, equinovarus deformities	Immature respiratory patterns, breathing irregularities, such as hyperventilation, apnea
Williams syndrome[30,33] (elfin facies)	Mild neurologic dysfunction, poor motor coordination	Hallux valgus	Variable congenital heart disease

Adapted with permission from McEwen I. Mental retardation. In: Campbell SK. *Physical Therapy for Children.* Philadelphia: WB Saunders; 1994.

Learning Impairment

Learning is impaired in children with mental retardation. Children with mental retardation demonstrate an impaired ability to handle advanced cognitive processes, simultaneous demands, and organization of information, with subsequent effects on task performance as well as task mastery.[44] Physical therapists must be able to adapt evaluation and treatment approaches to accommodate the coimpairment of deficient intellectual functioning. Clearly, the range of cognitive deficit and ability found in children with mental retardation is indicative of variant levels of performance, functioning, and potential.[45] It is the task and the challenge of the therapist to assist the child to maximize his or her potential for optimum functioning across environments.

Assessment of Physical Therapy Intervention

Key Elements of Assessment

A successful and effective physical therapy assessment of the child with mental retardation depends largely on the therapist's approach to the child. Four important elements should facilitate the process of assessment.

First, throughout the assessment, the therapist must analyze not only what the child can do but also the *processes underlying the observed skills and behaviors.*[46] Thus, the therapist must determine not only what tasks the child can do but also why the child can do those specific tasks and not others. Movements must be broken down into components, and basic mental, physiologic, and physical processes must be analyzed in relation to those tasks.

Second, evaluative procedures used for children, particularly mentally retarded children, often differ from the more rigid clinical procedures used for adults. As in all of pediatrics, much information can be gathered by interacting with the child through observation and during play. Standard evaluative tests and procedures may be used as rapport is established, depending on the functional level of the child. Owing to the attention deficits and associated problems of the mentally retarded child, the evaluation should be done serially, and should be ongoing. Consistent with the functional approach to curriculum planning, the physical therapist should perform an evaluation with as many *functional aspects,* using age-appropriate materials, as is reasonable.

The third important element necessary for an appropriate evaluation is related to the basic orientation of the therapist. As with other areas of physical therapy, but more importantly with the multiply handicapped child, the therapist must be able to identify not only the disability but also the child's abilities, however minimal. The skilled therapist will identify even the smallest of abilities and effectively communicate the importance of those abilities to the child, parents, and other professionals working with the child. A major focus of treatment involves attempts to increase those abilities. This *"positive" orientation and approach* will have a beneficial effect on the child's self-image and on those people working with the child.[47] If our actions suggest a true concern and expectation for progress, however limited that progress may be, the effect of this attitude should encourage the child, the teachers, and the family to strive toward goals that have been identified.[47]

The fourth important element in evaluation is that the therapist must always concurrently assess *sensory processes and attention.* Children experience their world through sensory (afferent) pathways and the feedback received from sensory input. They assimilate the information; they take action; and they consequently modify subsequent actions. Because the sensory or receptive abilities must be intact for normal movement to occur, the therapist must include assessment of the sensory systems as a major component in the overall evaluation of the child.[46] The therapist must understand by what means—or even whether—the child is perceiving the world, including you, the evaluator, before continuing with the evaluation.

Sensory Assessment and Treatment

The therapist must determine the basic responsiveness of the child before deciding on an appropriate interaction strategy for the rest of the evaluation. Kinnealy distinguished two broad categories of children with mental retardation on the basis of their reactions to various sensory stimuli.[48] She described one group as having difficulty monitoring the intensity of sensory input and, therefore, difficulty in modulating the response. The other group was described as having reduced perception of the incoming stimuli. This group required more intense input for arousal or elicitation of a response. This initial difference in perception of sensory stimulus is a critical point of departure that the therapist must ascertain during the first attempt at interaction with the child.

VISUAL

When assessing the child's visual sense, the therapist should note the ability of the child to orient to, focus on, and track a visual stimulus. A flashlight, or some other illumination, or a brightly colored, patterned toy should be placed approximately 7 to 15 inches from the child's face for this assessment.[49] This range of distance affords optimal visual clarity in early development. Getman and associates have suggested that horizontal tracking is easier than vertical tracking, and that diagonal tracking is the most difficult.[50] Notable responses include difficulty in tracking across the midline and resting eye movements (nystagmus). The term *cortical blindness* describes an inability to interpret visual information owing to severe brain damage or occipital lobe atrophy.

During treatment, visual stimulation activities can be used to provide practice in both focusing and tracking. Children who have poor head control may have an inadequate base of support for eye movements. Treatment aimed at improving postural mechanisms may improve visual skill.[46] Adaptive aids to ensure proper body positioning should be used as needed. Vestibular input may also improve visual focusing and processing because vestibular reflexes, in combination with optic and tonic neck reflexes, maintain a stable image on the retina while the head and body are in motion.[46] The vestibulo-oculomotor pathways contribute to skilled movements of the eyes that can be used for educational skills, including reading and writing.[51]

AUDITORY

The child's response to auditory stimuli may range from an absence of response, to simple orientation to and movement toward the stimulus, to a startle response.[46] Although it is difficult to assess hearing loss in a child with mental retardation or multiple handicaps, referral for a complete audiologic evaluation is indicated when- ever there is a possibility of a hearing loss. Audiologic testing can be used to identify a hearing loss, to differentiate between conductive and sensorineural loss, and to quantify the degree of loss. Tympanometry (an objective measure of eardrum function) helps identify a conductive loss when behavioral testing is unreliable. Testing for brain stem–evoked response traces the passage of an auditory stimulus from the ear to the brain stem. Central or cortical deafness describes a lack of interpretation of auditory information owing to brain damage.

Vestibular stimulation is a component of treatment aimed at enhancing auditory integration. Although the vestibulocochlear nerve (cranial nerve VIII) has been described as comprising two separate entities (vestibular and auditory), it developed phylogenetically as a unit, and its portions appear to be related functionally.[46] There is clear clinical evidence that difficulties in hearing interfere with equilibrium responses. Vestibular input may not only improve equilibrium reactions but may also sometimes enhance auditory attention and integration.[52]

TACTILE

The tactile system is the largest sensory system, and it plays a major role in both physical and emotional behavior.[53] The tactile system develops earliest in utero, and the ability to process tactile input is important for neural organization.

As early as 1920, Head described two cutaneous systems: the "protopathic" and the "epicritic" systems.[54] The primitive protopathic system was described as protective, causing a person to react to tactile stimuli with increased affect and alertness.[54] The protopathic system may be synonymous with the spinothalamic system described by Poggin and Mountcastle.[55] The epicritic system was described as having a more discriminative function, and is synonymous with the described lemniscal system.[55] This epicritic system allows a person to respond to light touch with a well-localized sensation. The dualism of these systems may actually be more of an intermingling of the two, or portions of a continuum, rather than a strict dichotomy. Normal neural organization is likely characterized by a continuous gradient of functional organization of the two paths.[56] The systems are normally in balance. When threatened, there is a predominant response of increased alertness and increased affect. When not challenged, however, the person is free to explore and manipulate the environment.[57]

Many children with brain damage show an imbalance between the two pathways. With neurologic impairment, many children show an aversive response to some types of tactile stimulation. This aversion to tactile stimuli, called *tactile defensiveness,* is often manifested by such behavior as hyperactivity or distractibility.[56] Children who show tactile defensiveness may display avoidance reactions around the hands, feet, and face. This behavior has obvious implications for the manner in which a child explores the environment, appreciates tactile sensation, and thus learns. Tactile defensiveness in the oral area may cause the child to reject textured or flavored food in preference to smoother, blander foods.

Although no data are available to support the idea, some professionals suggest that tactile defensiveness is part of a generalized "set" of the nervous system by which the child interprets stimuli as "danger."[56] Tactile functions were among the first means by which the child received information about his or her environment in order to adapt appropriately. The result of neurodevelopmental disorders is often behavior that appears to be less completely evolved and less discriminatory than normal. Tactile defensiveness or overresponsiveness may be seen in this context as poorly developed mechanisms for the interpretation of information. Clinically, the child may appear anxious, emotionally labile, or threatened and unable to cope. Compensatory behavior may be characterized by withdrawal, irritability, or distractibility.[56]

Ayres has suggested various treatment regimens designed to alter the balance of the two systems in favor of increased discrimination. The postulate on which treatment is based is that certain types of sensory input will normalize the neural process and will elicit a protective response. This response will promote a balance between the protective and discriminative aspects of the total system. The sensory input that appears to be particularly effective in influencing the modulating mechanism operates through the tactile system. The proprioceptive system serves a cooperative role in this functional scheme.[56]

The physical therapist can easily incorporate into treatment, appropriate activities for both the tactile and proprioceptive systems. Heavy touch and pressure or weight bearing are excellent activities for decreasing tactile hypersensitivity and promoting proximal joint stability. Light touch or stimuli that tickle or irritate the child should be avoided in favor of activities that offer deep pressure.

The response of the child with mental retardation to tactile input must be observed and monitored during evaluation and treatment. The therapist must note whether the child responds to the stimulus (i.e., the touch of the therapist's hand), and if a response is noted, the therapist must identify the type of response. If the input is noxious, does the child respond with a grimace, or does the child move actively to avoid the stimulus? One might surmise that the child who actively removes or withdraws from the noxious stimulus is not only aware of the stimulus but also has some proprioceptive sense by which to locate and remove the stimulus. Conversely, the therapist must be aware of the child who is so totally unaware of sensory input that the therapist is unable to penetrate and reach the child by any means. Clearly, knowing the level of awareness of the child will direct the therapist through subsequent stages of the evaluation process.[46]

VESTIBULAR

Along with the tactile system, the vestibular system is one of the earliest developing sensory systems in the human being. The tracts within the vestibular system are fully myelinated by 20 weeks of gestation.[56] Information from the vestibular system tells us our position exactly in relation to gravity, whether or not we are moving, and our speed and direction of movement.[53] Semicircular canals within the inner ear are the vestibular receptors that provide dynamic information regarding angular acceleration around the body's axis. The utricles are receptors that provide static information concerning the position of the body in relation to gravity.[58] The vestibular system is so sensitive that changes in position and movement have a powerful effect on the brain, and this effect changes with even the most subtle adjustments of movement or posture.[56]

Vestibular sensations are produced mainly within the vestibular nuclei and the cerebellum.[56] Stimuli are sent caudally in the spinal cord and into the brain stem, where they serve a powerful integrative function. Some stimuli are also sent rostrally from the brain stem to the cerebral hemispheres.[53]

The vestibular system has a strong effect on muscle tone and movement. This influence is mediated through the lateral and medial vestibular nuclei and affects efferent transmission down the spinal cord. Vestibular influence usually exerts a facilitatory effect on the gamma motoneuron to the muscle spindle and may influence the alpha motoneurons supplying skeletal muscle. By activating the gamma efferent to the muscle spindle, the afferent flow from the spindle is maintained and regulated for assistance with motor function. This basic role in muscle function and mobility gives the vestibular system an important role in the development and maintenance of body scheme that depends on interpretation of movement.[56] Impulses ascending to higher brain stem and cortical levels synapse with tactile, proprioceptive, visual, and auditory impulses to provide both perception of space and orientation of the body within that space.[53] Vestibular input seldom enters conscious thought or awareness except when the stimulus is so intense that we are rendered dizzy.

Vestibular function can be assessed clinically by noting the presence of and duration of nystagmus after vestibular stimulation, such as spinning. Nystagmus is a slow movement of the eyes in one direction, followed by a rapid movement in the opposite direction.[46,59] It is important to know whether the child overreacts to or is threatened by movement, or has difficulty in attending to and assimilating movement experiences.

The physical therapist may choose to include various movement or vestibular activities in a child's program with the hope of achieving several goals. With a knowledge of the child's response to vestibular stimulation, activities can be chosen to improve balance, simulate experience of movement, influence muscle tone (specifically, antigravity extensors), promote awareness and eye contact, and increase spatial awareness and perception. Examples of equipment used in these movement activities include swings, barrels, and scooter boards.

SELF-STIMULATION

Self-stimulation in some children with mental retardation is an area of concern. This type of behavior can take many forms, including self-abuse. Examples of self-stimulation include constant mouthing of objects or the hand, spinning, head banging, hand or arm flapping, teeth grinding, rocking, and self-biting. Evaluation of the sensory status of the child may identify the reason for self-stimulation. The child may be performing self-stimulation to fulfill a basic sensory need, or he or she may be overstimulated and may be reacting out of frustration or an inability to cope with sensory overload.[46]

In educational programs, the tendency is to discourage self-stimulation, especially when the stimulation is abusive or socially unacceptable. An appropriate sensory input must be substituted or the child may substitute another form of self-stimulation. A child who cannot cope with the sensory stimuli in the environment and is being overstimulated needs to have sensory input graded to tolerance.[46] As in all other areas of evaluation and treatment, the therapist must look beyond the behavior to the processes that are initiating it. Underlying sensory abnormalities or deficiencies must be recognized and treated before a change in behavior can be expected.[60]

The manner in which the child provides self-stimulation can suggest strategies that may be effective in improving or eliminating the behavior. Slow, rhythmic rocking may be the distractible child's method of calming himself or herself, whereas violent, irregular rocking may be the hypotonic child's method of providing sensory input that will increase muscle tone and alertness. The type of behavior must also be considered in light of the developmental age of the child. Constant mouthing of objects and hands is socially unacceptable for a school-aged child. If, however, that child is functioning at a lower developmental and functional level than age would dictate, oral exploration is a primary component of the learning process.[46] Rather than restricting such oral exploration and stimulation, the child must be provided means of oral stimulation, such as tooth brushing, and foods of various textures, in order to help facilitate progression to the next developmental and functional level.

To summarize, the physical therapist assessing the child with mental retardation must have various skills and must approach the evaluation with a flexible but organized strategy. Assessment must include not only developmental testing, functional assessment, goniometrics, posture, and strength but also a complete evaluation of the sensory systems. Because the main goal of treatment is to enhance basic developmental processes and to improve function, there must be a thorough examination of all sensory and motor components of development. It is challenging and rewarding to evaluate such a complex group of skill areas and still have a concise picture of the whole child.

Key Elements of Physical Therapy Intervention

General Principles

Treatment and management of the child with mental retardation must be directed toward the development of the child's full potential in all areas of learning: motor, cognitive, and affective. The child's ability to respond appropriately and effectively in terms of movement, intellectual function, and attitudes and feelings serves as the major long-range goal of treatment. This concept of treatment applies to the total function of the child. A deficit in one type of behavior may influence all other types. The child who needs motor stability may also benefit from psychological stability. Influences used to change the former may also have an effect on the latter and vice versa.[47] Although the physical therapy setting is structured to provide mainly for the acquisition of motor skills, the environment should facilitate development in all areas of behavior.

There are several important elements to remember when designing effective treatment programs for children with mental retardation. The therapist must recognize the importance of choosing activities that accommodate the mental age of the child but that are also as age-appropriate as possible. Display 8-3 offers several examples of how purely developmental activities can be translated into functional activities.

Activities in the treatment program should be interesting, fun, and meaningful. Because children with mental retardation often have a poor attention span, therapeutic activities should be chosen that most effectively and efficiently meet the identified goal. Rather than asking a child to do a standard exercise regimen for strengthening, the necessary therapeutic activities can be translated into a functional task or social game. This approach not only sustains interest, cooperation, and enthusiasm, but it emphasizes carryover into activities of daily living. It may also promote achievement of goals in other areas, such as social, emotional, self-help, and cognitive skills. The therapist must be imaginative and should integrate many different

DISPLAY 8-3

Examples of Functional Activities that Incorporate Developmental Skills

Assessment Item	Underlying Skill	Examples of Alternative Materials/Activities
Walks on balance beam	Balance	Walking on bleachers, walking between rows of chairs
Holds rattle for 5–10 seconds	Can hold an object for 5–10 seconds	Cup, spoon, book, hairbrush, coin, pencil and ball
Stacks 3 wooden blocks	Perceptual-motor coordination of stacking	Glasses, bowls, dishes, trays, records, and cassette tapes
Strings 3 1-inch beads	Perceptual-motor coordination of inserting and pushing/pulling through	Lace shoes
Places peg in pegboard	Eye-hand (or hand-hand) coordination of placing an object in another object	Straw in milk carton, sock in shoe, toast in toaster, coin in vending machine slot, key in lock, pencil in sharpener
Picks up raisin with pincer grasp	Uses pincer grasp to pick up items	Food, table game pieces, coins, pages of book, vocational items (nails, hooks)
Anticipates being picked up	Anticipates routine event	Being fed, bathed, tickled, greeted, and being put to bed

From Downing J, Bailey B. Presented at the TASH Annual Conference; December 9, 1988; Washington, DC.

approaches in order to develop an effective treatment approach for a particular child in a particular situation.

Repetition and consistency are crucial aspects of any treatment plan in which learning is expected to occur. Because repetition is important for learning any task, the therapist must design several activities that teach the same component task but do so in different ways. For example, if the treatment goal is to improve extension of the trunk, the therapist may use activities such as a basketball drop or scooterboard games. These activities are varied but enjoyable methods of attaining the same goal. This approach to treatment planning ensures not only the necessary repetition of activities, but also offers the dimensions of interest and fun for a child with limited comprehension or attention.

One of the most important yet most difficult skills for the therapist to master is the ability to delineate priorities for treatment and to establish effective and appropriate long-term plans. When the therapist is faced with the challenge of a child with numerous deficits in many areas of development, it is easy for the therapist to become overwhelmed. When developing treatment plans, it is important to consider the child as a whole person. All pieces of the evaluation puzzle should merge to provide the therapist with a composite picture of how the child is or is not functioning within the child's world. The priorities for treatment should become clear by looking at the child's overall development in this functional sense.

Learning Characteristics

Differences in the Child with Mental Retardation

An overview of cognitive development is necessary in order to understand the cognitive limitation of the child with mental retardation and to design effective treatment programs to overcome those cognitive limitations.

Piaget's Theory of Intellectual Development

Jean Piaget, in order to explain normal and abnormal intellectual development, divided the developmental process into four stages: the sensorimotor period (0–18 months); the preoperational stage (2–7 years); the stage of concrete operations (7–12 years); and the period of formal operations (12 years and older).[61] The delineations offered by Piaget's stages provide a basis for understanding the sequence of normal development and the limitations consistent with various degrees of mental retardation.

Children learn mainly through exploration of the senses and through movement during the sensorimotor stage. The ability to coordinate sensorimotor activity to reach certain goals is apparent in primitive forms of intelligence. During this early stage, exploration of the environment includes much experimentation. Learning cannot be generalized to new situations during this period, and most discoveries are made by trial and error. A child who is severely impaired may never progress beyond this stage of intellectual development.[61]

The preoperational stage is characterized by the development of language and the beginnings of abstract thought. Children at this stage can use symbols to represent objects that are not present, and may be able to classify and group objects, although not proficiently. A child with an IQ between 35 and 55 may not develop beyond this stage.[61]

During the concrete operations stage, the ability to order, classify, and relate experience to an organized whole begins to develop.[62] The child can solve some mathematical problems and can read well. The child can generalize learning to new situations and can begin to recognize another person's point of view. There is still an inability to deal with hypothetical problems. Persons with mild cognitive impairments often remain at this level of development.[61] Piaget's final stage—formal operations—normally begins at 12 years of age and continues throughout life. The abilities to reason and hypothesize are characteristic of this stage. The child with mental retardation seldom reaches this level of development.

Intervention to Limit Cognitive Impairment

Concrete Concepts Compared with Abstract Concepts

Children with mental retardation are less able to grasp abstract concepts than concrete concepts.[63] When working with children with mental retardation, the therapist must present treatment concepts using meaningful, concrete directions. Activities are best understood when demonstrated, done passively first, or translated into familiar activities pertaining to daily life.

Memory

The literature regarding the mentally retarded person's ability to remember shows that that ability is related to the type of retention task involved.[62] Use of short-term memory is consistently difficult for the child with mental retardation.[64–66] Smith indicates that a high level of distractibility by external, irrelevant stimuli is associated with these short-term memory deficits. With this knowledge in mind, some of the following strategies can be used during physical therapy sessions.

1. Remove irrelevant, distracting material from the treatment area. Do not work with the child in distracting surroundings, even if room dividers or curtains must be used to separate a small space from a larger, busy area.
2. Present each component of the task clearly and separately.
3. Begin with simple tasks and then progress to more difficult tasks.
4. Explain your expectations of the child at each stage.
5. Give immediate and consistent positive reinforcement.
6. Repeat directions as often as necessary.
7. Check the accuracy of performance frequently.
8. Keep the child informed of progress, and give the child an opportunity to demonstrate or practice the new skill independently.

Most researchers agree that practice, review, and overlearning help the child with mental retardation with long-term retention of skills. The therapist can promote learning and retention by providing ample opportunity to use the newly learned material. Physical therapists inform parents and teachers of a child's progress and should encourage practice of the newly learned task at home or in the classroom. Learning cannot occur or be retained when the physical therapy sessions are an isolated segment of the child's day. Extended practice, and communication with other team members are both vital.

TRANSFER OF LEARNING

Transfer of learning is regarded as the ability to apply newly learned material to new situations having components that are similar to those of the material that was newly learned.[65] The literature on transfer of learning suggests that two factors, in particular, be considered when formulating a plan for treatment.

Meaningfulness is an important element in transfer of learning for the cognitively impaired child. A meaningful task is both easier to learn at the outset and easier to transfer to a second setting than one that has no meaning for the learner. This concept strongly supports the use of functional activities during physical therapy as opposed to meaningless "splinter skills."

Moreover, learning can be transferred best when both the initial task and the transfer task are *similar*. If, for example, the therapist is working on the ability to push rather than to pull on crutches, all of the therapy tasks, such as pushing in a prone position, sitting push-ups, and other tasks, can be transferred more readily to the task of pushing on crutches. *Consistency* also helps the child see the connection between therapy tools and their function.

Knowledge of basic learning concepts and an understanding of cognitive development are crucial for the physical therapist working with an intellectually impaired child. Physical therapy is a learning situation, and some modifications in approach will be necessary to accommodate the differences in performance seen in the child with mental retardation.

Intervention to Limit Physical and Functional Impairments

Pediatric physical therapists traditionally have focused their efforts on interventions designed to limit musculoskeletal, neuromuscular, and cardiopulmonary impairments; reduce functional limitations; and prevent secondary impairment.[43] Early identification of these musculoskeletal, neuromuscular, and cardiopulmonary problems and anticipation of their recognition as associated within specific diagnoses, gives the therapist an insight into appropriate lifespan management of the child with mental retardation. A glance again at Display 8-2 gives the therapist familiarity with some of the specific musculoskeletal, neuromuscular, or cardiopulmonary risks associated with common types of mental retardation. Within this chapter, a focus on physical therapy management for the child with Down syndrome will offer the entry-level therapist a strategy for applying this management model to any child with any type of mental retardation diagnosis. The child's needs as they change throughout the lifespan will determine the level of support intervention required by physical therapy.

The Team Concept

When working with the child with mental retardation, physical therapists must view themselves and their treatment goals as part of a total management plan. Use of an interdisciplinary team of professionals is the standard approach for children with special needs. Comprehensive delivery of services for the child with mental retardation is beyond the scope of any one professional discipline. One of the main values of an interdisciplinary approach is the pooling of knowledge so that a composite and relevant course of action can be made. Because the child with mental retardation will have delays in many areas of development, the skills of many professionals can be used. No single professional has the necessary scope of expertise nor the resources to effectively provide care and education throughout the life of the child with mental retardation.[67]

In order to be effective, each professional on the team must understand the periodic shift of authority and emphasis at different times and different stages of development. Input from the physical therapist will sometimes be of paramount importance, whereas at other times, the priorities will lie in other areas of care. During these latter periods, the physical therapist may play a consultative or advisory role. Success of the team in its primary purpose of helping the child achieve his or her maximum potential will depend on each professional considering the whole child, while offering the needed expertise to alleviate specific problems or handicaps.[47] Communication among team members and respect for one another's unique knowledge and skills are keys to making the team process work.

Effective use of all team members will ensure that consistency and reinforcement are present throughout the child's total program. For example, if certain sounds are being taught in speech therapy, the learning of these sounds can be reinforced by using them during physical therapy sessions. The physical therapist and special education teacher must work as partners in caring for the child. The teacher must be taught handling techniques, positioning, and simple techniques of stimulation. The therapist is uniquely qualified to assist the teacher in understanding the impact of abnormal sensorimotor function on the achievement of cognitive milestones. For example, consider the child with extensor hypertonus, average head control, and obvious interference from tonic neck reflexes. In such a case, knowledge of the basics of muscle tone management could be invaluable to the teacher when working on a cognitive skill with the child, such as performing a simple cause-and-effect activity (e.g., manipulating a "busy-box"). A simple suggestion from the therapist that the child be side-lying rather than supine could reduce the influence of the extensor tone and enable the child to reach for and manipulate the "busy box." Such a cooperative approach both facilitates the child's accomplishment of the educational goal and reduces the frustration of the teacher. In addition, were the teacher unaware of the physical therapy goal to reduce the influence of the extensor tone and the influence of the tonic neck reflex, postures that would be inconsistent with physical therapy goals might be used unknowingly.[68] The physical therapist must communicate and work with all members of the team, including the nurse, occupational therapist, psychologist, physician, teacher, physical education teacher, speech therapist, and parent (Fig. 8-1).

Whenever they work with children, physical therapists must recognize the importance of the

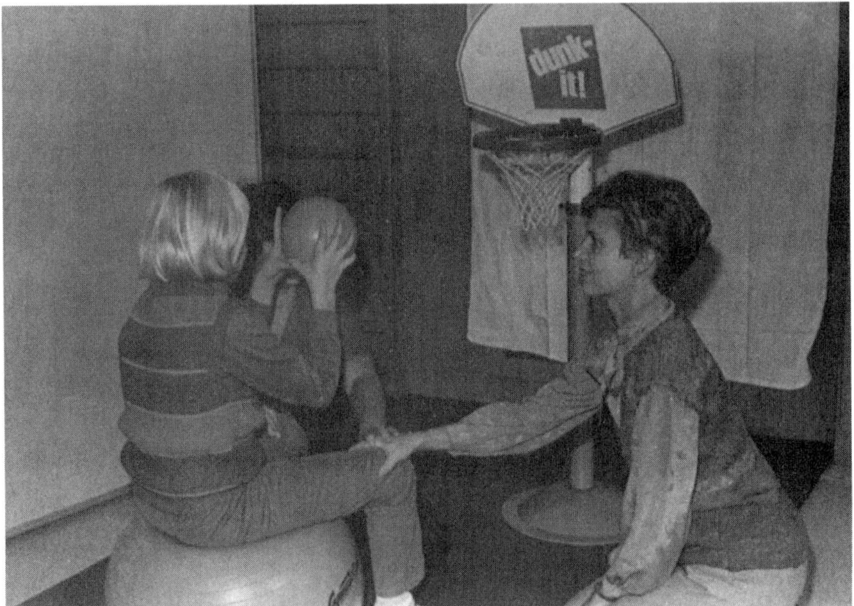

Figure 8-1 ▪ Adapted physical education activity used for therapeutic endeavors in a recreational mode. It is important for the adapted physcial education teacher to have a thorough understanding of the sensory and motor skills being developed.

parents as part of the therapeutic team. Program carryover into the home is important for maximum treatment effectiveness. The parents must learn how to handle the child and must be able to help achieve the goals of the program (Fig. 8-2). This concept is true not only for physical therapy, but for all areas of treatment and education. When asking parents to participate in a home program of care, physical therapists must be able to assess the abilities of the parent. The therapist must recognize problems or conditions in the home that may limit the successful participation of the parents.[68] Referral to appropriate agencies may help parents alleviate or resolve those problems or conditions. Several books that discuss the special needs of families of children with mental retardation may be useful for physical therapists.[69–72] The long-term nature of problems associated with mental retardation and management of those problems usually require a major commitment from the family.

A Management Model for Physical Therapists for the Child with Down Syndrome

Definition

Down syndrome is a chromosomal disorder resulting in 47 chromosomes instead of 46.[73–75] Commonly called trisomy 21, Down syndrome results from faulty cell division affecting the 21st pair of chromosomes, either owing to a nondisjunction (95%), translocation (3% to 4%), or least commonly, as a mosaic presentation (1%).[76]

History and Incidence

Down syndrome is the most common cause of mental retardation and is a diagnosis frequently encountered by pediatric physical therapists. Approximately 5000 infants with Down syndrome

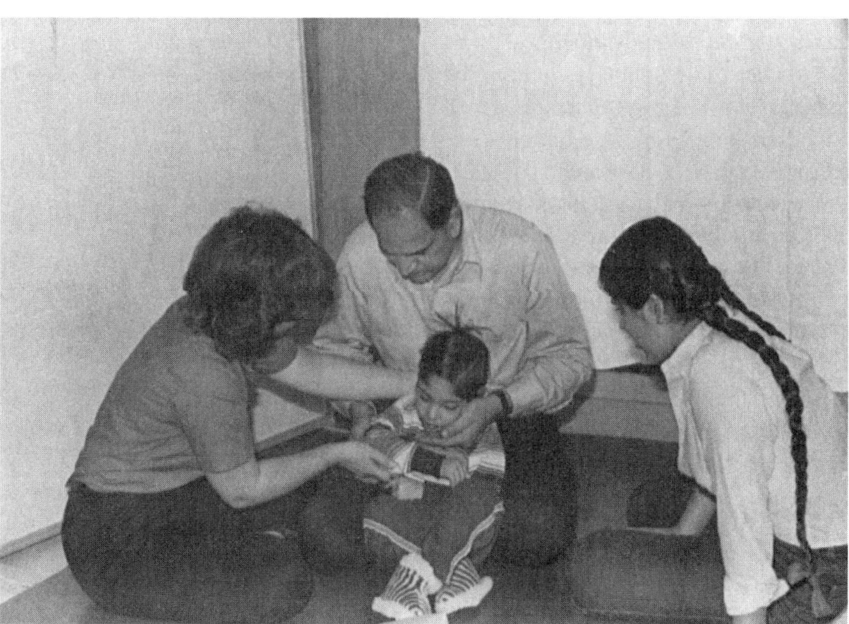

Figure 8-2 ▪ A physical therapist teaches proper handling techniques and proper positioning skills.

are born annually in the United States with an incidence of one in 700 live births.[9,77]

Evidence of an awareness of Down syndrome dates back to early times, with the earliest anthropologic record stemming from excavations in the 7th century of a Saxon skull that had many of the structural changes associated with Down syndrome.[76] Artwork throughout the Middle Ages contains depictions of children with the now-recognized facial characteristics of Down syndrome. Despite these early historical conjectures, there are no published documented reports of Down syndrome until the 19th century. This is understandable from a historical perspective because of the prevalence of infectious diseases and malnutrition that overshadowed research into genetic problems. Also, until beyond the mid-19th century, only half of the mothers survived beyond their 35th birthday (and it is well known that there is an increased incidence of Down syndrome in mothers of advanced maternal age), and many children who indeed were born with Down syndrome probably died in early infancy.[76]

In 1846, Edouard Sequin described a patient with features suggestive of Down syndrome. In 1866, John Langdon Down published a paper describing the characteristics of the then-recognizable syndrome, which has since borne his name.[76] It was not until the mid-1950s that progress in methodologies to visualize chromosomes allowed more accurate studies of human chromosomes, leading to Lejeune's discovery that an alteration in the 21st chromosomal pair is the characteristic hallmark of Down syndrome.[78]

Pathophysiology and Associated Impairments of the Child with Down Syndrome

Down syndrome results in neuromotor, musculoskeletal, and cardiopulmonary pathologies, which all require management by pediatric physical therapists. As with any etiology of mental retardation, an awareness of the pathologies and impairments indigenous to that specific etiology will offer the practicing therapist a model for lifespan management for the child.

Neuropathology

The primary neuropathology causing CNS disorder in children with Down syndrome is owing to several well-documented brain abnormalities. Overall brain weight in individuals with Down syndrome is 76% of normal, with the combined weight of the cerebellum and brain stem being even smaller—66% of normal. There is also microcephaly, and the brain is abnormally rounded and short with a decreased A-P diameter, specifically called microbrachycephaly.[79–80] The number of secondary sulci is reduced, resulting in a simplicity of convoluted patterns in the brains of children with Down syndrome.[81] Several cytologic distinctions of the brain in Down syndrome include a paucity of small neurons, a migrational defect involving small neurons, and decreased synaptogenesis owing to altered synaptic morphology.[81] There are also structural abnormalities in the dendritic spines in the pyramidal tracts of the motor cortex that possibly underly the motor incoordination so often seen in children with Down syndrome.[82] Research also shows evidence of a lack of myelination as well as a delay in the completion of myelination between 2 months and 6 years of age, which may explain the overall developmental delay typically seen in children with Down syndrome.[83] Some studies claim that up to 8% of children with Down syndrome also have some form of seizure disorder.[84]

Sensory Deficits

Visual and hearing problems are common in children with Down syndrome and have a direct impact on physical therapy assessment and intervention. Visual deficits include congenital as well as adult onset cataracts, myopia (50%), farsightedness (20%), strabismus, and nystagmus.[84] Other ocular findings of less clinical significance include the presence of Brushfield spots in the iris and the classic presence of epicanthal folds.

Many children with Down syndrome (60% to 80%) are found to have a mild to moderate hearing loss.[84] Otitis media is a frequently occurring medical problem that may contribute to intermittent or persisting hearing loss in children with Down syndrome.[73]

Cardiopulmonary Pathologies

Forty percent of children with Down syndrome are born with congenital heart defects; most commonly, atrioventricular canal defects and ventriculoseptal defects.[73] Although usually repaired in infancy, heart defects not corrected by age 3 are highly associated with greater delays in motor skill development.[85]

Musculoskeletal Differences

Children with Down syndrome demonstrate many musculoskeletal differences that are of concern to the physical therapist. Linear growth deficits are observed, including a decrease in normal velocity of growth in stature, with the greatest deficiency between 6 and 24 months of age,[86–88] leg length reduction,[89] and a 10% to 30% reduction in metacarpal and phalangeal length. Muscle variations may also be present including an absent palmaris longus and supernumerary forearm flexors. There is also a lack of differentiation of distinct muscles bellies for the zygomaticus major and minor and the levator labii superior,[90] which may account for the typical facial appearance of the child with Down syndrome.

The most significant musculoskeletal differences, however, are owing in large part to the hypotonia and ligamentous laxity characteristic of this disorder. Ligamentous laxity is thought to be owing to a collagen deficit and commonly results in pes planus, patellar instability, scoliosis (52%), and atlantoaxial instability.[86,91,92] Atlantoaxial subluxation with risk for atlantoaxial dislocation is caused by laxity of odontoid ligament, whereby there may be excessive motion of C1 on C2 (12% to 20% incidence).[93–96] Hip subluxation is also commonly seen in children with Down syndrome.

Generalized hypotonia, found in all muscle groups of extremities, neck, and trunk, is a hallmark feature in children with Down syndrome. It is a major contributing factor to developmental motor delay.[97,98] Grip strength, isometric strength, and ankle strength have all been found to be deficient in studies on school-age children with Down syndrome.[99,100]

Additional Physical Characteristics

The back of the head is slightly flattened (brachycephaly), and the fontanels are frequently larger than normal and take longer to close. There may be areas of hair loss, and the skin is often dry and mottled in infancy, rough in the older child. The face of the child with Down syndrome has a somewhat flat contour, primarily because of the underdeveloped facial bones, facial muscles, and a small nose. Usually, the nasal bridge is depressed and the nasal openings may be narrow. The eyes are characterized by narrow, slightly slanted eyelids, with the corners marked by epicanthal folds. The mouth of the child with Down syndrome is small, the palate narrow, and the tongue may take on a furrowed shape in later childhood. Dentition is often delayed and may be spotty. The abdomen may be slightly protuberant secondary to hypotonia and the chest may take on an abnormal shape secondary to congenital heart defect. More than 90% of children with Down syndrome develop an umbilical hernia. Hands and feet tend to be small, and the fifth finger is curved inward. In about 50% of children with Down Syndrome, a single crease is observed across the palm on one or both hands (simian crease). The toes are usually short, and in the majority of children with Down syndrome, there is a wide space between the first and second toes, with a crease running between them on the sole of the foot.

Physical Therapy Assessment and Treatment for the Child with Down Syndrome

Physical therapy assessment of the child with Down syndrome should be holistic, viewing the child from multiple perspectives. The therapist must be aware of coexisting medical problems and especially alert to those typically associated with Down syndrome such as cardiac status, atlantoaxial stability, hearing and visual status, and the presence of seizure disorders. The therapist must also integrate the child's cognitive capabilities into the evaluation process, including discussion of formal intelligence tests with appropriate team members and parent interviews, as well as conducting a brief cognitive assessment as part of a comprehensive developmental test battery. Evaluation includes any or all of the following measures as appropriate for the age and setting within which the child is evaluated: comprehensive developmental testing, component testing of gross and fine motor skills including qualitative observational assessment of movement, musculoskeletal assessment, assessment of automatic reactions and postural responses, and ultimately, a functional assessment. These pediatric evaluation procedures are discussed elsewhere in this text. Evaluation of the child with any type of mental retardation disorder, including Down Syndrome, additionally encompasses assessment of the musculoskeletal, neuromotor, and cardiopulmonary impairments associated with the specific diagnosis (see Display 8-3) and knowledge of the coexistence of the cognitive deficit associated with mental retardation and how that affects physical therapy assessment and treatment.

Learning Differences

Generally, children with mental retardation have been found (1) to be capable of learning a fewer number of things; (2) to need a greater number of repetitions to learn; (3) to have greater difficulty generalizing skills; (4) to have greater difficulty maintaining skills that are not practiced regularly; (5) to have slower response times; and (6) to have a more limited repertoire of responses.[101,102]

The levels of cognitive impairment seen in children with Down syndrome vary, from profoundly to mildly impaired, with a mild to moderate impairment being most common. As with any child with coexistent visual or hearing deficits, therapists must adapt interaction, assessment and teaching to accommodate these coimpairments. Children with mental retardation typically demonstrate attentional difficulties and difficulties with information processing. Research also shows a myriad of specific cognitive problems encountered in children with Down syndrome, including difficulties in sequential verbal processing, social-cognitive skills, auditory memory, and motor planning.[103–107] Children with Down syndrome appear to have significant impairments in verbal–motor interactions, with learning least proficient when the mode of response or reception calls for auditory or vocal skill.[108] It is important, therefore, for therapists to utilize frequent visual demonstration, practice and rehearsal, and perhaps multimodal sensory avenues in order to best interact with the child with Down syndrome. The child with Down syndrome is more likely to remember the rules and patterns of a new activity if he or she is presented with input over many modalities—visual and kinesthetic as well as verbal.[109]

Associated Motor Deficits

The ligamentous laxity and generalized hypotonia associated with Down syndrome contribute the most to the motor delays and secondary musculoskeletal impairments that are of utmost concern to pediatric physical therapists. The degree to which hypotonia is present will vary, but most investigators agree that it is the most frequently observed characteristic in children with Down syndrome.[75,110–113] Hypotonia is distributed to all major muscle groups including neck trunk, and all four extremities.[114]

Developmental Delay

Clinically, hypotonia has been well established to be highly correlated with developmental delay, including delay in attainment of gross motor and fine motor milestones,[85,115] as well as with delay in other areas of development such as speech acquisition and cognitive development.[98,116–118] Studies also have shown the persistence of primitive reflexes beyond the time when they should disappear.[98] Consistent with delayed integration of primitive reflex patterns, a slower rate of development of postural reactions has been noted in children with Down syndrome.[119] Additional studies by Harris and Rast and Shumway-Cook also demonstrated difficulties in postural control, antigravity control, deficits in postural response synergies when balance perturbations were introduced, and consequently, the development of compensatory movement strategies as children with Down syndrome attempted to learn to move and stabilize themselves.[119–121] These investigators attribute the movement deficiencies seen in children with Down syndrome primarily to disturbances in postural control and balance.

Not only is developmental delay to be anticipated when evaluating children with Down syndrome, but there is also some evidence to suggest that the underlying hypotonia, ligamentous laxity, and postural difficulties contribute to some of the movement differences frequently observed in children with Down syndrome. Examples include "W" sitting, where the child will characteristically spread his or her legs to a full 180-degree split while in prone and then advance to a sitting posture by pushing up with his or her hands into sitting.[122] Gait acquisition is delayed and is immature, characterized by a persistent wide base and out-toeing.[122,123] It has been suggested that these differences in movement qualities are caused by hypotonia, ligamentous laxity, and a resultant lack of trunk rotation. Hypotonia has also been shown to contribute to slower reaction time and depressed kinesthetic feedback.[124] Children who have motor impairments are at subsequent risk for secondary impairments because of their restricted ability to explore the environment, especially cognition, communication, and psychosocial development.[125–127]

PHYSICAL THERAPY EVALUATION AND TREATMENT IMPLICATIONS

1. Evaluation should include administration of a comprehensive or component test to measure and track the developmental delay.
2. Qualitative assessment of movement will alert the therapist to movement differences and possible emergent compensatory strategies.
3. Treatment must include an understanding from a functional, dynamic systems perspective; the control parameters most likely to cause a responsiveness shift when attempting to influence developing motor strategies.[128]
4. General Goal: Anticipate gross and fine motor delay and provide interventions to minimize it.
   a. Utilize positioning and handling activities throughout early infancy and childhood to promote antigravity control and weight-bearing.
   b. Facilitate antigravity extension in prone and weightshifting within and as transition from prone.
   c. In supine and supported sitting, encourage midline orientation, antigravity bimanual activities including eye-hand coordination,

and activities to promote anterior neck and trunk antigravity strength.

d. Emphasize trunk extension and extremity loading, which tend to increase axial tone.[129]
e. Encourage emergence of righting and postural reactions through use of rotation within and during movement.
f. Allow for dynamic rather than static exploration of movement.
g. Introduce developmental milestones when chronologically appropriate, including supported sitting and standing, when trunk control and alignment are able to be established.
h. Anticipate delay in postural control responses and provide functional opportunities to enhance development in areas of cognition, language, and socialization.
i. Teach parents and other team members activities and position choices that will enhance the child's overall development.

Musculoskeletal Problems

In addition to generalized hypotonia, ligamentous laxity is a hallmark musculoskeletal characteristic of Down Syndrome and commonly results in pes planus, patellar instability, scoliosis (52%), and atlantoaxial instability.[86,91,92] The previously noted atlantoaxial relationship is identified by sagittal plane radiographs of the cervical spine in three different positions: flexion, neutral, and extension.[130–132] A joint interval of 6 to 10 mm is considered symptomatic. A joint interval of more than 4.5 mm carries precautions with it. Early signs of atlantoxial dislocation include gait changes, urinary retention, reluctance to move neck, and increased deep tendon reflexes (DTRs).[96] In cases of dislocation with symptomatic atlantoaxial instability, posterior arthrodesis or fusion of C1 and C2 is recommended.[130] In addition to atlantoaxial instability, thoracolumbar scoliosis is also an associated vertebral column musculoskeletal impairment frequently seen in children and adolescents with Down syndrome, usually defined as of a mild to moderate degree.[92]

In the lower extremities, hip instability, patellar instability, and foot deformity are the most common musculoskeletal concerns for the physical therapist managing the child with Down syndrome. Hip subluxation is secondary to developmental acetabular dysplasia and long, tapered ischia that result in decreased acetabular and iliac angles as well as laxity of ligamentous support.[91] Pes planus and metatarsus primus varus are the major foot deformities seen in children with Down syndrome.[92]

PHYSICAL THERAPY EVALUATION AND TREATMENT IMPLICATIONS

1. Ligamentous laxity makes any joint less resistant to any trauma, malalignment, or uneven forces. Alignment and support are crucial. At the atlantoaxial joint, this laxity makes the joint less resistant especially to superimposed flexion, where the joint interval is already widened.
2. Therapists should avoid exaggerated neck flexion, extension, rotation, and positions or movements that may cause twisting or undue forces. With caution, joint approximation or compression of the cervical spine should be performed gently with all children with Down syndrome and is contraindicated in children with identified atlantoaxial instability. Therapists should also use caution when placing a child in the inverted position or in other positions that increase risk of a fall onto the head.[96]
3. In the infant and child under the age of 2 years, a radiograph will not reliably detect atlantoaxial instability. Extreme caution must be taken and any activity that may result in cervical spine injury may be contraindicated.
4. Physical therapists must closely monitor children with Down syndrome for changes in neurologic status and be vigilant in assessing

risk of atlantoaxial instability. Parent education should include issues of atlantoaxial instability, symptoms of neurologic compromise, periods and activities that may carry increased risk, and activities to avoid if instability is identified.[96]

5. The Committee on Sports Medicine of the American Academy of Pediatrics recommends an initial set of cervical spine radiographs at 2 years of age and follow-up radiographs in grade school, at adolescence, and adulthood.[130]
6. Contact sports and physical activities that may result in cervical spine injury may be contraindicated.[133] The following activities are considered to be restricted for children with even asymptomatic atlantoaxial intervals of greater than 4.5 mm: gymnastics (somersaults), diving, high jump, soccer, butterfly stroke in swimming, exercises that place pressure on the head and neck, high-risk activities that involve possible trauma to the head and neck, and participation in pentathalon.[130,134]
7. Screening for scoliosis should be a routine part of lifespan management of the child with Down syndrome, especially during periods of increased risk such as growth spurts, puberty, and throughout adolescence. Parents should be taught to perform routine screening for scoliosis. Activities and exercises should promote symmetry and alignment.
8. Musculoskeletal assessment also should include biomechanical assessment of the lower extremity and orthotic management, if indicated, for pes planus. In the infant, assessment of hip stability is a routine part of a physical therapy evaluation and referral is indicated for orthopedic assessment if hip instability if suspect. Supported standing in a stander should not be instituted unless hip stability and proper alignment has been established.
9. General Goal: Maintain alignment and encourage normal movement forces in order to promote optimal biomechanical forces for best musculoskeletal development and prevention of anticipated malalignments and instabilities.
   a. Use of aligned compression or weight-bearing forces in order to stimulate longitudinal bone growth as well as thickness and density of the bone and shaft;
   b. Aligned, supported weight bearing in order to promote joint stability and formation;
   c. Facilitation of normal cocontraction, force production, and increased muscle tone.

In summary, the impact of all of these associated motor deficits in Down syndrome on physical therapy can be viewed as how they affect the child's development and overall functioning. Most of these movement problems have their bases in CNS pathology or primary musculoskeletal differences, which then often lead to secondary impairments, in flexibility, stability, force production, coordination, postural control, balance, endurance, and overall efficiency. The specific intervention used will depend on the identified problems and on the consequences that can be predicted and perhaps prevented.

Neuromuscular Impairments	**Functional Implication**
Hypotonia, low force production	Motor delay, poor contraction Movement paucity
Slow automatic postural reactions	Balance limitations
Slow reaction time	Decreased speed
Joint hypermobility	Instability, movement anxiety
a-a Instability, scoliosis, foot deformities	May preclude access to activities or limit participation level in activity

Cardiopulmonary Fitness

General physical fitness is often below desired levels in children with mental retardation, and specifically, in children with Down syndrome,[135] Children with Down syndrome are at risk for restrictive pulmonary disease with concomitant decreased lung volumes and a weak cough, because of generalized trunk and extremity weakness.[136–138] Reduced cough effectiveness may contribute to high incidence of respiratory infections.[139] Decreased lung volumes including vital capacity and total lung capacity may contribute to a deficiency of the pulmonary system to oxygenate the mixed venous blood or remove the carbon dioxide from the same blood.[140] If there is a reduction in the maximum amount of oxygen available for transport, the energy available for activities is lowered, and consequently a poorer level of physical fitness is achieved.

PHYSICAL THERAPY EVALUATION AND TREATMENT IMPLICATIONS

The implications for lifespan management of the child with Down syndrome are obvious.

1. Greater emphasis on physical fitness may increase cardiopulmonary endurance and muscular strength. Programming should begin with children of primary age in order to prevent a slowing of activity and the subsequent onset of obesity and long-term atherosclerotic risk profiles.[135] Knowledge of improvement reported from training programs for children with Down syndrome supports the ability of these children to respond to early intervention.[141,142]
2. Physical therapists have an excellent opportunity to impact on the health of children with Down syndrome through direct intervention or in consultation with special educators or physical/recreational educators.
3. General Goal: Encourage commitment to wellness by promoting cardiopulmonary endurance, overall physical fitness, and parent/caregiver/client education.

Summary

In the management of the child with mental retardation, the physical therapist is challenged to use various skills. The many complex and persistent difficulties encountered by children with mental retardation often require innovative methods of physical therapy evaluation and treatment. It is easy to understand that physical therapists may feel overwhelmed by the complexity of this population.

This chapter has attempted to give therapists a "user-friendly" strategy for physical therapy management, including evaluation and intervention, for *any* child with a diagnosis of mental retardation. Therapists are reminded to view the mental retardation itself as only a partial description of that child's learning impairment, which may vary in severity from having anywhere from a mild to a profound influence on that child's functional learning capabilities. This may be further confounded by other concomitant sensory deficits, including visual, hearing, or sensory organizational problems. Physical therapy evaluation and treatment methods must incorporate not only the basic principles of pediatric physical therapy but also an understanding of the principles of teaching and learning as they relate to the child with mental retardation.

Additionally, although there are at least 350 known etiologies for mental retardation,[26] the therapist can easily investigate any of those specific etiologies and acquaint themselves with any commonly associated neuromuscular, musculoskeletal, or cardiopulmonary impairments. This investigative approach will sharpen the therapist's assessment skills and alert the PT to the presence of likely coimpairments or associated medical problems. An understanding of the primary pathology and associated motor deficits readily assists the therapist in establishing treatment goals and priorities. Effective lifespan physical therapy management of the child can then encompass the anticipation of secondary deformities and risks for that child, which can then be shared with parents and other team members. This chapter illustrated the application of this investigative strategy to the physical therapy management of a child with Down syndrome. This same investigative strategy can be utilized for any mental retardation diagnosis encountered in pediatric physical therapy practice.

Communication of the changing needs of children with mental retardation to parents and other professionals requires not only technical expertise on the part of the therapist but also the ability to be a sensitive listener and creative teacher. Through an effective interdisciplinary approach to the child and his or her family, we can strive to help the child with mental retardation to function at his or her best in society.

ACKNOWLEDGMENTS

I wish to gratefully acknowledge the children and parents from whom I have learned so much. I congratulate all of them for their courage, spirit and unconditional love.

REFERENCES

1. Nichtern S. *Helping the Retarded Child.* Grosset and Dunlap; 1974.
2. Sebelist RM. Mental retardation. In: Hopkins HL, Smith HD, eds. *Willard and Spackman's Occupational Therapy.* 9th Ed. Philadelphia: JB Lippincott; 1996.
3. National Institute on Mental Retardation: Orientation Manual on Mental Retardation. Ontario, Canada: York University; 1981.
4. Itard J. *The Wild Boy of Aveyron.* Englewood Cliffs, NJ: Prentice-Hall; 1962.
5. American Association on Mental Retardation (AAMR). 1719 Kalorama Road, NW, Washington, DC, 20009-2683.
6. Reynolds MC, Birch JW. *Teaching Exceptional Children in All America's Schools.* Reston, VA; The Council for Exceptional Children; 1977.
7. American Association on Mental Retardation. *Mental Retardation: Definition, Classification, and System of Supports.* 9th Ed. Washington, DC: American Association on Mental Retardation; 1992.
8. Ginsburg L. *Social Work Almanac.* 2nd Ed. National Association of Social Workers Press; 1995.
9. Berkow R, ed. Mental illness and developmental disabilities. In: Ginsberg L. *Social Work Almanac,* 2nd ed. Washington, DC: National Association of Social Workers Press; 1992.
10. Thorndike RL, Hagen E, Sattler J. *Stanford-Binet Intelligence Scale.* Chicago, IL: Riverside, 1985.
11. Wechsler D. *Wechsler Intelligence Scale for Children-III*. San Antonio, TX: Psychological Corp; 1991.
12. Wechsler D. *Wechsler Preschool and Primary Scale of Intelligence.* San Antonio, TX: Psychological Corp; 1967.
13. Kaufman AS, Kaufman NL. *Kaufman Assessment Battery for Children.* Circle Pines, MN: American Guidance Service; 1983.
14. Doll EA. *Vineland Social Maturity Scale.* Minneapolis: American Guidance Service; 1953.
15. Nihara K, Foster, R, Shelhaas, M, et al. *Adaptive Behavior Scales.* Washington, DC: American Association on Mental Deficiency; 1974.
16. Lambert NM, Windmiller MB. *AAMD Adaptive Behavior Scale,* School edition. Monterey, CA: Publishers Test Service; 1981.
17. Sparrow SS, et al. *Vineland Adaptive Behavior Scales.* Circle Pines, MN: American Guidance Service; 1984.
18. Adams GL. *Comprehensive Test of Adaptive Behavior.* Columbus, OH: Merrill; 1984.
19. Sloan W, Birch JW. A rationale for degrees of retardation. *Am J Ment Defic.* 1955;60:262.
20. World Health Organization. International classification of impairments, disabilities, and handicaps. Geneva, Switzerland: World Health Organization; 1980.
21. Nagi SZ. *Disability and Rehabilitation.* Columbus, OH: Ohio State University Press; 1969.
22. Bertoti DB. Physical therapy for the mentally retarded child. In: Tecklin JS. *Pediatric Physical Therapy.* Philadelphia: JB Lippincott; 1993.
23. Chinn PC, Drew CJ, Logan DR. *Mental Retardation: A Life Cycle Approach.* St. Louis: CV Mosby; 1979.
24. *Diagnostic and Statistical Manual of Mental Disorders.* 4th Ed. Washington, DC: American Psychiatric Association; 1994.
25. *International Classification of Diseases* (ICD). Ann Arbor, MI: World Health Organization; 1992.
26. Carter CH. *Handbook of Mental Retardation Syndromes.* Springfield, IL: Charles C Thomas; 1970.
27. Nyhan WL, Sakati NO. *Genetic and Malformation Syndromes in Clinical Medicine.* Chicago: Year Book Medical Publishers; 1976.
28. Bergsma D. *Birth Defects: Atlas and Compendium.* Baltimore: Williams & Wilkins; 1973.
29. Berg JM et al. *The de Lange Syndrome.* New York: Pergamon Press; 1970.

30. Jones KL. *Smith's Recognizable Patterns of Human Malformation.* 5th Ed. Fletcher J, ed. Philadelphia: WB Saunders, 1996.
31. Harris SR, Shea AM. Down syndrome. In: Campbell SK. *Pediatric Neurologic Physical Therapy.* 2nd Ed. New York: Churchill Livingstone; 1991.
32. Shumway-Cook A, Woollacott MH. Dynamics of postural control in the child with Down syndrome. *Phys Ther.* 1985;65:1315–1322.
33. Bloom AS et al. Developmental characteristics of recognizable patterns of human malformation. In: Berg JM. *Science and Service in Mental Retardation: Proceedings of the Seventh Congress of the International Association for the Scientific Study of Mental Deficiency* (LASSMD). New York: Methuen, 1985.
34. Keenan J et al. A statewide public and professional educational program on fragile x syndrome. *Ment Retard.* 1992;30:355–361.
35. Rinck C, Fragile x syndrome. *Dialogue on Drugs, Behavior and Developmental Disabilities.* University of Missouri. 1992;4(3):1–4.
36. Anderson LT, Ernst M. Self-injury in Lesch-Nyhan disease. *J Autism Dev Dis.* 1994;24:67–81.
37. Aughton DJ, Cassidy SB. Physical features of Prader-Willi syndrome in neonates. *Am J Dis Child.* 1990;144:1251–1254.
38. Dykens EM, Cassidy SB. Prader-Willi syndrome: Genetic, behavioral and treatment issues. *Child Adolesc Psychiatric Clin North Am.* 1996;5: 913–927.
39. Guidera KJ et al. Orthopaedic manifestations of Rett Syndrome. *JL Pediatr Orthop.* 1991;11: 204–208.
40. Holm VA, King HA. Scoliosis in the Rett syndrome. *Brain Dev.* 1990;12:151–153.
41. Nomura Y, Segawa Y. Characteristics of motor disturbance in Rett syndrome. *Brain Dev.* 1990;12: 27–30.
42. Stewart KB et al. Rett syndrome: A literature review and survey of patents and therapists. *Phys Occup Ther Pediatr.* 1989;9(3):35–55.
43. McEwen I. Mental retardation. In: Campbell SK. *Physical Therapy for Children.* Philadelphia: WB Saunders; 1994.
44. Detterman DK, Mayer JD, Canuso DR, et al. Assessment of basic cognitive abilities in relation to cognitive deficits. *Am J Ment Retard.* 1992;97: 251–286.
45. Horvat M, Croce R. Physical rehabilitation of individuals with mental retardation: Physical fitness and information processing. *Crit Rev Phys Rehabil Med.* 1995;7(3):233–252.
46. Montgomery PC. Assessment and treatment of the child with mental retardation. *Phys Ther.* 1981; 61:1265–1272.
47. Pearson PH, Williams CE, eds. *Physical Therapy Services in the Developmental Disabilities.* Springfield, IL: Charles C Thomas; 1972.
48. Kinnealy M. Aversive and nonaversive responses to sensory stimuli in mentally retarded children. *Am J Occup Ther.* 1973;27:464–472.
49. Robb R. Approach to a child with visual problems. In: Avery ME, First LE, eds. *Pediatric Medicine.* 2nd Ed. Baltimore: Williams & Wilkins; 1994.
50. Getman GN, Kone ER, et al. *Developing Learning Readiness.* St. Louis: McGraw-Hill; 1966.
51. DeQuiros JB. Diagnosis of vestibular disorders in the learning disabled. *J Learn Disabil.* 1976;9:50–58.
52. Moore J. Cranial nerves and their importance in current rehabilitation techniques. In: Henderson A, Coryell J, eds. *The Body Senses and Perceptual Deficit.* Boston: Boston University; 1973:102–120.
53. Ayres AJ. *Sensory Integration and the Child.* Los Angeles: Western Psychological Services; 1979: 34–35.
54. Head H. *Studies in Neurology.* Vol. 2. London: Oxford University Press; 1920:396–397.
55. Poggin GF, Mountcastle VB. A study of the functional contributions of the lemniscal and spinothalamic systems to somatic sensibility. *Johns Hopkins Med J.* 1960;106:266–316.
56. Ayres AJ. *Sensory Integration and Learning Disorders.* Los Angeles: Western Psychological Services; 1972.
57. Ayres AJ. Tactile functions: Their relation to hyperactive and perceptive motor behavior. *Am J Occup Ther.* 1964;18:6–11.
58. Clark RG, Gilman, S, Wilhaus-Newman, S. *Essentials of Clinical Neuroanatomy and Neurophysiology.* 9th Ed. Philadelphia: FA Davis; 1996.
59. Westcott SL, Lowes LP. Richardson PK. Evaluation of postural stability in children: Current theories and assessment tools. *Phys Ther.* 1997;77:629–645.
60. Lemke H. Self-abusive behavior. *Am J Occup Ther.* 1974;28:94–98.
61. Batshaw NL, Perret YM. *Children with Handicaps: A Medical Primer.* 2nd Ed. Baltimore: Paul H. Brookes; 1986.
62. Hardy RD, Cull JB. *Mental Retardation and Physical Disability.* Springfield, IL: Charles C Thomas; 1974.
63. Weiner H. *Comparative Psychology of Mental Development.* New York: International University Press; 1948.
64. Bird EKR, Chapman RS. Sequential recall in individuals with Down syndrome. *J Speech Hearing Res.* 1994;37:1369–1381.
65. Smith R. *Clinical Teaching: Methods of Instruction for the Retarded.* New York: McGraw-Hill; 1968.

66. Hale CA, Borkowski JG. Attention, memory, and cognition. In: Matson JL, Mulick JA, eds. *Handbook of Mental Retardation.* New York: Pergamon Press; 1991.
67. Scheerenberger RC. Mental retardation: Definition, classification, and prevalence. *Ment Retard Abstr.* 1964;1:432–441.
68. Connolly BH, Anderson RM. Severely handicapped children in the public schools—A new frontier for the physical therapist. *Phys Ther.* 1978;58: 433–438.
69. Odel SJ, Greer JG, Anderson RM. The family of the severely retarded individual. In: Anderson RM, Greer JG, eds. *Educating the Severely and Profoundly Retarded.* Baltimore: University Park Press; 1976:251–261.
70. Barsch RH. *The Parent of the Handicapped Child.* Springfield, IL: Charles C Thomas; 1968.
71. Roos P. Parents and families of the mentally retarded. IN: Kauffman JM, Payne JS, eds. *Mental Retardation: An Introduction and Personal Perspectives.* Columbus, OH: Charles E. Merrill; 1975.
72. Farber B. *Family Organization and Crisis: Maintenance of Integration in Families with a Severely Retarded Child.* Lafayette, IN: Child Development Publication, Society Research Child Development, 1960.
73. Coleman M. Down's syndrome. *Pediatr Ann.* 1978;7:90.
74. Kirman BH. Genetic errors: chromosome anomalies. In: Kirman BH, Bicknell J, eds. *Mental Handicap.* Edinburgh: Churchill Livingstone; 1975.
75. Harris SR, Shea AM. Down syndrome. In: Campbell SK, ed. *Pediatric Neurologic Physical Therapy,* 2nd Ed. New York: Churchill Livingstone; 1991.
76. Pueschel SM. Cause of Down syndrome. In: Pueschel SM. *A Parent's Guide to Down Syndrome: Toward a Brighter Future.* Baltimore: Paul H Brookes Publishing Co.; 1990.
77. Huether C. Demographic projections for Down syndrome. In Pueschel SM, Tingey C, Rynders CE, et al., eds. *New Perspectives on Down Syndrome.* Baltimore: Paul H Brookes Publishing Co.; 1987.
78. Lejeune J, Gauthier M, Turpin R. Les chromosomes humain en culture de tissus. *CR Acad Sci (D).* 1959;248:602.
79. Roche AF. The cranium in mongolism. *Acta Neurol.* 1966;42:62.
80. Penrose LS, et al. *Down's Anomaly.* London: Churchill Livingstone; 1966.
81. Scott BS, et al. Neurobiology of Down's syndrome. *Prog Neurobiol.* 1983;21:199.
82. Marin-Padilla M. Pyramidal cell abnormalities in the motor cortex of a child with Down's syndrome. *J Comp Neurol.* 1976;67:63.
83. Wisniewski KF, et al. Postnatal delay of myelin formation in brains from Down's syndrome. *Clin Neuropathol.* 1989;6(2):55.
84. Pueschel SM. Medical Concerns. In: Pueschel SM. *A Parent's Guide to Down syndrome: Toward a Brighter Future.* Baltimore: Paul H Brookes Publishing Co.; 1990.
85. Zausmer EF, Shea A. Motor Development. In: Pueschel SM. *The Young Child with Down syndrome.* New York: Human Sciences Press Inc.; 1984.
86. Shea AM. Growth and development in Down syndrome in infancy and early childhood: implications for the physical therapist. In: *Touch Topics in Pediatrics,* Lesson 5. Alexandria, VA: American Physical Therapy Association; 1990.
87. Castells S, Beaulieu I, Torrado C, et al. Hypothalamic versus pituitary dysfunction in Down's syndrome as a cause of growth retardation. *J Intellect Disabil Res.* 1996;40:509–517.
88. Cronk CE, Crocker AC, Pueschel SM, et al. Growth charts for children with Down syndrome; 1 month to 18 years of age. *Pediatrics.* 1988;81: 102–110.
89. Rarick GG, Seefeldt V. Observations from longitudinal data on growth and stature and sitting height of children with Down syndrome. *J Ment Defic Res.* 1974;18:63–78.
90. Bersu ET. Anatomical analysis of the developmental effects of aneuploidy in man: The Down syndrome. *Am J Med Genet.* 1980;5:399.
91. Dummer GM. *Strength and flexibility in Down's syndrome.* In American Association for Health, Physical Education an Recreation: Research Consortium Papers: Movement Studies, vol. 1, book 3. Washington, DC; American Association for Health, Physical Education and Recreation, 1978.
92. Diamond LS, et al. Orthopedic disorders in patients with Down's syndrome. *Orthop Clin North Am.* 1981;12:57.
93. Giblin PE, Michele LJ. The management of atlantoaxial subluxation with neurological involvement in Down's syndrome: a report of two cases and review of the literature. *Clin Orthop.* 1979;140:66.
94. Whaley WJ, et al. Atlantoaxial dislocation and Down syndrome. *Can Med Assoc J.* 1980;123:35.
95. Brenneman S, Stanger M, Bertoti DB: Age-related considerations: pediatric. In: Saunders RM. *Saunders Manual of Physical Therapy Practice.* Philadelphia: WB Saunders; 1995.
96. Gajdosik CG, Ostertag S. Cervical instability and Down syndrome: Review of the literature and implications for physical therapists. *Pediatric Phys Ther.* 1996;8:1:31–36.

97. Carr J. Mental and motor development in young Mongol children. *J Ment Defic Res.* 1970;14:205.
98. Cowie VA. *A Study of the Early Development of Mongols.* Oxford: Pergamon Press; 1970.
99. Morris AF, Vaughan SE, Vaccaro P. Measurements of neuromuscular tone and strength in Down syndrome children. *J Ment Defic Res.* 1982;26:41–47.
100. MacNeill-Shea SH, et al. Relationship of ankle strength and hypermobility to squatting skills of children with Down syndrome. *Phys Ther.* 1985; 65:1658–1666.
101. Brown L, et al. A strategy for developing chronological age appropriate and functional curricular content for severely handicapped adolescents and young adults. *JI Spec Educ.* 1979;12: 81–90.
102. Orelove FP, Sobsey, D. Designing transdisciplinary services. In: Orelove, et al. *Educating Children with Multiple Disabilities: A Transdisciplinary Approach.* Baltimore: Paul H Brooks; 1991.
103. Horvat M, Croce R. Physical rehabilitation of individuals with mental retardation: Physical fitness and information processing. *Crit Rev Phys Rehabil Med.* 1995;7(3):233–252.
104. Hartley XY. Lateralization of speech stimuli in young Down's syndrome children. *Cortex* 1981; 17:241.
105. Marcel MM, Armstrong V. Auditory and visual sequential memory of Down syndrome and nonretarded children. *Am J Ment Defic.* 1982;87:86.
106. Edwards JM, Elliott D, Lee TD. Contextual interference effects during skill acquisition and transfer in Down's syndrome adolescents. *Adapt Phys Act Quart.* 1986;3:250.
107. Elliott D, Weeks DJ. A functional systems approach to movement pathology. *Adapt Phys Act Quart.* 1993;10:312.
108. Griffiths MI. Development of children with Down's syndrome. *Physiotherapy* 1976;62:11–15.
109. Hagen C. A approach to the treatment of mild to moderately severe apraxia. *Top Land Dis.* 1987; 34:8.
110. Cummins H, Talley C, Platou RV. Palmar dermatoglyphics in mongolism. *Pediatrics* 1950;5: 241.
111. Levinson A, Friedman A, Stamps F. Variability of mongolism. *Pediatrics* 1955;16:43.
112. McIntire MS, Dutch SJ. Mongolism and generalized hypotonia. *Am J Ment Defic.* 1964;68:669.
113. Wagner HR. Mongolism in orientals. *Am J Dis Child.* 1962;103:706.
114. McIntire MS, Menolascino FJ, Wiley JH. Mongolism—some clinical aspects. *Am J Ment Defic.* 1965;69:794.
115. Harris SR. Relationship of mental and motor development in Down's syndrome infants. *Phys Occup Ther Pediatr.* 1981;1:13.
116. Canning CD, Pueschel SM. Developmental expectations: an overview. In: Pueschel SM. *A Parent's Guide to Down Syndrome: Toward a Brighter Future.* Baltimore: Paul H Brookes Publishing Co.; 1990.
117. LaVeck B, LaVeck GD. Sex differences in development among young children with Down syndrome. *J Pediatr* 1977;91:767.
118. Cicchetti D, Sroufe LA. The relationship between affective and cognitive development in Down's syndrome infants. *Child Dev.* 1976;47:920.
119. Haley SM. Postural reactions in children with Down syndrome. *Phys Ther.* 1986;66(1):17–31.
120. Rast MM, Harris SR. Motor control in infants with Down syndrome. *Dev Med Child Neurol.* 1985;27:682–685.
121. Shumway-Cook A, Woollacott M: Dynamics of postural control in the child with Down syndrome. *Phys Ther.* 1985;65:1315–1322.
122. Lydic JS, Steele C. Assessment of the quality of sitting and gait patterns in children with Down's syndrome. *Phys Ther.* 1979;59(12):1489–1494.
123. Parker AW, Bronks R. Gait of children with Down syndrome. *Arch Phys Med Rehabil.* 1980;61:345–351.
124. O'Connor N, Hermelin B. *Speech and Thought in Severe Subnormality.* London: Oxford Press; 1963.
125. Hays RM. Childhood motor impairments: Clinical overview and scope of the problem. In: Jaffe KM. *Childhood Powered Mobility.* Washington, DC: RESNA; 1987; 1-10.
126. Affoltier FD. *Perception, Interaction and Language: Interaction of Daily Living: The Root of Development.* New York: Springer-Verlag; 1991.
127. Kermonian R, et al. Locomotor experience: a facilitator of spatial cognitive development. *Child Dev.* 1988;59:908–917.
128. Ulrich BD, Ulrich DA, Collier DH, et al. Developmental shifts in the ability of infants with Down syndrome to produce treadmill steps. *Phys Ther.* 1995;75:20–29.
129. Long TM, Cintas HL. *Handbook of Pediatric Physical Therapy.* Baltimore: Williams & Wilkins; 1995.
130. American Academy of Pediatrics, Committee on Sports Medicine: Atlantoaxial instability in Down syndrome. *Pediatrics.* 1984;74:152–154.
131. Pueschel SM, Scola FH. Atlantoaxial instability in individuals with Down syndrome: Epidemiologic, radiographic, and clinical studies. *Pediatrics.* 1987;80:555–560.

132. Singer SJ, Rubin IL, Strauss KJ. Atlantoaxial distance in patients with Down syndrome: Standardization of measurement. *Radiology.* 1987;164:871–872.
133. Giblin PE, et al. The management of atlanto-axial subluxation with neurological involvement in Down syndrome. *Clin Orthop.* 1979;140:66.
134. Cooke RE. Atlantoaxial instability in individuals with Down syndrome. *Adap Phys Act Q.* 1984;1: 194–196.
135. Dichter CG, Darbee JC, Effgen SK, et al. Assessment of pulmonary function and physical fitness in children with Down syndrome. *Pediatr Phys Ther.* 1993;5(1):3–8.
136. Polacek JJ, Wang PY, Eichstaedt CB. *A Study of Physical and Health Related Fitness Levels of Mild, Moderate, and Down Syndrome Students in Illinois.* Normal, IL: Illinois State University Press; 1985.
137. DeCesare J. Physical therapy for the child with respiratory dysfunction. In: Irwin S, Tecklin JS. *Cardiopulmonary Physical Therapy.* 3rd Ed. St. Louis: Mosby–Yearbook; 1995.
138. Connolly BH, Michael BT. Performance of retarded children, with and without Down syndrome, on the Bruinicks Oseretsky Test of Motor Proficiency. *Phys Ther.* 1986;66:344–348.
139. Harris SR, Tada WL. Genetic disorders in children. In: Umphred DA. *Neurological Rehabilitation.* Princeton, NJ: CV Mosby; 1985.
140. Ruppel G. *Manual of Pulmonary Function Testing.* 3rd Ed. St. Louis: CV Mosby; 1982.
141. Skrobak-Kaczynski J, Vavik T. Physical fitness and trainability of young male patients with Down syndrome. In: Berg K, Eriksson BO. *Children and Exercise IX.* Baltimore: University Park Press; 1980.
142. Weber R, French R. *The Influence of Strength Training on Down Syndrome Adolescents: A Comparative Investigation.* Texas Women's University.

Adaptive Equipment for Physically Challenged Children

Emilie Kallenbach Aubert, M.A., P.T.

Physical therapists have many products at their disposal to help provide the physically challenged child with better means for positioning, achieving mobility, and performing activities of daily living (ADLs). New products are being developed every year in an attempt to satisfy the needs of children with disabilities. Products and materials are available in both standard, commercially produced forms and custom-fabricated forms to meet individualized specifications for each child.

The great variety of products and materials available and the constantly changing and expanding market present a formidable problem for the therapist who tries to give parents useful suggestions regarding equipment. How can students or recent graduates acquaint themselves with these products in order to feel confident in guiding families who need adaptive equipment for their children? What conditions should be evaluated before making decisions regarding adaptive equipment? What is the true role of adaptive equipment for children with physical disabilities, and are there particular dangers or contraindications to adaptive equipment? These questions are addressed in this chapter, the main goal of which is to provide the student and the therapist who is inexperienced in pediatrics with a theoretical construct to facilitate decision making about adaptive equipment, regardless of familiarity with any particular piece of equipment. Commonly used equipment—prone standers, side-lyers, and wheelchairs—are evaluated, and case studies are used to further delineate approaches to practical decision making. There are few, if any, clear, scientific, objective guidelines on which to base a decision about adaptive equipment. The selection of adaptive equipment for children is still an art, rather than a science. As physical therapists, our goal is to try to meet the needs of physically challenged children by using a critical approach to document our successes and failures in the hope of consequently transforming this "art" into a science.

Role of Adaptive Equipment

Adaptive equipment is becoming increasingly necessary as an adjunct to direct treatment. No child can realistically receive the constant handling needed throughout the day to prevent abnormal movement patterns and postures. Although the physical therapist may teach families, day-care providers, and teachers about methods of handling the child to encourage optimal development, the child must be allowed time to move, explore, and relax without constant help. The increased cost of direct care and the crowded conditions often found in therapeutic programs suggest a need for alternatives to direct patient handling.

One alternative is the judicious use of adaptive equipment to allow correct positioning during free, independent time for the child. Adaptive equipment can also provide for the reinforcement and use of positions and movements introduced to the child during treatment sessions. Similarly, abnormal or undesirable positions or movements can often be prevented by use of correct equipment.

Adaptive equipment may make possible functional skills that the child may otherwise be unable to do. These uses of adaptive equipment not only promote motor and sensory development but concurrently improve cognitive, perceptual, emotional, and social development.

Adaptive equipment, in addition to its direct therapeutic benefits, may serve an important role by assisting in the daily management of the child at home. Some indispensable items include bathtub seats, hydraulic lifts, and adapted high chairs. Adaptive items that facilitate safe and effective transportation may include many types of car seats, strollers, and wheelchairs.

Although adaptive equipment should be prescribed with the goal of achieving maximum benefits with the least restriction, this ideal approach may occasionally need to be compromised. For example, some families may be unwilling to adjust the routines of all family members to meet the needs of only one member. Also, ideal goals may not be possible because of architectural barriers that prohibit the use of certain adaptive devices. When barriers (behavioral, architectural, or financial) exist, the therapist must analyze the short-term needs of the family and the long-term goals of the child before making a decision or recommendation. Whenever adaptive equipment is recommended, its use must be monitored to ensure that therapeutic goals and family needs are being met.

Precautions When Using Adaptive Equipment

Can adaptive equipment be dangerous? This is a difficult question to answer, especially because most equipment has a design that is inherently free of dangers. Problems may arise from the way in which equipment is used by various caretakers. Although a particular piece of equipment may have been prescribed, fitted, and properly explained, its overuse or misuse may cause difficulties.

Misuse

Adaptive equipment is often static and, although beneficial, may not provide a rich environment for learning new movements or transitions from one position to another, or for exploration. Gross motor development in normal children is known to require learning through doing, moving, and feeling. Sensory, vestibular, and tactile input are all required to produce varied and competent motor output. Static positioning, which occurs when some adaptive equipment is used excessively, can retard motor development by modifying sensory input and limiting spontaneous movement activity.

A carefully developed plan for therapeutic use of a piece of adaptive equipment must take into consideration not only the potential benefit but also the potential deleterious effects. Normal motor development relies on coordination of both agonist and antagonist muscle groups to complete a pattern of movement. Adaptive equipment tends to "fix" a child into one pattern, albeit therapeutic, while denying the opportunity to experience the competing or antagonist pattern. For example, a side-lyer provides an opportunity for the child to play while placed in a neutral, midline orientation. Although a neutral, midline orientation may be an appropriate goal, it is important to note that an asymmetric orientation is not inherently bad or undesirable. An asymmetric orientation is a normal precursor to weight shifting, lateral flexion, and lateral rotation. The pathologic or abnormal pattern or orientation may compete with the pattern facilitated by the equipment. Although the competing pattern may be abnormal, the therapist is responsible for teaching normal or "balanced" movement patterns.

The person who places the child in a position must be aware of the benefits of various positions and must avoid constant and unchanging positioning habits. Inappropriate use of equipment, which places the child in static postures, can also lead to other complications, such as joint contracture, which may eventually require surgical repair, or skin breakdown. Anyone who has responsibility for the child must understand the therapeutic goals and must monitor equipment use to maximize the benefits and minimize the deleterious effects.

Poor Planning

Poor planning for growth can lead to misuse of equipment. With the current difficulty experienced in receiving authorization for third-party payment for expensive equipment for the physically challenged child, the therapist must anticipate and plan carefully for both the physical and developmental growth of the child. The inexperienced therapist may overlook the changing needs of the child. A child who requires positioning in sitting during the early years may be given an expensive chair that will provide fine positioning and optimal use of the upper extremities for fine motor skills. However, despite the initial advantages of the chair, it may be inappropriate for future mobility and socialization needs. Predicting the child's needs in the areas of growth and development, education, and recreational alternatives (e.g., wheelchair sports) is a monumental task, but one in which physical therapists must often participate at the request of insurers and local and state funding agencies.

Therapists must learn how various agencies and providers prefer to reconcile those requirements and reimbursement patterns with the patient's needs. Some providers prefer devices that, although more frequently replaced than costlier items, are more cost-effective at the outset. Other providers prefer an initial, larger expenditure for a device that will last for 3 to 5 years. These considerations must be addressed in order to meet the child's best interest. The consequences of miscalculations in these decisions will be a child who is poorly accommodated in an ill-fitting device that does not meet his or her current needs. In such instances, the therapist must then explore difficult alternatives, such as borrowing or adapting old equipment, until the patient is eligible for new equipment. The growth potential of various pieces of equipment is discussed later in this chapter. Clearly, growth and developmental considerations are a critical aspect when selecting adaptive equipment.

Equipment Use Versus Facilitation

The use of equipment in place of facilitation of the development of nonassisted skills is a concern relating to adaptive equipment. We have already discussed how positioning devices may not allow for "balanced" development. Unfortunately, many therapists and parents are biased toward the idea that, because there are so many equipment options, equipment is equivalent to therapy. The child is thus "plugged into" many types of equipment (e.g., progressing from high chair to car seat to side-lyer to stander). Although each piece of equipment allows the child to challenge current patterns and to develop alternative patterns, the equipment is not a substitute for treatment. Equipment restricts the two types of experiences of learning—active motor transitions and movement for exploration—which are the ultimate goals of normal motor development. Some therapists believe that a child who is poorly fitted for adaptive equipment or a child who uses no adaptive equipment receives more treatment through oral feedback and handling (to reposition) than the child who is "well-equipped." That belief advocates neither malpositioning nor denial of needed equipment to maximize therapeutic input; rather, it suggests that, just as appropriate equipment can be useful for satisfying the overall needs of a child, overuse or misuse of equipment can be detrimental.

Safety Issues

Ensuring the safe and correct use of the equipment is a top priority. Caregivers, and the child when he or she is age appropriate, must be taught the correct methods of donning and doffing equipment. Strategies such as color coding and numbering straps (to make sure they are fastened to the proper end point and in the proper sequence) help avoid mistakes in donning the device. This is particularly helpful when caregivers in addition to the parents are involved, such as grandparents, babysitters, day-care staff, teachers, and teacher's aides.

Another safety issue relates specifically to mobility equipment. Equipment that gives a nonlocomotive child the ability to locomote requires attention to the environment in which the equipment is used as well as attention to the child's cognitive and judgment abilities. If the equipment makes it possible for the child to maneuver in an area of the home in which he or she could not maneuver previously, is the area adequately childproofed? Or in the case of a motorized wheelchair instead of a manual wheelchair, does the child exhibit sufficient judgment to use the motorized chair safely, regarding both his or her own safety and the safety of others?

Psychosocial Issues

Although carefully selected and fitted adaptive equipment can open many otherwise closed doors and increase a child's independence, the use of equipment can be psychosocially disadvantageous. Often equipment, especially extensive equipment, has a way of drawing attention to a child's disabilities and therefore his or her differences. Children tend to be honest, sometimes brutally so. Adaptive equipment, or anything else that separates a child from peers, can be emotionally and socially challenging for the child with a disability.

In addition to socially and psychologically separating a child from others, adaptive equipment can actually physically separate a child. A child who is strapped into plastic, vinyl, wood, and metal seems to be the recipient of fewer hugs and physical affection. This may be simply because of the physical barriers provided by the equipment, but it may also be the result of adults who are intimidated by the equipment and the child and are fearful of "disturbing something" if they get too close to the child.

Determining a Child's Equipment Needs

The therapist who provides routine, continuing care for the disabled child is often not the same therapist responsible for purchasing adaptive equipment. Sometimes, because of the size or nature of the facility at which the child receives routine treatment, a referral to a larger, more well-equipped institution may be appropriate to determine equipment needs. Whether the child is referred to a children's hospital, to a wheelchair clinic in a major medical center, or directly to the vendor's establishment, the provision of appropriate apparatus depends mainly on detailed and accurate information about both the child and the child's environment. The primary therapist should be present during the evaluation for equipment to give an accurate assessment of the child's needs. If the therapist is unable to attend, a report with an assessment of the child's needs and a recommendation for choices of equipment must be included in the referral.

A standardized initial assessment is required whether a therapist is serving in a primary care or a consulting role. The therapist should assess the child in relation to a specific piece of apparatus. Because of time restrictions, the assessment may concentrate on one specific type of equipment or functional need (e.g., sitting), and additional assessments may be required for other equipment needs. Once a piece of equipment has been received, the therapist must examine the child to ensure that the apparatus suits the child, that it meets the identified goals, and that those people who will be using the equipment understand its correct use.

Initial Evaluation

The parameters to be considered when evaluating a child's need for adaptive equipment are similar to those of most other evaluations. The goal of such an evaluation, however, is to clarify and direct the therapist to the most appropriate equipment options available. The following specific items should be considered in the evaluation.

RANGE OF MOTION

Range of motion (ROM) is important in selecting almost all equipment because accommodating the patient in most apparatuses will depend on adequate ROM and joint mobility. The device being considered will dictate the motions that are necessary for success.

Critical ranges of motion for using adaptive devices include adequate head and neck rotation to bring head to midline, trunk rotation to achieve trunk symmetry, a minimum of 90 degrees hip and knee flexion for functional sitting, and plantigrade feet (neutral dorsiflexion/plantarflexion) for standing and use of footrests or the floor when sitting.

MUSCLE TONE, CONTROL, AND STRENGTH

Muscle tone, control, and strength deserve careful consideration when selecting equipment. The degree of strength or motor control needed for functional use of the device must be determined. For example, use of a manually controlled wheelchair requires strength and coordination of the upper extremities. If the child does not have adequate upper extremity function, or if the child is functioning asymmetrically, a manually controlled wheelchair is an inappropriate choice. A motorized device that does not require the strength needed for a manually controlled chair may be more useful for the child. A motorized chair also has options for control that do not require any upper extremity function. A specific, detailed assessment by an experienced technician can help the therapist identify alternative methods to attain optimal management of the equipment. In the example of a motorized device, strength is only one determinant of success. One must also evaluate cognitive, visuomotor, perceptual, and social functions as well as child's judgment abilities.

Positioning devices, such as standers, sidelyers, and seats, require little strength or motor control but often have a modifying effect on muscle tone that must be examined. The child's orientation to gravity will have significant bearing on muscle tone when the child tries to assume an upright position. Therefore, in addition to active muscle control and strength, the therapist must assess patterns of involuntary movement and evaluate the child with regard to spasticity, athetosis, flexor predominance, or extensor predominance.

Is the movement pattern of mild, moderate, or severe magnitude? Does the patient have cortical control manifested by a voluntary ability to initiate and complete the pattern of motion? A child positioned in a prone stander and tilted slightly forward from a vertical position may show increased extensor tone in an attempt to achieve an upright position against the force of gravity. Increased scapular retraction and hyperextension of the neck may have detrimental side effects in the patient with hypertonia. The child who has a strong extension pattern may show reduced tone when sitting in a chair that is reclined 15 degrees from an upright position. Although the child may not demonstrate optimal upper extremity function when tipped back, this position may suit him or her better for transportation in a car or bus. Appreciation of particular short-term goals for such a child is important for proper selection of positioning. The tilted chair would be unacceptable for use in the classroom but very useful for improving mobility.

REFLEXES

A change of position with respect to gravity will also influence the child whose motor patterns are dominated by reflexes. The prone or supine position may increase or decrease the tonic labyrinthine reflex. Side-lying may facilitate the asymmetric tonic lumbar reflex. Because inadvertent facilitation of primitive reactions may create a block in the normal developmental pattern, each piece of equipment should be evaluated for its effect on reflexes. For example, some devices for mobility, such as bicycles, may aggravate a persistent asymmetric tonic neck reflex. As the child pushes the pedal with the right foot, the head is turned toward the right side to enhance the effectiveness of the push. The child reverses this pattern when pushing with the left foot. Only in unusual circumstances would a therapist choose to use a technique that encourages using obligatory reflexes. The use of devices to restrict or inhibit primitive reflexes is more common, thus providing an opportunity for the development of more normal and symmetric patterns of movement.

SENSATION

Although it is unusual for a child with cerebral palsy to have a major sensory deficit, children with myelomeningocele, or other impairments with compromised sensation to touch in the lower extremities and trunk, offer tremendous challenges to the therapist attempting to develop a program involving the use of adaptive equipment. Priorities for the child with myelomeningocele include providing safe, pressure-tolerant seating and upright positioning. The therapist must have a thorough knowledge of the patient's sensation in order to achieve these goals. The patient and family should be consulted with regard to sensation, as they usually have a keen awareness of the sensory loss, as well as potential danger zones. This situation is particularly true for the older child. Particular attention must be paid to bony prominences, including the ischial tuberosities, greater trochanters, sacrum, knees, and heels, as well as the skin over the spinal lesion. These bony prominences also must be monitored in a child with intact sensation but limited ability to reposition him- or herself because of poor motor control, weakness, or severe spasticity.

PERCEPTION, COGNITION, AND SOCIAL/EMOTIONAL FACTORS

Most physical therapists are not trained specifically to assess perception, cognition, or social/emotional development; as a result, these areas are often ignored. This is a serious omission for the pediatric patient, whose prognosis for function with adaptive equipment often depends more on perception, cognitive function, and social/emotional skills than on physical abilities. Motivation, intelligence, and normal perception often overcome even severe physical impairments. The opposite is also true. Limitations in perception, cognition, or social/emotional skills may result in function that is lower than would be predicted by physical findings alone. In order to develop realistic goals for a child, the therapist must know the "whole" child and must integrate information from the teacher, social worker, occupational therapist, and psychologist into the therapeutic plan.

FUNCTION

Functional skills are both important and difficult to assess because they require integration of all other information in an attempt to determine why a child behaves in a certain manner. The therapist must discover what the child does and how he or she achieves a goal, and why the child does not do more. If the therapist does not evaluate the child in this manner, it is probably impossible to develop appropriate goals for treatment and to select appropriate adaptive equipment. For example, some children tend to "bunny hop" rather than creep. It is important to know if this tendency to "bunny hop" is secondary to a strong symmetric tonic neck reflex, weakness in the extensors of the hip and knee, or both. Treatment would be different for the two problems.

A similar thought process should be used when deciding whether or not the child needs equipment. For example, if a 2-year-old child is not rolling or exploring the environment, is a device aimed at improving mobility an appropriate goal? The therapist must first assess whether the child is cognitively disabled and, therefore, disinterested in the environment; whether the child is afraid of mobility because of visual impairment; whether the child has a strong neck reflex or hypertonia that poses physical limitations; or whether the child has been placed in devices that limit the opportunity to develop independent mobility at home. If this information is not acquired and assimilated, realistic recommendations for equipment cannot be made. Only when working with a child who is severely limited by tone and reflexes would it be appropriate to turn immediately to adaptive devices for remediation.

The child with profound cognitive deficits may not gain from the use of equipment because the child will need to deal with both the device and the environment. In order to allow the visually impaired child to manipulate the environment, we need to improve methods for exploration of that environment. Equipment may add another obstacle that the visually impaired child must overcome. When the child lacks experience in exploring the environment, the therapist must offer as much freedom of movement and equipment-free mobility as is possible. Although equipment may eventually play a role in each of these situations, adaptive equipment should not be the first type of treatment used. Adaptive equipment should supplement and complement function with the least amount of restriction of the child.

The child who is physically limited may show great improvement in cognitive ability, social interaction, and independence when mobility is improved. When adaptive equipment or devices are used judiciously, this improvement in mobility should occur without increases in abnormal reflexes or patterns of movement.

Evaluation of ROM, muscle tone, motor control, strength, reflexes, perception, cognition, and social/emotional status is an integral component of the assessment of the child. Only when these parameters are considered and we understand why a child is behaving in a particular manner can we treat the child effectively, including recommending appropriate adaptive equipment.

Once the goals for the device and the type of device being considered are identified, the therapist should evaluate the family and school environments. Goals for the child must be compatible with the goals of the caregivers at home and school. Because adaptive equipment is often used in several settings, there may be many conflicts and problems to solve while trying to achieve the short- and long-term goals for the child. Problems may arise for the child who is institutionalized or in a school placement. For example, the ability to teach the correct use of equipment to members of a changing or rotating staff is a major consideration. Ease of maintenance and minimizing the number of easily lost parts are additional considerations in institutional care.

Assessment of the Home and Family

Useful information can be obtained by asking the family about its expectations for the apparatus being considered. This opportunity for members of the family to express their opinions promotes a dialogue between family and therapist whereby the therapist can determine whether the family goals are realistic or whether compromises are necessary. Objective data about the family should encompass the following categories and questions:

1. *Physical layout of the dwelling.* The therapist should seek to answer the following questions:
   - Is the dwelling a house or apartment?
   - How many steps are found in the home?
   - Is there easy access to the home from the outdoors (i.e., no stairs, availability of an elevator, etc.)?
   - How large are the rooms?
   - Can equipment for mobility be used in the home?
   - Is there space for equipment use and storage?
   - How wide are the doorways?
   - Are the floors carpeted?
   - Are bathrooms, tubs, and toilets accessible?
2. *Community.* The therapist should determine whether the family lives in an urban, suburban, or rural community in order to assess the availability of and options for transportation and socialization. Knowing the availability of privately owned vehicles and/or public transportation is important when the therapist is considering mobility equipment. Also important are such issues as the weight of the device, its versatility on various surfaces, and its ease of transport, all of which must be tailored to the child's living conditions.
3. *Socioeconomic factors.* The cost of equipment may have a serious impact on the final decision regarding apparatus for the physically challenged child. When making a decision about buying adaptive equipment, the therapist, in conjunction with the social worker, must examine insurance coverage, other third-party payment systems, funding agen-

cies within the community, and potential rental options. Size of the family, daily routine, and the time available for the child with special needs as well as potential options for additional help, must be considered. Compliance with the suggested use of adaptive equipment may ultimately be the main issue to be considered in the decision to obtain the equipment. If there is little realistic expectation, based on many of the aforementioned issues, that the child will benefit from having the equipment, there may be little justification for its purchase.

School Assessment

When assessing a child's need for equipment, the physical therapist must consider the school setting in which the child may spend a large portion of the day. It is important to determine whether the child is enrolled in a special school or mainstreamed into a regular classroom. In a special school, teachers and staff are usually very open to suggestions and are well-equipped to handle any devices being considered. It is often these teachers who initiate the purchase or procurement of the equipment, and they are eager to learn and work with the child.

When the child is mainstreamed—attending a regular school—teachers and other staff may be reluctant to accept adaptive equipment because of their limited experience with special apparatus. This reluctance of the staff may be related not only to the health and developmental needs of the child, but also to concerns about the time, space, liability for, and acceptability of these devices in a classroom of children without handicapping conditions. A thoughtful compromise is often necessary in order to meet the physical, educational, emotional, and social goals of the disabled child.

Examples of equipment that might be recommended for use in the classroom include the following:

1. Special chairs, seating devices, or adaptations to the regular desk chair
2. Wheelchair lapboards
3. Wheelchair or desk easels
4. Standing frames, tables, and prone standers
5. Wedges for seating in chairs
6. Wedges or bolsters for positioning on the floor

The physical therapist can be a valuable resource person for teachers and other staff by making suggestions and helping procure equipment that can enhance a child's educational experience. Often, a piece of adaptive equipment can make the difference between a child feeling fully included in, rather than excluded from, classroom work and activities.

Summary

Clearly, there are many aspects to consider in determining a child's need for adaptive equipment. The following case study should clarify both the dynamics of the problems involved in selection of equipment and the thought processes and compromises involved in developing rational solutions to these problems.

Equipment Selection

When the evaluation of the child is completed and goals are established, the types of equipment available, or alternatively, the practicality of making equipment, are determined.

Purchasing Equipment

Many companies make devices and equipment that are identical in concept. Criteria that must be considered in choosing a specific device include the following:

1. *Dimensions of the apparatus.* The device should not only be adequate when purchased

Case Study—Ellen, 5 Year Old with a Spastic Diplegia Pattern of Motor Function Secondary to Cerebral Palsy.

Ellen is a 5-year-old girl with a spastic diplegia pattern of motor function secondary to cerebral palsy. She was integrated into a normal elementary school. Ellen is intelligent and alert, and she enjoys all aspects of her school routine. Ellen's classroom teacher has two main concerns about Ellen. First, although Ellen is ambulatory, her gait is slow and labored, making it difficult for her to walk to classes in distant locations in the school building. Class trips have also been a problem for Ellen. The teacher's second major concern is Ellen's socialization during recess. Because mobility is a large part of the recess activity, Ellen's limited mobility makes socialization difficult. Ellen's mother was notified of the teacher's concerns, and she sought help from Ellen's physical therapist. Ellen receives treatment twice a week from her therapist, who is aware of Ellen's strengths and limitations. Ellen's mother presented to the physical therapist the concerns of the teacher and her own personal concerns. These additional concerns included the fact that Ellen recently had a growth spurt and has become increasingly difficult to lift and carry. This new difficulty occurs mainly when the family goes on outings. It has also become difficult for Ellen to keep up with her active older brother and with her 3-year-old sister. Although mobility in the family's split level home in the suburbs has not been a problem. Ellen rarely plays outside because the children who live closet to her and who are the same age live several blocks away. Therefore, the family car is needed to transport Ellen almost everywhere she needs to go.

Ellen's therapist must satisfy the needs of the child, the family, and the school. Although the school's needs suggest that independent mobility is important and could be achieved with a properly fitted wheelchair, the family does not presently need this equipment. Because Ellen is ambulatory within the home and has help when she goes out with her family, a large, lightweight, easily folding modified umbrella stroller should be adequate. The difference in price between the two items is several hundred dollars, but each device has advantages and disadvantages. Ellen's therapist chose a systematic approach to the problem. She re-evaluated Ellen and added to her own list of goals those concerns expressed by the school and family. The list was as follows:

Problems

1. ROM—presently within normal limits. Tightness in hip and knee flexors is increasing as Ellen grows taller.

Intervention Strategies

a. Daily ROM exercises
b. Night splints to maintain ROM
c. Frequent positional changes; avoidance of long periods of sitting

Problems

2. Tone, control, and strength—inadequate antigravity back extensor and abdominal control for normal gait, causing trunk reversal. Poor endurance; moderate spastic extensor pattern in lower extremities; poor control when movement is isolated out of pattern; asymmetry of involvement, with right side more spastic and shortened.

Intervention Strategies

a. Weakly outpatient treatments
b. Training in upright and other positions to use more normal movement pattern
c. Positioning to avoid asymmetry
d. Avoidance of positions or activities that increase fixing and extensor pattern
e. Family education and home program

Problems

3. Social and emotional development—copes well with disability; unable to participate in many group activities at home and school, especially those requiring mobility; encouragement and facilitation of progress in social and emotional development will be both the problem and the goal.

(continued)

Case Study—Ellen, 5 Year Old with a Spastic Diplegia Pattern of Motor Function Secondary to Cerebral Palsy. (Continued)

Intervention Strategies

a. Provide alternative means of mobility
b. Educate and support patient in developing strategies for coping with and compensating for disability

Problems

4. Functional ability—able to ambulate functionally and independently but with poor endurance; poor reciprocal movement of the lower extremities secondary to abnormal extensor tone; poor weight shifting as a result of weak antigravity trunk muscles; independently makes transition from prone→supine→sitting→standing.

Intervention Strategies

a. Treatment to reduce extensor tone and maintain adequate ROM
b. Improve strength and control of trunk musculature
c. Gait training
d. Home training in proper movement pattern for gait
e. Avoidance of activities that will increase asymmetry and tone of extensor muscle groups

After the reevaluation and generation of this list of problems, Ellen's therapist was more confident about the decision to purchase the modified umbrella-type stroller with adequate support to achieve proper positioning and alignment.

1. With ROM a potential problem for Ellen, increased sitting time had to be discouraged and positional changes encouraged. Because the stroller does not offer independent mobility, Ellen would not enjoy sitting in the stroller for a long time.
2. Although a wheelchair provides more options for positioning in symmetric alignment using lateral pads, these attachments provide passive positioning and do not encourage active work on righting and equilibrium. Because Ellen was able to right herself with facilitation by verbal feedback or light tapping, Ellen's therapist believed that lateral supports were excessive and not indicated. The stroller must provide a firm seat and back support in order to allow Ellen to align herself properly.
3. When Ellen was tested for upper extremity function using a loaner wheelchair, the results suggested that a wheelchair would not be useful. The result of attempts at propulsion with the upper extremities was an overflow of tone into the lower extremities. This overflow increased extensor tone in the lower extremities and caused increased asymmetry in Ellen's trunk. This response was considered to be counterproductive to gait, and the possibility of propulsion in a wheelchair was ruled out for the present time.
4. Because Ellen has not complained of feeling left out or rejected in classroom activities and because she appears to be well adjusted to school without a wheelchair, independent mobility does not seem to be an important issue to her. Although the teacher has a valid concern about Ellen's mobility, the issue does not interfere with Ellen's social or emotional wellbeing. Periodic reevaluation, however, is necessary.
5. Because Ellen's family transports her in the family car where she is stable and comfortable wearing a standard seatbelt, a wheelchair is probably too heavy and cumbersome for their needs. The modified umbrella-type stroller is more practical for transporting Ellen. The stroller tends, however, to infantilize Ellen, who deserves to be treated as an increasingly mature and responsible person. Should Ellen's parents show signs of having difficulty accepting her disability or should they treat her as an infant or overprotect her unnecessarily, reconsideration of the stroller compared with the wheelchair might be appropriate. Ellen's family realizes that, although she is ambulatory and intelligent, she will continue to be restricted by her physical limitations and will require special considera-

(continued)

Case Study—Ellen, 5 Year Old with a Spastic Diplegia Pattern of Motor Function Secondary to Cerebral Palsy. (Continued)

tions. They also realize that her emotional health and development require that the family relate to Ellen as often as possible, and in the same manner as the other children. The umbrella-type stroller meets both Ellen's needs and the needs of the family without jeopardizing her normal social and emotional development.

6. Ellen's physical therapist had a final insight after reevaluating the child's equipment needs. The therapist realized that a possible third option—a three-wheeled motorized scooter (see below) might be most appropriate for Ellen's future mobility. The three-wheeled scooter is often used as an outdoor mobility device for ambulators with limited endurance or difficulty negotiating rough surfaces and terrain. This device is lighter in weight than standard motorized devices and is much more manageable (i.e., it can be placed in a car). The physical effort required to use the scooter is less than the effort required to propel a manual wheelchair, and so the undesirable asymmetry and increased tone observed when Ellen propelled a standard wheelchair could be avoided. By introducing this device to Ellen and her family, the therapist could help clarify whether the scooter would be acceptable to all concerned. If the scooter was deemed acceptable, the umbrella-type stroller would still be a valuable addition for short excursions or as a back-up device should the scooter malfunction (as from a dead battery).

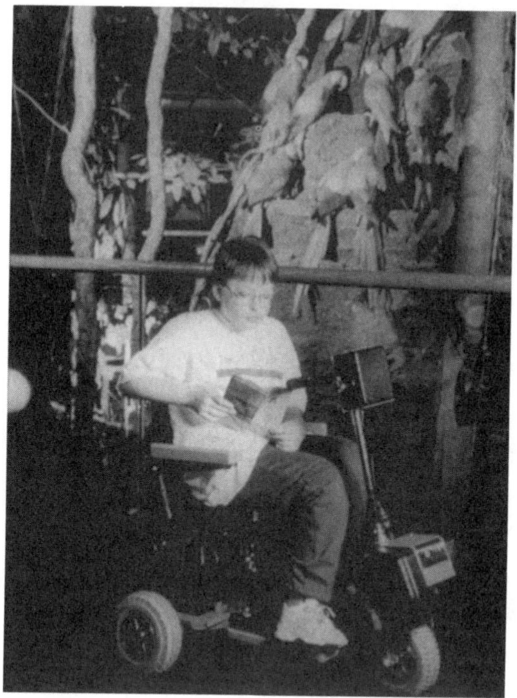

Ellen's therapist telephoned the classroom teacher to discuss the reasons for using an umbrella stroller both at school and at home. After an appropriate explanation, the teacher agreed with this solution on a temporary basis. The teacher reserved the right to present the issue again, if necessary. Constant reevaluation of all aspects of Ellen's physical, cognitive, psychological, and social development was agreed on. Any significant changes would require a reassessment of the decision.

but should also, if feasible, allow for some future growth. Some equipment have a built-in system for extending or enlarging the device. The therapist must determine which company makes the particular size best suited for each child.

2. *Availability of optional adaptations:* Are there parts that help improve the fit and specificity of the device? Are these options cost-effective, easily adjusted, and durable?
3. *Reputation of the manufacturer.* Is the product covered by a guarantee? Has the company

previously provided support when problems with equipment have arisen? Is service readily available and is equipment for trial use available? Will a company representative train or instruct the staff in optimal use of the device?

4. *Promptness of delivery.* Is the product kept in stock by most local vendors or medical supply houses? Is there a backlog of orders that will delay the equipment's delivery? Is the product custom-made?
5. *Cost.* Is the price reasonable for the anticipated use of the product, or will less expensive alternatives provide the same benefits?
6. *Aesthetics.* Is the device cosmetically acceptable to the patient and family, or will it be rejected on this basis?
7. *Weight, size, and manageability.* Is the device easy to use, and can it be stored? Can it be transported if necessary? (That is, does it fold or disassemble in some way?)

Brochures or catalogs available from the manufacturer or vendor will provide much of this information. Local vendors who may have extensive experience with the equipment can help in answering many questions. Physical therapists in local hospitals or in the community can recommend vendors or specific salespeople. The therapist should not feel obligated to order from any person in particular. Although one salesperson might be knowledgeable about wheelchairs, another person may have more experience with positioning devices or self-help equipment.

Anyone procuring or fabricating equipment on a regular basis should keep records on the various devices, manufacturers, and vendors they use. Records should indicate ease of fit, wear of the device (how well it holds up over time), acceptance or criticism from patients and family, and the efficiency of customer service, including the elapsed time from placement of an order to delivery of equipment. Records may be kept on computer or in card catalog form (or some similar system), and may be a useful resource for future recommendations and orders. In addition, the catalog file may provide the basis for quantitative data regarding benefits and deficits of various adaptive devices. Perhaps the compilation of these data can serve to help the profession evolve from an art to science.

Making Equipment

The decision to make equipment is based on many variables that must be considered carefully.

PERSONNEL

Will physical therapists be building the equipment themselves, or will they be serving as consultants to other builders? Other people who might build equipment for children include commercial woodworkers, woodworking hobbyists, volunteer organizations with appropriately skilled members, and the child's parents. If the therapists build the apparatus, how will their schedules allow for this time expenditure? Will patients be canceled or will special time be allotted? Will overtime hours be needed? If the physical therapist is a consultant, how will this time be allocated and at what expense? If other people are building the equipment, will they be compensated, and if so, by whom? Will parents pay directly, or will insurance companies pay the cost? Will the facility offering the services assume the cost? Will permission be given to build the equipment only after approval by third-party payers of the needed funding, or will the facility assume the cost in the hope that funds will be forthcoming? Who will bear the cost if funds are unavailable?

SPACE

Is adequate space available for building the apparatus on the premises? If space is available, will the safety and comfort of patients be compromised by this building site? Building is noisy, dirty, and potentially dangerous because of the tools and materials used. Ventilation must be provided if fumes from toxic paint or varnish are expected. This item may be a major problem when working with children with lung disease.

COST

A decision must be made initially about the cost-effectiveness of making equipment. Items that must be accounted for include tools, space needs, building materials, time for planning and designing, time for measuring and building, and time away from patient care. In making a decision, the advantages of customized equipment must be weighed against the expense of designing, planning, and building the apparatus. Will adapting a commercially available device be the best compromise?

FAILURES

Can and will the facility absorb the loss in revenue that accrues from equipment that is inadvertently incorrectly fitted or that appears to be inappropriate when completed? This issue of equipment failure must be considered, because even the most experienced equipment technician will make mistakes.

TIMING AND SETTING

An advantage of custom-made devices is evident when equipment is needed immediately. Therapist-fabricated equipment is usually available in days or weeks rather than the months often required for bureaucracies to approve, fund, order, and receive the equipment. Building the equipment might also be an attractive alternative when the device is required only for one specific setting, such as the classroom, but not for transport or home use.

SUMMARY

Despite the potential drawbacks, many therapists still choose customized equipment. Customization may be particularly useful for the young child who is growing rapidly and for the child whose need is only temporary. In each of these situations, a simply made piece of equipment could satisfy the short-term needs of the patient. The child could use the fabricated equipment until he or she outgrows it, at which time another piece could be made, or if growth has slowed, a commercially available piece could be substituted. One of the main reasons for building equipment is that commercially available equipment often does not satisfy the needs of a child with unique problems. Recently, however, manufacturers have shown an increased interest in children with physical impairments, which has resulted in a wider variety of and improvements in apparatuses.

Selection of Materials

Adaptive equipment can be built using various materials, each of which has unique qualities, advantages, and disadvantages. Personal preference often plays a major role in the decision to use a particular type of material. Although each material has its specific properties, most can be adapted to various uses. Some materials are lighter in weight, some are easier to use, some are easier to wash and keep clean, and some are more durable. Because none of the products is perfect, the therapist should have knowledge of several different materials. The therapist can try to match the material's advantages to the specific needs of the child. Wood, triwall, and Adaptafoam are materials used commonly by pediatric therapists.

WOOD

Wood is inexpensive, durable, and available, but requires a moderate measure of skill. Large work areas are required because wood has a "messy" quality and requires many different hand and power tools, some of which are expensive. Many therapists prefer to have professional carpenters construct adaptive devices from wood because of the level of skill required. Parents, however, are

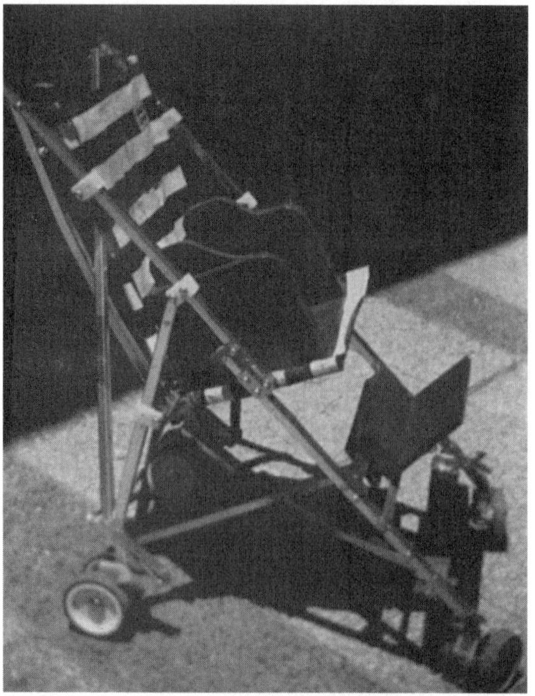

Figure 9-1 ▪ Umbrella-type stroller with a triwall insert and foot support.

often familiar with woodworking, and a therapist may enlist the help of such a parent, providing plans and specifications for the equipment needed. Fabrication by family members can be a rewarding and satisfying means of helping in the care of their child. Wooden equipment is often heavy, but it is also durable. Strength and durability are important qualities when material is to be used by a larger child. Wooden devices often need padding for comfort, and either painting, varnishing, or sealing for protection against liquids. Wood is often used for making inserts for seats, side-lyers, prone standers, and various ingenious mobility toys.

TRIWALL

Triwall consists of triple-thickness corrugated cardboard that is lightweight, firm, and inexpensive. Triwall is fast and easy to use, although its use requires an electric sabre saw (or other saw), glue gun, and hand tools, such as a hammer, screwdriver, and utility knife. Although it is not waterproof, triwall can be treated with acrylic latex paint or fabric for sealing and preservation. Triwall is less durable than wood, which makes it most appropriate for temporary or trial pieces of equipment, or for children who are growing rapidly (Fig. 9-1). Like wood, triwall is a firm, solid medium and may require padding for comfort. Many therapists consider triwall useful for making customized chairs that must be measured precisely for the child. A "bolster-type" chair available commercially and a similar chair made from triwall are shown in Figures 9-2 and 9-3. Although selection of a design and measuring the child and the triwall are time-consuming chores, actual building with triwall is a fast process. Working with this material is noisy, messy, and potentially dangerous because of the tools. A separate workplace

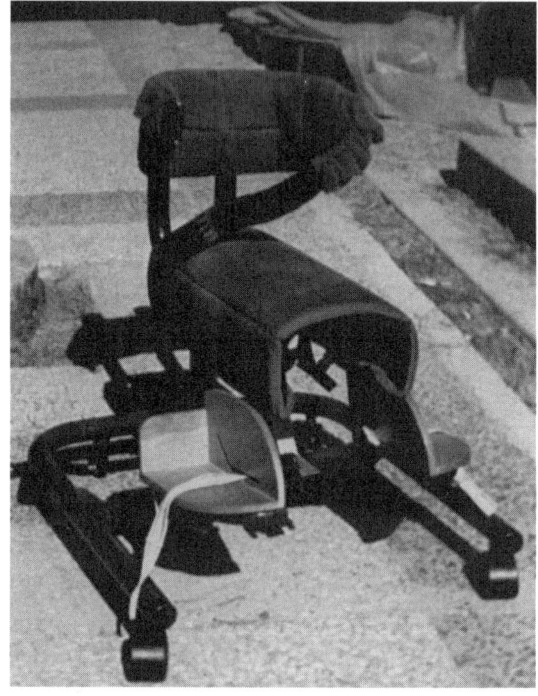

Figure 9-2 ▪ Commercially made "bolster" chair.

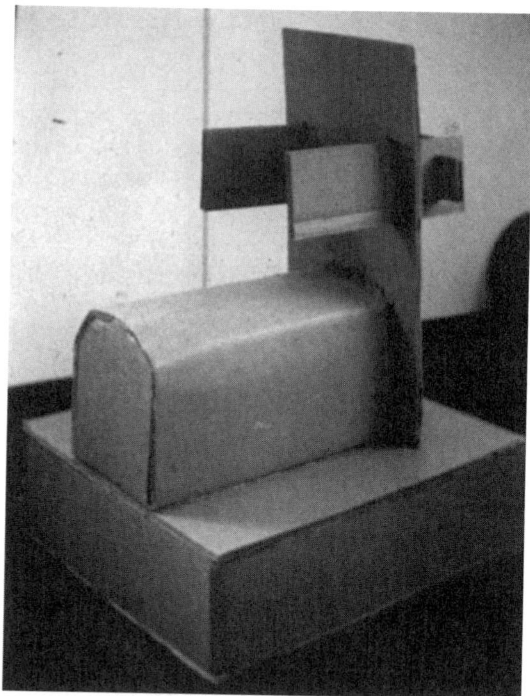

Figure 9-3 ▪ Triwall alternative to the commercially made bolster chair shown in Figure 9-2.

is recommended. As with wood, family members and volunteers can be recruited to make apparatuses from triwall. Special training is usually necessary, and many parents are reluctant to try because of fear of mistakes and failure. Some judicious support and praise for the family member can help overcome reluctance, and the parent may become an essential part of the team that is making the adaptive equipment for the child. A seating insert made from triwall is shown in Figure 9-4.

ADAPTAFOAM

Adaptafoam is another commonly used medium for pediatric equipment because it is a dense, nonporous, nontoxic foam that is both fast and easy to use, but is more expensive than wood or triwall. The need for tools is minimal (e.g., heat gun, electric knife, and utility knife). Although a work area is useful, Adaptafoam is less messy than wood or triwall and poses less risk because of the limited use of tools. A special coating—Adaptavinyl—is the only paint that can be used, and its safe application requires excellent ventilation. However, because Adaptafoam is nonporous, it can be left unpainted and cleaned with soap and water when it becomes soiled. Covers can be made for the apparatus if the family prefers. Adaptafoam is available in several dimensions and different densities. With some experience, a physical therapist can determine the best use of the various types of Adaptafoam. Adaptafoam is easy to use because it bonds to itself when heated for a short time. Glue and nails are unnecessary. However, this self-bonding property loses some attractiveness when Adaptafoam is used with other material, such as wood, to which Adaptafoam will not bond.

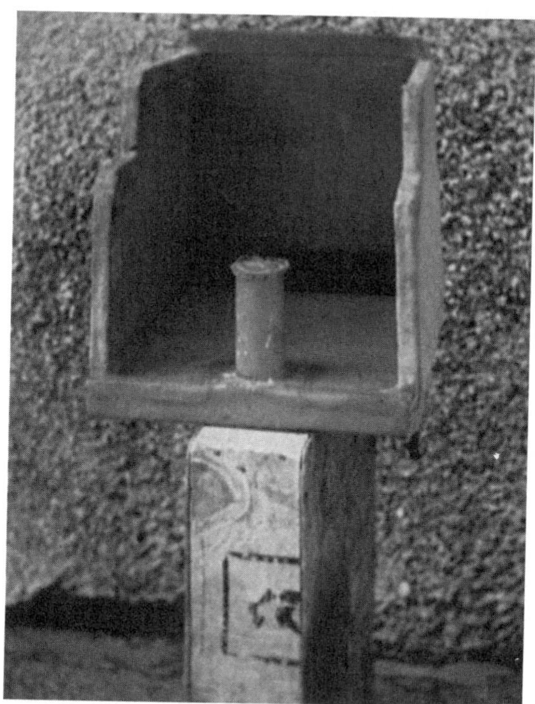

Figure 9-4 ▪ Triwall seat insert.

Adaptafoam is commonly used to make prone-lyers, seats, inserts, small standers, and various components, including headrests and utensil handles for other apparatuses. Adaptafoam, unlike triwall, is easy to adjust for growth by inserting an additional piece of material when necessary. Like wood and triwall, Adaptafoam provides a firm surface and may need to be padded or covered to improve comfort.

Commonly Used Equipment for Various Positions

We have already discussed general uses for equipment as adjuncts to treatment. We have noted that physiologic benefits will accrue when equipment is properly conceived and frequent changes of position are used. Among those benefits are inhibition of pathologic tone, reduction of abnormal reflexes, and prevention of soft tissue contractures. Let us now look more specifically at some of the issues involved in providing children with equipment to support various positions and activities—sitting, standing, and side-lying.

Sitting

GENERAL CONSIDERATIONS

The sitting position is optimal for function and, therefore, is important for the older child and adult. Although maintained sitting posture is a goal achieved by most normal infants before 1 year of age, sitting is used for prolonged function much later in life. By watching children in preschool and kindergarten, it is apparent that a goal of many teachers is maintenance of sitting for group activities. Children in the early school years who are younger than 7 years of age require frequent changes in position. They prefer to play and work in the prone position, standing by a table, and in other positions that easily allow for transitional movements and change. Sitting, as a position for optimal function, occurs only after the children "learn" to sit for prolonged periods of time. Sitting is defined as ". . . a position in which the weight of the trunk is transferred to the support area mainly by the ischial tuberosities and surrounding tissues."[1] Proper alignment in sitting is thought to improve patient function by providing an adequate and secure base, inhibiting abnormal tone, and improving perception of the environment. There are also significant social benefits to being upright and mobile.

Although there is a large body of literature devoted to seating for the pediatric age group, most of the material reports clinical experience and empirical data rather than controlled scientific data. The result of this lack of scientific documentation is poor standardization when evaluating and providing adaptive seating devices. Conflicts regarding the value of various positioning options could be more easily and completely resolved if a scientific basis existed for each option. Because the literature on pediatric seating is limited, we can, as an alternative, examine the adult literature and attempt to apply it to the pediatric age group. The factors that follow should be considered when evaluating a chair.

The first concern is the purpose of the chair. We know that chairs can be "function-specific." A lounge chair is uncomfortable when a person is eating a meal, yet a straight-backed chair with little padding is undesirable for relaxation. Similarly, a physical therapist must consider function when designing chairs for children with special needs. Many therapists believe that a custom-built chair is always preferable, but whether one is buying or making a chair, the following parameters, established for adults, should be considered.

SEAT

HEIGHT. The height of the chair seat should allow the feet to be placed flat on the floor or a foot rest. Height should be such that with feet flat, hips are flexed to at least 90 degrees. Slightly more hip flexion is even more desirable to prevent children from going into extensor posturing. Comfortable placement of the feet should prevent excessive pressure on the popliteal fossa caused by the front edge of the seat.[1,2]

DEPTH. The seat should be shallow enough to provide for flexion of the knee without pressure in the popliteal area and without slouching. Slouching negates contact of the lumbar region with the backrest, thus nullifying any gain offered by backrest options. The seat should be deep enough to allow maximal distribution of weight.[2]

Shallow-depth seats allow for hips to drop into less than 90 degrees flexion and also increase pressure per square inch on the posterior thighs where they are in contact with the seat. When hip flexion is less than 90 degrees, extensor spasticity may increase in some patients. Increased pressure means increased risk of skin breakdown.

PADDING. Padding helps to distribute pressure away from the 6-mm^2 surface of each ischial tuberosity that normally bears weight in sitting. This allows for increased sitting tolerance.[3,4] However, surfaces that are too soft increase the difficulty with which postural changes are made during sitting, and this lack of postural change can lead to back strain. Akerblom judged movement while sitting to be the most important requirement of a comfortable chair.[3] He designed a chair that allowed for various conditions (i.e., the trunk off of the support surface, sitting with lumbar support, or reclining back with both lumbar and thoracic support). These options reduce muscle strain and increase tolerance.[3]

BACK

Consideration must be given to trunk musculature and spinal ligaments in order to avoid back discomfort. The anterior and posterior longitudinal ligaments provide their best support with the back in neutral position. Increasing the normal lordosis may stretch the anterior longitudinal ligament, whereas exaggerated kyphosis will stretch the posterior longitudinal ligament and may cause posterior protrusion of degenerating intervertebral discs. These changes produce low back pain and cause difficulty in achieving the back extension needed to rise from sitting. In addition to the need for movement in the chair to prevent muscular fatigue, support for the weight of the trunk will reduce the muscular work of sitting. This support can be provided by a reclining backrest. Support for the lumbar curve and allowance for the posteriorly protruding sacrum and buttocks are also recommended. The height of the backrest need not extend above the shoulder. Freedom to change position and improved mobility are provided by limiting the height to this level.[5]

ARMRESTS

Armrests should be positioned to bear approximately 50% of the weight of the patient's arms. Armrests are also used by a person to change from a sitting to a standing position.

ANGLE OF THE BACK OF THE SEAT

The angle formed between the seat and backrest is most comfortable between 95 and 110 degrees. This angle may cause the person to slide forward, particularly a problem with increased extensor tone in the hips and back musculature. Using a wedged cushion, with the greatest height in the front, may help counteract this problem. Alternatively, the entire chair can be tilted back so that gravity pushes the patient back into the chair to avoid the problem of sliding. Attention to avoidance of pressure in the popliteal area is important when the chair is reclined.[1] Lumbar supports are also recommended for the reclined chair.

Not only the orthopedic and biomechanical needs of the child must be considered, but the effects of those needs on muscle tone, reflexes, and function must also be considered. Most therapists use an empirical or trial-and-error approach to determine good positioning for a particular child. Because most therapists agree that the pelvis is important for correct stabilization, the pelvis serves as the keystone for seating. Once the pelvis is aligned properly, the trunk, head, and lower extremities will have a more stable base. The specific approaches, options, and adaptations are too numerous to review here. However, the objectives of providing seated weight-bearing on the ischial tuberosities, as occurs with adults, and maintaining a slight lumbar lordosis, are reasonable expectations for the child.

Hip flexion of at least 90 degrees (slightly more being even better) during seating is advocated by many physical therapists, especially when seating the child with cerebral palsy.

The 90+ degree angle at the hips and knees will aid stabilization by providing solid weight-bearing on ischial tuberosities and feet. Furthermore, this position corrects sensory input and decreases the likelihood of posterior pelvic tilt that may result in increased dorsal kyphosis, scapular protraction, and hyperextension of the neck. Bergan suggests that normal wheelchair seats provide sensory feedback and a spatial orientation that the child is "backward."[6] One of the problems associated with this unusual sensory feedback and orientation is an increase in extensor tone thought to accompany the "sling" effect of most wheelchair seats. A firm seat and back should reduce the unwanted feedback and orientation.

In addition to altering the hip angle, the chair may be tilted, anteriorly or posteriorly, until the desired results of positioning are achieved. The issues of concern when making these adjustments continue to be pelvic alignment for stability while in a sitting position and the effects on tone of the various angles of the hip and of the seat itself. Nwaobi and colleagues, using electromyograms, found that orientation of the body and head in relation to gravity plays a significant role in controlling extensor activity.[7] Perception and hand function will also be altered as differing angles and positions are used. Therefore, an individualized approach, examining the effects of each change in position, will be necessary in determining optimal seating arrangements for children.

Once it appears that the various angles of hips, seat, and chair have been established and pelvic stability with minimal abnormal tone and reflexes has been achieved, the therapist must consider the trunk, head and neck, and the lower extremities of the child. Ninety degrees of knee flexion and good weight bearing on the feet should be encouraged to enhance stability. Too much weight-bearing on the plantar surface can result in a primitive extensor thrust pattern that will significantly reduce stability. Alignment of the trunk should encourage maximal symmetry, yet provide for movement and active postural adjustment. A headrest or supports should be used only if needed to improve positioning or to protect the child during mobility. The ultimate goal of the sitting position should be to align the child without restricting the movements and postural adjustments available to the child. Reassessment of the seating device is necessary when the patient's postural tone improves and skills are acquired.

CONSIDERATION OF THE SPECIFIC DISABILITY

The criteria and limits described for seating are applicable to all types of seating systems and for all disabilities. The emphasis changes with the disability, but the concepts are constant. Appropriate seating for the child with cerebral palsy, for instance, must take into consideration the effects on tone and abnormal reflexes. Padding and pressure relief warrant increased attention in the child with myelodysplasia. Height of armrests and enhancement of function are of great concern for the child with myopathy. The limitation of the seating devices and concerns regarding their use will be reasonably constant across disability groups. These limitations and precautions include limitation of joint motion secondary to static positioning; poor skin tolerance as a result of prolonged use of the seating device and a limited ability to change position; and reduced independent functional mobility resulting from abuse of seating devices.

WHEELCHAIRS

Providing a wheelchair for a patient requires an understanding and application of all the criteria previously discussed about proper alignment and positioning. It is also beneficial to know about the options available in purchasing a wheelchair and the compromises involved when selecting certain options over others.

Before continuing, it is worth stating that the wheelchair industry is in constant flux. This is why a well-informed and capable vendor or manufacturer's representative is critical to the rehabilitation team. The representative can provide information about changes and innovations in durable medical equipment (DME), as well as about the comparative adaptability, durability, cost, and features of wheelchairs and other equipment supplied by competing manufacturers.

It may be easiest to discuss options by looking at a typical order form for a pediatric chair (see Display 9-1). These forms are traditionally completed by the vendor, patient, and physical therapist working together to meet the patient's needs.

The first consideration is chair design. For independent mobilizers, two basic options exist—a *rigid frame or folding X-frame wheelchair*. Most people are familiar with a cross-braced folding wheelchair and opt for this type as it is easiest to transport in cars and store in home closets. The rigid-frame chair does not fold, but the wheels are removable and the back drops down, leaving a small box-type structure. The rigid-frame chair offers increased stability and ease of rolling, and it is always the chair of choice in sports and recreation. In many instances, once the child adjusts to it, families find the rigid chair to be as manageable as the folding chair. The disadvantage of the rigid-frame wheelchair is its limited growth adjustability resulting in it often being overlooked for the pediatric population. If properly fitted, however, in many instances it can provide years of use.*

In patients who are not independently mobile owing to cognitive function, upper extremity involvement, asymmetry, or other problems, a standard wheelchair may not be the best option. The vendor should be consulted regarding alternatives, which are beyond the scope of this chapter. For older, more intelligent, but more involved individuals with asymmetry or significant tone, a motorized device may be considered. *Three-wheeled scooters* are becoming increasingly popular and are often a wonderful alternative to motorized chairs. The scooters (Fig. 9-5) are much less expensive than a standard motorized wheelchair (approximately $2200+ versus $6000 to $15,000),† they break down to components that are lighter and easier to move from home to car, and they are relatively simple to learn to operate and maintain. Any seating system—from a simple standard molded plastic seat to the most elaborate custom-made system—can be adapted to the scooter. Of concern, however, is that the patient must have bilateral hand use and some degree of reach in order to hold the scooter's handle bars, push the accelerator, and steer. *Traditional motorized wheelchairs* are extremely heavy, do not dis-

*Modified rigid wheelchairs have now been devised that combine rigidity but allow for some growth. Additional information can be obtained from an informed vendor.

†Prices vary dramatically based on the seating and positioning options required and the need for additional electronic options.

DISPLAY 9-1

A Sample Order Form for a Pediatric Wheelchair

Effective July 5, 1993 **ORDER FORM**

Date: ____________ P.O.#: ____________
Buyer: ____________ Customer#: ____________

Bill To:
Name ____________
Mailing Address ____________
City ____________ State ______ Zip ______
Phone (______) ____________

☐ **Drop Ship/Ship To:**
Name ____________
Street Address ____________
City ____________ State ______ Zip ______
Phone (______) ____________ Marked For ____________

QUICKIE 2 ☐ ***Adult*** ☐ ***Kids***

COLOR ☐ ***Blue*** ☐ ***Black*** ☐ ***Red*** ☐ ***Midnight Purple*** ☐ ***Silver***
☐ ***Sky White*** ☐ ***Teal*** ☐ ***Hot Pink*** ☐ ***Ultra Yellow*** ☐ ***Lavender***
☐ Blue Sapphire ☐ Blk Diamond ☐ Candy Red

FRAME DIMENSIONS
Frame Width ☐ ***11"**** ☐ ***12"*** ☐ ***13"*** ☐ ***14"*** ☐ ***15"*** (Seat Width 1/2" Narrower)
☐ ***16"*** ☐ ***17"*** ☐ ***18"*** ☐ ***19"*** ☐ ***20"*** (*11" Wide by Upholstery)
Sling Depth ☐ 10" ☐ 11" ☐ ***12"*** ☐ 13"
☐ 14" ☐ 15" ☐ ***16"*** ☐ 17"[1] ☐ 18"[1]
Cushion ☐ ***2"*** ☐ ***3"*** ☐ ***4"***
☐ Solid Seat[3] ☐ Omit Cushion ☐ Omit Seat Sling

BACKREST (Push Handles Std.) ☐ ***Low*** (8 1/2"-12")[17] ☐ ***Med*** (12"-15 1/2")[17] ☐ ***Tall*** (15 1/2"-19")[17]
Backrest Options ☐ 8° Bend (Med & Tall)[17] ☐ Omit Push Handles[17] ☐ Depth Adjustable[18, 11]
☐ Omit Depth Adj Solid Back & Hardware ☐ Omit Depth Adj Solid Back Include Hardware
☐ Swing-Away Adj Stroller Handles (Avail w/ Depth Adj Back Only) ☐ Solid Back[3, 17]
☐ Backrest Cushion[17] ☐ Adj Upholstery (Avail w/14"-20" Frame Widths and Med or Tall Back Heights)[17]
☐ Omit Back Upholstery[17] ☐ Omit Back Post & Upholstery[17]

FRAME SPECIFICATIONS
Frame Length ☐ Kids ☐ ***Reg*** ☐ Long ☐ Hemi[5] ☐ Long Hemi (17"-18" Deep)[5]
Hanger Type ☐ ***60°*** ☐ ***70°*** ☐ ***90°*** ☐ ***70° V***[19] ☐ Hemi (60°) ☐ Omit Hangers
☐ Articulating-Adult (15"-20" Widths)[2]
☐ Articulating-Kids (11"-16" Widths; Std w/2" Footrest Ext Tubes and Adj Flip-Up Footplates)[2]
☐ Impact Guards - Plastic ☐ Impact Guards - Neoprene
Footplates ☐ ***Composite***[9] ☐ Plastic Cover ☐ Reverse ☐ High Mount[6]
☐ Foam[4] ☐ Angle Adj[9] ☐ Angle Adj High Mount[9] ☐ Omit Footplate
☐ 90° Adj Flip-Up[4, 8] ☐ 90°/90° Footboard[4, 7] ☐ Extended[9]
☐ Heel Loops ☐ Omit Leg Strap
Footrest Ext Tubes[20] ☐ ***Short*** (14"-16 1/2"; N/A w/Articulating Legrest) ☐ ***Med*** (16 1/2"-19") ☐ ***Long*** (19"-21 1/2")
☐ Omit Ext Tubes

CASTERS ☐ ***8" Pneumatic*** ☐ 8" Polyurethane ☐ 5" Low-Profile Polyurethane
☐ 6" Pneumatic ☐ 6" Polyurethane ☐ Aluminum Caster Rim
Caster Options ☐ 3/4" Longer Fork Stem Bolt ☐ 1 1/2" Longer Fork Stem Bolt
☐ Caster Pin Locks ☐ Omit Caster Wheels ☐ Quick-Release Caster Stems[21]

ARMRESTS ☐ ***Padded Swing-Away***[17] ☐ Omit Armrests
☐ Adult - Height Adjustable w/Std Pad (10") ☐ Adult - Height Adjustable w/Full-Length Pad (14")
☐ Kids - Height Adjustable w/Std Pad (10") ☐ Kids - Height Adjustable w/Full-Length Pad (14")
Stroller Handles ☐ Stroller Handles (Reg)[10, 17] ☐ Stroller Handles (Tall)[10, 17]

AXLE PLATE ☐ ***Std*** ☐ Amputee[11] ☐ Quad Release Axle Nuts
☐ One-Arm Drive (Attach One-Arm Drive Supplemental Order Form)

REAR WHEELS
Rim ☐ Mag[12] ☐ ***Spoke*** ☐ Omit Rear Wheels/Axles
Size ☐ 20" ☐ 22" ☐ ***24"*** ☐ 26" (3/4" Stem Bolt Std w/26" Wheels)
Tire ☐ ***Pneumatic*** ☐ Full-Profile Polyurethane[12] ☐ Airless Insert[12]
☐ Low-Profile Polyurethane[13] ☐ Kevlar[13] ☐ High-Pressure Clincher (24", 26" Only)[16]
Handrim ☐ ***Aluminum*** ☐ Plastic Coated ☐ Long Tabs ☐ Omit Handrims
Projections ☐ Vertical[14] 20"/22" 24"/26"
☐ Oblique ☐ 6 ☐ 8 ☐ 10 ☐ 12

WHEEL LOCKS ☐ ***High-Push*** ☐ Low ☐ Omit
☐ High-Pull ☐ Do Not Mount
Wheel Lock Options ☐ 6" Ext Handles ☐ 9" Ext Handles
☐ Grade Aids (N/A w/ Polyurethane High-Pressure Clincher Tires or Kids Length Frames.)

ACCESSORIES
☐ Anti-Tip Tubes
☐ Armrest Pouch (Hgt Adj)
☐ Caddy
☐ Crutch Holder
☐ Front-End Stabilizer
☐ Leg Strap
☐ Leg Strap-Double
☐ Spoke Guards
☐ Transfer Board
☐ Tool Kit

Backpack & Seat Pouch (Specify Color)
☐ Adult ________
☐ Kids ________
☐ Seat Pouch ________

Clothing (Specify Color and Size)
☐ Long Sleeve Shirt __
☐ Sweatshirt ________
☐ Golf Shirt ________
☐ T-Shirt ________
☐ Jacket ________
☐ Barrel Bag
☐ Hat ________
☐ Eyeglass Holders ___

Lifting Straps
☐ Q2 Low[10, 17]
☐ Q2 Medium[10, 17]
☐ Q2 Tall[10, 17]

Positioning Belts
☐ Long Velcro® Style (67")
☐ Short Velcro® Style (57")
☐ Long Buckle (64")
☐ Short Buckle (54")

Side Guards
☐ Fabric Kids
☐ Fabric Regular
☐ Plastic Kids[15]
☐ Plastic Reg[15]

Touch-Up Paint
☐ Color: ________

Wheelchair Tray Table
☐ Extra Small 10"-12"
☐ Small 13"-14"
☐ Medium 15"-17"
☐ Large 18"-20"

Special Instructions ____________

Items in *Bold Italic* Print are Standard

1. Available only on long frame.
2. N/A w/high-push wheel locks.
3. 8° bend not available; 11"-15" wide, 10"-15" deep only.
4. Not available with heel loops; single leg strap standard.
5. Hemi hangers only.
6. Only available on 60° hangers and hemi hangers.
7. Available only with 11"-16" frame widths.
8. Available only with 11"-16" frame widths and 90° hangers.
9. Available on 14"-20" widths.
10. Omit push handles.
11. Not available with swing-away armrest; height adj. available at swing-away price.
12. Not available on 26" wheels.
13. Only available on 24" wheels.
14. Not available with low-profile polyurethane tires.
15. Not available with height adjustable armrests.
16. Not available with mag wheels.
17. Not available with depth adjustable back.
18. Standard with 20" solid back height and stroller handles.
19. Available with 16"-20" frame widths and composite footplates only.
20. Not available with 90° hangers or articulating legrest-kids.
21. Not available with caster pin locks; not available with 3/4", or 1 1/2" fork stem bolt;

Specifications Subject to Change without Notice

930004 7/93

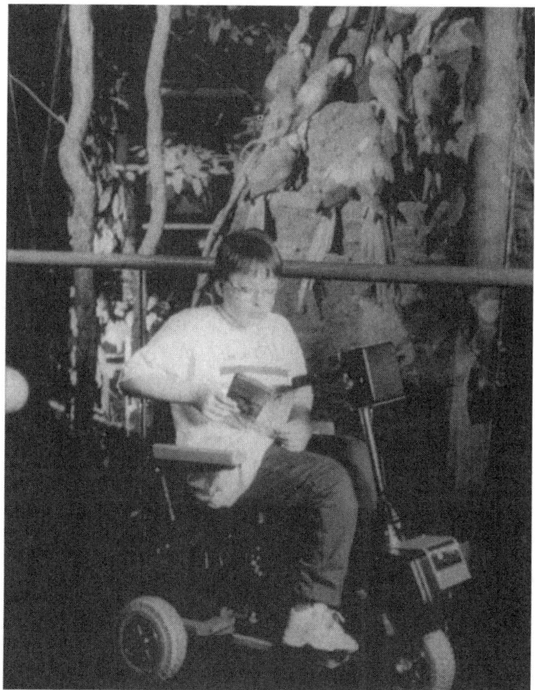

Figure 9-5 ▪ The three-wheeled scooter.

assemble easily into component parts, and generally require a van for transport and ramps or a stair-free entrance to the home. Additionally, they are usually quite sophisticated electronically, which may mean frequent fine tuning and adjusting. They usually accommodate environmental control systems, allow for changes in position (e.g., reclining), and can be operated with any number of switches. Traditional motorized wheelchairs require more of a trial-and-error approach to perfect fit and to train the patient, and maintenance may be more involved. The scooter is preferred for a marginal ambulator who requires a device for long distances, whereas the traditional motorized wheelchair is usually reserved for the individual who requires a more extensive mobility system for full-time use. Specialists should be consulted if a traditional motorized wheelchair system is being considered, and one should never be ordered casually by an inexperienced clinician.

Once the chair style has been selected, the size, fit, and options must be determined.

1. Seat width should allow for growth and should be able to accommodate outerwear for cold winter climates. Most vendors consider 1 inch on each side to be appropriate. Too much room makes it very difficult to propel the wheelchair effectively, especially when armrests are used. In most pediatric models, chairs can be ordered in 1-inch increments to custom-fit any child. In an X-frame wheelchair, growth for width is achieved by replacing the cross braces and upholstery of the wheelchair. (No growth adjustment is available in a rigid chair.) In the pediatric population, almost all patients are provided with a solid seat, used with a cushion, to avoid the slinging effect of upholstery. Cushions made of 2-inch foam are standard with many wheelchair companies, but many alternatives exist, including gel and air cushions.

   Cushions can be used not only to protect skin, but to change the patient's placement and alignment within the chair. Increasing the cushion height decreases the back height and armrest height, lowers the foot plates relative to the patient, and changes the patient's effective arm length and access to the wheels. This technique is often used to extend the use of a chair for several months for a patient who is growing tall but who has not outgrown the width of the chair. It is important, when measuring a chair, to remember to account for changes relating to cushion use (Fig. 9-6).
2. Seat depth should permit comfortable knee flexion without popliteal pressure. In the pediatric population, a solid seat back with hardware placed between the uprights often allows for several inches of growth. The insert is placed forward of the uprights and is

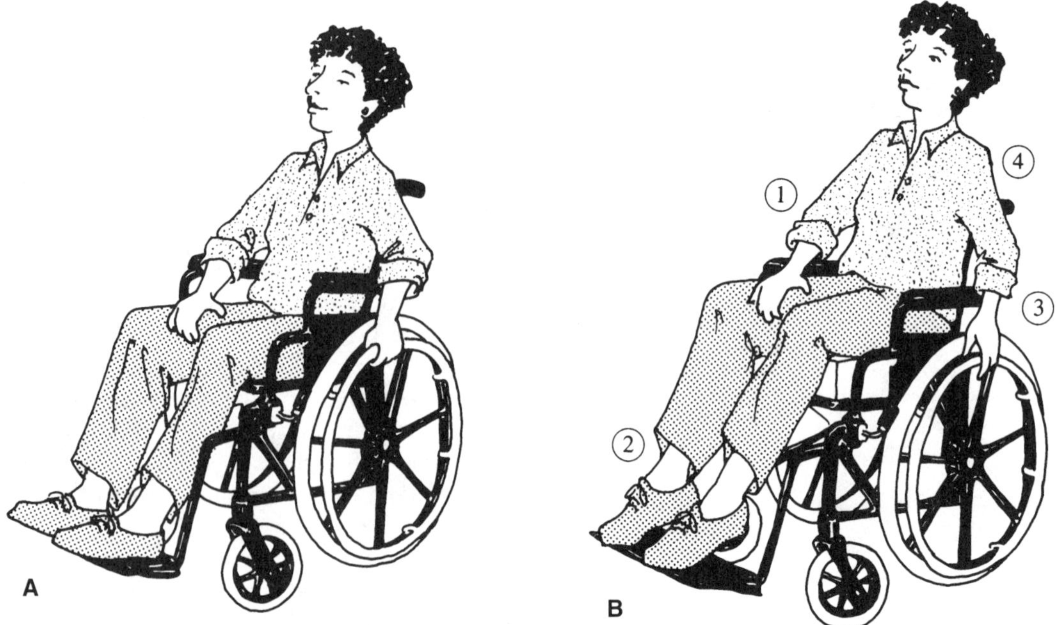

Figure 9-6 ■ (**A**) Patient is accommodated without cushion. (**B**) Use of a cushion will change: (1) Position of arm on armrest; (2) relative leg length; (3) relative arm length in relation to the wheel; and (4) the amount of back support (decreased).

moved back as the child grows. However, the most energy-efficient alignment of a patient for propulsion places the greater trochanter over the axis of the back wheel and only 40% of the combined weight of the wheelchair and occupant on the front casters. It is, therefore, unwise to use cushions or allow for excessive seat depth. Axle plate adjustments are available, but the extent of improvement depends on many factors, including the frame size of the chair. A sling back, for any patient who can tolerate it without being poorly positioned or aligned, can improve mobility, increase sitting tolerance, and decrease the weight of the wheelchair by eliminating heavy inserts and hardware.

3. The preferred backrest height is below the scapulae, but many patients require additional support. A serious dilemma arises when using a head support for bus transport to school. Automobile safety standards require headrests, and a patient is often safer using a headrest for transportation only (i.e., the patient who has fair head control when in a static position but who experiences fatigue or becomes compromised with excessive movement). It is difficult to mount a headrest on a sling back chair; thus, selection of even a removable headrest often implies changing to a solid back. In certain instances, this combination may be contraindicated for independence and energy-efficient mobility. This problem remains unresolved unless the patient can transfer into a federally approved car seat when in the bus, thus negating the need for a headrest mounted on the wheelchair itself.
4. Foot plates and leg rests are often dictated by patient size and the wheelchair caster

wheel size. Although many therapists believe that 90-degree knee flexion is optimal for weight bearing through a flat foot, this position may not be feasible. Vendors are the best resource for determining which options are available considering the frame size, wheel size, and the patient. More companies are becoming aware of the need for multiple-angle foot plates to allow for the braced and nonbraced foot, but this has proved to be a serious and difficult problem to solve in the past. It is always best to get removable leg rests, and elevating foot gear should only be requested if absolutely necessary, as it is both heavy and difficult to fit properly.

5. Wheel size is critical in achieving the most energy-efficient propulsion. Ideally, the elbow should be extended 120 degrees when the handrim is grasped at the highest point.[8] Pneumatic tires give a smoother ride (adding some shock absorbency) but require maintenance. For small children, the weight of the patient may not justify the need for the extra work; in older, heavier patients, however, the ride on rough terrain is clearly better on pneumatic tires.
6. Caster size is the ultimate compromise. In the small-framed chair, adjustability of the rear axle is lost if the caster is too big, as the clearance between the two wheels is minimal. Small tires add maneuverability but get stuck in cracks, ditches, and the like. The author recommends the smallest tire that will still allow wheelchair management on the terrain that is navigated most often. The options range from 5- to 8-inch diameter wheels.
7. Armrest height should be comfortable, should allow the patient to take some weight off the shoulders, and should allow easy access to the wheels. Essentially, the type of armrest should be dictated by ease of management. Many experienced wheelchair users prefer to be without armrests; however, bus drivers, parents, and other caregivers often rely on them for added support when transferring the chair into and out of vehicles.
8. Brakes should be placed for easiest management and can be operated either by pushing or pulling, depending on the patient's preference. Many companies also offer high- or low-mount options for brakes.
9. A seat belt is essential on a child's wheelchair. The seat belt should not come around the child from the middle of the back of the wheelchair. Rather, the belt should originate at the angle of the seat and back on both sides, closing over the child low on the pelvis.
10. Anti-tippers are also a must on a child's wheelchair, especially the young child and the novice wheelchair user.
11. Lapboards or trays are particularly helpful for children, especially the school-age child. The lapboard, if used, must be carefully fitted to the chair so as not to increase the overall width of the chair. Lapboards that are made of clear Lucite or a similar material are preferable to opaque lapboards. The see-through lapboard helps facilitate positive body image by allowing the child to see his own lower extremities and lower trunk. Likewise, the ability of others to see the whole child through the lapboard tends to have a positive impact on the child's interactions with others.

Children with special needs such as a deformity that must be accommodated in the wheelchair will benefit from a wheelchair that is customized to the child's shape by a foam product. The child sits on or back against a container filled with foam. The foam takes approximately 2 minutes to solidify. The foam forms around the deformity. Once hardened, the foam is padded as necessary and covered (Fig. 9-7).

Once a wheelchair prescription is complete, the therapist should feel satisfied that the deci-

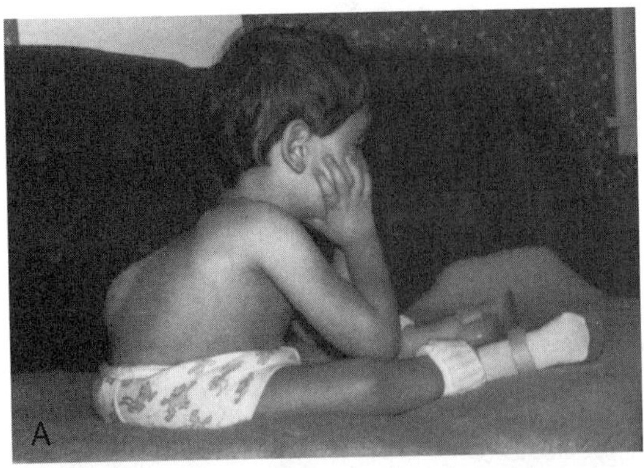

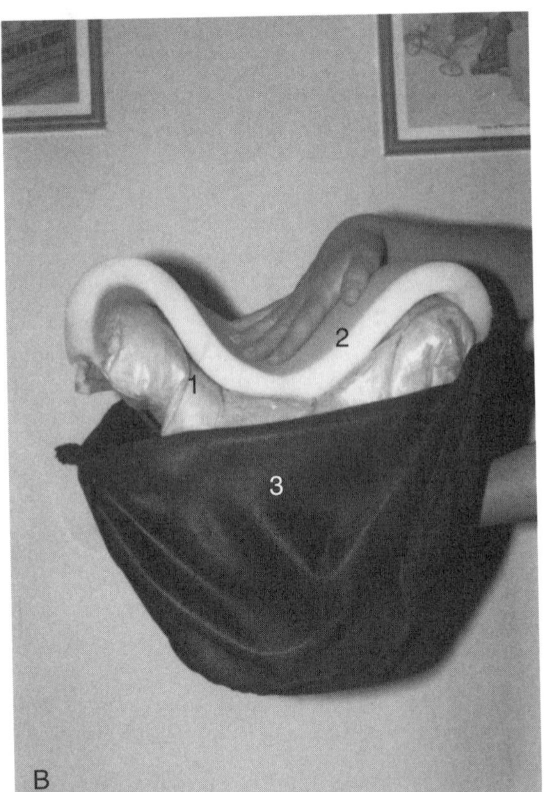

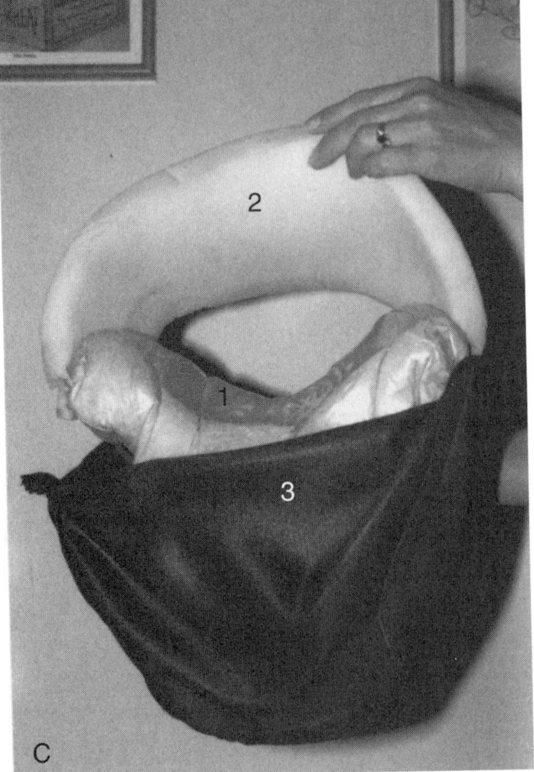

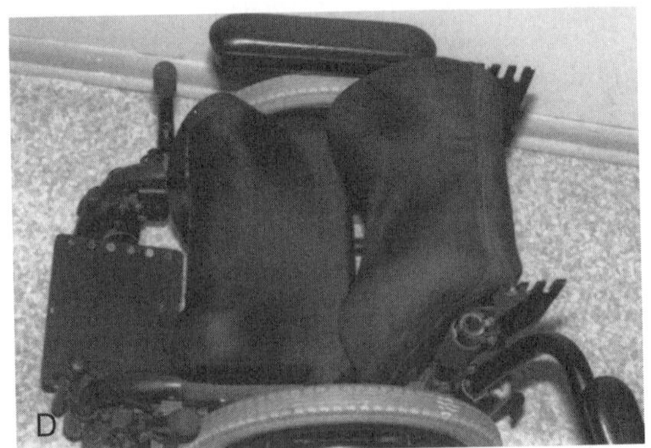

Figure 9-7 ▪ (**A**) Child with myelomeningocele with gibbus on back may require a custom-fitted wheelchair back. (**B**) (1) Solidified foam that conforms to child's back during fitting; (2) soft foam for added protection from pressure; (3) wheelchair back upholstery. (**C**) (1) Solidified foam; (2) soft foam; (3) wheelchair back upholstery. (**D**) Finished wheelchair with custom conformed back.

sions made are the best for a given patient. Any misgivings should be discussed with more experienced therapists, another vendor, or a manufacturer's representative. Therapists should always remember that they are ordering expensive equipment and, more importantly, that the equipment selected will affect the quality of the patient's life for the next 3 to 5 years.

SPECIAL SEATS

A variety of special chairs are available commercially or can be constructed for specific seating problems. Chairs that incorporate the basic principles of seating as discussed in this chapter can have many adaptations to facilitate a desired posture.

The corner chair (Fig. 9-8) is a chair that has lateral supports for the upper trunk. These supports position the child in shoulder girdle protraction, a strategy that tends to decrease extensor spasticity in children with tone problems such as cerebral palsy.

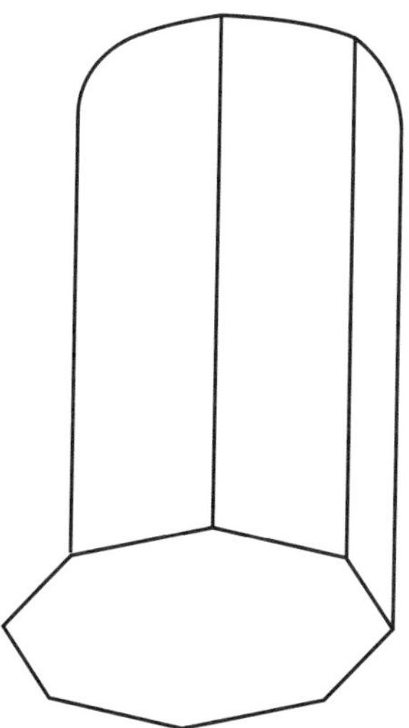

Figure 9-8 ▪ Corner chair. The angled sides aid in protraction of the shoulder girdle, inhibiting extensor hypertonia.

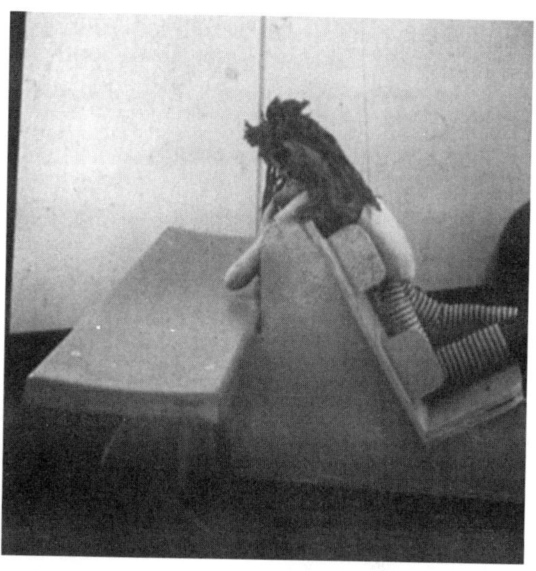

Figure 9-9 ▪ A triwall prone stander covered with enamel paint is used for kneeling.

Bolster chairs are chairs with a bolster type seat (see Figs. 9-2 and 9-3). These chairs also aid in inhibiting excessive extensor tone by flexing and abducting the hips.

Standing

PRONE STANDERS

Prone standers are used frequently for children who require, but cannot achieve, the position of upright standing or its approximation. The child is placed in a prone position on the device. The trunk, buttocks, and lower extremities are all supported. The angle of the board is then increased toward a vertical position, depending on the child's tolerance and the therapist's goals. When the board is at its maximal angle, usually slightly less than 90 degrees, weight bearing is optimal through the lower extremities and feet, although sometimes a kneel-standing position is used. A prone stander is shown in Figure 9-9. The patient benefits from the physiologic changes associated with weight bearing and from the social and perceptual opportunities afforded by an upright position. As the angle of the prone stander decreases to less than upright, the benefits of lower extremity weight bearing will decrease because weight is borne more completely by the trunk.

Several other aspects of the use of the prone stander should be considered. Upper extremity function may range from almost total weight bearing in the child whose prone stander is less than 45 degrees above horizontal to completely free use of the upper extremities in the child who is in an upright position.

When the prone stander is less than 45 degrees above the horizontal, activities involving not only bilateral weight-bearing in the upper extremities but also weight-shifting, unilateral weight-bearing, and reaching can be performed. Extensor muscle function of the neck and back will also vary significantly with various angles. As the patient approaches the upright position, the muscular effort for head righting will decrease. The physical therapist can either facilitate or inhibit muscle activity in various muscle groups by varying the angle of the prone stander.

The therapist must assess the quality of movement shown by the child in the prone stander. The function of the head, neck, scapulae, and upper extremities should be included in this assessment, as should trunk alignment and positioning of the lower extremities. Hyperextension of the neck, exaggerated retraction of the scapulae and holding the upper extremities in the "high-guard" position, and poor symmetry and midline position of the trunk secondary to muscle imbalance are all common postural problems of the child placed in a prone stander. The therapist must consider that proper weight bearing for normal standing requires dynamic pressure through the heels, with the center of gravity passing posterior to the ankle joint; this position is not feasible in a prone stander. Therefore, the use of the prone stander must be evaluated carefully. The prone stander is useful if the physiologic benefits of weight bearing are the major goal or if it is being used to accommodate hands-free standing. If the prone stander is considered for preambulation skills and conditioning, its use may be inappropriate and counterproductive.

When the prone stander is introduced into the patient's program, the entire treatment regimen should be reevaluated. Although the child may appear to adapt well to use of the prone stander for 1 hour each day, longer use or abuse may cause undesirable changes. Increased extensor tone is an example of a change commonly seen with prolonged use of a prone stander. The increased tone may reduce the previously adequate position for sitting and may create difficulties at home and school. This negative effect might require adjustments in the amount of time spent in the prone stander, or it may require a different approach to positioning in the stander.

One of the most important benefits of using a prone stander is to allow the child to interact with peers in play or school situations. Being able to work at a table or play at an elevated sandbox with peers has important social and emotional benefits.

SUPINE STANDERS

A supine stander is an alternative to the prone stander and may better meet the needs of some children whose goal is to achieve an upright position. Similar to a standard tilt table, a supine stander allows weight bearing through the trunk and lower extremities, with the degree of weight-bearing proportional to the angle of the supporting surface. The child is secured around the trunk, hips, and knees with those areas in as close to neutral alignment as is possible. With those criteria achieved, the supine stander is angled toward a 90-degree upright position. Unlike the prone stander, the supine stander does not provide for weight bearing for the upper extremities, and lower extremity weight bearing occurs through the heels rather than the forefeet. The supine stander affords the numerous physiologic benefits of upright weight bearing provided by the prone stander and allows the child to perceive and interact with the environment from an upright posture. Variations of the supine stander are shown in Figures 9-10 and 9-11.

As with all adaptive devices, use of the supine stander must include a careful assessment of the child for compensations, some of which may be pathologic. Commonly noted deviations that occur with a child in a supine stander include thoracic kyphosis with protrusion of the head, hyperextension of the cervical spine, and asymmetry secondary to imbalanced muscle control. If tolerance for an upright position is limited and the child is reclined, increased evidence of asymmetric tonic neck reflex and the Moro reflex may occur. These abnormal reflexes may occur in a supine or semireclined position for any patient with poorly integrated reflex activity. The patient will push into or fix against gravity. Because normal development requires the acquisition of antigravity control, the increased reflex activity in a supine position is counterproductive. Upper extremity function for the child in a supine stander usually requires a special table or easel, thus restricting the child's participation in group activities. The supine stander, although used less commonly than the prone stander, has become popular in recent years. As with other pieces of adaptive equipment, periodic evaluation is necessary to

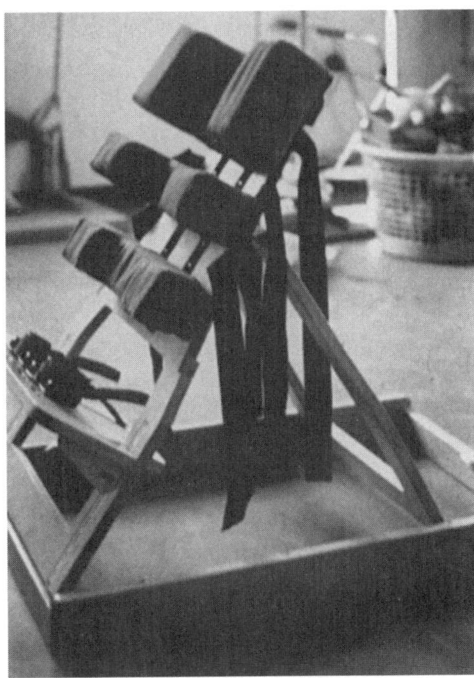

Figure 9-11 ▪ Supine stander made of wood. It is padded for comfort and was designed and built entirely by parents.

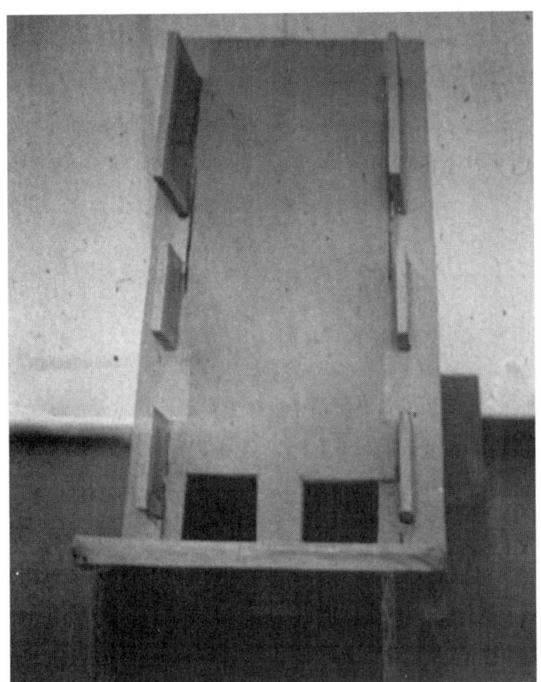

Figure 9-10 ▪ A supine stander made of triwall.

determine the long-term benefits and hazards associated with the supine stander.

Side-Lying

SIDE-LYERS

Side-lyers are particularly useful for young children or large people of low developmental function who may require an alternative to sitting and lying in bed or on the floor. Side-lyers can be elaborately constructed or be very simple devices with pillows, straps, and other makeshift items. A typical fabricated side-lyer is shown in Figure 9-12. When using a side-lyer, the objective is to place the child in a side-lying position according to the following criteria:

1. The trunk should be as symmetric as possible.
2. The head should be supported in alignment neutral to the trunk.
3. Weight-bearing limbs (upper and lower) should be slightly flexed.
4. Non–weight-bearing limbs should be free to move.

This position encourages play in the midline, dissociation between the limbs, and neutral head and trunk alignment. It is also a position that is relatively neutral regarding most abnormal reflex activity. Straps are commonly used to support the trunk, pelvis, and occasionally, the weight-bearing leg. Pillows or pommels usually support the upper leg in a neutral position for abduction/adduction and for internal/external rotation. The device should accommodate the child on either side unless circumstances prevent the child from lying on both sides.

Frequent reassessment is required to ensure that no compensations occur either when using or after being removed from the side-lyer. Areas of potential problems include hyperextension of the neck from pushing against the head support, and flexion and retraction of the shoulder on the non–weight-bearing side. When using a side-lyer, the therapist must be careful when aligning the child with chronic hyperextension of the neck or a tracheostomy. Positioning in either of these cases must not cause an airway obstruction or compromise the child's ventilation.

Although the side-lyer allows for easy manipulation of toys and objects because one hand is

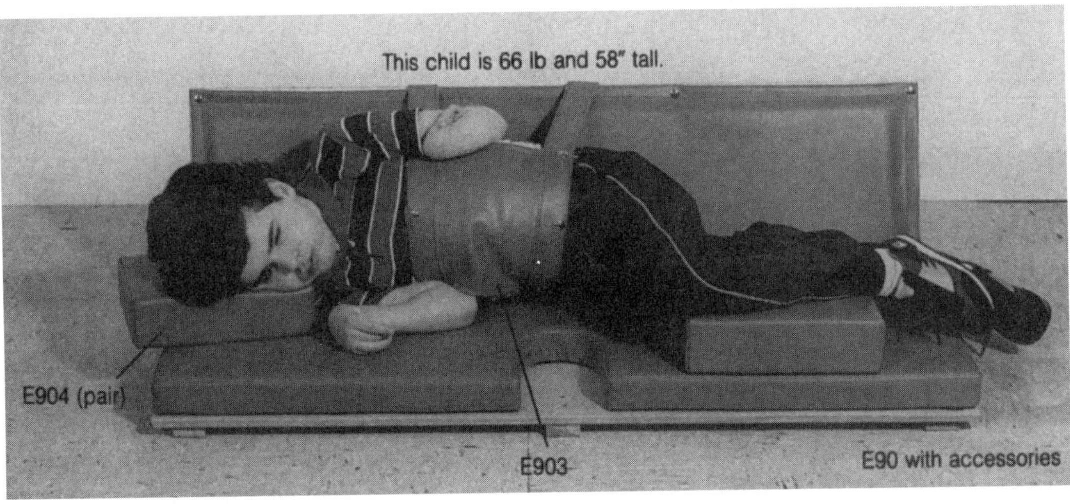

Figure 9-12 ▪ A commercially available side-lyer.

fixed in good alignment, the position is not optimal for perceptual development because the child must play with objects in a horizontal plane when the environmental backdrop is vertical (i.e., toys are rotated 90 degrees with respect to the visual field). This ironic occurrence is not a contraindication to using a side-lyer unless the child has obvious or suspected difficulties with perception or cognition. Most children compensate easily for the problem, especially when sides are alternated, and enjoy these changes of position.

Overall Considerations

Although not a complete list of positioning devices, examples have been provided to illustrate the issues to be considered in choosing and using equipment and the negative consequences that may occur. Negative consequences can be minimized by periodic reassessment of the child and by education of the family and staff. When people who work with the child are aware of the potential negative effects of the equipment, they are more likely to anticipate and recognize early signs of those effects.

Because all physical therapists who work with children and adaptive equipment will be required to suggest the frequency and duration of use, it seems appropriate to discuss the issue of endurance. Unfortunately, a uniform answer rarely exists. Endurance depends on variables that change daily. Rather than suggesting specific times for use, the therapist may choose to let the warning signs of fatigue guide the usage. Those warning signs include difficulty maintaining the desired posture, increased asymmetry, complaints of discomfort, and verbal requests to be moved. The therapist recommends that the device be used until any one of those signs is apparent. It may be worthwhile to encourage attempts to increase endurance gradually over the course of several weeks or months, with the realization that minor variations in tolerance will occur daily. Because daily variations in activity level are normal for everyone, we should acknowledge these variations in the physically challenged child.

Prolonged positioning in any one posture is contraindicated. In addition to fatigue, negative effects of prolonged positioning include pressure ulcers, joint stiffness, and decreased passive and active range caused by hypertonus.

Mobility Equipment

In addition to providing assistance with positioning, adaptive equipment can supplement a child's existing manner of independent locomotion or offer mobility to children who otherwise have no form of locomotion. Some devices, such as a scooter board or a "sit and propel" device, are appropriate only within the home or classroom, whereas other devices such as wheelchairs (already discussed in this chapter) make it possible for the child to be mobile within the community.

Scooter Boards

A scooter board is a flat, padded board with casters (Fig. 9-13). Prone on the board, a child propels himself or herself using hands on the floor. Scooter boards are especially helpful for the toddler or young child who has no prone locomotion and is therefore limited in floor play and exploration. Sometimes a scooter board is incorporated into a prone stander.

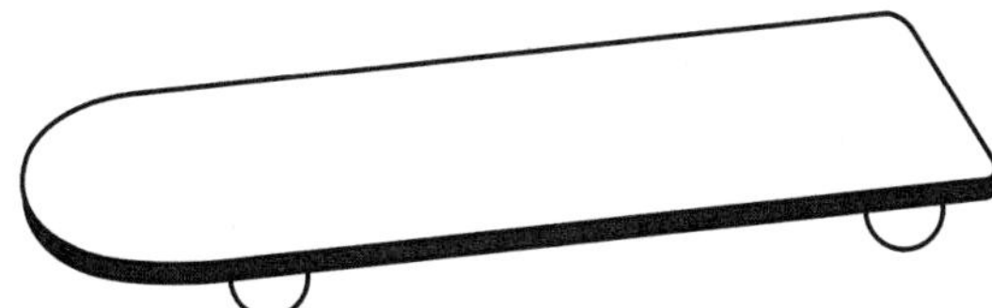

Figure 9-13 ▪ The scooter board is a wheeled mobility device that allows the child to locomote on the floor with his or her peers.

Pre-Wheelchair Devices

These devices allow children 18 months to 5 years to play at peer level. A child long-sits on this device and propels himself or herself by moving the large wheels with the upper extremities. Several commercial designs are available or one could be constructed (Fig. 9-14).

Tricycles

Tricycles are a fun and functional way for some small children to locomote. Specially adapted tricycles are available commercially, or a standard tricycle can be modified. Modifications may include vertically turned handgrips (to inhibit flexor hypertonia of the trunk and facilitate antigravity trunk extension), abduction pommels, back supports, and foot straps. Foot straps are usually applied at the angle of the foot and lower leg, rather than across the toes, thereby preventing a stimulus to the ball of the foot, which could cause uncontrolled plantarflexion and generally increase abnormal extensor tone in the lower extremities and trunk.

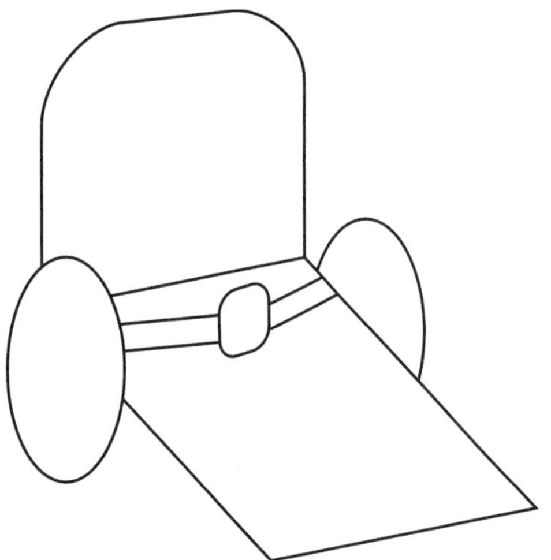

Figure 9-14 ■ The pre-wheelchair device allows the child to be mobile on the floor and teaches the use of the upper extremities for propelling the wheelchair.

Tricycles, although sometimes awkward to transport, are appropriate for use within the community and can be an important adjunct to a child's independence.

Other Mobility Aids

A variety of other aids to mobility may be used, depending on the child's impairments and degree of involvement. Mobility aids commonly used with adults can be used with children and include the following:

1. Lofstrand, platform, or axillary crutches
2. General lower extremity orthoses (SMO, AFO, KAFO, HKAFO)
3. Specific orthotic devices (parapodiums, Orlau Swivel Orthosis, reciprocating gait orthosis)

Equipment for Infants and Toddlers

Let us now examine the needs of the infant and toddler, and the availability of devices for these younger children. Children in this age group are often undiagnosed, or they may show a developmental delay that may or may not result in a long-term disability. Children who require long periods of hospitalization for cardiac, pulmonary, gastrointestinal, and other disorders are also included in this group, as are children who are normal but whose parents request information about various types of apparatus to aid development.

Hospitalized Children

Normal motor development is an integrated process that requires sensory input and freedom to respond to that input through motor exploration and play. Normal patterns of movement develop when agonist and antagonist muscles learn balanced and synergistic cooperation. Because equipment may disrupt or interfere with this process by limiting or restricting sensory input as well as movement, its use in infants and toddlers is almost always discouraged.

Movement in hospitalized children is often restricted by monitors, telemetry devices, and therapeutic medical equipment. It would be counterproductive to the child's motor development to add to these necessary devices other types of apparatus. The objective for the hospitalized child is often to provide optimal freedom of movement within the limits imposed by medical equipment and practice. Physical therapy for these hospitalized children should encourage increased activity, if safe, and should facilitate movement patterns that, because of the external limitations, are difficult for the child to initiate. As the child's medical status improves, or when the child returns home, equipment use should still be limited, except when indicated to promote physical control or safety.

In the United States, car seats for the transport of infants and young children are required in all 50 states. Unfortunately, few guidelines exist for disabled individuals who are unable to use standard car seats or seat belts. This oversight is of serious concern for many parents and professionals working with children. A few car seats for this special population are available commercially. Check with equipment vendors regarding seats that could meet specific needs. Also, simple modifications, such as adding an abduction pommel or a small seat wedge to a standard car seat can be made, as long as the integrity of the seat and safety are not compromised by the adaptation.

Standard strollers and high chairs should be used sparingly, and the child should be in a stable position to allow for optimal oral motor function, head righting and control, and freedom of movement of the upper extremities.

Concepts of seating and positioning already discussed in this chapter should be applied to the use of strollers and high chairs. For example, the toddler who is able to sit in a high chair should have adequate hip flexion (90 degrees) and enough support to facilitate trunk symmetry and midline use of the hands. Umbrella strollers are not suitable for many infants and toddlers because they encourage adduction and internal rotation of the hips and posterior tilt of the pelvis in a "pseudo" sitting posture.

Physical therapy for the infant and toddler should concentrate on encouraging normal, controlled, and motor patterns, and devices should not predominate. The therapist working with the young child should make recommendations to the parents about facilitating movement and avoiding static positioning when the child is left alone to play.

As these children grow older, some will outgrow their temporary disability, but others will develop additional symptoms, and a diagnosis may become more evident. Children in the latter group are likely to have continued treatment and equipment needs, and should be evaluated as previously outlined.

Ventilator-dependent children represent a small but growing population with major equipment needs. With increasing frequency, the physical therapist will be called on to assist in the discharge planning and management of ventilator-dependent children. Technologic advances have prolonged life expectancy for many children with chronic illnesses, including those with myelomeningocele with symptomatic Arnold-Chiari malformation. New, portable ventilators and third-party funding have aided in transforming these once chronically hospitalized children into active members of the community. These children often return home, attend their local schools, and participate in recreational and social activities. Such participation requires a transport system for essential life-support equipment, which includes a portable ventilator and battery, electric cascade humidifier (if the patient will be in one setting for many hours), oxygen source, airway suction unit with catheters and hoses, a bag of supplies, and other items. An innovative approach must be taken with this population in order to address their developmental, orthopedic, and respiratory needs. It is essential to find a vendor who is interested in working with the family and who is able to tailor the specific apparatus to the child's unique requirements. A great deal of trial-and-error effort often is extended in an attempt to resolve the problems presented by the weight of the ventilators, unusual balance points, difficult maneuverability, and the child's need to be in close proximity to these devices.

The two systems shown in Figures 9-15 and 9-16 were designed to meet the specific needs of both child and family. Figure 9-15 shows a commercially available double stroller that has been reinforced to house the ventilator in the rear seat with the battery suspended between the seats. The child can recline or sit upright and has use of an age-appropriate and cost-effective device that is both aesthetically pleasing and manageable. Figure 9-16 shows an Alvena frame adapted for a Snug Seat with the battery on the front foot plate and the ventilator positioned behind the seat. The patient is positioned high enough to allow easy access to the equipment stored underneath and to accommodate the comfort of caregivers who may perform suctioning and other procedures. The Snug Seat tilts 45 degrees in space

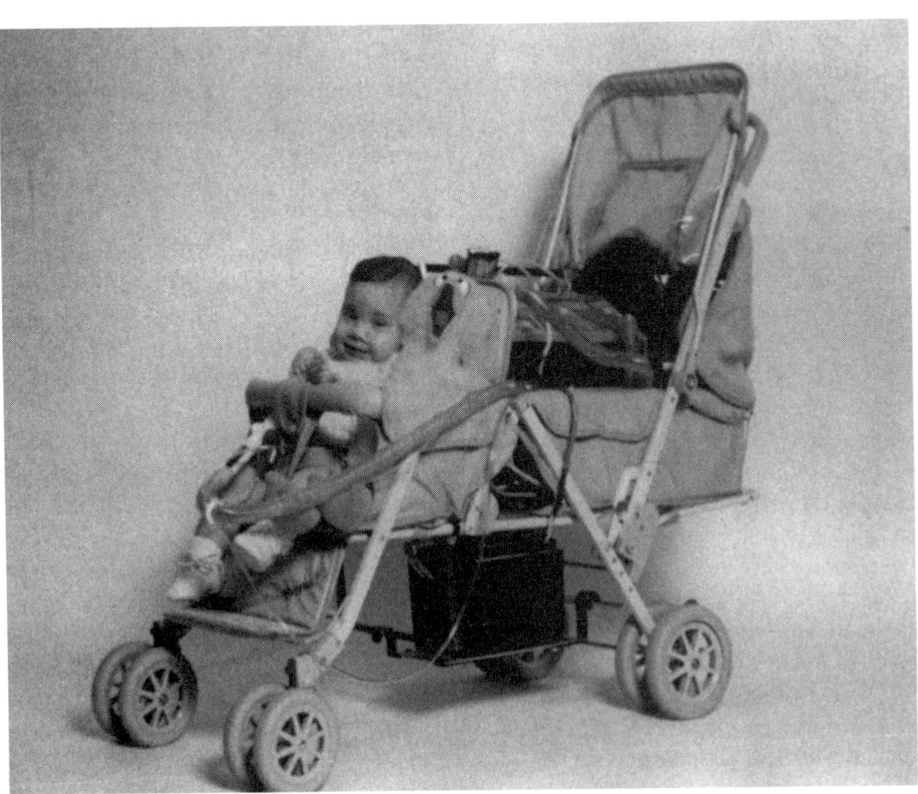

Figure 9-15 ▪ A commercially available double stroller.

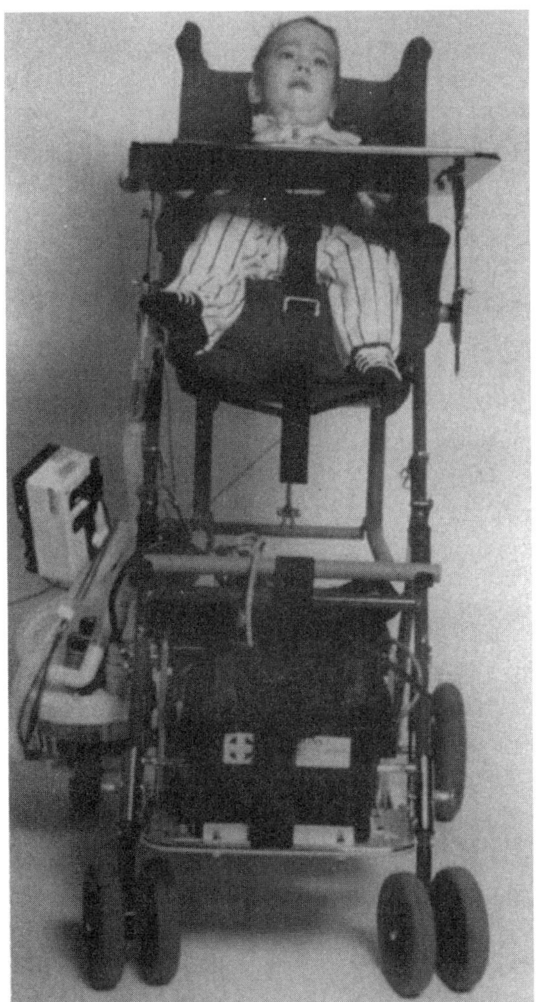

Figure 9-16 ▪ An Alvena frame adapted for a Snug Seat.

and allows for easy adjustments for postural changes or growth. As the child grows and independent mobility becomes a concern, manual or motorized wheelchairs can be adapted for the child's use.*

*A very special thank you to the DME Shoppe and Joe Thieme (Naperville, IL), for creating these units and many more similar devices.

Infants and Toddlers with Normal Neuromotor Development

Let us consider the equipment used frequently for babies and toddlers without special needs, including swings, jumpers, and walkers. It has become common practice for families to purchase these devices for their children, despite little knowledge of their advantages or disadvantages.

Swings are probably the most benign device of the three mentioned. There is little evidence to indicate that swings are unsafe during this period, but must be used with supervision. Although swings are pleasant for the child and family, they should be used sparingly because they lack significant stimulation for motor growth and development.

Jumpers are devices that are suspended from doorways by large cables, springs, and clamps. The jumper enables the child to bounce up and down by extending the lower extremities and pushing against the floor. Although the child may enjoy the vestibular stimulation provided during such an activity, caution must be exercised. The child must be supervised constantly to ensure that he or she does not fall, bang against the doorframe, or become entrapped in the cables or springs when reaching out for a toy. Even restricted use of the jumper may lead to the development of patterns of exaggerated extensor activity with components of strong internal rotation of the hips and plantarflexion of the ankles. As a result, some children develop a tendency to toe-walk. Also, the high impact loading on the child's young bones and joints may be injurious. In addition to these potential hazards the jumper, like other devices, impedes development of normal motor skills by eliminating the opportunity to make transitions from one pattern to another and by restricting the learning of new sequences of movement. For reasons of safety as well as the potential for the development of abnormal movement patterns, physical therapists generally discourage the use of these jumpers by all children.

Unlike swings and jumpers, walkers have been implicated in injuries severe enough to be fatal. In 1993 more than 23,000 walker-related injuries, mostly to children between the ages of 5 and 15 months, were seen in hospital emergency rooms.[8] The number of injuries is most likely significantly higher when one considers those injuries that are never reported or are treated in clinics or at home. During the period of 1989 through 1993, 11 walker-related deaths occurred.[8] Most injuries have been the result of the walker tipping over, falling down stairs, collapsing because of poor structural design, or finger entrapment. Injuries have included abrasions, lacerations, fractures, burns, poisonings, severe head trauma, and death.[8]

Many facilities recommend walkers under the mistaken impression that walking skills are helped by these devices. Not only are baby walkers potentially dangerous but they do not facilitate the development of normal walking and, in fact, may actually impede motor development. Ridenour studied the effects of frequent and regular use of a walker on bipedal locomotion in human infants. She found that walkers modified the mechanics of infant locomotion in several ways. Infants who used walkers were able to commit numerous mechanical errors while succeeding in bipedal locomotion.[9] The patterns of locomotion with an infant walker are neither normal nor advantageous. Children who use these walkers are in poor weight-bearing alignment, holding their trunk and lower extremities in flexion. There is also frequent asymmetry as the child leans, and toe-walking is common. Additionally, a 1986 study by Crouchman found prone locomotion to be delayed in many normal babies who spent excessive time in infant walkers.[10]

These observations suggest that walkers may have a significant adverse effect on motor development, even though the adverse effects may be of short duration once walker use is discontinued.[10,11] Although further study is needed to confirm findings relative to infant walker use and the development of motor skills, particularly ambulation, most physical therapists discourage the use of walkers by infants with apparent normal neuromotor development and strongly discourage their use in infants with documented or suspected neurologic deficits.

Activities of Daily Living

Although not strongly emphasized in this chapter, activities of daily living (ADLs) should be mentioned briefly. ADLs are not major concerns for infants or toddlers with impairments, but they grow increasingly important as these children grow older and become more capable of caring for themselves. Because families can usually manage the ADL needs of a young child, the issue of ADLs as a therapeutic goal may be overlooked or not considered as the child grows older.

Equipment for ADLs, particularly for toileting and bathing, should be assessed according to guidelines similar to those used for other pieces of apparatus described in this chapter. Toilets may be modified by adding abduction pommels, vertical handgrips (to keep the child symmetric and decrease flexor hypertonia), corner style backrests, and foot rests. Essential to good positioning on the toilet is for the child's hips and knees to be flexed to 90 degrees with feet flat on the floor or foot rests. This position helps limit extensor spasticity in those children affected by hypertonia and also helps all children relax their abdominal muscles and feel secure. If the child feels secure, confident, and relaxed, toileting may proceed more rapidly and easily.

When choosing a bathtub seat, both ease of management in the tub and safety of the child are the major objectives. Although many bathtub seats exist, seats that are completely satisfactory for both use and safety are difficult to find for all children, but they are particularly difficult to find when the child becomes older and heavier. Vendors should provide sample bathtub seats for both inspection and mock usage trials. The family must decide which tub seat provides the safest and most suitable solution depending on the particular environmental barriers of the home and the physical needs of the child.

Communication Aids

Although most of this chapter has focused on adaptive equipment relative to positioning, mobility, and ADL needs, that is to say the physical needs of the child, it is important that we give brief consideration to another category of adaptive equipment used with our pediatric clients. Augmentative communication strategies frequently involve equipment.

As physical therapists we must be familiar generally with communication devices for two reasons. First, out interaction with children in the therapeutic environment necessarily requires our ability to communicate with them. This brief synopsis is intended to broadly familiarize the reader with various types of communication devices that may be encountered.

A second reason for physical therapists to have an understanding of augmentative communication is that many of these strategies require controlled movement as a means of communicating. Knowing about these systems can help the physical therapist address movement issues that can facilitate the child's successful use of a communication strategy. In fact, the physical therapist at times may work closely with a Speech and Language Pathologist in developing appropriate motor control for a communication system.

Augmentative communication strategies are classified as gestural, gestural-assisted, or neuro-assisted.[13]

Gestural Strategies

Gestural strategies are unaided strategies, requiring no instrumentation and therefore no "adaptive equipment." Movement, generally of the face and upper extremities is used to transmit messages visually. Smiling, nodding, or shaking of the head and other head and eye movements and hand gestures are typically used gestural communication strategies.

Additionally, several gestural communication systems may be used. These include American Sign Language (Ameslan), American Indian Hand Talk (Amer-Ind), manual shorthand, left-hand manual alphabet (a left-hand variation of the American Manual Alphabet used in Ameslan), eye-blink encoding, and gestural Morse code.[13]

Gestural-Assisted Strategies

These aided communication strategies require adaptive equipment in the form of a communication board or display that is activated by gesture or movement. Users of this type of strategy point to components on the display to transmit their messages.[13]

Gestures may be direct muscle gestures of the head, upper extremity, or eyes. If head movements are used, a headpointer is required. Indirect use of muscle gestures occurs when the display is controlled by an electronic switching device activated by muscle gestures and includes the use of microcomputers. Muscle gestures used to activate switches include finger, head, foot, and eyebrow movements. Switches may be controlled by joysticks, pushbuttons (such as keyboards), pads, squeeze bulbs, and blowing or sucking on the end of a tube (sip and puff switches). Gestural-assisted communication aids may simply be visual symbol sets such as photographs, drawings, the alphabet, and printed words on the display. This classification of communication strategies also includes several specific systems of symbols such as Picsyms, Sigsymbols, Blissymbolics, and Rebuses.[13]

Gestural-assisted communication devices are available commercially. However, they are generally most effective functionally when custom-made for a specific child.

Neuro-Assisted Strategies

These aided communication strategies also use a display, but unlike the gestural-assisted strategies that rely on gestural manipulation of a switching mechanism, the display is activated by bioelectrical signals from the body such as muscle action potentials. This type of device is most needed in the child who has motor impairments so severe that he or she is unable to control body movements adequately for gesturing. The same displays are used as in the gestural-assisted systems, but the switches are controlled by surface electrodes on the brain (EEG) or a selected muscle (EMG).[13]

Summary

The purchase, building, and use of adaptive equipment are complex and time-consuming aspects of pediatric physical therapy. These processes are further complicated by the lack of scientific documentation to help with the appropriate and objective choice of equipment. The available options are so numerous that even the most experienced physical therapist is unlikely to feel that all equipment has been considered before making a choice. The safest and most realistic approach to the selection of adaptive devices for children lies in a theoretical construct based on careful evaluation of the child. The goals and status of the child must be known before therapeutic needs can be met with various types of equipment. When this information is known, the therapist can develop a therapeutic program that includes safe and effective use of equipment without unwanted negative effects. When the child's needs and goals are considered, the specific details of the numerous devices available become less intimidating or confusing. Frequent reevaluation by the therapist will ensure that the child receives continuing benefits from adaptive equipment. Input from teachers, aides, and parents will provide invaluable feedback regarding the child's use of the equipment. The scheme suggested in this chapter provides the therapist with the opportunity to document the needs of the child, to select or make the equipment, to evaluate the effects of the equipment, and to reassess the child's status periodically.

REFERENCES

1. Marks A. On making chairs more comfortable—how to fit the seat to the sitter. *Fine Woodworking.* 1981;31:11.
2. Keegan J. Alterations in the lumbar curve related to posture and sitting. *J Bone Joint Surg.* 1973;35A:7.
3. Akerblom B. *Chairs and Sitting.* Presented at the Symposium on Human Factors in Equipment Design; 1954; Sweden.
4. Knutsson B, Lindh K, Telhag H. Sitting: An electromyographic and mechanical study. *Acta Orthop Scand.* 1966;37:415–426.
5. Keegan J. Evaluation and improvement of seats. *Industr Med Surg.* 1962;31:137–148.
6. Bergan A. *Positioning the Client with Central Nervous System Deficits: The Wheelchair and Other Adapted Equipment.* 2nd ed. New York: Valhalla Press; 1985.
7. Nwaobi O, Brubaker C, Cusick B, et al. Electromyographic investigation of extensor activity in cerebral palsy children in different seating positions. *Dev Med Child Neurol.* 1983;25:175–183.
8. Brubaker C. Ergonomic considerations. *J Rehabil R D* [Clin Suppl]. 1990;27:37–48.
9. Ridenour M. Infant walkers: Developmental tool or inherent danger? *Percept Mot Skills.* 1982;55: 1201–1202.
10. Consumer Product Safety Commission. Baby walkers: Advance notice of proposed rulemaking. *Fed Reg.* 1994;59:39306–39311.

11. Crouchman M. The effects of babywalkers on early locomotor development. *Dev Med Child Neurol.* 1986;28:757–761.
12. Kauffman I, Ridenour M. Influence of an infant walker on onset and quality of walking pattern of locomotion: An electromyographic investigation. *Percept Mot Skills.* 1977;45:1323–1329.
13. Silverman F. *Communication for the Speechless.* 3rd ed. Needham Heights, MA: Allyn & Bacon; 1995.

BIBLIOGRAPHY

Bull M, Stroup K, Stout J, et al. Establishing special needs care seat loan program. *Pediatrics.* 1990;85: 540–547.

Hulme JB, Shaver J, Acher S, et al. Effects of adaptive seating devices on the eating and drinking of children with multiple handicaps. *Am J Occup Ther.* 1987;41:81–89.

Mazur MD, Shurtleff D. Orthopedic management of high-level spina bifida—early walking compared with early use of a wheelchair. *J Bone Joint Surg.* 1989; 71A:56–61.

Stout J, Bull M, Stroup K. Safe transportation for children with disabilities. *Am J Occup Ther.* 1989;43: 31–36.

Trefler E, ed. *Seating for Children with Cerebral Palsy—A Resource Manual.* Memphis: University of Tennessee; 1984.

Zacharkow D. *Posture: Sitting, Standing, Chair Design and Exercise.* Springfield, IL: Charles C Thomas; 1988.

Pediatric Oncology

Christine R. Morgan

For each of the common childhood cancers, the survival rate has increased over the past several decades. In the 1960s, for example, less than 20 percent of children with acute lymphoblastic leukemia survived for more than 5 years, whereas currently more than 70 percent survive.[1] Along with the physical problems directly related to the oncologic diseases, the various forms of medical management cause side effects that often require intervention by several disciplines. Thus, increasing numbers of pediatric physical therapists will be treating these children, not only in acute care hospitals, but also in rehabilitation, outpatient, home care, and school settings as well. For these reasons, pediatric physical therapists need to be informed about the wide range of pediatric oncologic diseases, current medical management, and the resultant side effects of these treatments.

Treatment of children with cancer is performed at pediatric cancer centers throughout the United States. These centers enroll patients in clinical trials that are monitored by the National Cancer Institute to ensure consistency of treatment across the country. These cancer centers are often associated with one of two national groups: the Children's Cancer Study Group (CCSG) and the Pediatric Oncology Group (POG). Each of these groups meets biannually to review results of current studies and to develop plans for new treatment strategies.[2]

Incidence

Cancer is the chief cause of death by disease and the second leading cause of death overall, following trauma, in children ages 1 to 14 years. An estimated 8800 new cases of cancer in children will occur in the United States in 1997, with an estimated 1700 deaths, one third of which will be attributable to leukemia.[3]

Etiology

The causes of childhood cancer are largely unknown. However, several environmental and genetic factors have been associated with an increased risk of cancer in children. One environmental factor is *ionizing radiation*. Exposure to radiation in infancy and childhood can be the result of atomic bomb explosions, nuclear fallout, or more commonly, the use of irradiation for medical treatment. Chemical agents, including some types of hormones and chemotherapeutic agents, have also been implicated as carcinogens in humans.

Certain pediatric cancers may have both a hereditary and nonhereditary form, including Wilms' tumor and retinoblastoma. Also, certain hereditary diseases or chromosomal disorders such as neurofibromatosis, which has an increased association with several forms of pediatric cancer, or Down syndrome, which has an increased link to childhood leukemia, may predispose children to cancer.[4]

Signs and Symptoms

Common signs and symptoms of cancer in children can include fever, pain, a mass or swelling, bruising, pallor, headaches, neurologic changes, and visual disturbances.[3] Children may often be misdiagnosed initially, as these signs and symptoms are frequently seen in other common pediatric disorders.

Types of Cancers

Childhood cancers generally vary from those seen in adults. The most frequently seen cancers of adulthood involve the lung, breast, colon, and skin, whereas those in children most often include the leukemias, embryonal tumors, and sarcomas. Common types of pediatric cancers include the following:

- Leukemia
- Central nervous system (CNS) tumors
- Lymphomas
- Neuroblastoma
- Wilms' tumor
- Bone cancer
- Rhabdomyosarcoma
- Retinoblastoma

Leukemia

Leukemia is a malignant disease of the blood that originates in the bone marrow, the gel-like substance that fills the inner cavities of bones.[5] The marrow produces various blood components, including erythrocytes or red blood cells, thrombocytes or platelets, and leukocytes or white blood cells. In leukemia, undifferentiated or immature white blood cells, called blasts, tend to proliferate in the bone marrow. The accumulation of these nonfunctional cells eventually inhibits the production of normal blood cells, thus resulting in the typical signs and symptoms related to deficiencies of these cells (Table 10-1). Leukemia cells may also begin to invade various organs of the body, causing enlargement and dysfunction.[5]

TYPES OF LEUKEMIA

Acute

Leukemia is the most common form of cancer in children, comprising approximately 2500 cases per year. There are two major types of leukemia in children; acute lymphoblastic leukemia (ALL) and acute myelogenous leukemia (AML). The ratio of occurrence of ALL to AML is 4:1.[1]

ALL, also called acute lymphocytic or acute lymphatic leukemia, is the most common form of pediatric leukemia. It is slightly more common in boys than in girls, and occurs more frequently in Caucasians than in non-Caucasians.[6] The peak age of occurrence is 3 to 4 years.[1] (See Case Study [M.B., Caucasian Female with Diagnosis of ALL].)

AML, also called acute granulocytic leukemia or acute nonlymphocytic leukemia, primarily affects adults but is the second most common form of leukemia in children. Like ALL, AML also occurs slightly more frequently in males than in females.[1] It is more common in teens than in children ages 1 to 10 years, although no peak age is evident.[7]

Chronic. Chronic forms of leukemia, including chronic myelogenous leukemia (CML), also exist but are rare in the pediatric population.[1]

Symptoms of leukemia include fever, pallor, bone pain, lethargy, anorexia, and bleeding.[8] The diagnosis of leukemia in children is made initially on the basis of an abnormal complete blood count (CBC), and definitively by a bone marrow biopsy.

TABLE 10-1
Explanation of the Complete Blood Count (CBC)*

	Red Blood Cells (Erythrocytes)	**White Blood Cells (Leukocytes)**	**Platelets (Thrombocytes)**
Function	Contain hemoglobin, which carries O_2 to the body and returns CO_2 to the lungs	Mobilize body's defense system against infection	Prevent and stop bleeding by clumping together to form a clot at the site of injury
Normal values	Hemoglobin: Infant/child, 12 g/dL Adult female, 12–16 g/dL Adult male, 13–18 g/dL	7000–11,000 (off chemotherapy) 1500–4000 (on chemotherapy)	150,000–400,000/mm^3
Name for low value	Anemia	Neutropenia	Thrombocytopenia
Low value	<8 g/dL	ANC† <500	<20,000/mm^3
Signs and symptoms associated with low values	Fatigue, pale lips, pale skin, loss of appetite	No obvious signs	Bleeding gums, nose bleeds, increased bruising. petechiae

*Information adapted from Children's Hospital of Philadelphia Information for Parents Instructions for Home Management of a Child with Cancer

†Absolute neutrophil count

Case Study—M.B., Caucasian Female with Diagnosis of ALL.

M.B. is a Caucasian female who was diagnosed as having ALL in 1984 at 3 years of age. Initial treatment included a 2 ½ -year chemotherapy protocol of vincristine, methotrexate, and Adriamycin. Following the completion of the protocol, remission was maintained for approximately 9 months, at which time M.B. suffered a relapse. A more intense treatment protocol was initiated, including CNS irradiation and chemotherapy. Concurrently, M.B.'s family underwent HLA testing to determine the availability of a compatible bone marrow donor.

At 7 years of age, M.B. underwent an allogeneic BMT using marrow donated from her 9-year-old brother. Following the transplant, she was confined to the LAF room for 7 weeks. The physical therapy department was consulted during this admission for maintenance of her general activity level and strength, as well as for prevention of contractures, skin breakdown, and pulmonary complications.

Subsequently, M.B. developed chronic GVH disease that severely affected her joints, necessitating consultation for home physical therapy services owing to pain, decreased ROM, and significantly impaired function. Treatment consisted of a stretching program, general strengthening and mobility activities, as well as progressive ambulation as improvement occurred. Equipment was also needed, including a wheelchair, walker, and MAFOs. Once M.B. became ambulatory, physical therapy was continued at an outpatient facility for gait training and promotion of higher level gross motor skills.

In October of 1990, M.B. developed a serious blood infection, prompting admission to an acute care facility and treatment with amphotericin. During this admission, an IV infiltration occurred, resulting in a large, open wound on the dorsum of M.B.'s left foot. Following skin grafting, M.B. was discharged to home, where she developed extreme pain attributable to graft rejection. She was readmitted and treated with hyperbaric oxygen twice a day for 2 weeks, then returned home to allow healing to occur. Physical therapy services were reinitiated in the home because M.B. was nonambulatory again. Treatment consisted of wound care and, later, scar management techniques, and ROM activities to the left foot, ankle, and other joints owing to the residual effects of GVH disease. General strengthening and mobility activities were also performed, along with ambulation training using a non–weight-bearing pattern with a walker, and later, progression to partial and then full weight-bearing for the left lower extremity.

M.B. is now 11 years old and is demonstrating no recurrence of her leukemia. She has, however, required heelcord releases as a result of the effects of her GVH disease. She remains mildly limited in her higher level gross motor skill ability, including running and jumping, owing to joint problems as well as scarring on her left foot. She has been able to return to school this year and otherwise remains healthy and active.

TREATMENT

Initial treatment of leukemia is generally a 2- to 3-year process that includes the following stages:

- Induction Phase—An attempt to eradicate all malignant cells from the body
- Remission—An apparent disappearance of disease symptoms and abnormal cells in the bone marrow
- Consolidation/Maintenance Therapy—Continuation of treatment despite remission, because a significant number of undetectable cells may persist and could proliferate without further therapy

A relapse is a reappearance of leukemic cells in the bone marrow with a recurrence of all signs and symptoms.[5]

Generally, treatment protocols vary according to the type and severity of the leukemia, and may include any or all of the following:

- Combinations of chemotherapeutic agents
- Intrathecal injections of chemotherapeutic drugs into the CNS*
- CNS irradiation*

Bone marrow transplantation (BMT) may be performed if a compatible donor is available. BMT is generally performed after the first relapse in patients with ALL, but in those with AML, it may be performed as soon as the first remission is achieved because the prognosis is significantly poorer.[10]

Brain Tumors

Brain tumors are the most common form of solid tumors in children, and the second most common form of pediatric cancer overall.[6,11] Brain tumors are occasionally congenital, occur most frequently in children ages 1 to 10 years of age, and are slightly more common in males than in females.[6] Signs and symptoms of brain tumors in children vary widely according to the size and location of the tumor. Common symptoms include headaches, nausea, vomiting, irritability, balance disturbances, ataxia, hemiparesis, and visual problems.[12,13]

TREATMENT

Treatment of brain tumors may include surgical resection (if possible), including total resection or tumor debulking. Irradiation is also a primary treatment for CNS tumors, although it must be used cautiously in young children owing to the late effects of decreased IQ and learning problems seen in patients who have received cranial irradiation.[14] Chemotherapy may be utilized to treat CNS tumors, although its effectiveness is often significantly decreased owing to difficulty in crossing the blood-brain barrier.[9] Shunt placement may be necessitated by blockage of cerebrospinal fluid (CSF) flow by the tumor, which may result in increased intracranial pressure.[15] Prior to shunting, however, it is important to ensure that no malignant cells are present in the CSF, because otherwise, the procedure may increase the risk of spread to other parts of the body.

Some postoperative problems commonly associated with CNS tumors include limited range of motion of the neck, hemiparesis, ataxia or dysmetria, weakness, and speech and/or visual problems.

COMMON TYPES OF BRAIN TUMORS

The most common pediatric brain tumors are listed in Display 10-1. Following is a more detailed discussion of these specific types of brain tumors.

MEDULLOBLASTOMA. Medulloblastomas comprise 10 to 20 percent of primary CNS tumors, occurring predominantly in the cerebellum.[12] Early signs are those of increased intracranial pressure[16] (Display 10-2), as well as ataxia.[15] Treatment includes surgical resection (if possible), followed by irradiation, because medulloblastoma is very radiosensitive.[12] Metastases may occur throughout the meninges and involve areas outside the CNS.[16]

DISPLAY 10-1
Most Common Pediatric Brain Tumors

- Medulloblastoma
- Astrocytoma
- Ependymoma
- Brain-stem glioma
- Craniopharyngioma

Heideman RL, Packer RJ, et al. Tumors of the central nervous system. In: Pizzo PA, Poplack DG, eds. *Principles and Practice of Pediatric Oncology*. Philadelphia: J.B. Lippincott; 1989:505–554.

*Specific treatment of the CNS may be necessary because many chemotherapeutic agents do not readily cross the blood-brain barrier.[9]

DISPLAY 10-2
Symptoms of Increased Intracranial Pressure*

Classic traid
- Morning headaches
- Vomiting without nausea
- Diplopia or other visual disturbances

Subacute signs
- Declining academic performance
- Fatigue
- Personality changes
- Complaints of vague intermittent headaches

In infants and toddlers
- Irritability
- Anorexia
- Developmental delay

*Adapted from Heideman RL, Packer RJ, et al. Tumors of the central nervous system. In: Pizzo PA, Poplack DG, eds. *Principles and Practice of Pediatric Oncology*. Philadelphia: J.B. Lippincott; 1989: 505–554.

ASTROCYTOMA. Two primary forms of astrocytomas occur in childhood, including cerebellar astrocytomas and supratentorial astrocytomas. Cerebellar astrocytomas comprise 10 to 20 percent of childhood CNS tumors,[15] with the most common symptoms being those associated with increased intracranial pressure, as well as ataxia. The primary treatment is surgery with the goal of total resection.[16]

Supratentorial astrocytomas comprise 35 percent of CNS tumors in childhood. Signs and symptoms of supratentorial astrocytomas include those related to increased intracranial pressure, as well as visual disturbances and seizures. Histologic subtypes of these tumors include fibrillary and pilocytic tumors, which are well differentiated, as well as malignant anaplastic astrocytoma and glioblastoma multiforme, which are less differentiated, of a high grade, and very aggressive, widely invasive tumors.[15] The primary treatment of supratentorial astrocytomas is surgery, although total resection is frequently not possible owing to tumor location. Radiation therapy is also commonly utilized. Chemotherapy may be indicated for those patients with high-grade tumors.[12]

EPENDYMOMAS. Ependymomas comprise 5 to 10 percent of primary CNS tumors,[15] occurring in the posterior fossa and cerebral hemispheres.[17] Initial signs and symptoms relate to increased intracranial pressure in posterior fossa ependymomas, and include seizures and focal cerebellar deficits in supratentorial tumors.[15] Treatment includes surgical resection, if possible, followed by irradiation.[12]

BRAIN-STEM GLIOMAS. Brain-stem gliomas comprise 10 to 20 percent of CNS tumors in children, with signs and symptoms that include progressive cranial nerve dysfunction and gait disorders.[15] The primary medical treatment for brain-stem gliomas is irradiation because surgery is hazardous owing to tumor location and chemotherapy has not been found to be beneficial.[16] Treatment is generally palliative because the overall prognosis for these tumors is poor.[15]

CRANIOPHARYNGIOMAS. Craniopharyngiomas are histologically benign tumors that comprise 6 to 9 percent of primary childhood CNS tumors[15] and occur primarily in the midline suprasellar region.[12] Signs and symptoms of craniopharyngiomas include visual disturbances, headaches and vomiting, as well as endocrine disturbances.[16] Treatment of craniopharyngiomas includes total surgical resection, or subtotal resection with irradiation if total resection is not possible.[12]

Lymphomas

Hodgkin's disease and non-Hodgkin's lymphoma together comprise a heterogeneous group of malignant diseases arising from the lymphatic system.[17]

HODGKIN'S DISEASE

Hodgkin's disease is a malignant disorder that arises primarily in peripheral lymph nodes.[17] It is most common in young adults in their 20s and 30s, and is more common in males than females.[18] Initial symptoms of Hodgkin's disease include a painless swelling in the neck, groin, or axilla. Treatment generally includes radiation therapy and/or chemotherapy, depending on the extent of the disease.[17]

NON-HODGKIN'S LYMPHOMA

Non-Hodgkin's lymphoma is a group of disorders that most frequently involve the abdomen and mediastinum.[17] These malignant disorders occur most commonly in children 7 to 11 years of age,[19] and in males more frequently than females.[18] Initial symptoms may include abdominal pain or swelling, swelling of the face and neck, or difficulty swallowing.[17] Treatment of non-Hodgkin's lymphoma includes irradiation and chemotherapy, used individually or in combination, depending on the location and extent of disease.[20]

Neuroblastoma

Neuroblastoma is a tumor that develops from neural crest cells. It may arise anywhere in the sympathetic nervous system, with the most common sites of origin being the adrenal glands or paraspinal glanglion.[21] Neuroblastoma occurs early in life, with 25 percent being diagnosed by 1 year of age and 75 percent by 5 years of age.[17] Males are affected slightly more frequently than females.[18] The initial symptoms of neuroblastoma vary according to the location of the tumor, but most commonly include pain, an abdominal mass, or persistent diarrhea. Total surgical resection offers the best chance for cure, although chemotherapy and irradiation are both utilized in cases of subtotal resection.[17] A significant feature of neuroblastoma is its ability to regress spontaneously in some cases.[4]

Wilms' Tumor

Wilms' tumor or nephroblastoma is a tumor that originates in the kidney and occurs in both hereditary and nonhereditary forms.[17] The hereditary form is autosomal dominant, may be bilateral or multifocal, and generally occurs at an earlier age than the nonhereditary form.[4] Wilms' tumor is most common in children from birth to 15 years of age,[17] with the peak age being 1 to 4 years.[6] Signs and symptoms of Wilms' tumor include an abdominal lump or mass, hematuria, fatigue, low-grade fever, or abdominal pain.[17] Certain developmental anomalies are associated with Wilms' tumor, including aniridia, hemihypertrophy, and genitourinary abnormalities.[4] Treatment for Wilms' tumor includes a radical nephrectomy with removal of surrounding tissue and lymph nodes, followed by chemotherapy and possible irradiation.[17]

Bone Tumors

The two most common forms of bone cancer in pediatrics include osteogenic sarcoma or osteosarcoma, and Ewing's sarcoma.[6]

OSTEOGENIC SARCOMA

Osteogenic sarcoma, the most common form of bone cancer in children,[6] arises from the epiphyses of the long bones where active growth is occurring. The most common sites of disease are the long bones of the extremities, including the femur, humerus, and tibia.[22] Osteogenic sarcoma occurs most frequently in individuals 10 to 25 years of age, and affects males more frequently than females.[17] Symptoms include pain, swelling, and possible pathologic fracture.[4] Metastases, especially to the lungs, may arise rapidly.[22]

TREATMENT. Treatment of osteogenic sarcoma generally includes amputation with excision of a wide margin of tissue above the proximal aspect of the tumor to ensure total disease removal. Types of lower extremity amputations performed for osteogenic sarcoma include above-knee (AK) or below-knee (BK) amputations, hip or knee disarticulations, or hemipelvectomy. A limb salvage procedure, involving removal of the tumor and surrounding tissue without severing of the limb, may be performed as an alternative to amputation in order to preserve limb function or improve cosmesis. Limb salvage procedures vary according to the extent of tissue involvement, but always include the resection of a wide margin of unaffected tissue around the tumor in order to prevent recurrence of the malignant lesion. Bone replacements used in limb salvage procedures may include cadaver allografts as well as autologous or vascularized grafts. Metal endoprosthetic devices may also be utilized for bone and joint replacements.[23]

The decision to perform amputation versus a limb salvage procedure involves many factors, including the age and level of musculoskeletal development of the patient, the size and location of the tumor, the possibility of metastases, and the lifestyle and preference of the patient and family. Poor candidates for limb salvage procedures include those with distal tibial lesions or those with extensive proximal tibial lesions, as a wide margin of tissue is unavailable for excision.[23] No difference in survival rates has been found between the two procedures.[24,25]

Another surgical option for children with osteogenic sarcoma, primarily those with distal femoral tumors, is rotationplasty. In this procedure, the distal femur, knee joint, and proximal tibia and fibula are resected. The remaining portion of the distal lower extremity is then rotated longitudinally 180 degrees and the residual distal tibia is fused to the proximal femur. The reversed ankle joint is then able to act as the knee joint, with the foot encompassed in the prosthetic shank. The primary advantage of this procedure is the increase in residual limb length from an AK to a BK level, with a resultant increase in overall function.[26,27]

Radiation therapy has not been found to be effective in the treatment of osteogenic sarcoma, primarily because of the radioresistance of the tumor.[5,22]

EWING'S SARCOMA

Ewing's sarcoma is a tumor of the bone that arises most frequently in the bone shaft. It may originate from the long bones, such as the femur and humerus, but it may also be found in the ribs and pelvis as well. Ewing's sarcoma is seen primarily in individuals 10 to 25 years of age, most commonly affecting teens. Symptoms include pain or tenderness, swelling, fever, chills, and weakness. Common metastatic sites include the lungs and other bones. Because of the tumor's significant radioresponsivity, the *treatment* most frequently utilized for Ewing's sarcoma is irradiation. Chemotherapy may be utilized as well.[17]

Rhabdomyosarcoma

Rhabdomyosarcoma is a soft tissue tumor that arises from muscle cells. The most common sites of occurrence include the head and neck, pelvis, and extremities. Rhabdomyosarcoma is generally not a well-encapsulated tumor and may spread rapidly. It occurs most commonly in children ages 2 to 6 years, and more frequently in males than in females. The initial symptom of rhabdomyosarcoma is a noticeable mass. *Treatment* generally includes surgery, followed by irradiation and chemotherapy.[17]

Retinoblastoma

Retinoblastoma is a tumor of the eye that may or may not be hereditary. One third of the cases are bilateral.[17] Retinoblastoma generally appears before the age of two,[4] and tends to remain localized for long periods before metastasizing.[17] Males and females are fairly equally affected by retinoblastoma.[18] Irradiation is the *primary treatment* for tumors that are diagnosed at an early stage. However, for tumors diagnosed later, removal of the eye may be necessary. Chemotherapy and/or irradiation may be used to treat metastases.[17]

Treatment

Medical Management

The primary forms of medical treatment utilized for children with cancer include surgery, chemotherapy, and irradiation. These treatments may be used individually or in combination, depending on the type of cancer and its location in the body.

Surgery

Surgery for children with solid tumors is performed to eradicate the tumor by removing as many cancerous and precancerous cells as possible. A wide margin of normal tissue along the tumor's edge may also be excised because of the possibility of transitional cells. Care is taken during tumor resection to remove the tumor as one mass, if possible, in order to prevent "seeding" of cancerous cells into normal tissue. If complete resection of the tumor is impossible, surgery may also be utilized for tumor debulking or diagnostic biopsy. Irradiation and/or chemotherapy may be used preoperatively to shrink a tumor, or postoperatively to treat residual tumor, metastases, or micrometastases.

Chemotherapy

Chemotherapeutic agents are chemical substances, used alone or in combination, to control or palliate cancer processes. These agents disrupt the reproductive capabilities of cancer cells, resulting in tumor death.[5] Different chemotherapy drugs affect cells in different stages of the cell cycle. Most chemotherapeutic agents do not readily cross the blood-brain barrier. Thus, unless injected intrathecally, these drugs have little effect on malignant cells in the CNS.[9] The major chemotherapeutic agents are grouped according to their effect on cell chemistry and include alkylating agents, antimetabolites, antitumor antibiotics, plant alkaloids, hormonal agents.[28] Additional drugs continue to be tested. Two newer families of chemotherapy drugs currently showing promise in the treatment of cancer include the taxanes and camptothecan derivatives.[29]

Goals of chemotherapy include:

- Preoperative shrinking of tumor
- Curative therapy
- Adjuvant therapy to treat residual tumor or metastases
- Palliative therapy for symptom relief

Chemotherapeutic drugs are typically administered by oral, intramuscular, intravenous, subcutaneous, or intrathecal methods.[17] Newer methods for the delivery of chemotherapy medications also continue to be developed, such as injection directly into a body cavity or through the use of prolonged intravenous infusion pumps.[29]

Irradiation

Radiation therapy is the directing of high energy electromagnetic emissions at a tumor in order to cause cell death. The ionizing radiation acts to disrupt the DNA of the cell, compromising the cell's reproductive capacity and causing the death of the tumor. The amount of radiation that may be utilized is limited by the patient's *radiation tolerance,* which is the ability of surrounding normal tissue to resist the effects of irradiation. Certain organs, such as the liver, kidney, and lung, have a poor radiation tolerance, whereas other organs, such as the brain and the extremities, are relatively radioresistant. To increase normal tissue tolerance, *fractionated treatments* may be administered, which involve the use of multiple, smaller doses of radiation as opposed to one large dose[5] (Fig. 10-1).

Recent advances in radiation therapy include *conformal radiotherapy,* which provides an improved ability to adapt each treatment more specifically to a patient's particular cancer. Thus, the tumor is able to be targeted more precisely and with increased levels of radiation while less of the surrounding tissue is destroyed. Protons and neutrons are also now being used in addition to x-rays and gamma rays.[29]

The goals of radiation therapy include the following:

- Reducing tumor size preoperatively
- Destroying residual tumor postoperatively
- Destroying tumor that is unable to be removed surgically
- Decreasing tumor size for palliative relief of symptoms

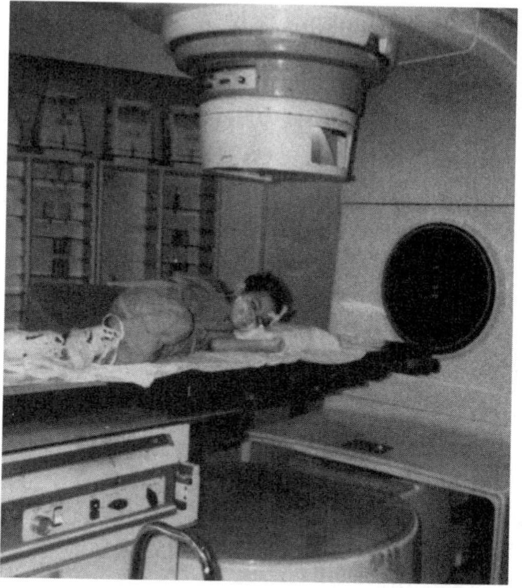

Figure 10-1 ▪ Three-year-old child with a brain tumor positioned for radiation therapy.

Side Effects of Chemotherapy and Radiation Therapy

When considering the mechanisms by which chemotherapy and irradiation work, it is evident that both treatments act to disable the reproductive capacity of rapidly growing cancer cells. However, because targeting only cancer cells is impossible, these treatments also affect normal, fast-growing cells, such as hair follicles, gastrointestinal tract cells, and bone marrow cells, resulting in side effects, such as alopecia, nausea and vomiting, and myelosuppression. Other common side effects of chemotherapy and irradiation include musculoskeletal, cardiovascular, and respiratory problems, as well as nervous system toxicity.[30]

Within the past several years, numerous advances in cancer diagnosis and treatment have been made. Significant progress is anticipated within the next decade as well. At this time, the most promising new areas of cancer research and treatment appear to be immunotherapy and gene therapy.

Immunotherapy

Within the field of immunotherapy, researchers are currently investigating the immune system's ability to resist the initial development and progressive growth of cancer, as well as how best to manipulate the immune response to maximize this resistance.[31] Current approaches for its application to cancer treatment include five major areas (Display 10-3). The first involves the use of *recombinant hematopoietic growth factors,* or colony stimulating factors, which may be used to stimulate the proliferation of blood cells. This action may permit more rapid recovery after marrow-suppressive treatments, or may stimulate the growth of cells that have the capabilities of enhancing tumor destruction.

Adoptive immunotherapy involves the use of supplanted immune-competent cells to promote a response brought about by these cells.

DISPLAY 10-3
Immunotherapy

Current approaches to cancer treatment include:

- Recominant hematopoietic growth factors—stimulate proliferation of blood cells
- Adoptive immunotherapy—use of supplanted immune–competent cells
- Active specific immunotherapy—use of vaccines to augment immune reaction or prevent development of cancer
- Biologically derived chemotherapy—use of cells (intreferon or TNF) to evoke toxic reactions to cancer cells
- Passive immunotherapy—use of monoclonal antibodies to target tumor cells

One example of this form of immunotherapy already well-established for use with certain pediatric cancers is allogeneic bone marrow transplantation, which uses a genetically nonidentical donor as a source of marrow cells.

The third area of immunotherapy that may be applied to cancer treatment is *active specific immunotherapy,* which involves the use of vaccines, given either to augment the immune reaction against tumor cells or to prevent the initial development of cancer. *Biologically derived "chemotherapy"* involves the use of cells generated by the immune system, such as interferons or tumor necrosis factors (TNF), to evoke toxic reactions against cancerous cells.

Last, *passive immunotherapy* involves the use of monoclonal antibodies to target tumor cells. However, because these antibodies may locate but not necessarily destroy tumor cells, modifications of this technique are also being explored, including the linking of radionuclides, potent toxins, or antineoplastic agents to the antibodies.[32]

Several of the preceding techniques are currently being investigated or utilized with pediatric oncology patients. However, much more extensive research is required to reveal the maximum potential of immunotherapy as it relates to cancer in children.

Gene Therapy

Gene therapy, which is predicated on the biochemical foundation of cancer originating in the genetic material of the cell, also appears to show significant promise in the fight against cancer. Two major categories of genes affecting the cell cycle are primarily involved: (1) proto-oncogenes that promote cell growth; and (2) tumor suppressor genes that inhibit abnormal growth (Display 10-4). As a result of either somatic or germ line mutations to these cells, their normal action is lost, resulting in proto-oncogenes driving excessive, abnormal multiplication and/or tumor suppressor genes no longer arresting inappropriate growth.

Gene therapy is thus designed to replace the mutated gene in order to halt the abnormal function and allow the cell to resume normal proliferation and differentiation. This is theoretically done by the insertion of a normally functioning gene into the patient's cells to replace the mutated gene. Methods currently under investigation to deliver genes to tumor cells include the use of weakened viruses to act as couriers.[33,34]

An alternate form of gene therapy, prodrug therapy, is also currently under investigation

DISPLAY 10-4
Gene Therapy

Two major categories affecting cell cycle are:

- Proto-oncogenes, which promote cell growth
- Tumor suppressor genes, which inhibit cell growth

Alternate forms of gene therapy are:

- Prodrug therapy
- Gene-directed enzyme prodrug therapy (GDEPT)

(see Display 10-4). Prodrugs are initially inert chemicals that convert in the body to highly toxic substances when activated by specific enzymes. In gene-directed enzyme prodrug therapy (GDEPT), the gene encoded for an activating enzyme is inserted into malignant cells. An inert prodrug is then administered to the patient. When the prodrug encounters the enzymes in the malignant cells, it becomes activated, resulting in death of the tumor cells.[35,36] In addition, this treatment may result in the "bystander effect," whereby surrounding cancer cells are also destroyed, possibly as a result of the release of toxins from the dying tumor cells.[34,36] As opposed to other forms of cancer therapy, this treatment has the advantage of allowing for greater specificity, targeting only malignant cells while avoiding the harmful side effects caused by damage to normal tissue.[36]

Although gene therapy techniques remain highly experimental at this time, considerable advancements in this area are anticipated in the near future. It is hoped that these developments will result in significant progress in the battle against cancer in children.

Bone Marrow Transplantation

The high doses of chemotherapy and radiation required to kill cancerous cells also cause death of the bone marrow cells. Thus, new marrow cells unexposed to the powerful therapy must be provided. This is accomplished by harvesting healthy marrow from a histocompatible donor and transfusing it into the affected patient. The donor marrow then disseminates into the patient's bone and, unless rejected, begins to produce healthy blood cells once again.

The primary types of bone marrow transplants include:

- Autologous—using the patient's own marrow
- Allogeneic—using marrow from a histocompatible donor

In order to find a compatible donor for an allogeneic transplant, *human leukocyte antigen* (HLA) typing is performed to determine whether tissues from a donor, usually a sibling, will be accepted by the recipient. There is a one-in-four chance that two siblings will match perfectly.[10]

The entire transplantation process lasts a minimum of 6 to 8 weeks if minimal complications occur, and includes the following phases:

- Pretransplantation—begins approximately 10 days before the actual transplant, when preliminary total body irradiation (TBI) and chemotherapy are administered to eradicate residual disease and to immunosuppress the patient for the greatest opportunity for graft acceptance. The patient is placed in a sterile or laminar airflow (LAF) room at this time.
- Transplantation—donor marrow is harvested in the operating room (OR) through multiple aspirations from the anterior superior iliac spine (ASIS) and posterior superior iliac spine (PSIS). The marrow is filtered, treated, and then administered to the patient.[10]
- Posttransplantation—the patient remains in strict isolation until the graft has been accepted and the bone marrow begins to produce blood cells, thus enabling the patient to fight off infection. During this phase, supportive care is generally required, including multiple blood transfusions and antibiotics.

Numerous complications may occur during the transplantation process, including:

- Failure of engraftment/rejection
- Interstitial pneumonia
- Infection
- Hepatic veno-occlusive disease
- Drug treatment side effects[10]

Another major complication of bone marrow transplantation is graft-versus-host (GVH) disease, which may occur in allogeneic transplants when donor graft cells recognize the host tissue as foreign and react against it. The acute form of the disease generally occurs soon after transplantation and may include diarrhea, skin rash, and hepatic dysfunction. The extent of disease may be mild to life-threatening. Chronic GVH disease generally occurs 4 to 6 months posttransplant and is often a generalized multisystem disease which may have a profound effect on immune function and may lead to death.[37,38]

Physical Therapy Management

Chart Review

When initially consulted regarding a pediatric oncology patient, the physical therapist should conduct a thorough chart review prior to the physical therapy evaluation. Significant information obtained from the chart includes the type and location, as well as the stage, or extent of spread, of the disease. Although criteria vary with each form of cancer, general staging guidelines identify stage I as an area of localized disease that generally offers the best chance for cure; the stages progress through stage IV, which refers to widespread or metastatic disease and generally indicates a very poor prognosis.

Additional information obtained from the chart should include past and present medical management, such as surgical procedures, irradiation, and chemotherapy. For patients who have undergone surgical excision of a tumor, it is important to note the extent of the resection, because partial resection may indicate the need for further medical intervention. Ventriculoperitoneal shunt placement, as well as placement of a central line or indwelling catheter, used to withdraw blood or administer intravenous (IV) medications, are also significant factors in the past surgical history. For children undergoing radiation therapy, the duration of treatment is important to note. Similarly, for patients receiving chemotherapy, the types of drugs are significant, because many have side effects that impact on the child's physical status and treatment program.

For hospitalized patients, the results of the CBC should be listed daily in the chart. These blood cell counts are significant to physical therapists, because abnormal levels require modifications in the approach to the child as well as to the treatment program (see Table 10-1). A patient's nutritional status is also important to note because it may have an effect on the child's activity level and performance in therapy.

Physical Therapy Evaluation

While conducting the initial evaluation, the physical therapist must be aware that the child may not tolerate a lengthy initial session. Thus, the elements of the evaluation must be individually prioritized for each patient. Specific limitations should be considered, as they influence the child's overall function. Components of the physical therapy evaluation are detailed along with specific information and precautions for each of the areas as they relate to pediatric oncology. Also, Display 10-5 outlines the important information and steps in a physical therapy evaluation.

MUSCULOSKELETAL EVALUATION

A thorough musculoskeletal examination should be performed, including tests of range of motion (ROM), muscle strength, posture, sensation, and pain. When performing the ROM evaluation, particular attention should be given to cervical mobility in those children who have undergone brain tumor resection, because these patients tend to guard or restrict movement at the incision site because of fear and/or pain. Special consideration should be given to ROM of the involved extremity or residual limb of patients who have undergone limb salvage or amputation procedures. Hamstring and heelcord

DISPLAY 10-5
Physical Therapy Evaluation

	Comments
A. Patient/Parent History	
B. Observation	
C. Musculoskeletal Evaluation	
▪ Range of motion	▪ Monitor cervical mobility in children following brain tumor resections ▪ Complete thorough evaluation of limb following limb salvage procedure or amputation
▪ Muscle strength	▪ Use caution when using resistance testing with children with a low platlet count
▪ Posture	▪ Monitor for lateral head tilt in children with brain tumors ▪ Monitor for scoliosis, kyphosis, and leg length discrepancies in children following radiation owing to possible epiphyseal damage
▪ Pain	▪ Use various methods to assess according to child's age and ability to communicate
D. Neurologic Evaluation	▪ Complete thorough evaluation in children with CNS involvement
▪ Muscle tone	
▪ Sensory systems	▪ Include evaluation of cranial nerve function and vision (monitor for diplopia, field cuts, etc.)
▪ Reflexes	
▪ Balance and equilibrium	
▪ Coordination	
E. Respiratory Status and Cardiovascular Endurance	▪ May be affected by: Radiation to the mediastinum; Chemotherapy drugs; Prolonged bedrest
F. Functional Assessment	
▪ Transfers	
▪ Gait and mobility	▪ Common gait deviations may include: Asymmetry owing to hemiparesis; Ataxia secondary to cerebellar effects; High steppage owing to peripheral neuropathy
▪ Developmental/gross motor skills	
G. Activities of Daily Living/Self-Help Skills	

length may be limited in children who have been inactive or confined to bed for long periods of time. Limitations in joint ROM may also be present in areas where chemotherapeutic drug extravasation has occurred.

A general *strength and sensory evaluation* should be included in the physical therapy assessment. Caution should be used when providing resistance to evaluate strength in those patients who are thrombocytopenic owing to the potential for bruising as well as bleeding into a muscle or joint. Significant findings of the sensory evaluation may include asymmetry as seen with hemiparesis, or proximal versus distal discrepancies that may indicate peripheral neuropathy secondary to chemotherapy.

Deformities, such as scoliosis, kyphosis, and leg length discrepancies, may be detected during the *postural evaluation,* especially in those patients who have had epiphyseal damage as a result of radiation therapy.[30,39] Children with brain tumors may present with a lateral head tilt.

The *pain assessment* is an important component of the pediatric oncologic evaluation. Various methods of assessment may be utilized for different age groups according to the child's ability to identify and communicate feelings of pain. Examples of pain assessment methods/tools include the observation of pain-related behaviors in infants and toddlers, facial expression charts for younger children, and body-mapping or visual analogue scales for older children.[40]

NEUROLOGIC EVALUATION

The neurologic examination includes the assessment of muscle tone and reflexes, as well as *balance and coordination skills,* especially in those children with CNS involvement. Current theoretical models of sensory organization in balance testing are systems-mediated, incorporating visual, proprioceptive, and vestibular input. In patients with CNS involvement, it is important to distinguish among these systems, as the results will impact significantly on the treatment plan.[41] *Visual assessment* should also be performed to detect such problems as diplopia or visual field deficits. Facial paralysis may occur in patients with cranial nerve involvement.

Functional Assessment

The *evaluation of gait and overall functional status* is very significant for children with cancer. Common gait deviations include asymmetry secondary to hemiparesis, ataxia secondary to CNS/cerebellar effects, and high steppage resulting from peripheral neuropathy.[39] The functional assessment should also include evaluation of developmental skills in infants and toddlers, as well as transitional abilities and higher level gross motor skills in older children.

RESPIRATORY STATUS AND CARDIOVASCULAR ENDURANCE

Finally, *respiratory status and cardiovascular endurance* should be evaluated, especially in those patients who have undergone irradiation to the mediastinum, because they have an increased risk for adverse pulmonary effects.[30] Endurance may be significantly decreased in children who have been inactive or restricted to bedrest for long periods of time.

FUNCTIONAL ASSESSMENT TESTS

Because of current trends in health care and the need for objective documentation, the use of standardized tests to demonstrate functional status and/or gains may be indicated. Assessments that may be useful with this population include the Pediatric Evaluation of Disability Inventory (PEDI)[42] and the Functional Independence Measure for Children (WeeFIM).[43]

The PEDI is a tool that assesses functional status in infants and young children in three domains including self-care, mobility, and social function. It includes sections for caregiver assessment and modifications as well. The PEDI is designed for children ages 6 months to 7.5 years,[42] but may also be utilized for older children who, owing to the extent of their disability, may fall into this lower age range of skills. The PEDI is discussed in more detail in Chapter 2, Tests of Infant and Child Development.

The WeeFIM, a modified version of the adult Functional Independence Measure, is also designed for use with children ages 6 months to 7 years. This tool measures a child's actual performance in a functional setting in the areas of self-care, sphincter control, mobility, locomotion, communication, and social cognition. The test is scored on a seven-point scale according to the amount of assistance required to complete each task.[43]

Goals

From the results of the physical therapy evaluation, patient problems are identified. These problems then direct the development of patient goals, which should be functional, measurable, and able to be achieved within a stated time period.

When establishing goals for this patient population, it is vital to consider the child's needs, as well as those of the family. Specific goals will vary according to the nature of each child's actual or potential deficits. The categories of physical therapy goals for pediatric oncology patients are listed in Display 10-6.

Physical therapy in pediatric oncologic patients addresses not only the primary effects of the disease but also the side effects of medical interventions. The oncologic diseases most frequently requiring physical therapy intervention due to primary effects include bone cancers (owing to amputation or limb salvage procedures) and CNS tumors (because of their neurologic sequelae).

DISPLAY 10-6

Physical Therapy Goals for Pediatric Oncology Patients

- Preventive—avoiding disabling sequelae prior to their occurrence
- Restorative—maximizing motor return in patients with deficits
- Supportive—promoting the greatest level of functional independence possible when residual disease exists and progressive disability is anticipated
- Palliative—increasing or maintaining comfort and independence in patients with terminal disease

From McKenna RJ, Wellisch D, Fawzy FI. Rehabilitation and supportive care of the cancer patient. In: Murphy GP, Lawrence W, Lenhard RE, eds. *American Cancer Society Textbook of Clinical Oncology*. 2nd ed. Atlanta: American Cancer Society; 1995:635–654.

Physical Therapy Intervention: Disease-Related Disability

BONE CANCER

If at all possible, children undergoing amputation or limb salvage procedures for bone cancer should be referred to a physical therapist prior to surgery. The preoperative physical therapy session(s) should include instruction in ambulation with assistive devices, as well as exercises to be initiated immediately postoperatively. The physical therapist should also address postoperative expectations, providing an introduction to prosthetics as well as an explanation of the components of the rehabilitative process.

INTERVENTIONS. Immediately following amputative surgery, an initial prosthesis is placed on the residual limb in the operating room. This prosthesis remains intact for 6 to 8 weeks, assisting with the shaping of the limb as well as providing a surface for immediate weight-bearing. Gait training is generally initiated 1 to 2 days following surgery.[15]

After 6 to 8 weeks, the patient advances to a temporary prosthesis, which is necessary because frequent weight changes during postoperative chemotherapy may cause the volume of the residual limb to fluctuate. To accommodate the changes in size, varying thickness of lining material or stump socks should be used as needed. The physical therapist should monitor the residual limb size using circumferential measurements to determine when stabilization has occurred. With stabilization, the patient may then progress to a definitive prosthesis.[45]

Postoperative *physical therapy management of amputees* includes ROM exercises, a limb positioning program, strengthening activities, as well as gait training and postural exercises. The ROM program emphasizes stretching of the hip and knee flexors, as these muscle groups are most likely to develop contractures. The positioning program is developed to reinforce the stretching, with particular emphasis on prone-lying for periods throughout the day. Strengthening of all major muscle groups of the residual limb should be performed, with particular attention to the abductors in patients with AK amputations so as to avoid a Trendelenberg gait pattern,[45] and to hip elevators and abdominals in children with hip disarticulation so as to promote pelvic tilt.[46] Gait training activities also include instruction in the use of the prosthesis and assistive device, with the promotion of as normal a gait pattern as possible. Instruction in stair climbing and falling activities should also be provided. Postural exercises should focus on identifying the child's center of gravity as well as maintaining a level pelvis in weight-bearing positions. In order to promote independence, the child and family should be instructed in prosthetic mechanics and donning and doffing the device.

For patients who have undergone *limb salvage procedures,* the physical therapy program varies according to the area, the amount of tissue resected, and the types of endoprosthetic devices utilized. All programs should include ROM and strengthening exercises for surrounding joints and musculature, as well as skin care techniques for the involved region to promote incisional healing and to prevent skin breakdown. Orthoses may also be required to provide limb support and increase joint stability, as well as to minimize pain.

CENTRAL NERVOUS SYSTEM TUMORS

The scope of physical therapy for children with CNS tumors is extremely broad owing to the great variety of signs and symptoms that may occur, depending on the size and location of the tumor and the medical treatments utilized.

INTERVENTIONS. Most patients with brain tumors will initially undergo surgical resection.[39] Physical therapists should be consulted 1 to 2 days postoperatively to initiate a bedside program of passive ROM and positioning. Some patients, especially those with abnormal muscle tone, may require foot and ankle splints to prevent plantar-flexion contractures. A positioning program and splint schedule should be posted at the bedside for the nursing staff and other caregivers.

Patients may undergo intraoperative placement of a ventriculostomy to drain CSF externally following surgery. These children generally remain generally in the intensive care unit (ICU) confined to bedrest until the body is able to absorb the excess CSF independently, or until an internal shunt is placed. During this period of inactivity, active-assistive, active, resistive, or passive exercises are performed to prevent further musculoskeletal sequelae while the child's movement and function are restricted.

Once the child becomes medically stable and the ventriculostomy, if present, has been removed, the head of the bed is elevated to increase the child's alertness and promote increased orientation to upright positioning. The head elevation may cause headaches, nausea, and dizziness, requiring gradual increases in upright angles. Once the child tolerates a more erect position, sitting in a reclining wheelchair may begin for increasing periods of time, with a gradual raising of the seat back toward a more upright position. During this period, the patient should be performing active neck ROM exercises in all planes and participating in active exercises and functional activities. Depending on the need for monitors or ventilators, the child may soon progress to treatment sessions in the physical therapy department. These sessions may include sitting balance, transitional, mobility, and progressive ambulation activities. In patients functioning at a more advanced level, higher level gross motor and coordination skills may be incorporated into the treatment program. Handling and facilitation should be utilized with infants and very young children to promote age-appropriate motor skills following normal developmental sequences.

COMMON NEUROLOGIC SEQUELAE. Common neurologic sequelae of CNS tumors in both surgical and nonsurgical patients include hemiparesis, ataxia and dysmetria, balance disturbances, and visual problems. Children may also demonstrate cognitive sequelae, including poor judgment and attention to safety factors, as well as learning and motor planning deficits that impact on physical therapy treatment. Additional disorders, such as visual/perceptual problems, aphasia, dysarthria, and feeding/swallowing problems, may require input from other members of the rehabilitation team, including occupational and speech therapists (Fig. 10-2).

Physical therapy management of patients with hemiparesis as a result of a brain tumor should include activities to maintain the musculoskeletal status of the affected side, including passive ROM, positioning, and sensory education. Splinting may also be necessary to maintain or assist a joint and prevent deformity. Facilitation/inhibition techniques are utilized to promote motor recovery on the affected side. Functional skill instruction should be provided, including bed mobility, transitions, and ambulation. Once the patient reaches a plateau, compensatory strategies may be necessary if residual deficits persist. These strategies often include assistive devices, such as a walker with a platform attachment, cane, one-arm drive wheelchair, or orthosis. For patients with *ataxia and dysmetria,* physical therapy treatment should include activities that challenge the neuromuscular system. Provision of manual support, approximation, or resistance, as well as the addition of weights to the trunk or extremities, may provide increased proprioceptive feedback and improved proximal stability, resulting in an increased fluidity of distal movement. Weights and wheels may also be added to the walker to provide a fixed point of stability. Proprioceptive neuromuscular facilitation activities, such as rhythmic stabilization and slow-reversal-hold techniques, may be incorporated into the treatment session to promote increased stability.[46] The provision of verbal and visual feedback to the patient is a significant component of treatment activities with this patient population.

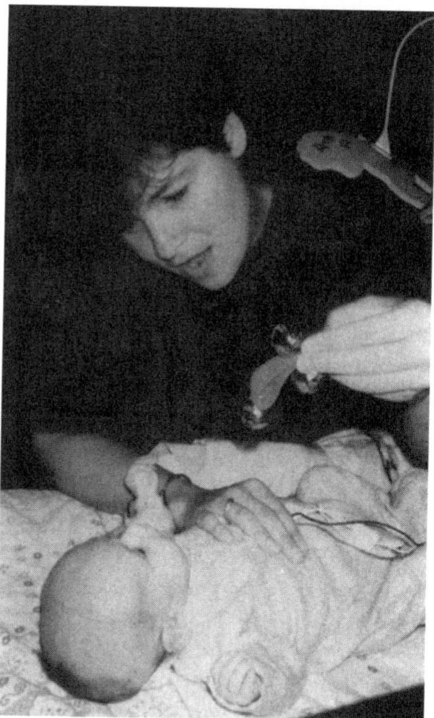

Figure 10-2 ▪ Sensory stimulation activities with a 6-week-old child who is status post brain tumor resection.

Balance disturbances may be addressed in both feedback and feedforward modes, including activities where displacements are unexpected as well as anticipated (Fig. 10-3). During feedforward activities, the patient is challenged to achieve the necessary postural set prior to performing a movement task or functional activity. The incorporation of functional tasks into balance activities may result in improved patient performance, as the child has a clearly defined goal around which to organize motor behavior. A variety of environmental contexts and varying surfaces should be incorporated into the treatment program to permit greater generalizability to normal environmental conditions. Balance beams, tilt boards, and "physioballs" are frequently utilized for the promotion of balance skills in children. Instruc-

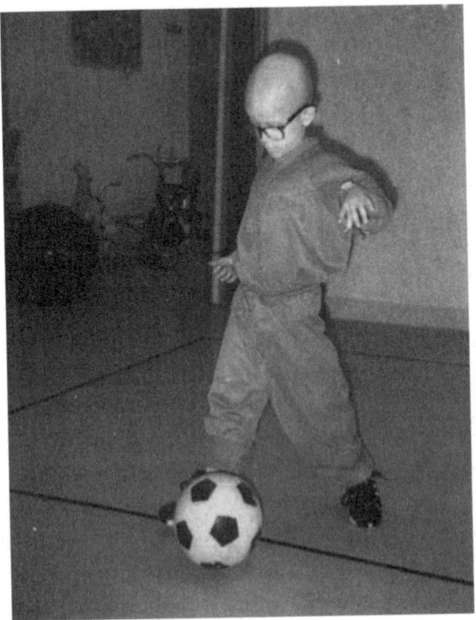

Figure 10-3 ■ Kicking a ball emphasizes balance and coordination as well as distal motor control for a child with peripheral neuropathy.

tion in compensatory techniques should also be provided, such as avoiding ambulation in dark areas and on uneven surfaces until adequate balance skills have been acquired.

Visual problems, such as diplopia and hemianopsia, are common in patients with CNS tumors. Compensatory strategies may be utilized until the disturbances resolve, including eyepatching for diplopia and increased visual scanning in patients with visual field deficits.

Physical Therapy Intervention: Medical Side Effects

Pediatric physical therapists may have only a limited role in minimizing the impact of some of the common side effects, such as alopecia, nausea and vomiting, and myelosuppression, caused by various cancer treatments. However, the role of the physical therapist is vital in the treatment of those children experiencing other problems secondary to disease and treatment side effects, such as musculoskeletal problems, cardiopulmonary effects, and neurotoxicity of medications.

ALOPECIA

The majority of children undergoing medical treatment for cancer will develop alopecia. Although younger children may not be concerned with this condition, older children and teens may be quite conscious of their physical appearance. Patients may elect to wear hats or wigs during treatment sessions. Physical therapists should work to promote a positive self-image in these patients, as well as to provide emotional support and reassurance that the hair loss is generally temporary.

NAUSEA AND VOMITING

The effects of nausea and vomiting may cause a decrease in the child's ability or motivation to participate actively in a physical therapy program. Fortunately, new and more powerful drugs are currently being utilized to decrease or prevent these effects.[29] However, if problems persist, the scheduling of treatment sessions at times during the day when these effects have subsided may increase participation in and compliance with therapeutic activities. A bedside program may also be developed for family members or other caregivers to carry out with the patient at times when side effects have decreased, such as in the evening.

MYELOSUPPRESSION

Myelosuppression in pediatric oncology patients may be caused by many factors, including chemotherapy, irradiation, infection, or bone marrow invasion by the malignant lesion. With chemotherapy, myelosuppression generally occurs within 10 to 14 days following drug administration. Medical management of immunosuppressed children may include multiple blood transfusions,[30] as well as isolation or sterile precautions. New growth factor medications are also now being tested and utilized to stimulate the proliferation of the various blood cells after immunosuppressive treatments.[29]

When treating children who are myelosuppressed, the levels of each particular type of blood cell are important to note, because decreased levels of each may impact on the treatment session differently. Patients with *anemia,* a decreased percentage of red blood cells, will also have a decreased hemoglobin level, which affects the oxygenation of tissues and return of CO_2 to the lungs. These patients may exhibit fatigue, pallor, shortness of breath, loss of appetite, and decreased endurance.[5] Packed red blood cell transfusions may be necessary for relief of symptoms. Physical activity must be graded according to patient tolerance until blood levels return to normal. Children may require frequent rest periods during therapy sessions, and vital signs should be monitored. Patients with severe symptoms may require instruction in energy conservation techniques.[47]

Thrombocytopenia, a decrease in platelets, indicates a diminished ability of the blood to clot, resulting in an increased potential for bleeding or hemorrhage. Common signs of thrombocytopenia include bleeding gums, nosebleeds, bruising, or petechiae. Physical therapy guidelines for patients with thrombocytopenia, as developed at the Sloan Kettering Cancer Center, are included in Table 10-2. Patients may require transfusions for very low platelet levels or if active bleeding occurs.

Of the five types of white blood cells, the most significant indicator of the ability to fight infection is the neutrophil. The level of neutrophils in the body, the *absolute neutrophil count (ANC),* is calculated by multiplying the total white blood cell count by the percentage of mature neutrophils.[47] A child with an ANC of less than 500 is considered to have *neutropenia,* which indicates a significantly impaired ability to fight infection. Guidelines for caregivers of children with neutropenia include strict adherence to sterile precautions as ordered by physicians, including the wearing of masks, gowns, gloves, and shoe covers. Frequent handwashing should be performed as well. Children with very low white blood cell levels may require bedside physical therapy treatment. Patients, if permitted to leave their rooms, may be required to wear a mask in hospital corridors and in the physical therapy department for their own protection. Neutropenic patients who are permitted in the physical therapy gym should be scheduled at those times when a minimal number of other patients are present in the treatment area. Physical therapists with infections of any type should not treat neutropenic patients. All precautions should be continued until neutrophil levels increase adequately to enable the patient to fight infection once again.

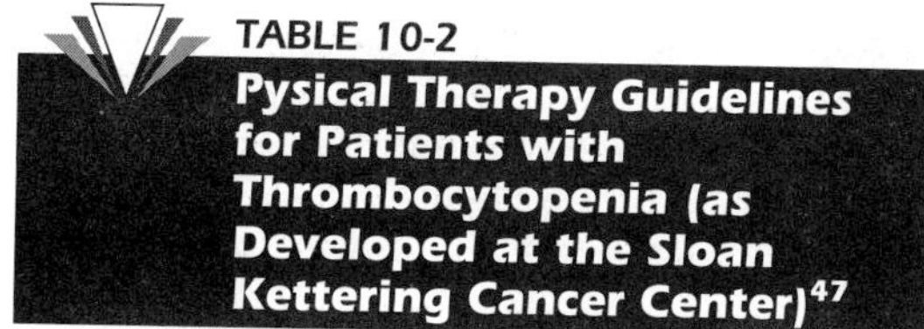
TABLE 10-2
Pysical Therapy Guidelines for Patients with Thrombocytopenia (as Developed at the Sloan Kettering Cancer Center)[47]

Thrombocyte Count	Appropriate Activity Level
30,000–50,000/mm^3	Active exercise only, no resistive exercise
20,000–30,000/mm^3	Gentle active or passive exercise only
<20,000/mm^3	Minimal exercise and essential activities of daily living (ADLs) only

MUSCULOSKELETAL SEQUELAE

Multiple musculoskeletal problems may occur in pediatric oncologic patients as a result of disease and medical intervention. Although the most effective treatment is prevention, physical therapy management is generally symptomatic if problems occur.

ROM limitations may occur owing to the effects of bedrest, guarding of a joint because of pain, skin and soft tissue fibrosis from irradiation, or drug extravasation into or near a joint. Treatment of contractures includes a passive ROM/stretching program although, because of the potential for bleeding, caution must be utilized with those patients who are thrombocytopenic. Equipment, including splints or serial casts, dynamic bracing, or continuous passive motion devices, may also be utilized for treatment of contractures.[39] In addition to the ROM program, in those patients with skin involvement, scar management techniques, such as compression dressings, may be indicated to minimize scarring effects.

Muscle weakness and atrophy are common in pediatric oncology patients, and may frequently be accompanied by a decrease in cardiovascular endurance as a result of inactivity or bedrest. The strengthening program may include isometrics as well as active-assistive, active, or resistive exercises. Cardiovascular fitness in children may be addressed with such activities as ball games, bicycle ergometry, progressive ambulation, or higher level gross motor activities such as hopping, jumping, skipping, and running.

The treatment of pain in pediatric oncology patients is a complicated issue. Whereas physical therapy techniques, such as transcutaneous electrical nerve stimulation (TENS), massage, and superficial thermal agents, may be effective in treating pain of muscular origin,[39] disease-related pain in children is customarily managed medically with nonnarcotic or narcotic analgesics. New methods to deliver pain medications to children continue to be developed, such as suppositories, skin patches, implanted pumps, and topical creams.[48] Older children and adolescents may also benefit from the use of patient-controlled analgesia (PCA), by which a predetermined amount of pain medication is delivered intravenously each time the patient pushes a button. This form of pain medication delivery may have the added benefit of providing a greater sense of control over the pain that accompanies many forms of cancer. The involvement of a pediatric pain team, which includes a physical therapist, is ideal for the pain management of children with cancer. Such teams are currently active in the several major pediatric treatment facilities in the United States.

Multiple skeletal sequelae may occur in children with cancer as a result of the disease and treatment effects. Bony instability may develop in patients who have undergone limb salvage procedures, as well as in children with metastatic bone disease. Treatment should include techniques to minimize stress on the bone, such as protective body mechanics, non–weight-bearing ambulation with an assistive device, and use of splints or bracing. Scoliosis, kyphosis, and leg length discrepancies may develop as late effects of cancer treatment.[30,39] Spinal deformities should be addressed with strengthening and mobility exercises for the trunk and associated musculature. Advanced deformities may require evaluation and intervention by an orthopedic physician. Leg length discrepancies may require the addition of a shoe lift or orthotic to prevent pelvic obliquity and permanent deformity. Postural exercises should be incorporated into the physical therapy program of all children with skeletal deformities.

Mobility or gait problems are common in this population owing to peripheral neuropathy, limb salvage and amputation procedures, and the effects of bedrest or bony abnormalities as described earlier. Progressive ambulation training should be utilized with these patients, including assistive devices and orthotics as needed.

Edema may occur as a result of an interruption in the lymphatic drainage system caused by tumor blockage or lymph node resection. Treatment should include gravity-assisted drainage using elevation, active muscle pumping and, if necessary, the use of compression garments.[39]

Equipment needs for these children may include wheelchairs and assistive devices for activities of daily living equipment (ADL), as well as prosthetics or orthotics.

CARDIOPULMONARY EFFECTS

Multiple cardiac and pulmonary complications may result from the medical interventions used in children with cancer. *Cardiomyopathy* may be caused by the anthracyclines, a group of chemotherapeutic drugs that includes doxorubicin (Adriamycin) and daunorubicin. Similarly, *pericarditis* may result from irradiation of the mediastinum, and may occur acutely as well as months to years after treatment. Both disorders may eventually result in congestive heart failure.[30] Grading activity programs in accordance with patient tolerance, as well as frequent rest periods and close monitoring of vital signs, is indicated for these children. Instruction in energy conservation techniques may be provided to patients exhibiting significant cardiac insufficiency.

Chemotherapy and radiation therapy, as well as metastatic lung disease, may result in pulmonary compromise. Common pulmonary problems in children with cancer include pulmonary fibrosis and interstitial pneumonitis, which lead to decreased chest wall mobility, dyspnea, and decreased exercise tolerance.[30] Physical therapy for these patients should incorporate respiratory activities to maintain lung expansion and chest wall mobility. Suggested activities include deep breathing exercises, incentive spirometry, pulmonary or breathing games, and cardiovascular conditioning activities.

NEUROTOXICITY

A common side effect of the chemotherapeutic vinca alkaloids, especially vincristine, is a progressive peripheral neuropathy[49] for which physical therapy is frequently indicated. Initial signs of vincristine neurotoxicity include loss of the Achilles tendon reflex, followed by paresthesias of the fingers and toes. Distal sensory loss may occur, accompanied by progressive distal weakness that initially affects wrist and finger extensors as well as ankle dorsiflexors. If the drug is continued at this point, generalized progressive weakness may follow, resulting in a significant decrease in overall function.

Once the drug is discontinued, reversal of the symptoms of neurotoxicity generally occurs fairly rapidly, beginning with the resolution of the paresthesias, followed by an increase in muscle strength. However, superficial sensory loss and depressed deep tendon reflexes may resolve more slowly, if at all. Overall, the symptoms of the neuropathy are largely reversible and cause minimal residual disability.[50]

Common initial physical sequelae of neurotoxicity include foot drop during ambulation, wrist drop, weak grasp, and decreased distal sensory feedback. Patients with more profound involvement may develop an inability to ambulate, with distal muscle weakness and atrophy.[51–53] An equinovarus deformity of the foot may develop owing to paralysis of the extensor muscles of the foot and ankle, which results in an unopposed flexor pull.[53]

The physical therapy program for patients with peripheral neuropathy should include ROM/ stretching as well as distal strengthening exercises. Orthotics, such as molded ankle-foot orthoses (MAFOs), may be indicated to maintain adequate foot and ankle position and to support the foot during ambulation. Wrist splints may also be required to maintain and assist the distal upper extremity. Patients should be instructed in compensatory strategies for altered sensation, such as using caution on uneven surfaces and using visual rather than tactile and kinesthetic cues to maintain balance.[39] Instruction in skin care techniques such as closely monitoring bath water temperature and checking daily for signs of skin breakdown when using an orthotic, especially in areas of decreased sensation, must also be provided to patients and families. Patients with more advanced peripheral neuropathies may require instruction in the use of assistive devices for ambulation, such as walkers or canes. Severely affected patients may require wheelchairs and other ADL equipment.

As symptoms begin to resolve, more aggressive use of facilitation techniques, such as proprioceptive neuromuscular facilitation, should be incorporated into the physical therapy program, along with continued strengthening exercises. Serial casting or heelcord lengthening procedures may be necessary for fixed contractures of the ankle.

Physical Therapy Intervention: Bone Marrow Transplantation

Physical therapy treatment should be an integral part of a BMT admission because of the significant potential for pulmonary, musculoskeletal, and neurologic problems. Common problems include decreased ROM, weakness, pneumonia, deconditioning, and muscle atrophy. These sequelae may occur as a result of long periods of confinement in the LAF room, the patient's general inactivity level, and/or the various procedures and side effects of treatment. The LAF room provides for air exchange in a manner to provide an environment that is almost free of microorganisms.

Physical therapists should be consulted on admission of the child. Initial treatment goals are generally preventive, and may include:

1. Maintenance of joint ROM and prevention of contractures
2. Maintenance of muscle strength and prevention of atrophy
3. Promotion of pulmonary hygiene and prevention of pneumonia
4. Maintenance of balance, coordination, and endurance
5. Promotion of overall physical and emotional well-being[54]

When treating a patient in the LAF room, the physical therapist is required to follow specific sterile isolation precautions that generally include handwashing, followed by the donning of a mask, gown, gloves, hat, and shoe covers. All items taken into the room must be sterilized, making the use of physical therapy equipment difficult. Thus, creativity is important in the development of therapeutic activities for these patients. Manual forms of resistance are frequently utilized for strengthening. Balls and other smooth pieces of equipment may be cleaned with disinfectant and used, provided no Velcro or other potential sources of bacteria are present. Some facilities will permit cardiovascular training equipment, such as a stationary bicycle, to remain in the BMT unit permanently. Specific rules and regulations of individual facilities should be investigated and strictly followed by physical therapists for the sake of the patient's health and well-being.

The physical therapy treatment program for BMT patients should include ROM, strengthening, pulmonary exercises, as well as balance and coordination activities. The ROM activities should emphasize the stretching of hamstrings, heelcords, and hip flexors, which may become particularly tight owing to positioning and general inactivity. Strengthening may include active and resistive exercises. Resistance may be provided manually by the therapist or by utilizing the patient's own body weight. Examples of strengthening exercises include sit-ups, bridging, push-ups, arm circles, straight leg raises, and short arc quadriceps exercises. Awareness of the patient's platelet count prior to each session is extremely important, because stretching and resistive exercises may cause bleeding or hemorrhage in those patients who are thrombocytopenic. Activities, such as bicycling in the supine position, jumping jacks, or jogging in place, will help maintain aerobic capacity and cardiopulmonary endurance. Balance and coordination may be addressed with one-foot balance activities; heel, toe, or line walking; as well as reaching and targeting games. Deep breathing exercises may be used to maintain aerobic capacity and chest wall mobility in an effort to prevent pneumonia and other pulmonary complications. Instruction in relaxation techniques may help children to deal with anxiety, pain, and the effects of treatment. Motivating these children to be active at a time when they may be quite ill and depressed is a particularly challenging task for the pediatric physical therapist.[54]

Initial physical therapy treatment should also include the development of a bedside exercise and activity program to be posted in the LAF room. Instruction regarding the program components should be provided to the child and family early in the hospitalization course when the patient is feeling fairly well. Then, if the patient is unavailable for physical therapy treatment at certain times during the day because of other procedures or illness, these activities may be carried out with the child at a later time.

Physical Therapy Intervention: Terminal Disease

The pediatric physical therapist may be consulted to assist in the management of homebound children with terminal cancer. Treatment of these patients may include passive ROM exercises, pain management techniques, and positioning to prevent skin breakdown as well as to increase the patient's comfort. Family instruction in positioning, transfers, skin care, and exercises is also a vital component of the physical therapy program. Wheelchairs, hospital beds, pressure relief cushions and mattresses, ADL and assistive devices, as well as commodes and bathing equipment, may be required. Psychological and emotional support of the patient and family must also be provided owing to the extreme stress and devastation associated with the impending death of a child from cancer.

Summary

The physical therapist is an essential member of the pediatric oncology team, which generally also includes physicians, nurses, occupational therapists, speech therapists, social workers, nutritionists, and child life therapists. With this population, each team member must focus not only on the issues relevant to his or her own

DISPLAY 10-7

Resource Agencies that Provide Literature, Brochures and Information for Professionals and Families

Agency	Means of Contact
The American Cancer Society	1-800-227-2345 http://www.cancer.org
The Oncology Section of the American Physical Therapy Association (APTA)	1-800-999-APTA
The American Brain Tumor Association	1-800-886-2282 http://www.abta.org
The National Cancer Institute	1-800-4-CANCER http://www.cancernet.nci.nih.gov
The Candlelighter's Childhood Cancer Foundation	1-800-336-2223 http://www.candlelighters.org
The Leukemia Society of America	1-212-573-8484 http://www.leukemia.org

discipline but must also address the whole child as well as the child's role within the family structure, school, and community. Thus, physical therapy for these patients must address not only the physical status of the child, but also the social and emotional issues associated with the diagnosis of cancer in children.

Several excellent resource agencies provide literature to professionals, as well as brochures and information that may be shared with patients and their families. These agencies are listed in Display 10-7.

REFERENCES

1. Pui CH. Childhood leukemias. In: Murphy GP, Lawrence W, Lenhard RE, eds. *American Cancer Society Textbook of Clinical Oncology.* 2nd ed. Atlanta: American Cancer Society; 1995:501–523.
2. Bleyer WA. The impact of childhood cancer on the United States and the world. *CA.* 1990;40(6); 355–367.
3. American Cancer Society: *Cancer Facts and Figures—1997.* Atlanta; American Cancer Society; 1997.
4. Marina NM, Bowman LC, Pui C-H, et al. Pediatric solid tumors. In: Murphy GP, Lawrence W, Lenhard RE, eds. *American Cancer Society Textbook of Clinical Oncology.* 2nd ed. Atlanta: American Cancer Society; 1995:524–551.
5. Link MP. Cancer in childhood. In: Bleck EE, Nagel DA, eds. *Physically Handicapped Children, A Medical Atlas for Teachers.* 2nd ed. New York: Grune and Stratton; 1982.
6. Young JL, Ries LG, Silverberg E, et al. Cancer incidence, survival, and mortality for children younger than age 15 years. *Cancer.* 1986;58:598–602.
7. Grier HE, Weinstein HJ. Acute nonlymphocytic leukemia. In: Pizzo PA, Poplack DG, eds. *Principles and Practice of Pediatric Oncology.* Philadelphia: J.B. Lippincott; 1989:367–382.
8. Pui C-H, Rivera G. Leukemia. In: Rudolph AM, Hoffman JI, eds. *Pediatrics.* 18th ed. East Norwalk, CT: Appleton and Lange; 1987:1096–1104.
9. Vietti T, Bergamini RA. General aspects of chemotherapy. In: Sutow WW, Fernbach DJ, Vietti TJ, eds. *Clinical Pediatric Oncology.* St. Louis: CV Mosby; 1984:210–243.
10. Quinn, JJ. Bone marrow transplantation in the management of childhood cancer. *Pediatr Clin North Am.* 1985;32:3.
11. Sutow, WW. General aspects of childhood cancer. In: Sutow WW, Fernbach DJ, Vietti TJ, eds. *Clinical Pediatric Oncology.* St. Louis: C.V. Mosby; 1984:1–13.
12. Association For Brain Tumor Research: *A Primer of Brain Tumors,* 4th ed. Chicago: Association for Brain Tumor Research; 1988.
13. Blossom B, Barnhart L. Brain tumors. In: Umphred DA, ed. *Neurologic Rehabilitation.* St. Louis: C.V. Mosby; 1985:442–451.
14. Duffner PK, Cohen ME, et al. Late effects of treatment on the intelligence of children with posterior fossa tumors. *Cancer.* 1983;51:223–237.
15. Heideman RL, Packer RJ, et al. Tumors of the central nervous system. In: Pizzo PA, Poplack DG, eds. *Principles and Practice of Pediatric Oncology.* Philadelphia: J.B. Lippincott; 1989:505–554.
16. Eys JV. Malignant tumors of the central nervous system. In: Sutow WW, Fernbach DJ, Vietti TJ. *Clinical Pediatric Oncology.* St. Louis: CV Mosby; 1984.
17. U.S. Department of Health and Human Services: *Young People with Cancer.* Bethesda, MD: National Cancer Institute; 1991.
18. Young JL, Miller RW. Incidence of malignant tumors in U.S. children. *J Pediatr.* 1975;86:2.
19. Murphy SB. Classification, staging and end results of treatment of childhood non-Hodgkin's lymphomas: Dissimilarities from lymphomas in adults. *Semin Oncol.* 1980;7(3):332–339.
20. American Cancer Society. *Cancer Manual.* 7th ed. Boston: American Cancer Society; 1986.
21. Hayes FA, Smith EI. Neuroblastoma. In: Pizzo PA, Poplack DG, eds. *Principles and Practice of Pediatric Oncology.* Philadelphia: J.B. Lippincott; 1989: 607–622.
22. Gahagan CA. Physical therapy management of patients with osteosarcoma. *Oncol Section Newslett.* 1984;2(2):6–7.
23. Link MP, Eilber F. Osteosarcoma. In: Pizzo PA, Poplack DG, eds. *Principles and Practice of Pediatric Oncology.* Philadelphia: J.B. Lippincott; 1989: 689–712.
24. Eilber FR, Morton DL. Limb-salvage for skeletal and soft tissue sarcomas. *Cancer.* 1984;53:2 579–2584.
25. Simon MA, Aschliman MA. Limb-salvage treatment versus amputation for osteosarcoma of the distal end of the femur. *Bone J Surg.* 1986;68:9.
26. Jaffee N. Advances in the management of malignant bone tumors in children and adolescents. *Pediatr Clin North Am.* 1985;32:3.
27. Murray MP, Jacobs PA. Functional performance after tibial rotationplasty. *J Bone Joint Surg.* 1985; 67:3.

28. Fleming ID, Brady LW, Mieszkajski GB, et al. Basis for major current therapies for cancer. In: Murphy GP, Lawrence W, Lenhard RE, eds. *American Cancer Society Textbook of Clinical Oncology*. 2nd ed. Atlanta: American Cancer Society; 1995:96–134.
29. Hellman S, Vokes EE. Advancing current treatments for cancer. *Sci Am*. 1996;275(3):118–123.
30. Mulne AF, Koepke JC. Adverse effects of cancer therapy in children. *Pediatr Rev*. 1985;6:9.
31. Heberman RB. Principles of tumor immunology. In: Murphy GP, Lawrence W, Lenhard RE, eds. *American Cancer Society Textbook of Clinical Oncology*. 2nd ed. Atlanta: American Cancer Society; 1995:135–145.
32. Frost JD, Sondel PM. Immunotherapy for infection and malignancy in children with cancer. *Adv Pediatr*. 1994;41:385–413.
33. Deisseroth AB. Current trends and future directions in the genetic therapy of human neoplastic disease. *Cancer*. 1993;72(7):2069–2074.
34. Jenkins J, Wheeler V, Albright L. Gene therapy for cancer. *Cancer Nurs*. 1994;17(6):447–456.
35. Connors TA. The choice of prodrugs for gene directed enzyme prodrug therapy of cancer. *Gene Ther*. 1995;2(10):702–709.
36. Marias R, Spooner RA, Light Y, et al. Gene-directed enzyme prodrug therapy with a mustard prodrug/carboxypeptidase G2 combination. *Cancer Res*. 1996;56:4735–4742.
37. Lenorsky C, Feig SA. Bone marrow transplantation for children with cancer. *Pediatr Ann*. 1983;12:6.
38. Ramsay NK. Bone marrow transplantation in pediatric oncology. In: Pizzo PA, Poplack DG, eds. *Principles and Practice of Pediatric Oncology*. Philadelphia: J.B. Lippincott; 1989:971–990.
39. Gerber LH, Binder H. Rehabilitation of the child with cancer. In: Pizzo PA, Poplack DG, eds. *Principles and Practice of Pediatric Oncology*. Philadelphia: J.B. Lippincott; 1989:957–970.
40. Shapiro B. The management of pain in pediatrics. Lecture Notes, as presented to the Delaware Valley Pediatric Special Interest Group at Children's Hospital of Philadelphia. Philadelphia; January, 1990.
41. Nashner LM. Sensory, neuromuscular, and biomechanical contributions to human balance. Proceedings of the American Physical Therapy Association Forum, Nashville, TN: June 13–15, 1989.
42. Haley SM, Coster WJ, Ludlow LH, et al. *Pediatric Evaluation of Disability Inventory: Development, standardization, and administration manual*. Boston: New England Medical Center Publications; 1992.
43. MS all ME, Braun S, Granger C, et al. *The Functional Independence Measure for Children (WeeFIM), Developmental Edition (Version 1.5)*. Buffalo, NY: Uniform Data Set for Medical Rehabilitation; 1992.
44. McKenna RJ, Wellisch D, Fawzy FI. Rehabilitation and supportive care of the cancer patient. In: Murphy GP, Lawrence W, Lenhard RE, eds. *American Cancer Society Textbook of Clinical Oncology*. 2nd ed. Atlanta: American Cancer Society; 1995:635–654.
45. Stanger M. Physical therapy intervention with pediatric oncologic amputees. Lecture, American Physical Therapy Association CSM, Orlando, FL, Feb., 1991.
46. Villaneuva R. Principles of total care—Rehabilitation. In: Sutow WW, Fernback DJ, Vietti TJ, eds. *Clinical Pediatric Oncology*. St. Louis: C.V. Mosby; 1984:319–331.
47. Iltis M. Cancer chemotherapy toxicity guidelines for the physical therapist. *Oncol Section Newslett* 1986;4(3):5–7.
48. Foley KM. Controlling the pain of cancer. *Sci Am*. 1996;275(3):164–165.
49. Rosenthal S, Kaufman S. Vincristine neuropathy. *Ann Intern Med*. 1974;80:733–737.
50. Holland JF, Scharlau C, et al. Vincristine treatment of advanced cancer: A cooperative study of 392 causes. *Ca Res*. 1973;33:1258–1264.
51. Allen JC. The effects of cancer therapy on the nervous system. *J Pediatr*. 1978;93:(6):903–909.
52. Casey EB, Jellife AM. Vincristine neuropathy: Clinical and electrophysiological observations. *Brain*. 1973;96:69–86.
53. Ryan JR, Emami A. Vincristine neurotoxicity with residual equinovarus deformity in children with adult leukemia. *Cancer*. 1983;51:423–425.
54. James MC. Physical therapy for patients after bone marrow transplantation. *Phys Ther*. 1987;67:6.

Orthopedic Management

Meg Stanger

Introduction

The term *orthopedics* in pediatric physical therapy is often used to refer to a specific group of pediatric diagnoses. Within the profession of physical therapy, orthopedics refers to a subspecialty of practice. Many of the medical professions have a tendency to compartmentalize their profession and the patients they see by body systems, such as children with orthopedic disabilities or children with neurologic disabilities. This practice lends itself to specialization or the development of clinical expertise in a well-defined area. However, this practice also may fragment the care of patients and even the thinking of the professionals involved.

The various systems of the body are intertwined and normal or atypical influences on one system almost always have an impact on other body systems. This is especially true of a young child whose musculoskeletal system is immature and susceptible to external and internal influences. The action of muscles working within a normal neurologic system is necessary for the development of joints and the shape and contour of a child's bones. When the neurologic or muscular systems are altered or impaired, many times secondary skeletal impairments develop.

This chapter discusses the growth and development of a child's musculoskeletal system and pediatric musculoskeletal assessment, introduces a classification system based on morphogenesis, and provides an overview of pediatric orthopedic diagnoses commonly encountered by pediatric physical therapists. This chapter contains the term *orthopedics* in the title and focuses on specific orthopedic diagnoses. However, the effects of normal and atypical forces on an immature musculoskeletal system and the secondary impairments that may develop, as well as the discussion of the components of a pediatric musculoskeletal assessment, can be applied to many children seen in pediatric physical therapy. For example, most children with a primary diagnosis of neurologic origin present with impairments of their musculoskeletal system that may impact on their overall function.

Musculoskeletal Development

The formation of the musculoskeletal system occurs during the embryonic period (2nd–8th weeks postconception). The limb buds arise from mesenchymal cells and appear during the 4th week, with the upper limb developing 2 days ahead of the lower limb. Mesenchymal cells begin to differentiate into cartilage within 4 to 5 days of the formation of the limb bud. The formation of a cartilaginous skeleton occurs rapidly and is completed during the first fetal month (3 months from conception). The cartilaginous template then begins to be replaced by bone with the appearance of primary ossification centers in the diaphysis of the long bones. Secondary ossification centers appear near the end of fetal development and remain until puberty when skeletal growth is complete.[1,2]

Joint formation begins as the cartilaginous template is being formed. An area of flattened undifferentiated cells forms between two areas of cartilage. The flattened area transforms into three layers, and the peripheral layers maintain contact with the cartilage and eventually become the joint capsule. The middle layer cavitates and forms the joint cavity. The original cartilage at the interface of the joint capsule remains and becomes the articular cartilage.[1,2]

The extremities are susceptible to major morphologic abnormalities during the embryonic period when the limb buds are developing. For example, exposure of the embryo to pharmocolgic agents while the limb buds are forming may result in congenital limb deficiencies. During the fetal period, structures increase in size and cartilage begins to be replaced by bone formation; however, minimal bone remodeling occurs. During this time, the fetus is more susceptible to minor morphologic abnormalities that are the result of position constraints and abnormal mechanical forces.[2] For example, torticollis or clubfeet may result from position constraints late in the pregnancy. Postnatally, much bone remodeling occurs at a rapid rate of 50% annually in the infant and toddler and gradually slows to the adult rate of 5% annually.

Bone grows in length through the continuation of the process of endochondral ossification begun during the fetal period. Endochondral ossification is often referred to as epiphyseal growth because longitudinal growth occurs at the epiphyseal plate. Increases in the diameter of bone or bone thickness occur through appositional growth or the laying down of new bone on top of old bone. These two types of bone growth respond differently to mechanical loading and the forces associated with weight bearing and muscle pull. Appositional bone growth is stimulated by increased compressive forces. Increased weight bearing results in increased thickness and density of the shaft of the tibia.[3,4] However, decreased weight bearing, as seen with immobilization, results in atrophy of the bone.[3]

The response of epiphyseal growth to mechanical forces is dependent on the direction, magnitude, and timing of the force. Intermittent compressive forces applied parallel to the direction of growth cause longitudinal bone growth; however, constant compressive forces of excessive or high magnitude retard bone growth.[5] A compressive force may be applied unevenly across the epiphyseal plate, resulting in slowing of growth on one side only. The uneven growth produces an angulation of the epiphyseal plate and changes the direction of growth.[3] Mechanical loads or forces that are applied perpendicular to the longitudinal growth of the bone result in a change of direction or deflection of bone growth. New growth is deflected and results in displacement of the epiphysis if the load is maintained. A torsional stress to the epiphyseal plate defects columns of cartilage around the circumference of the epiphyseal plate in either a clockwise or counterclockwise direction. New bone then grows away from the epiphyseal plate in a spiral pattern resulting in a torsional deformity.

In summary, the growth and development of the musculoskeletal system is dependent on the normal interplay of multiple factors including hormones, nutrition, and mechanical forces.[5,6] The immature musculoskeletal system is vulnerable to abnormal mechanical forces and pressures; alterations in the timing, direction, or magnitude of forces may have a deleterious effect on the growing and developing musculoskeletal system. Congenital deformities and secondary musculoskeletal impairments that are seen in children with neurologic diagnoses are examples of the vulnerability of the immature musculoskeletal system to abnormal extrinsic forces. However, the immaturity of a child's musculoskeletal system can also be an advantage and is often used as the rationale for many treatment interventions that will be discussed throughout this chapter.

Musculoskeletal Assessment

A thorough musculoskeletal assessment should be included as part of a comprehensive evaluation of a child seen by a physical therapist. Depending on the history or diagnosis, certain aspects of the musculoskeletal assessment should be performed and other aspects may be omitted. However, for those children with a diagnosis that includes multiple joint or system involvement, a complete musculoskeletal assessment should be performed. The assessment may begin as a postural screen with a more in-depth assessment dependent on the findings of the initial screen. The assessment should be completed in a timely and organized manner. The order of the assessment outlined in the following sections may need to be altered depending on the comfort and interaction of the child.

History

A thorough history should be obtained from the parents and the child if the child is able to convey the information to the examiner. The history should obtain information regarding onset or a history of the presenting complaint, if pain is present, what aggravates or alleviates the pain, and any changes in posture or activity noted. Useful information can often be obtained by asking the parents to report to you a typical day for their child. While talking with the parents, the physical therapist should be observing the child's posture, play, spontaneous movements, and activities with relevance to the child's posture, noted asymmetries, difficulty with age-appropriate skills, and so on.

Postural Screen

During the postural screen, the therapist assesses skeletal alignment in a variety of positions, depending on the age of the child. Skeletal alignment should include spinal and lower extremity alignment and limb length. Spinal alignment is viewed from both a sagittal plane and posterior view. The therapist looks for a normal kyphosis and lordosis of the spine relative to the age of the child. From the posterior view, the physical therapist visually assesses symmetry of shoulder, scapulae, and pelvic height. Any asymmetries in rib position, such as a rib hump, would indicate a rotational deformity of the spine.

Lower extremity alignment should also be screened from a sagittal view as well as an anterior and posterior view. The therapist looks at symmetry of pelvic height; rotational variations of the lower extremities, such as the knees or feet pointing in or out; and a valgus or varus position of the knees or feet. From a sagittal view, the physical therapist assesses pelvic position and alignment of the hip, knee, and ankle.

Limb length should be assessed in both a weight bearing and non–weight bearing position using the accepted bony landmarks of the anterior superior iliac spine and the medial malleolus. The postural screen will direct the physical therapist to where to focus the next portion of a more in-depth musculoskeletal assessment.

Range of Motion

Although the goniometric techniques used to measure active or passive joint range of motion (ROM) in children and adults are similar, several factors must be kept in mind when assessing range of motion in children. Age-related differences exist in ROM values between adults and infants and young children. For example, a full-term newborn will exhibit flexion contractures of the hips and knees secondary to intrauterine positioning.

Before any goniometric measurement is taken, attention must be given so that the child is relaxed and remains calm. Movements should be slow so as to limit anxiety and to avoid eliciting a stretch reflex in children with increased muscle tone. Slow movements should also be used if pain is present or suspected and for those children who may have more brittle bones or recent fractures.

Reliability studies of the use of goniometry in children are present in the literature and should guide physical therapists in their use of goniometric measures to document ROM. Haley et al. demonstrated acceptable levels of interrater- and intrarater reliability ($r = .77–.89$) of spinal mobility in normal young children.[7] Several researchers have investigated the reliability of goniometric measurement of children with Duchenne's muscular dystrophy and children with cerebral palsy. High intrarater reliability was present in those studies, but interrater reliability was shown to be variable throughout the studies.[8–10] When measuring ROM in children, the most reliable results are obtained when the same therapist assesses changes in ROM over time.

Muscle length tests should also be included in the overall joint motion assessment. Specific tests and their procedures do not differ from standard procedures used with the adult population; however, several tests may be used more frequently used in pediatrics. Hip flexor muscle length is assessed using the Thomas test or the prone hip extension test. Hamstring length is usually assessed in adults using the straight leg raise test; however, the passive knee extension test (PKE) is commonly used with pediatrics (Fig. 11-1). The PKE can be used in the presence of a knee flexion contracture; therefore, it is useful for children who present with involvement of multiple joints.[11] The PKE is also easier to perform and more reliable with smaller limbs than the lower extremities of large adults.[12]

Strength

An accurate assessment of strength requires careful consideration in the pediatric population but yields important information regarding deficits and changes over time. A variety of methods to assess strength are available, and their use may

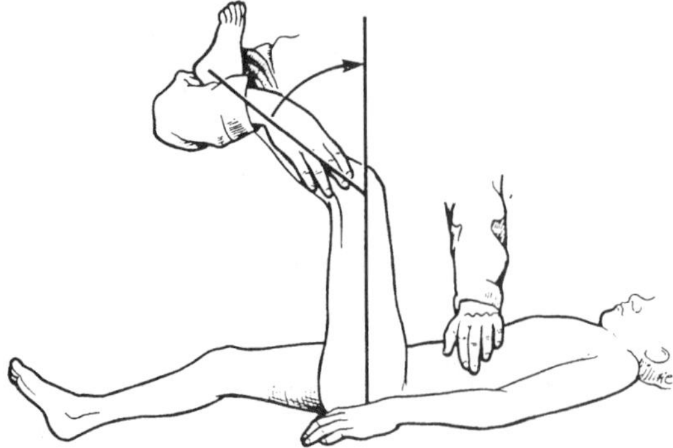

Figure 11-1 ▪ Passive knee extension test (PKE). Child is supine, hip is flexed to 90 degrees, and the knee is slowly extended until resistance is felt. The popliteal angle is recorded as a measure of hamstring contracture.

depend on the age and ability of the child. For infants and children younger than the age of 3 or 4 years, assessment of strength is most often accomplished through observation of movement and function. A child must be able to follow the directions of the testing procedure to ensure accurate results using either manual muscle testing (MMT) or dynamometry.[13]

MMT has the same inherent weaknesses with the pediatric population as with adults. The grades of Good and Normal are very subjective and do not account for any changes that may occur in a child over time secondary to maturation. Recent studies have demonstrated limited intertester and intratester reliability.[14] Other authors have determined the MMT may not identify strength deficits until they are greater than 50%.[15,16] Handheld dynamometry has been found to be a reliable and sensitive method of assessing strength in various populations of children.[17–19]

Lower Extremity Alignment (Rotational and Angular)

Normal skeletal development includes rotational or torsional and alignment changes of bones and joints. These normal developmental processes may be altered secondary to abnormal muscle pull or weight-bearing forces. Consequently, impairments that impact on function often result from the combination of abnormal forces on a developing skeletal system. The bones remain susceptible to deforming forces until growth is complete; therefore, the impairments may increase in severity over time.

Staheli has developed a rotational profile to assess lower extremity alignment and assist in determining which component of the lower extremity contributes to the rotational variation. The rotational profile consists of six measurements, including (1) foot-progression angle; (2) medial rotation of the hip; (3) lateral rotation of the hip; (4) thigh-foot angle; (5) angle of the transmalleolar axis; and (6) and the configuration of the foot. Normal values have been established for the first five measurements and can be used to determine whether the variation falls within the wide range of normal or if intervention is indicated.[20]

ROTATIONAL PROFILE

FOOT-PROGRESSION ANGLE (FPA). The Foot-progression angle is defined as the angle between the longitudinal axis of the foot and the line of progression of the child's gait. The FPA provides an overall summation of the child's rotation during gait but does not identify the contributing factors. A positive sign denotes out-toeing and a negative sign denotes in-toeing. The FPA can be objectively measured using a variety of footprint measures, including ink or chalk on the feet or more expensive commercially available methods. Many times in the clinic, the FPA is assessed subjectively to give the clinician an overall view of the child's rotation during gait. The procedures listed in the following sections assist the clinician with identifying the contributing factors to the overall rotational profile of the child (Fig. 11-2A).

HIP ROTATION. Medial and lateral hip rotation in prone are assessed to determine femoral

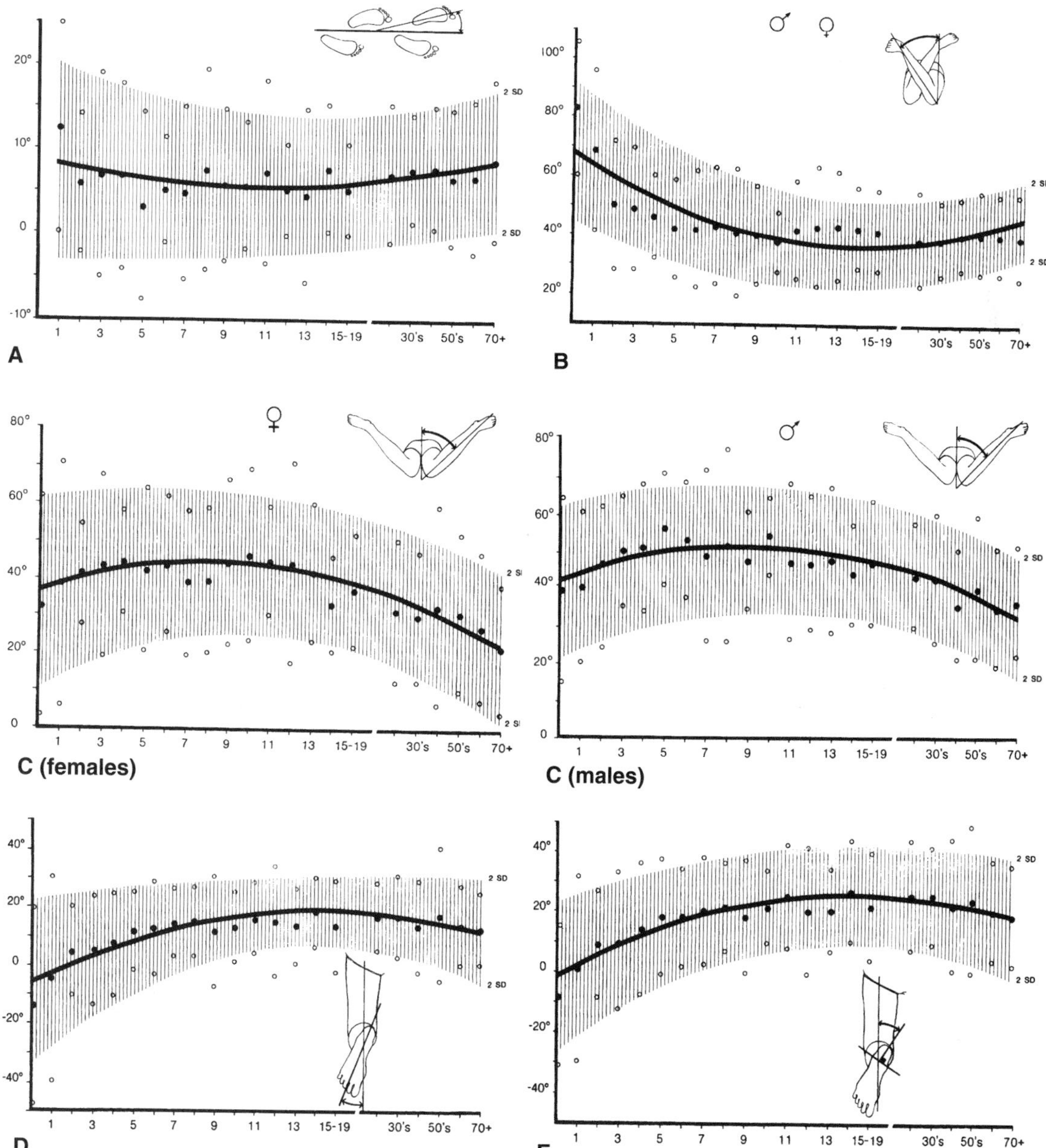

Figure 11-2 ▪ The five measurements in Staheli's rotational profile plotted as the mean values plus or minus two standard deviations for each of the age groups. The dark line indicates the mean values as they change with age, and the shaded areas indicate the normal ranges. (**A**) Foot-progression angle; (**B**) lateral rotation of the hip in males and females; (**C**) medial rotation of the hip in females and males separate; (**D**) thigh–foot angle; (**E**) angle of the transmalleolar axis.

torsion. The child is in prone with hips extended and knees flexed to 90 degrees, medial and lateral hip rotation measurements are then taken goniometrically. Soft tissue limitations may influence the final measure of hip rotation as well as the degree of femoral torsion. Normal medial hip rotation is less than 60 to 65 degrees. (Fig. 11-2B, C).

The literature also describes a second test of femoral torsion referred to as Ryder's test. The child sits with knees flexed to 90 degrees over the edge of a table. The greater trochanter is palpated while rotating the leg. When the greater trochanter is palpated most laterally, the angle of medial hip rotation is measured goniometrically (Fig. 11-3A, B). When the greater trochanter is palpated most laterally, the femoral neck should be parallel to the examining table and the measure of medial hip rotation correspond to the degree of femoral anteversion.[10,21]

THIGH–FOOT ANGLE (TFA). The child is in the prone position with the hips extended, the knee flexed to 90 degrees, and the foot in a natural resting position; do not attempt to align the foot. The angle formed from the bisection of the axis of the thigh and the axis of the foot is measured. This TFA is used to determine rotational variation of the tibia and the hindfoot. If the foot is in an out-toeing position, the value is positive; if the foot is in an in-toeing position, the value is negative (Fig. 11-2D).

TRANSMALLEOLAR AXIS (TMA). The child is positioned in prone, as previously described. A line perpendicular to the axis between the lateral and medial malleoli is drawn. The angle formed from between the perpendicular line and the axis of the thigh is measured. This angle assesses the contribution of the distal tibia to the rotational profile (Fig. 11-2E).

The contribution of the foot must also be included when assessing rotational variations. Assessing the alignment of the hindfoot and forefoot will determine whether a pronated or supinated position of the foot or metatarsus adductus is contributing to the FPA.

ANGULAR ALIGNMENT

If the initial postural screening revealed suspected lower extremity alignment deviations, such as a varus or valgus posture, an objective angular measurement should be performed. Expected values for genu varus and valgus will differ depending upon the age of the child. Genu varum is measured with the child in supine with legs extended and the patella facing upward and the medial malleoli touching. The distance be-

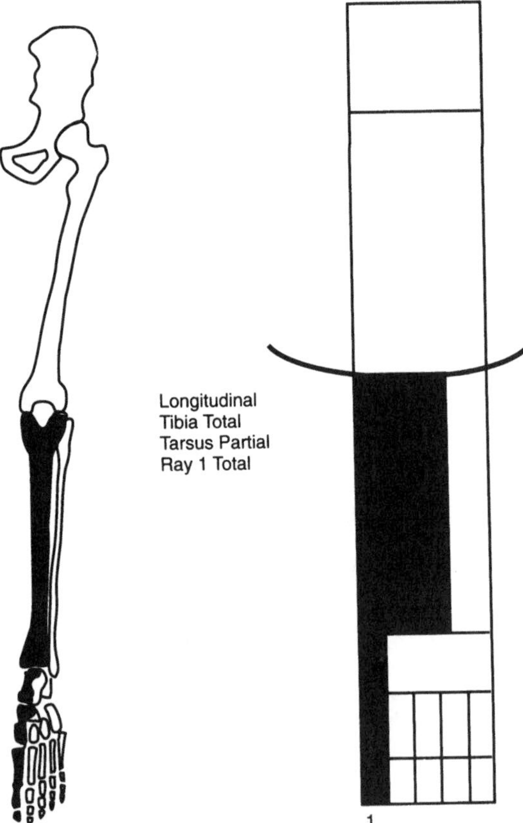

Figure 11-3 ■ (A) Example of a longitudinal deficiency of the lower extremity. (continued)

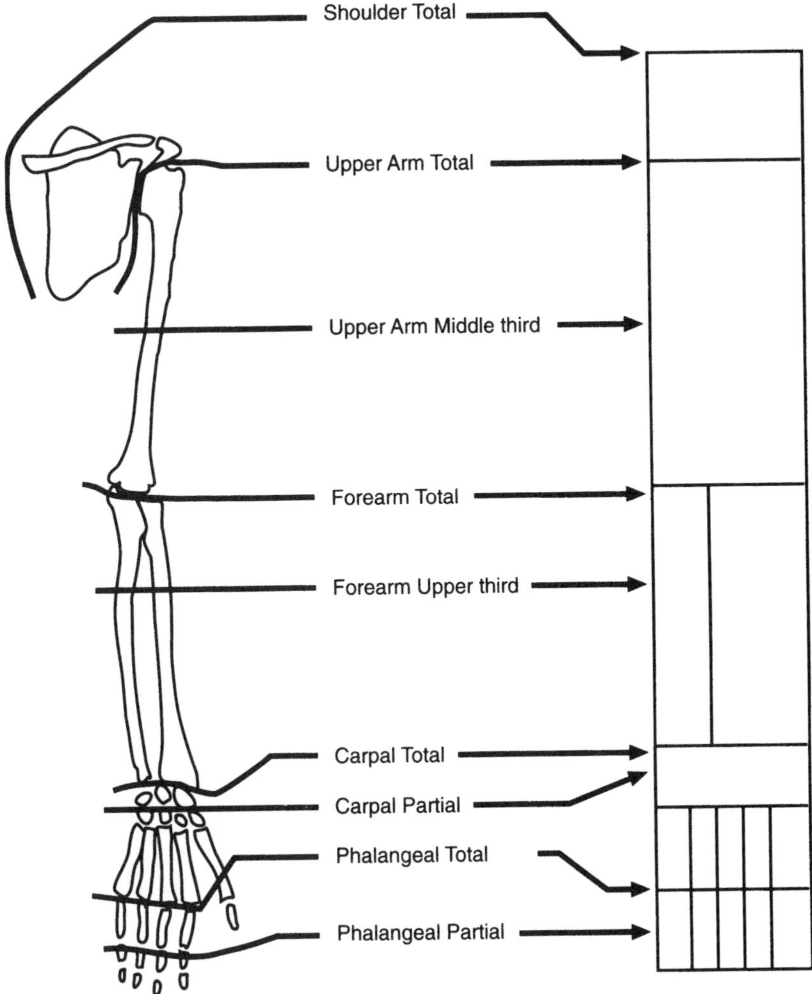

Figure 11-3 (Continued) ▪ (**B**) Example of transverse deficiencies at various levels of the upper extremity.

tween the femoral condyles is measured. Genu valgus is measured in the same position but with the knees touching. The distance between the malleoli is measured.[22] The contribution of angular variations must be delineated from rotational variations.

Additional areas that may be included in the musculoskeletal assessment include assessment of muscle tone, sensation testing, and developmental skill level. An assessment of muscle tone may reveal hypertonicity or hypotonicity of specific muscle groups and an imbalance of muscle forces around specific joints. These unbalanced muscle forces may produce impairments over time that cause pain or interfere with the child's functional abilities.

Sensation testing is performed with children just as with adults and incorporates the same rationale for inclusion of testing. Sensory testing is indicated when nerve involvement is suspected, such as with fractures or after an amputation or application of an external fixator.

Assessment of a child's developmental level is indicated if the orthopedic condition is suspected of delaying or interfering with development. For the ambulatory child, this includes an assessment of gait. Gait assessment is similar to assessing an adult and can be performed through systematic clinical observation or with more objective measures, ranging from video analysis to an instrumented gait laboratory. The age of the child must be considered when assessing gait and knowledge of the characteristics of early walking must be incorporated into the assessment (see Chapter 4, Cerebral Palsy).

Classification of Errors of Morphologic Development

In this chapter Spranger's classification of morphogenesis is used to introduce and discuss a multitude of diagnoses that fall under the category of pediatric orthopedics. This classification system provides a framework from which to understand the pathophysiology resulting in a particular diagnosis, the impairments and functional limitations that may develop as the child grows, and how physical therapy may have an impact.

The National Center for Medical Rehabilitation Research (NCMRR) has developed a five-dimensional model identifying the disabling process or continuum that may lead to societal limitations or handicap.[23,24] The first dimension is the pathophysiology or underlying medical or injury processes at the cellular or tissue levels. The second dimension is impairment or the organ or system disorders that could potentially impair function. An impairment may be permanent or susceptible to change and may or may not impact on function. Functional limitations is the third dimension of the model and is the result of a combination of multiple impairments in one or more systems. Functional limitations, as the term implies, limit a child's function with daily activities. Physical therapists usually intervene at the impairment or functional limitations level of the model. Persistent functional limitations that cannot be remediated or compensated for lead to disabilities. A child who is disabled is unable to participate in normal daily activities such as school or interacting with peers. The fifth and most severe dimension is societal limitations. Barriers that prevent a person from achieving his or her highest level of function are referred to as societal limitations and may include architectural barriers or specialized equipment or technology that is unobtainable through insurance coverage.

To illustrate the disabling process, a child with osteogenesis impefecta (OI) will be used as an example. For a child with OI, the pathophysiology is the abnormality in the connective tissue at the cellular level. One of the impairments that results is fragile bones susceptible to deforming forces and fracture. The child may sustain multiple lower extremity fractures resulting in malalignment, short stature, and weakness, resulting in a slow labored gait. The slow labored gait is a functional limitation that may lead to an inability of the child to keep up with his or hers peers during play or at school. The functional limitation has become a disability. The final dimension or societal limitation may result if the child is not permitted to attend a daycare of their peers owing to a fear of increased risk of fractures from the other children.

The use of Spranger's model provides a classification of pediatric orthopedic diagnoses by pathophysiology. With an understanding of the pathophysiology, the reader will be able to identify impairments that may be present or may develop and the impact of physical therapy on preventing or limiting the impairments, with the ultimate goal of minimizing the functional limitation and disability of the child.

Spranger's classification of disorders of morphogenesis consists of four divisions: malformations, disruptions, deformations, and dysplasias.[25] Malformations are morphologic defects of an organ or body part from an intrinsically abnormal developmental process. Because the abnormality is intrinsic from the moment of conception, the organ or body part never had the potential to develop normally. Examples of malformations include longitudinal limb deficiencies, cleft lip and palate, and septal defects of the heart.

Disruptions are morphologic defects of an organ or body part resulting from the extrinsic breakdown of an originally normal developmental process. Normal development is interrupted at the cellular level by an external factor such as a teratogen, trauma, or infection. Transverse limb deficiencies commonly seen with the use of thalidomide are an example of a disruption.

Deformations are abnormalities in form, shape, or position of a body part caused by mechanical forces. The deforming forces may be extrinsic to the fetus, such as intrauterine constraint, or intrinsic to the fetus, such as fetal hypomobility resulting from a neuromuscular defect. Examples of deformations include torticollis and metatarsus adductus. Deformations can be delineated into prenatal and postnatal deformities versus pathologic processes. Examples of postnatal deformities include tibial varum and rotational variations. Pathologic processes are usually deformities as the result of an insult to the epiphyseal plate or other area of the bone. These processes include the diagnoses of Legg-Calvé-Perthes disease, slipped capital femoral epiphysis, and limb length discrepancies resulting from insults or abnormal forces to the growth plate.

The final division in Spranger's classification is dysplasia. Dysplasias result from an abnormal organization of cells into tissues, which leads to abnormal tissue differentiation. Osteogenesis imperfecta (OI) is an example of a dysplasia.

The remainder of this chapter discusses specific orthopedic diagnoses and treatment interventions. When possible, treatment interventions are supported from evidence in the literature.

Congenital Limb Deficiencies

Using the International Society for Prosthetics and Orthotics (ISPO) classification system, congenital limb deficiencies are described as either longitudinal or transverse.[26] Longitudinal limb deficiencies are described as reduction or absence of an element or elements within the long axis of the limb. There may be normal skeletal elements distal to the affected bone or bones.[26] A longitudinal limb deficiency is an example of a malformation in which a morphologic defect of an organ or larger region of the body occurs when normal organogenesis is interrupted. Any combination of skeletal limb involvement is possible but certain distinct entities are more commonly seen than others. For this chapter, congenital longitudinal deficiency of the radius will be used as an example of upper extremity involvement and proximal femoral focal deficiency (PFFD) as an example of a lower extremity longitudinal limb deficiency. Both are examples of congenital malformations and are more frequent in their incidence as well as examples of children with limb deficiencies typically seen by therapists.

Longitudinal deficiency of the radius, often commonly referred to as radial clubhand, occurs in 1 per 100,000 live births, with bilateral involvement present in 50% of the children. Radial deficiencies can be defined as the failure of formation of parts of deficiencies on the radial side of the upper extremity, including the radius, carpals, metacarpals, and phalanges of the first ray and thenar musculature.[27,28] Heikel classified radial deficiencies into four types, ranging in severity from Type I (consisting of delayed appearance of the distal radial physis) to Type IV (involving complete absence of the radius).[29] Type IV is the most common presentation and is present in 50% of children with a radial deficiency.[22] Clinically, children with Type IV radial deficiency present with a shortened forearm of no greater than 50% of the length of the contralateral forearm, an elbow extension contracture, and radial deviation of the hand with an absent or deficient thumb.

The incidence of PFFD is 1 per 50,000 live births and is bilateral in 15% of children of children with PFFD. Aitken first described and classified four classes of severity of PFFD with Class A exhibiting the least involvement and Class D being the most severe (Fig. 11-4).[30] PFFD includes absence or hypoplasia of the proximal femur with varying degrees of involvement of the acetabulum, femoral head, patella,

TYPE		FEMORAL HEAD	ACETABULUM	FEMORAL SEGMENT	RELATIONSHIP AMONG COMPONENTS OF FEMUR AND ACETABULUM AT SKELETAL MATURITY
A	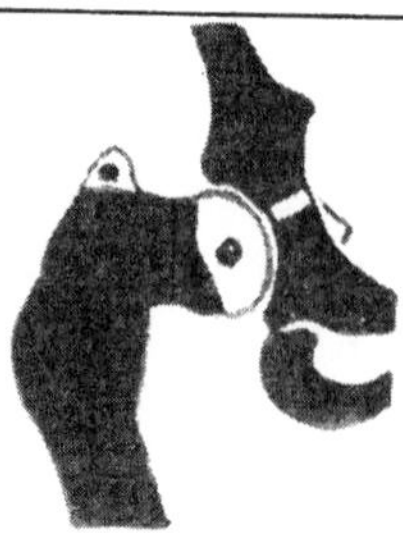	Present	Normal	Short	Bony connection between components of femur Femoral head in acetabulum Subtrochanteric varus angulation, often with pseudarthrosis
B	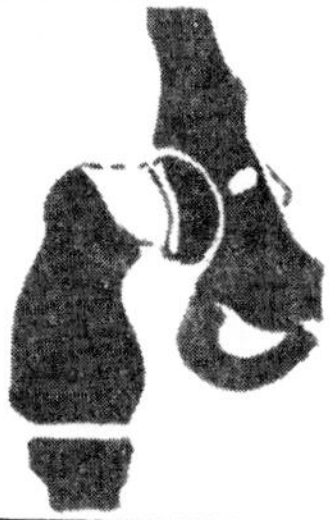	Present	Adequate or moderately dysplastic	Short, usually proximal bony tuft	No osseous connection between head and shaft Femoral head in acetabulum
C	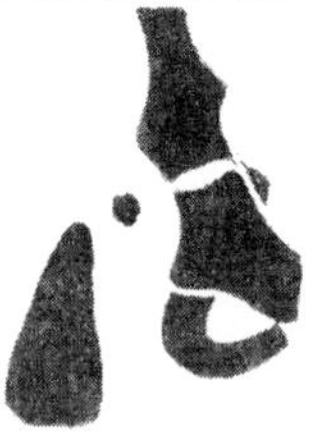	Absent or represented by ossicle	Severely dysplastic	Short, usually proximally tapered	May be osseous connection between shaft and proximal ossicle No articular relation between femur and acetabulum
D	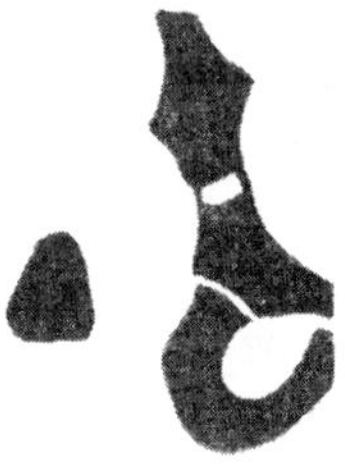	Absent	Absent Obturator foramen enlarged Pelvis squared in bilateral cases	Short, deformed	(none)

Figure 11-4 ▪ Aitken classification of proximal femoral focal deficiency.

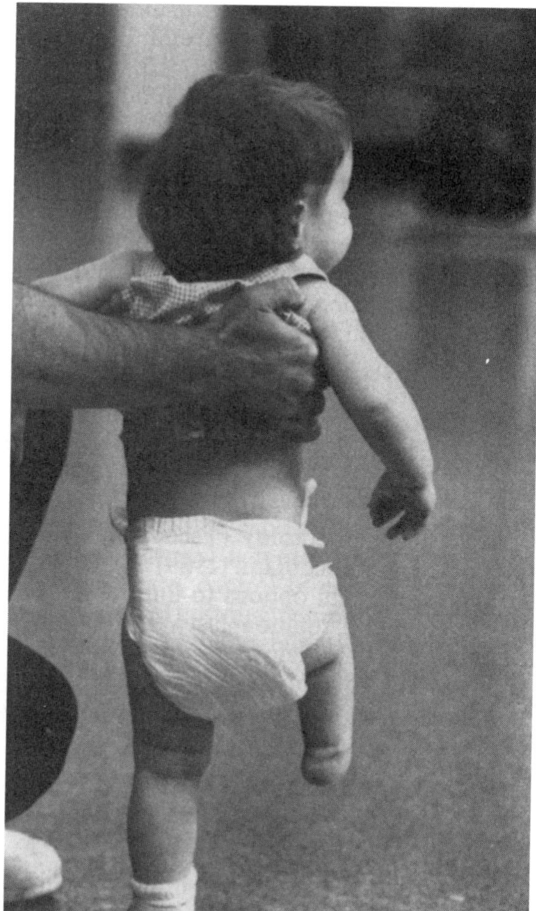

Figure 11-5 ▪ Child with unilateral proximal femoral focal deficiency who underwent a Boyd amputation of his right foot. Note popliteal crease near the diaper line indicating where his knee is located.

tibia, fibula, cruciate ligaments, and the foot. Clinically, infants with PFFD present with an abnormally short thigh held in hip flexion, abduction and external rotation (Fig. 11-5). Hip and knee flexion contractures are often present along with anterioposterior instability of the knee and a significant leg length difference, with the foot of the involved leg often at the height of the opposite knee.[31]

In transverse limb deficiencies, the limb develops normally to a particular level beyond which no skeletal elements exist.[26] Transverse limb deficiencies are an example of a disruption using Spranger's classification of morphogenesis and resemble in appearance a residual limb after surgical amputation. Most transverse deficiencies are unilateral, with a frequently seen scenario being a transverse forearm deficiency (Fig. 11-6).[27] This type of transverse deficiency occurs more frequently in females and exhibits a 2:1 left-sided predominance.[32]

Nonsurgical and Surgical Management of Congenital Limb Deficiencies

Children with longitudinal limb deficiencies often require multiple surgical procedures to obtain maximal function of the involved limb. Surgical procedures may include tendon trans-

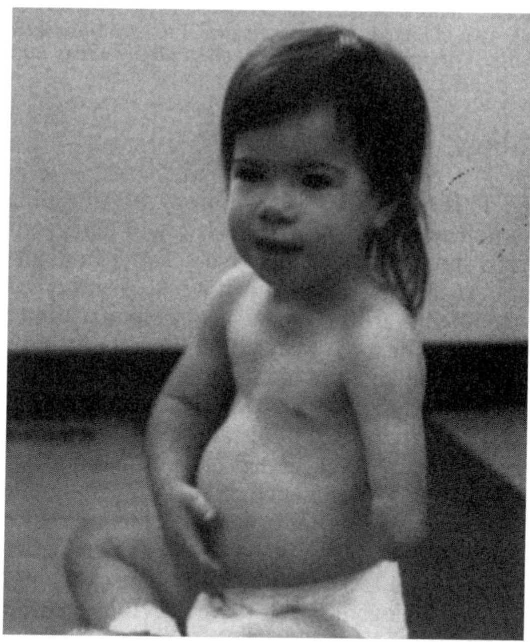

Figure 11-6 ▪ Child with congenital transverse below-elbow limb deficiency.

fers, realignment or repositioning of the hand and/or fingers, and osteotomies for the upper extremity and most commonly include a combination of amputation, fusion, limb lengthening, and osteotomies for lower extremity limb deficiencies. Surgical correction is rarely required for children with transverse limb deficiencies.

UPPER EXTREMITY: LONGITUDINAL RADIAL DEFICIENCY

Shortly after birth, the child's hand should be serially splinted or casted to stretch the shortened soft tissues and realign the hand as centrally as possible over the distal forearm. At the same time, therapy goals should also focus on increasing elbow ROM, especially elbow flexion. Stretching of the soft tissues is necessary before any surgical procedures. Between 6 months and 1 year of age, centralization of the hand by an orthopedic surgeon is often performed. The goal of centralization is a stable wrist centered on the distal ulna while maintaining functional wrist motion.[33]

Postoperatively, the child's hand is splinted in the newly aligned position on the distal ulna. Compliance with wearing of the splint is crucial for long-term success of the surgical centralization. The splint should be worn throughout the day and night during the healing phase. After the initial healing phase is complete, a splint should be worn at night until skeletal maturity is achieved. By skeletal maturity, the ulna has undergone epiphyseal adaptation to accommodate the centralized carpus to ensure stability of the wrist position and use of a night splint is no longer necessary.[33]

Centralization of the hand is contraindicated in older children or adolescents who have adapted to their hand position, when severe deformity of the hand is also present that would limit hand function and when elbow flexion is less than 90 degrees. Adequate elbow flexion is needed prior to surgery so that when the hand is realigned, the child is still able to bring his or her hand to the mouth.

LOWER EXTREMITY: PROXIMAL FEMORAL FOCAL DEFICIENCY

Surgical intervention for children with PFFD is varied, must be individualized, and can include any combination of amputation, reconstruction, fusion, or limb-lengthening procedures. Surgery addresses the issues of the unstable hip joint and the inequality of limb lengths; the two issues that interfere with the child's overall functional abilities. Many children require multiple surgical procedures; thought must be given early to develop a long-term surgical plan for family education and to condense surgeries into one procedure when possible.

The exception for surgery are those children with bilateral PFFD. Surgery is generally not recommended for children with bilateral PFFD, because their limb length is equal or near equal and they are able to ambulate with or without extension prostheses.[22,34,35]

Surgical options can be divided into those that involve amputation and reconstruction for eventual prosthetic fitting and those that involve limb-lengthening techniques. Three typical scenarios are discussed in the following. Before any surgical intervention, physical therapy should be initiated in early infancy to improve ROM at the involved hip, promote developmental activities (including symmetry of skills and weight bearing at the age-appropriate times), and assist with the development of age-appropriate balance skills.

Foot Amputation and Proximal Reconstruction. After this combination of a surgical procedures, the child's limb resembles and functions as an above-knee amputation. The foot is amputated at an early age, often before 8 months of age, so that the child may be fitted with a prosthesis. Proximal reconstruction, including forming a connection between the femoral head and the proximal femur and fusion of the knee, are usually performed when the child is between 2 and 6 years of age. Reconstruction of the proximal femur is only recommended if sufficient bone density is present and if gains in stability will be achieved. Fusion of the knee allow the limb to function as a single lever arm. This combination of surgical procedures is indicated for those children with the more severe manifestations of PFFD, including a very short femur and involvement of the femoral head and neck.

ROTATIONPLASTY. Rotationplasty, or the turnabout procedure, is a surgical technique that allows the child to function similarly to a child with a below-knee amputation. In children with PFFD the rotationplasty procedure is often performed as an amputation through the knee joint, the limb is rotated 180 degrees, and then reattached with a knee fusion. The neurovascular supply is left intact, and the lower leg muscles are reattached to corresponding muscles of the thigh. The child's ankle then functions as a knee joint, with ankle plantarflexion acting as knee extension and ankle dorsiflexion acting as knee flexion.[22,34] Indications for a rotationplasty procedure include (1) a normal ankle joint; (2) unilateral involvement; (3) a predicted limb length that would place the ankle of the involved limb at the knee of the uninvolved limb at skeletal maturity; and (4) a stable hip.[22]

Postoperatively, the child is casted until healing is complete. After cast removal, physical therapy must emphasize ROM of the ankle. Maximum plantarflexion range is needed to promote knee extension in the prosthesis and ankle dorsiflexion to neutral and beyond is necessary for sitting and other activities involving knee flexion. Strengthening of these muscle groups is also important; ankle plantarflexion and dorsiflexion strength provides stability in stance and powers the prosthesis during gait.

LIMB LENGTHENING. Limb lengthening may be indicated when more than 60% of predicted femoral length is present[34,36] or the discrepancy in femoral length is predicted to be less than 15 cm. Limb-lengthening procedures include unilateral frames such as the Wagner or circular frames, also called the Ilizarov. Limb-lengthening procedures for children with PFFD are often performed when the child is between 8 and 10 years of age. Contraindications include bilateral PFFD, unstable hip such as with Aitken Type C or D and poor carryover of care at home.[36,37] An in-depth description of limb-lengthening procedures is provided later in this chapter under Limb Length Discrepancies.

Prosthetic Training

Physical therapy intervention should begin before the fitting of the initial prosthesis. During infancy, physical therapy may be initiated on a weekly basis or a consultative basis, depending on the needs of the child and the family. Infants with a longitudinal limb deficiency have contractures or ROM limitations that must be addressed before surgery or prosthetic fitting. The infant with a radial deficiency requires stretching of the soft tissues, including passive exercises and splinting before surgery. The infant with PFFD requires ROM exercises to increase hip extension and adduction motions before surgery or prosthetic fitting. Infants with transverse limb deficiencies rarely exhibit contractures.

Infants with congenital limb deficiencies should also be monitored for their developmental skills. Symmetry of skills is emphasized as well as weight-bearing skills through both the upper and lower extremities. Early weight-bearing skills promote proximal joint stability that may be needed later to use a prosthesis. Children with an upper extremity transverse limb deficiency are usually fitted with a prosthesis by 6 months of age when they begin simple two-handed activities. Children with lower extremity limb deficiencies are generally fitted with a prosthesis between 8 and 10 months, when they begin weight-bearing skills.

When an infant or child first receives a prosthesis, the fit, alignment, and overall function are assessed. The child and family must be shown the proper donning and doffing techniques, instructed in a wearing schedule, and shown how to check the skin for redness or possible breakdown. The initial goal is for the infant or toddler to accept wearing the prosthesis and gradually increase the wearing time throughout the day. The prosthesis is usually removed for naps and should be removed when going to sleep for the night.

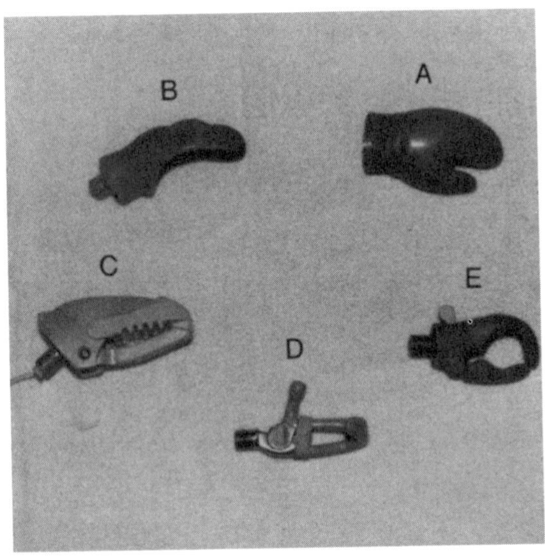

Figure 11-7 ■ Terminal device options: (**A**) Baby Mitt (Hosmer Dorrance, Campbell, CA); (**B**) Sport Mitt (Therapeutic Recreation Systems, Boulder, CO); an infant size may be suitable for crawling infants. (**C**) Child Amputee Prosthetics Project (CAPP) (Hosmer Dorrance) voluntary opening device. (**D**) Hosmer Dorrance 12p infant voluntary opening hook. (**E**) Anatomically Designed-Engineered Polymer Technology (ADEPT) (Therapeutic Recreation Systems) infant voluntary closing hook.

UE PROSTHETIC TRAINING

An infant's first prosthesis has a terminal device that is soft and cosmetically appealing but nonfunctional (Fig. 11-7). A more functional terminal device is added when the child begins to engage in bimanual play. Functional terminal devices are either voluntary-opening or voluntary-closing. Voluntary-opening terminal devices open as the child reaches forward with the arm, whereas voluntary-closing devices mimic reaching and grasping and close as the child reaches forward to grasp an object.

The initial goals for an infant or young toddler are to wear the prosthesis, become adjusted to the weight of the prosthesis, and begin to use the prosthesis for propping in prone or sitting and bimanual skills. By the age of 15 to 18 months of age, training on the use of an active terminal device should begin (Fig. 11-8). The child is taught to open the terminal device, grasp an object and then release the object.[38,39] This order of skill acquisition mimics the normal developmental sequence. The therapist must be familiar with the type of terminal device and how it operates before instructing the child. If the child has an above-elbow prosthesis, the elbow is locked when the child is initially learning to control the terminal device so that the child only learns one movement at a time. The child with an above-elbow limb deficiency activates the terminal device through scapular movements and a cable connected to the terminal device.

As the child progresses, the use of the terminal device should include manipulation of small objects and using the prosthesis as the helper hand to hold paper for writing or coloring, holding the handlebars of a tricycle, feeding, and dressing. Expectations need to be reasonable, because the child will use the uninvolved hand as the dominant hand. By school age, the child should be independent with self-care activities including dressing, toileting, and eating. Activities should always focus on independence with age-appropriate skills. By the time the child is in high school, he or she may want to

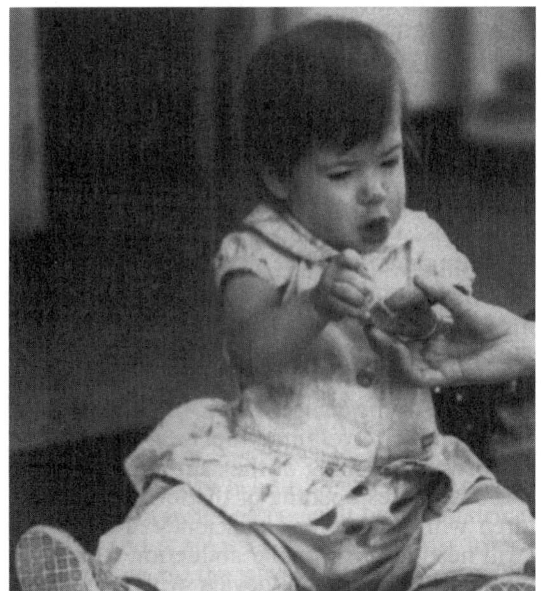

Figure 11-8 ▪ Child is wearing a right below-elbow prosthesis with an ADEPT voluntary closing hook. Therapist assisting child to operate the terminal device.

participate in various activities, including sports, driving, and social events. Various terminal device options are available to promote participation in numerous sports, to facilitate driving and control of the steering wheel, and cosmetic terminal devices are available for social times when cosmesis may be more important than function. The child, teenager, and young adult should always be a part of the discussion for therapy goals and prosthetic options.

LOWER EXTREMITY PROSTHETIC TRAINING

An infant or toddler younger than 2 years of age is usually fitted with a prosthesis without a knee joint (Fig. 11-9). The goals for initial prosthetic training are toleration of the prosthesis and to begin standing weightbearing activities. The prosthesis will interfere with the child's method of floor mobility and will require an adjustment period by the child. Initial standing activities should include transitions in and out of standing at a support, weight shift activities in preparation for gait and balance reactions, and protective skills. Gait training may be initiated with an assistive device; the assistive device is often discarded voluntarily by the child when it is no longer necessary. During the early preschool years, a prosthesis with a knee should be introduced to the child. Various prosthetic knee options are available that provide additional stability during the early years.

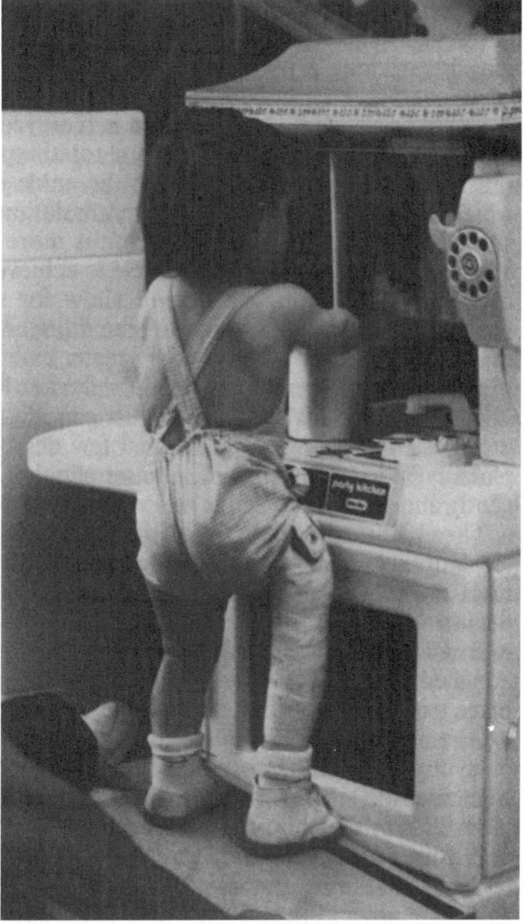

Figure 11-9 ▪ Fourteen-month-old child with lower extremity prosthesis without a knee component.

Growth is an issue with children and lower extremity prostheses. Young infants and toddlers can outgrow their prosthesis every 6 months. For this reason, fiberglass cast models for the socket are often used during these periods of rapid growth. For toddlers, spacers can be added to increase the length of the prosthesis and prolong the fit and use of the prosthesis. However, children will need to have their prosthesis replaced every 9 to 12 months because of growth and durability issues.

Many of the prosthetic options presently available for adults are available for children when they reach school age. Most of the prosthetic foot options, knee mechanisms, and lightweight materials are available and more practical for the preadolescent and young adult population. Some older children may require a second prosthesis for specific activities such as sports or water activities. Younger children may use their old prosthesis for water activities.

Prenatal Deformations

A deformation is an abnormal form, shape, or position of a part of the body caused by mechanical forces. Deformations are normal responses of the tissue to abnormal mechanical forces that may be extrinsic or intrinsic to the fetus. Intrauterine constraint is an example of an extrinsic force, whereas fetal hypomobility secondary to a nervous system impairment such as myelomeningocele is an example of an intrinsic force. If the deforming force is removed, normal development or maturation of the body part would be expected to occur.

This chapter discusses congenital muscular torticollis (CMT) as an example of an extrinsic deformation, and clubfeet as an example of either an extrinsic or intrinsic deformation. Both of these diagnoses may also have other causative factors; abnormal mechanical forces are only one of the possible contributing factors. Developmental dysplasia of the hip is an example of a deformation that probably begins prenatally, continues to progress if the deforming forces are not altered, and may not be recognized until much later in postnatal life. Last, this section discusses arthrogryposis as an example of an intrinsic deformation that begins very early in fetal development and consequently results in significant deformations at birth and throughout later life.

Congenital Muscular Torticollis

An infant with CMT presents with unilateral shortening of the sternocleidomastoid muscle, with subsequent limited cervical ROM. The infant's head is laterally flexed toward the shortened muscle, with the chin rotated to the opposite side. An infant with shortening of the right stenocleidomastoid muscle exhibits a posture of right lateral neck flexion with rotation of the head toward the left (Fig. 11-10). Facial asymmetry and plagiocephaly (flattening of the skull) are also often noted.

CMT is usually noted in the first 2 to 3 weeks after birth, with a reported incidence of .4 to 1.9%.[40,41] The etiology of CMT is not clearly understood at this time. Intrauterine malposition and birth trauma have been hypothesized as causative factors. Infants with CMT have a higher incidence of breech presentations[42,43] and associated congenital musculoskeletal diagnoses, such as hip dysplasia and foot deformities.[42,44]

A palpable mass or fibrotic tumor is often observed or is palpable within the belly of the sternocleidomastoid muscle and appears within the first few weeks after birth and then gradually disappears. The exact cause of the fibrotic tumor within the sternocleidomastoid muscle is not known. Researchers have hypothesized that occlusion of blood vessels with resultant anoxic injury to the sternocleidomastoid muscle may produce the fibotic changes observed within the muscle. The occlusion could result from intrauterine malposition or trauma at birth.[48] Several authors propose that fibrosis of the ster-

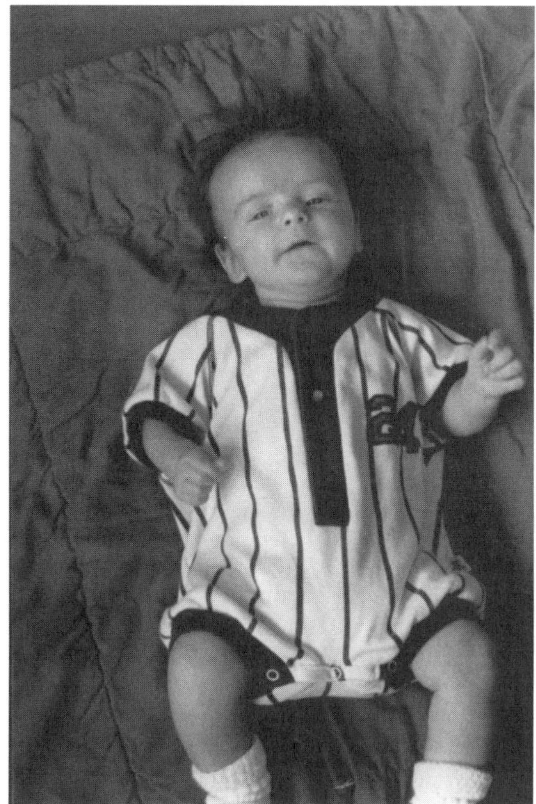

Figure 11-10 ■ Infant with a resolving congenital muscular torticollis. Note the facial asymmetry in the region of his mandible.

nocleidomastoid muscle is present in all children with CMT and ranges on a continum of no palpable mass to a firm palpable mass.[42,44]

CONSERVATIVE MANAGEMENT

Conservative management of CMT is generally recommended during the first 12 months. Conservative management includes passive stretching exercises of the sternocleidomastoid muscle, active ROM with subsequent strengthening exercises, and positioning and handling techniques to correct the infant's head position. Several studies have demonstrated the success of conservative management during the first year. Morrison achieved good to excellent results in 84% of patients diagnosed before 1 year of age.[43] Binder reported complete resolution in 70% of children treated before 1 year of age regardless of the severity or the presence of a fibrotic mass. Of the 15 children who underwent surgery, seven had severe CMT and were referred for treatment after 12 months of age.[42] Persistent facial asymmetry, intermittent head tilt with fatigue or illness, and functional asymmetry resembling hemiplegia but with a normal neurologic examination have been observed in children with full resolution, indicating the complexity of this disorder as well as possible long-lasting implications.[42] Emory's study of 101 infants with CMT further supports the use of conservative management in children younger than 1 year of age, with full recovery reported for 99% of the infants. Further delineation was made for duration of treatment in which infants with a fibrotic mass required 6.9 months of treatment compared with 4.7 months for children without a mass to achieve full resolution.[44] None of these studies included a control group to assist with determining the extent of time and maturation on the resolution of the CMT. Other authors report the spontaneous resolution of CMT without any intervention.[40,45]

Conservative management consisted of specific physical therapy intervention in both Binder's and Emory's studies. Physical therapy intervention included passive stretching of the sternocleidomastoid and upper trapezius muscles on the involved side, active rotation of the head toward the involved side, and handling and positioning during feeding and sleeping to promote active rotation or stretch of the sternocleidomastoid muscle. At 3 to 4 months of age, lateral neck flexion to strengthen the lengthened sternocleidomastoid muscle on the uninvolved side was initiated through developmental activities such as head righting and rolling.

SURGICAL MANAGEMENT

Sixteen percent of children who receive conservative management before 1 year of age will require surgical correction of the torticollis.[46] Surgery is generally indicated for children who are older than 12 months and have not responded to physical therapy, children initially referred for treatment after 12 months of age, and when cervical rotation is restricted greater than 30 degrees and facial asymmetry is present.[22,47] Surgical intervention usually involves release of the muscle distally at one or both of the heads, depending on the severity; excision of a portion of the muscle may also be indicated.[22] Postoperatively, physical therapy is indicated for achieving and maintaining cervical ROM and for strengthening of musculature to maintain newly achieved alignment of the head.

CMT, if left untreated, either by conservative management or surgical intervention, may lead to increased facial and cranial asymmetries secondary to abnormal growth of soft tissues, including the sternocleidomastoid muscle and surrounding fascia and vessels. The development of a cervical scoliosis with compensatory thoracic curvature has been reported in cases of unresolved CMT as well as occular and vestibular impairments.[22,48]

Congenital Metatarsus Adductus and Clubfoot Deformity

Metatarsus adductus is characterized by adduction of the forefoot in relation to the midfoot and hindfoot. The lateral border of the foot is convex with the curve beginning at the base of the fifth metatarsal.[49] Metatarsus adductus is an example of a deformation caused by intrauterine positioning and is associated with other positional deformations, such as congenital muscular torticollis and dysplasia of the hip.[50]

Metatarsus adductus is classified as mild with clinical correction of the forefoot to neutral and beyond, moderate with correction of the forefoot to midline, or severe when the forefoot is rigid and any correction toward midline is not possible.[51] Severe metatarsus adductus may also be referred to as metatarsus varus and may include medial subluxation of the tarsometatarsal joint.[22]

Mild metatarsus adductus resolves spontaneously without treatment by 4 to 6 months of age.[52,53] Infants with moderate or severe metatarsus adductus should be treated with serial casting until a flexible forefoot with proper alignment is achieved.[52] The height of the serial cast may need to extend above the knee to control any tibial rotation.

Clubfoot, or congenital talipes equinovarus, is a complex deformity involving ankle plantarflexion, hindfoot varus, and forefoot adduction. The incidence is 1 per 1000 live births, but the etiology is unclear.[49] Intrauterine positioning may be a causative factor in milder forms or when a primary neuromuscular impairment, such as myelomeningocele or arthrogryposis, is present. In the latter cases, decreased or absent fetal movement secondary to the primary neuromuscular impairment could lead to prolonged abnormal fetal positioning and the resultant clubfoot deformity at birth.

In the severe forms of congenital talipes equinovarus, pathologic deformities in the anatomy and alignment of the bony and cartilaginous structures of the foot are present. The muscles are also hypoplastic, giving an overall smaller appearance to both the foot and lower leg on the involved side. The etiology may be a defect in the mesenchymal cells forming the template for the cartilaginous model of the hindfoot structures indicating a dysplasia rather than a deformation.[22,54]

The goal of treatment for congenital clubfoot is to restore alignment and correct the deformity as much as possible and to provide a mobile foot for normal function and weight bearing. Initial treatment is begun shortly after birth and consists of splinting or casting. The cast must address the forefoot adduction, hindfoot varus, and ankle plantarflexion deformities but differing opinions exist as to which deformity should be addressed first.[22,52,55] Ideally, the cast extends above the knee to limit any rotary compensation from the tibia. Casting should continue until the foot is plantigrade and adequate alignment is documented by radiograph, improvement in foot position has ceased, or progress is very slow. Approximately one-third of infants with clubfoot deformity can be successfully managed with serial casting alone.[53] However is dislocation of the talocalcaneonavicular joint is present, surgical reduction is warranted.[22]

Surgical correction is usually performed before 6 months or age to limit the extent of secondary deformities from developing. The surgical procedure is dependent on the age of the child and the severity of the deformity but typically includes releases of the tight structures to promote realignment of the foot and ankle. Postoperatively, the infant or child may wear a night splint to maintain correction.

Developmental Dysplasia of the Hip

Developmental dysplasia of the hip (DDH) is a term used to cover a broad spectrum of hip anomalies in infants and young children that result from abnormal growth and development of the joint. The etiology of DDH most likely includes multiple factors, such as malposition and mechanical factors in utero, hormone-induced ligamentous laxity, genetics, and cultural or environmental factors. Malposition and mechanical factors include breech presentation in which the fetus hip lies against the mother's sacrum and a small intrauterine space. Cultures that swaddle their infants or use cradle boards that maintain the infant's hips in extension have higher incidences of DDH.[2] The incidence of DDH is very variable and is dependent on environmental factors, age of diagnosis, and inclusion criteria for the diagnosis of DDH.[22] However, the incidence of DDH increases in infants with other congenital deformations, such as torticollis or metatarsus adductus.[50,56]

During early fetal development, the acetabulum is very deep and the femoral head is spherical. Consequently, the femoral head is well covered by the acetabulum and the hip is a stable joint. With fetal growth and development, the acetabulum increases in diameter and becomes shallower, providing less coverage for the femoral head. The shallow acetabulum, less rounded femoral head, and increased femoral anteversion values present normally in infants at birth result in a very unstable hip. In the immediate postnatal period, depth of the acetabulum increases relative to diameter, producing a more stable ball and socket joint. The increased movement available to the newborn creates modeling forces that deepen the acetabulum as growth occurs. The most significant acetabular growth occurs during the first 18 months and minimal acetabular growth occurs after 3 years of age.[2]

Any interference with the normal growth and development of the hip joint may result in DDH. Interference can include abnormal forces resulting from positioning and confined space in utero, positioning that restricts normal kicking movements postnatally, and abnormal or absent muscle pull in utero and postnatally. The timing of these factors impacts on the severity of the joint changes. DDH, which results from malpositioning late in the last trimester, shows less anatomic changes and responds quickly to intervention compared with an infant whose hip development was affected early in fetal life. DDH in a newborn can be classified as subluxatable, dislocatable, subluxed, or dislocated (see Table 11-1).

ASSESSMENT

Newborn screening for DDH includes the Ortolani test and the Barlow maneuvers (Fig. 11-11A, B). Both of these tests are more reliable when the infant is calm and not crying and before 2 months of age. A crying infant tenses the soft tissues surrounding the hip joint and pre-

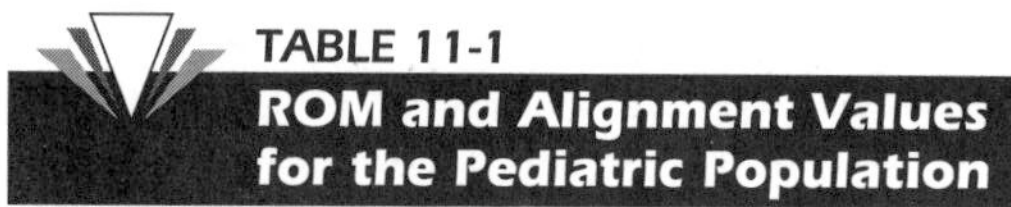

TABLE 11-1
ROM and Alignment Values for the Pediatric Population

Classification	Criteria
Normal	No instability of hip joint
Subluxatable	Femoral head within the acetabulum but can be partially displaced out from under the acetabulum
Dislocatable	Femoral head within the acetabulum but can be fully dislocated using the Barlow maneuver
Subluxed	Femoral head rests partially out of the acetabulum but can be reduced
Dislocated	Femoral head is completely out of the acetabulum

vents the examiner from observing any joint laxity or instability. As the infant grows, the unstable hip either remains in the acetabulum through normal development or remains outside the acetabulum and is prevented from relocating. Therefore, the Ortolani and Barlow maneuvers are much less reliable for infants older than 2 to 3 months of age.[22,52] Additional signs that may be noted in the newborn period include asymmetry of thigh or gluteal folds, marked limitation of hip abduction ROM or unequal femoral lengths, referred to as Galeazzi's sign. These signs become strong indicaters of DDH in the older infant when the Ortolani or Barlow maneuvers are no longer reliable. In older children who are ambulatory, DDH is usually diagnosed by an abnormal gait pattern. Children with unilateral DDH exhibit a positive Trendelenberg sign, and children with bilateral DDH walk with a waddle.[22,52]

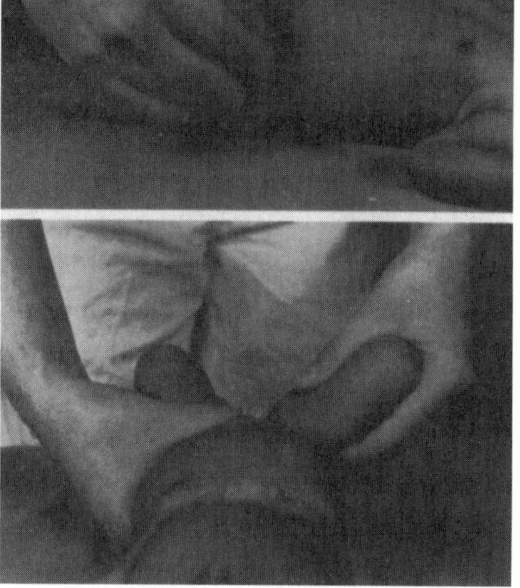

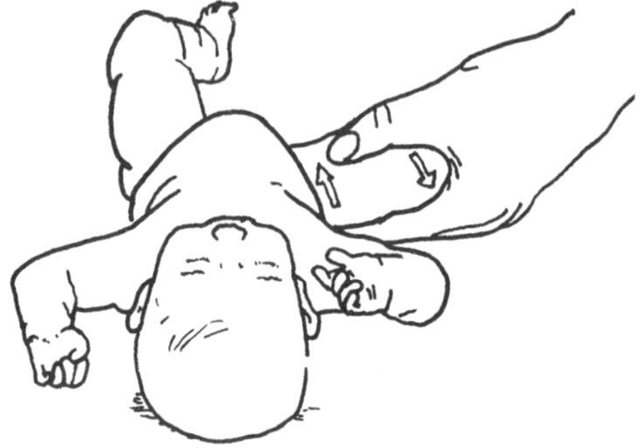

Figure 11-11 ▪ (*A*) The Ortolani maneuver. From a flexed and adduced position, the hip is abducted; the examiner feels a clunk as the femoral head moves into the socket. The examiner's other hand stabilizes the infant's pelvis.

When DDH is suspected from your assessment, the infant is referred for an ultrasound or radiography dependent on his or her age. Ultrasound is used for young infants when ossification of the femoral head is minimal and would not be detected on radiography. Any time an infant is referred for physical therapy, regardless of diagnosis, hip stability should be assessed. If risk factors are present, such as breech presentation or other congenital deformities, and your assessment is normal, the infant may still benefit from a referral for an ultrasound to confirm that DDH is not present.

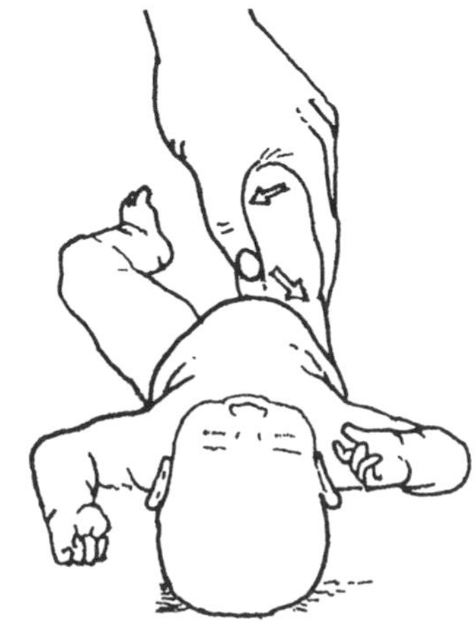

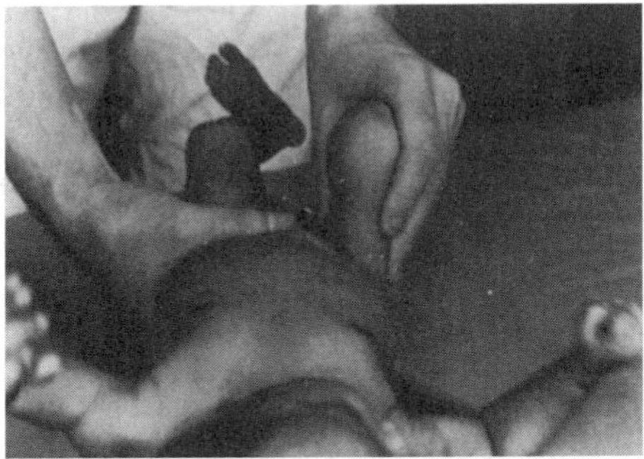

Figure 11-11 ▪ (**B**) The Barlow test. The examiner holds the infant's hip in flexion and slight abduction. The infant's hip is adduced while applying pressure in a posterior direction. Dislocation of the femoral head with pressure indicates an unstable hip.

MANAGEMENT

The aim of treatment is to return the femoral head to its normal relationship within the acetabulum and to maintain this relationship until the abnormal changes reverse.[56] The earlier the treatment is initiated, the less abnormal changes are present in the structures of the hip joint and the less time needed for the structures to return to their normal relationship. Treatment regimens will vary slightly between facilities and preference of the physician, but the same general concepts are followed in the management of infants and children with DDH.

Newborn to 6 Months. The goal of treatment is to maintain the femoral head within the acetabulum. An orthosis, typically the Pavlik harness, is used to maintain the infant's hips in a flexed and abducted position.

The Pavlik harness consists of a shoulder harness with two anterior and two posterior straps, stirrups for the legs, and booties to secure the feet (Fig. 11-12). In the Pavlik harness the infant's hips are flexed 90 to 100 degrees, which locates the femoral head in the acetabulum. With the infant in supine, the hips are allowed to fall into abduction, they are not forced into abduction. The abducted position stretches the hip adductor muscles and allows the femoral head to slide over the posterior rim into the acetabulum. The anterior and posterior straps permit active hip flexion and abduction but limit hip extension and adduction. Therefore, the Pavlik harness has a dynamic component that promotes active movement and modeling of the hip joint.

The Pavlik harness is worn 24 hours a day until the hip is stable; full-time use of the harness is continued after stability is achieved, and then a period of weaning out of the harness is instituted. The child's progress must be closely mon-

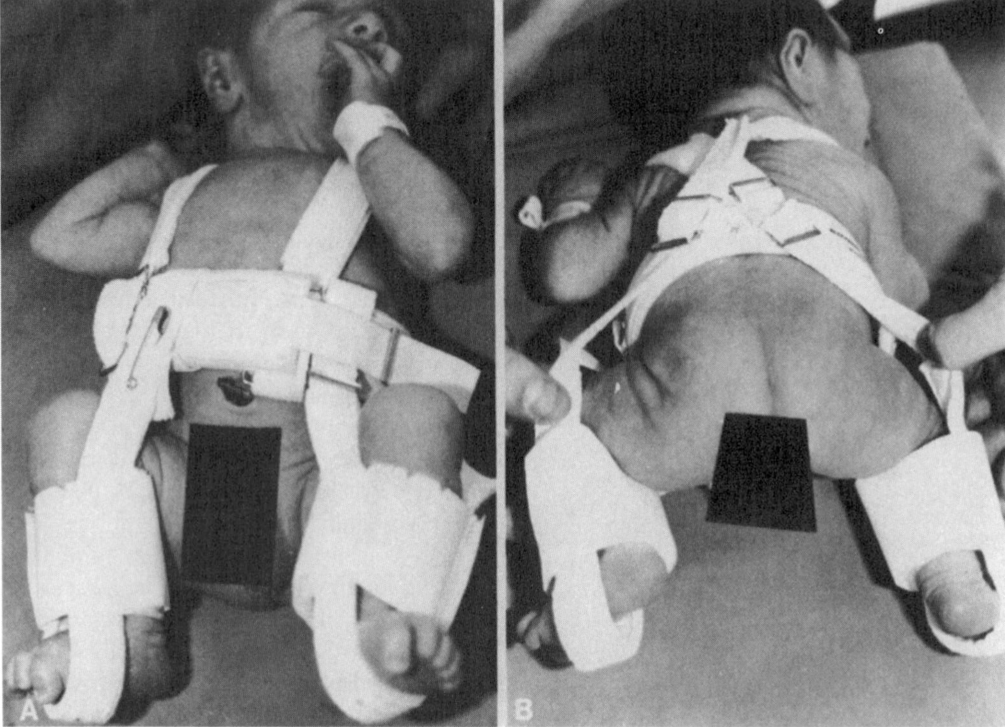

Figure 11-12 ▪ The Pavlik Harness maintains the infant's hips in flexion and allows active movement of the hips into abduction.

itored to detect complications or decide alternative treatments if hip stability is not developing.

Complications that can develop with the use of the Pavlik harness include avascular necrosis of the femoral head, femoral nerve palsy, and inferior dislocation.[22,57] These complications can be avoided through regular monitoring of the child's hips, parent or caregiver education, and proper fit of the harness. At many centers, the physical therapist works with the orthopedist and instructs the family in proper donning and doffing of the Pavlik harness. In an outpatient facility, an infant you are treating for another impairment may be wearing a Pavlik harness. It is imperative that the physical therapist be knowledgeable in the fitting of the Pavlik harness and recognize signs of ill-fit when they are working with these infants.

6 to 12 Months. After 6 months of age, it may become more difficult to relocate the femoral head in the acetabulum. Traction for a period of time may be attempted to relocate the hip and then institute wearing of the Pavlik harness. Closed reduction under anesthesia may be required with the application of a hip spica cast to maintain the hip in the located position.[22]

After 12 Months. Rarely will the child's hip be able to be relocated without surgical intervention. Conservative methods, such as home traction followed by closed reduction, may be attempted before a surgical procedure. Surgical correction may include release of tight soft tissue structures or osteotomy of the proximal femur to allow the femoral head to move into the acetabulum. Older children may require removal of a portion of the femoral shaft to reduce the forces on the femoral head when it is relocated in the acetabulum, femoral osteotomy, or acetabular osteotomy to aid in relocating the femoral head.[22,52,58]

Arthrogryposis Multiplex Congenita

Arthrogryposis multiplex congenita (AMC), also referred to as multiple congenital contracture (MCC), is a nonprogressive disorder characterized by multiple joint contractures and muscle weakness or imbalance. The reported incidence of AMC varies from 1 in 3000 to 1 in 4000 live births.[59,60] The disorder is related to a paucity of movement early in fetal development, leading to multiple contractures at birth. The exact etiology is unknown but is probably multifactoral. AMC is associated with multiple neurogenic or myopathic disorders that exhibit a defect in the motor unit including the anterior horn cells, roots, peripheral nerve, motor end plates, or muscle, resulting in weakness and decreased fetal movement early in development. Fetal immobility results in multiple joint contractures, fibrosis of muscles, and fibrosis of the periarticular structures.[60,61]

There is much variability among infants with AMC; however, common clinical features are generally present. These features include (1) featureless extremities that are often cylindical in shape with absent skin creases; (2) rigid joints with significant contractures; (3) dislocation of joints, especially the hips; (4) atrophy and even absence of muscle groups; and (5) intact sensation, although deep tendon reflexes (DTRs) may be diminished or absent.[60,62] The infant's contractures are usually symmetrical and typically include shoulder internal rotation, elbow flexion or extension, wrist flexion with ulnar deviation, hip flexion with either internal rotation or a frog-legged posture, knee flexion or extension, and equinovarus deformities of the feet (Fig. 11-13).[22]

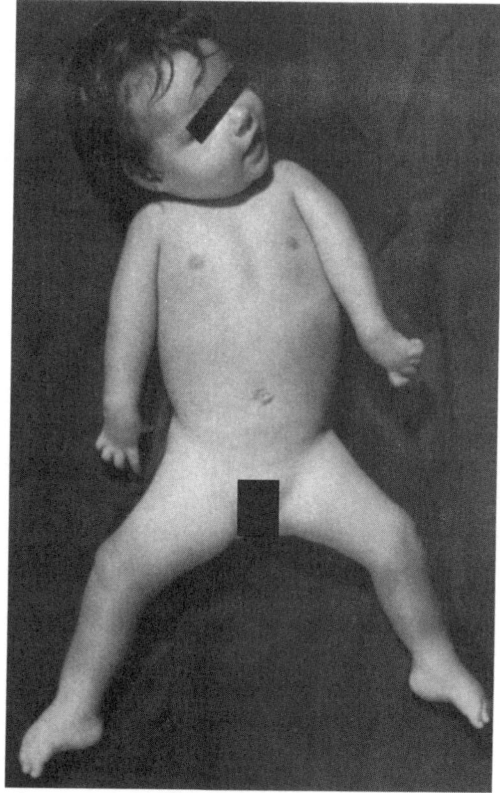

Figure 11-13 ■ *Arthrogryposis multiplex congentia in an infant. The shoulders are internally rotated and adduced, and the elbows and wrists are extended. The hips are flexed, externally rotated and abducted, and the feet demonstrate talipes equinocavus.*

MANAGEMENT

Intervention requires multiple disciplines working toward the same goal and timeline. The goal of intervention is to achieve the maximum functional level for each child. Treatment techniques include passive stretching through positioning, casting and splinting, strengthening activities, developmental skills, surgical procedures, and the use of adapted or rehabilitation equipment. The family is crucial in planning the long-term goals for the child and assisting with the carryover of activities.

INFANCY. Positioning and passive stretching exercises should begin shortly after birth. Serial casting begins in the first few months for foot deformities, knee flexion contractures, and wrist flexion contractures. Caution must be used to stretch only to the end range and maintain the stretch with a cast or splint. Forceful aggressive stretching of a rigid joint can result in damage to the joint capsule and surrounding soft tissues.[22] Any gains in ROM must be maintained with a splint or positioning device, or the contracture will recur.

Usually between 6 and 12 months of age, residual contractures at the feet and knees are surgically corrected.[52] Surgical correction involves release of the tight joint capsule and soft tissues. Surgical correction is maintained by splinting, strengthening exercises, and active functional movement. For example, a child who had a bilateral release of posterior structures of the ankle to correct an equinovarus deformity should have a splint fabricated to maintain the ROM as well as begin a standing program with the use of a standing device or ambulation aid.

The goals of intervention for the child's upper extremities must be well planned. For optimum function and independence with self-care skills, the child should have the ability to flex and extend the elbows. If this is not possible, treatment should aim to ensure that one elbow is able to flex for feeding activities and that the other elbow is able to extend for reaching and toileting activities (Fig. 11-14).

During this age range, the child should develop some mobility skills. Rolling is often difficult secondary to the lower extremity contractures. Some children may learn to scoot on the floor on their belly or their back initially. Most children can learn to sit but have difficulty achieving the sitting position independently. From sitting, floor mobility should be encouraged. Creeping on hands and knees is often difficult, and children often learn to scoot on their bottom. Pulling to stand may be limited by contractures of the lower extremity. Surgical techniques should be timed to prepare the child to stand when the child is developmentally ready. Preambulation activities should begin before 1 year of age.

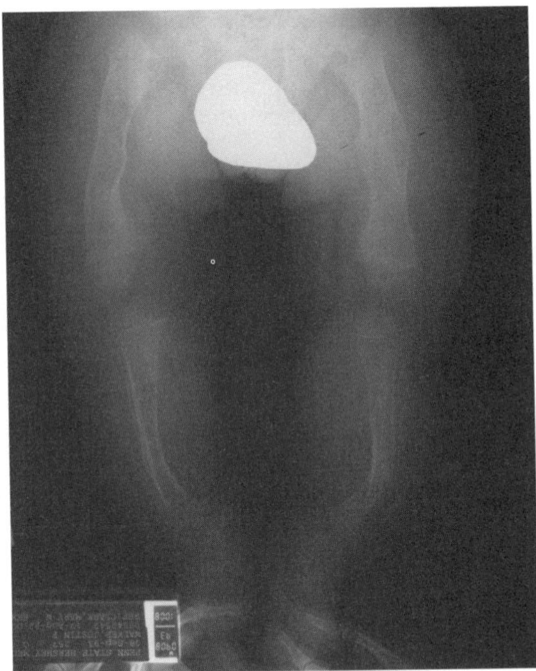

Figure 11-14 ■ Radiograph of 13-month-old child with Type III osteogenesis imperfecta. Note the poor bone density, previous fracture sites, bowing of the bones, and the length of the femurs in relation to the tibias.

12 MONTHS THROUGH PRESCHOOL. The goal of treatment during this age range is to develop the maximum level of independence with mobility and self-care skills. Ambulation is possible for many children with AMC and should be considered a viable goal until proven otherwise. Upper extremity skills focus on feeding and dressing activities. Maintenance of acquired ROM is crucial, as are continued gains in ROM. Strengthening exercises through age-appropriate activities, as well as specific mobility training, are incorporated into the program.

SCHOOL-AGE. The school-age time period often highlights the functional impairments that may exist for a child with AMC. The child's ambulation speed may be slow compared with his or her peers, and fine motor difficulty may interfere with writing speed and clarity. Adaptive and rehabilitation equipment may be necessary to assist the child with functioning independently in the school setting and maintaining social interaction with his or her peers.

Postnatal Deformations

Deformations can also occur postnatally secondary to the immaturity of the musculoskeletal system of a growing and developing child. The effect of growth on the musculoskeletal system can be used to correct prenatal deformities, such as seen in the treatment rationale for congenital muscular torticollis or metatarsus adductus. However, the effect of growth can also produce additional deformities postnatally if a force is abnormal or unopposed.

Rotational Deformities

The variation of a child's rotational profile that occurs with normal growth and development produces many questions for parents and subsequent visits to an orthopedist or a physical therapist. The child with a rotational variation presents with either an in-toed or out-toed gait. Clarification on what is a true normal rotational variation, when the rotation becomes a deformity, and appropriate assessment and intervention are necessary to answer parents' questions, recognize true problems, and possibly impact on those problems. The causative factors of the in-toeing or out-toeing must be evaluated and the rotational components measured using Staheli's rotational profile outlined earlier in the chapter. Staheli's rotational profile includes foot progression angle as an overall measure, hip rotation ROM to assess femoral torsion, TFA assessing tibial torsion and the hindfoot, angle of the TMA to assess the distal tibia, and the configuration of the foot. The measurements can then be compared with the normative values to determine whether the child falls within the range of normal for his or her age and which component or components of the lower extremity are contributing to the in-toed or out-toed gait pattern (See Fig. 11-2).

FPA shows the greatest variability in infancy before leveling off to a mean of 10 degrees with a range of –3 to 20 degrees in childhood. Hip rotation ROM is divided into medial and lateral rotation of the hip and is a clinical measure to assess femoral torsion. The sum of medial and lateral hip rotation is approximately 100 degrees and slightly more in infants.[63] Lateral rotation of the hip is greater than medial rotation in infants secondary to tightness of soft tissues from intrauterine positioning. Femoral anteversion is present in infancy but is not as noticeable because of the infant's position of lateral rotation. Femoral anteversion is usually noticeable in young children but continues to decrease from infancy throughout childhood. Persistent femoral anteversion may be classified as a rotational deformity when the following values exist: mild if medial rotation is 70 to 80 degrees and lateral rotation is 10 to 20 degrees, moderate if medial rotation is 80 to 90 degrees, and lateral rotation is 0 to 10 degrees and severe if medial rotation is greater than 90 degrees and no lateral rotation is present.[63] The TFA increases from a negative angle in infancy to a positive angle throughout childhood. The angle of the TMA also increases from infancy through childhood. The tibia is medially rotated in infancy secondary to intrauterine positioning. Derotation of the tibia toward the normal lateral tibial torsion values in adulthood occurs normally through growth and development.

Infants and young children exhibit greater femoral anterversion and medial tibial torsion that gradually decreases through normal growth and development. An in-toeing gait is most common during the second year after the child begins to walk. If the measured values fall outside the two standard deviation values for normal, a rotational deformity exists. Intervention is necessary only if that rotational deformity is cosmetically unappealing for the child or adolescent or if the deformity interferes with function.[63]

Previously, treatment has included exercise, bracing, shoe modifications, and orthpedic correction. Studies have shown that shoe modifications are ineffective in correcting in-toeing problems.[22,64] Various orthotic devices, such as the Denis Browne bar or twister cables, have not been shown to be effective and may actually cause secondary deformities at the knee.[53] Orthopedic surgery consisting of a femoral or tibial osteotomy may be indicated for children who exhibit deformities greater than three standard deviations from the normal values and when the deformity interferes with function or is cosmetically an issue for the child.

Dysplasias

A dysplasia is an abnormal organization of cells into tissue that leads to abnormal tissue differentiation.[6,25] Children born with a dysplasia exhibit widespread involvement because the abnormal tissue differentiation is present wherever the tissue is present.

Osteogenesis Imperfecta

OI is a congenital disorder of collagen synthesis that affects all connective tissue in the body and occurs with an incidence of from 1 in 20,000 to 30,000.[65] The musculoskeletal involvement is diffuse and includes brittle bones with excessive fractures, bowing of long bones, spinal deformities, muscle weakness, and ligamentous laxity (Fig. 11-15).[65–67] In addition to the musculoskeletal involvement, other clinical features of children with OI may include blue sclera, dentinogenesis imperfecta, hearing loss, growth deficiency, cardiopulmonary abnormalities, easy bruising, excessive sweating, and loose or dislocated joints.[65]

The clinical presentation of children with OI varies greatly and may be of genetic origin or a spontaneous mutation. Sillence developed a classification system based on genetic, clinical, and radiographic findings that broadly divides OI into four groups, Type I through Type IV.[68] Type I and Type IV are both autosomal dominant and milder in their presentation. Type I is the mildest form of OI with less incidence of fractures, growth deficiency and long bone deformities compared with the other forms. Individuals with Type I OI have blue sclera that persists throughout life, presenile hearing loss, and, may or may not exhibit dentinogenesis imperfecta.[65,68] Type II and Type III are both autosomal recessive and present with severe bone fragility and fractures at birth. Type II is often fatal in utero or the first few years of life. The skull, ribs, and long bones of infants with Type II OI are extremely osteoporetic and fragile. The infants may die from an intracranial hemorrhage during the birth process or respiratory complications in later infancy.[65] Children with Type III OI also exhibit very fragile bones with fractures and deformities present at birth. However, greater ossification is present in their skull than infants with Type II.[68] Children with Type III develop progressive deformity of their bones that include bowing of long bones and spinal deformities. Children with Type III OI exhibit significant growth retardation and functional limitations with mobility and self-help skills.

MANAGEMENT

Pharmacologic. Several pharmacologic and vitamin supplements have been studied in an attempt to decrease the fragility of the bones of children with OI. These agents have included calcitonin, flouride, hormones, and vitamins C and

D. All of these interventions have been shown to be ineffective in preventing fractures.[65,69]

ORTHOPEDIC. Fractures are managed with a soft splint or fiberglass cast for immobilization. The period of immobilization is kept short to minimize the bone demineralization that normally occurs with inactivity. Frequent fractures can lead to further demineralization, refractures, and bony deformity, specifically bowing of the long bones. Muscle pull on long bones can also cause significant anterior bowing of the long bones of the lower extremity.[65] Osteotomy and intramedullary rod fixation may be used to correct bowing deformities to facilitate use of orthotic devices and standing programs as well as to provide support to the bones to decrease the fracture rate.

REHABILITATION MEDICINE. Several practitioners from Children's Hospital Medical Center, Washington, DC, and National Institutes of Health have developed and revised a rehabilitation protocol over the past 10 to 15 years.[65–67,70] This protocol and the results of their follow-up studies will be discussed in the following section. Because of the wide variability among children with OI, the protocol is meant to serve as a guideline and must be indivualized for each child and family. The goals for the child with severe OI are to (1) prevent deformities of the head, spine and extremities; (2) avert cardiorespiratory compromise by avoiding constant positioning in supine; and (3) maximize the child's ability to move actively.[66] These goals are based on the theory that muscle strengthening and weight-bearing programs for upper and lower extremities promote active earlier use of the extremities and may lead to increased bone mineralization and less severe musculoskeletal deformities.[66,70]

Instruction in handling of an infant with OI is crucial for all parents and caregivers. The infant should be held with the head and trunk fully supported. For infants with severe OI, caregivers may be more comfortable holding the child on a pillow. Careful positioning of an infant with OI should begin in the first few days after birth with instruction from a knowledgeable physical therapist. Positioning aims to align the infant's head, trunk, and extremities and to protect the infant from hitting hard surfaces with activity. Emphasis is on midline orientation of the head and position changes to prevent the development of a laterally tilted head and misshapen skull. Active movement is encouraged as beginning strengthening exercises.

Strengthening activities progress from active movement to playing with lightweight toys and rattles. Active movement can be further encouraged in water either at bathtime or in a swim program with the parent present. Standard active-assistive and resistive exercises can be incorporated as the child becomes a little older. Emphasis is also on the development of head control and head righting in a variety of positions because children with OI often have a very large head. Developmental activities such as prone skills and rolling are encouraged. Independent sitting is encouraged when developmentally appropriate, as is some type of floor mobility. Those children who do not have the ability to develop independent sitting skills should be fitted for a custom-molded seat to promote head and trunk alignment and afford the child the opportunity to play in an upright position. Throughout the developmental progression, increasing or maintaining ROM and strength, especially of the pelvic girdle, is incorporated into activities.

Children should be fitted with orthoses when they have developed independent sitting skills and balance and are beginning to pull to stand. Those children who cannot sit independently but have developed head control should be fitted for a standing frame. The orthoses recommended in the protocol are containment or clamshell hip-knee-ankle-foot orthoses (HKAFOs).[66,71] Clamshell orthoses are similar to standard

HKAFOs except that a contoured anterior shell is present to support the thigh and lower leg. Gait training begins with an assistive device and may or may not progress to independent ambulation without an assistive device. With ambulation and upright positioning, attention must be directed to the pelvic girdle. Hip flexion contractures often develop, and children with OI typically require ongoing strengthening of their hip extensors and abductors.

Children who may not develop independent functional ambulation should be fitted with a manual or power wheelchair as appropriate. Positioning remains a key with any seating system and attention is given to head and trunk alignment.

In a 10-year follow-up report, Binder emphasizes the need for rehabilitation to focus on the child's functional needs.[67] She reports progress with functional skills in all groups of children with OI, ranging from improved head control to community ambulation. Progress appears related to severity of the disease but should be expected for all children with OI if the goals address functional needs. Those factors that impair independence include joint contractures and muscle weakness for those children with severe forms of OI and endurance capabilities for those children with less severe forms of OI.

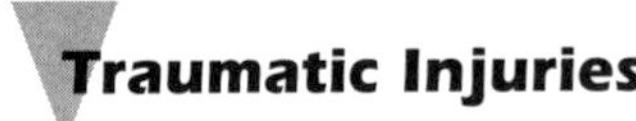

Traumatic Injuries

Fractures

Fractures in children differ from those in adults in multiple ways including the increased malleability, thicker periosteum, remodeling ability, open physis, and faster healing rate that are seen in children's bones (Table 11-2).[22,53,72] The malleableness and thicker periosteum allow bending types of fractures to occur in children that are not seen in adults. Children heal at a faster rate than adults secondary to the thicker periosteum and abundant blood supply. The younger the child, the faster the healing rate. For example, a femoral shaft fracture heals in an infant in 2 to 3 weeks, in a preschooler in 4 weeks, in a 7- to 10-year-old in 6 weeks and 8 to 10 weeks in an adolescent.[22] Nonunion fractures are rare in children because of the increased osteogenic activity of the thicker periosteum. Many fractures in children do not require reduction and realignment secondary to the remodeling ability of the bones in response to weight bearing and muscle pull forces. The physis is a weak area of a child's bone and, when it is disturbed, may result in a growth disturbance.

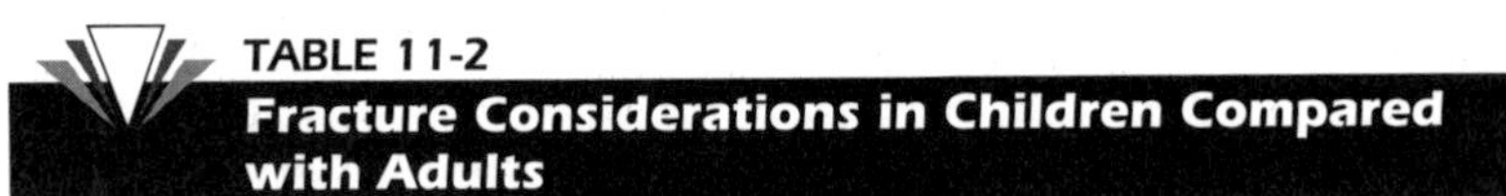

TABLE 11-2
Fracture Considerations in Children Compared with Adults

Features of Bone	Children	Adults
Bone Structure	Malleable	Firm
Periosteum	Thick	Thin
Blood Supply	May result in overgrowth in diaphysis/metaphysis	Overgrowth does not occur
Remodeling Ability	Significant	Minimal
Healing Rate	Rapid	Slower than child
Physis	Open	Closed
Nonunion	Rare	More frequent than children

Fractures may involve any portion of the bone including the epiphysis, physis, and shaft, and may be defined as complete or incomplete. Incomplete fractures may be further differentiated as a bend, buckle, or greenstick fracture (Fig. 11-15). A bend or bowing of the bone is seen in response to a deformation force, but a fracture line is not present. Buckle or torus fractures occur in response to a compressive force. Buckle fractures are often seen in the metaphyseal region of the bone and often resemble a bulge on the cortex of the bone. A greenstick fracture occurs when the bone exhibits a complete fracture on the tension side, but the cortex and periosteum are intact on the concave side. Greenstick fractures are common in children and must be converted to a complete fracture to avoid the complication of developing an angular deformity.[22] Fractures may also be defined by the direction of the fracture lines such as transverse, oblique, spiral, and comminuted (Fig. 11-16).

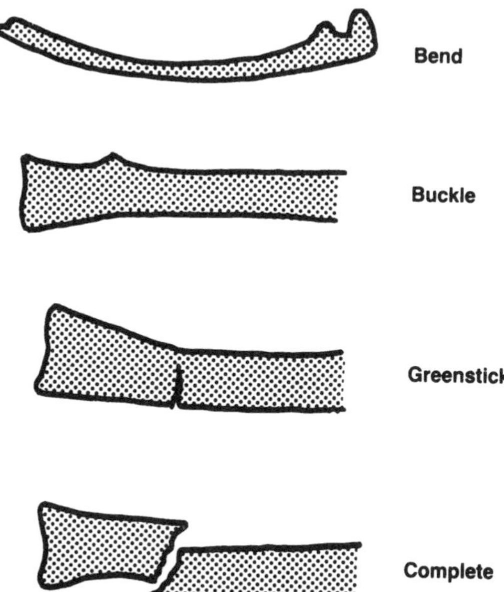

Figure 11-15 ▪ Incomplete and complete fractures in children. Buckle and greenstick fractures are unique to children.

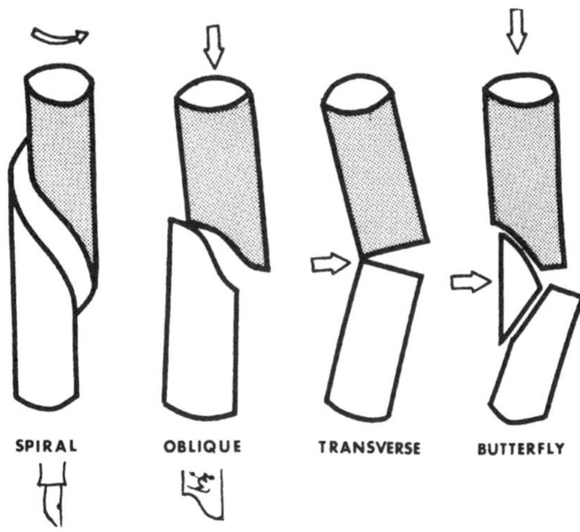

Figure 11-16 ▪ Fractures may also be defined by the direction of the fracture line.

Fractures involving the physis are unique to children and occur in approximately 15% of injuries to the long bones.[72] Fractures that involve the physis may cause growth retardation with resultant angular deformities. Physeal injuries are seen more frequently during times of rapid growth, such as preschool or prepubertal ages, and occur in physes that provide the most longitudinal growth. The distal radius is the most common site, followed by the distal ulna, distal humerus, proximal radius, distal tibia, distal femur, proximal humerus, proximal femur, proximal tibia, and phalanges for involvement of the physis.

Physeal injuries are commonly classified into five types according to the Salter-Harris classification system (Table 11-3).[22,53] The severity of involvement ranges from Type I with separation of the epiphysis from the metaphysis and no growth disturbance to Type V, which is a compression injury and results in a growth disturbance. Type V fractures may not be diagnosed until the growth disturbance is apparent. Type I and Type II fractures can be treated with closed

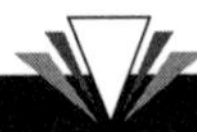

TABLE 11-3
Salter-Harris Classification of Physical Injuries

Type	Involvement	Treatment	Prognosis
I	Separation of epiphysis from metaphysis	Closed reduction	Good—no growth disturbance
II	Fracture line runs along physis through metaphysis; bony fragment	Closed reduction	Good—no growth disturbance
III	Vertical fracture line from epiphysis through physis, parallel to physis to periphery	Open or closed reduction	Good if circulation is not interrupted and good alignment is obtained
IV	Vertical fracture line from epiphysis, through physis and metaphysis; may be displaced bone fragment	Open reduction	May have disturbance of growth
V	Crushing of physis from severe compression force	Often not detected until arrest of growth is later detected	Arrest of growth, usually angular deformity

reduction, and a good outcome with no disturbance of growth is expected. Type III and Type IV fractures require open reduction with internal fixation. The outcome of Type III and IV fractures is related to the severity of involvement and the reduction of the fracture.

MANAGEMENT

Physical therapy following cast removal for incomplete fractures or physeal fractures Type I or II is rarely required. Children will often present with near-normal ROM after cast removal and will quickly gain strength through normal activities. Depending on the age of the child, a fiberglass shell may be used to protect the child's extremity for 1 to 2 weeks after-cast removal. This approach is especially important for young toddlers who fall frequently and may have just had a cast removed for a radial or ulnar fracture.

Children with fractures requiring open reduction and internal fixation or external fixation may require physical therapy for initial gait training and then later to gain ROM and strength. Aggressive stretching is rarely indicated for children post-fracture healing. Good communication between the physical therapist and orthopedist is necessary to develop appropriate goals and intensity of therapy.

Amputation

The causes of traumatic amputations in the pediatric population varies according to age and geographic location. Accidents involving farm machinery and power tools are the leading causes of traumatic amputations in pediatrics, followed closely by vehicular accidents, gunshot wounds, and railroad accidents.[73] Lawn mowers and household accidents account for most amputations in the 1- to 4-year-old population, whereas vehicular accidents, gunshot wounds, and power tools and machinery are common causes of traumatic amputations in the older child. As a comparison, acquired amputations from both trauma and disease account for 40% of childhood amputations, whereas congenital limb deficiencies account for 60% of childhood amputations. The highest incidence for traumatic amputations is in the 12- to 16-year-old age range.[73]

MANAGEMENT

The general management principles utilized with adults with amputations can be applied to children with amputations, with a few exceptions. The immature musculoskeletal system of the child offers advantages and disadvantages when managing traumatic amputations. Children tolerate surgical procedures that include skin grafts or closure of the wound under tension because they present with an adequate blood supply as compared with an adult with peripheral vascular disease. The use of skin grafts may allow preservation of limb length rather than amputation at a higher level without use of a skin graft.

Preservation of limb length is crucial not only for use of a prosthesis but to ensure continued growth of the limb. Amputation results in loss of physes and therefore limits the amount of possible growth from the affected limb. The physes at the shoulder and wrist account for the majority of growth in the upper extremity, whereas the physes around the knee contribute to the majority of growth in the lower extremity.[34]

Amputation through the midshaft of a long bone may result in terminal overgrowth. Terminal overgrowth is a painful, spikelike prominence of appositional bone growth on the transected end of the residual limb. The result is significant pain that interferes with weight bearing and use of a prosthesis. Terminal overgrowth occurs most frequently in the humerus, followed by the fibula, tibia, and femur.[34,74] When a child or adolescent complains of pain at the distal end of their residual limb, immediate consideration should be given to terminal overgrowth. On palpation, the body prominence may be felt and will elicit increased pain. The child should be referred to their orthopedist; the use of the prosthesis may need to be temporarily stopped to avoid further pain and the development of skin breakdown. Surgical correction for terminal overgrowth includes revision of the residual limb and, at times, capping of the distal end with an allograft for frequent recurrences.

PROSTHETIC TRAINING

Most children are fitted with an immediate-fit prosthesis in the operating room to control edema and begin early gait training. For those children who sustained significant trauma to the surrounding tissue or if a skin graft was necessary, an immediate-fit prosthesis is not used. Without an immediate-fit prosthesis attention must be given to wrapping of the residual limb to control edema and help shape the distal end. Immediately postoperatively, education must begin for positioning to prevent contractures, especially hip and knee flexion and hip abduction contractures.

Gait training begins postoperatively, and weight-bearing status is dependent on the physician. Initial gait training may be begun with a walker but should progress to crutches for most children over 6 years of age. Crutches will allow the development of a reciprocal gait pattern easier than most walkers. Many children will progress to ambulation without an assistive device depending on the level of their amputation.

Many prosthetic options are now available for the pediatric population ranging from passive terminal devices to myoelectrics for upper extremity amputations to energy-storing feet and modular component systems for the lower extremity. An in-depth review of prosthetics is beyond the scope of this introductory discussion of pediatric amputations. Refer to the earlier section in this chapter on congenital limb deficiencies for general guidelines regarding prosthetic training for various ages.

Pathologic Processes

Pathologic processes is a broad category of conditions that are abnormal and may impact on the developing and growing musculoskeletal system of a child. These processes are varied in their origin and may include vascular, infectious, metabolic, mechanical, traumatic, or structural.

Legg-Calvé-Perthes Disease

Legg-Calvé-Perthes disease is a self-limiting disease of the hip initiated by avascular necrosis of the femoral head. The precise cause of the avascular necrosis that disrupts blood flow to the capital femoral epiphysis in not known. Trauma, transient synovitis, infection, congenital or developmental vascular irregularities, and thrombotic vascular insults have all been theorized as producing the avascular necrosis of the femoral head.[75,76] The disease typically occurs between 3 and 13 years of age, with boys affected three to five times more frequently than girls. Legg-Calvé-Perthes disease is most commonly seen in boys between 5 and 7 years of age. Bilateral presentation is seen in 10% to 20% of children with the disease.[22,77]

Legg-Calvé-Perthes disease progresses through four clearly defined stages: (1) condensation; (2) fragmentation; (3) reossification; and (4) remodeling. During the initial phase a portion of all of the femoral head becomes necrotic and bone growth ceases. The necrotic bone is resorbed and fragmented; at this time revasucularization of the femoral head is initiated. During this second stage, the femoral head often becomes deformed and the acetabulum becomes flattened in response to the deformity of the femoral head. With revascularization, the femoral head begins to reossify. As the femoral head grows, remodeling of both the femoral head and the acetabulum occur.[75,78] The stage of the disease at the time of diagnosis, sex of the child, and age at onset impact on the final outcome and congruency of the hip joint.

Catterall developed a classification system to assist with predicting outcomes of children with Legg-Calvé-Perthes disease (Fig. 11-17 A–D).[78] Catteral's classification is divided into four categories and is based on the severity of femoral head involvement. Type I involves the anterior portion of the femoral head with no collapse and no sequestrum or fragmentation of necrotic bone. Type II involves a greater portion of the anterior portion of the femoral head and collapse of the involved portion. With Type III, a large portion of the femoral head is involved with collapse and sequestration of the involved portion. Metaphyseal involvement is seen with Type III. Type IV involves the entire femoral head, including collapse and sequestration and displacement of the femoral head and extensive metaphyseal involvement.

Clinically, children with Legg-Calvé-Perthes disease present with a limp and pain referred to the groin, thigh, or knee.[22,77] If the condition is undetected, hip ROM limitations may develop with restrictions in hip internal rotation and abduction, a hip flexion contracture may be present and a Trendelenburg-type gait may be observed. Muscle spasm of the hip adductors and ilopsoas may also be noted.[75,77] Children who may present to a physical therapist with the preceding symptoms and unknown etiology should be referred to a pediatric orthopedist.

MANAGEMENT

The goals of treatment are to relieve the symptoms of pain and muscle spasm, contain the femoral head in the acetabulum while bone remodeling occurs, and restore of ROM. Treatment for relief of pain includes anti-inflammatory medications, traction, and partial weight bearing with the use of crutches. Containment of the femoral head may be achieved through the use of traction, orthotic devices such as a

(text continued on page 415)

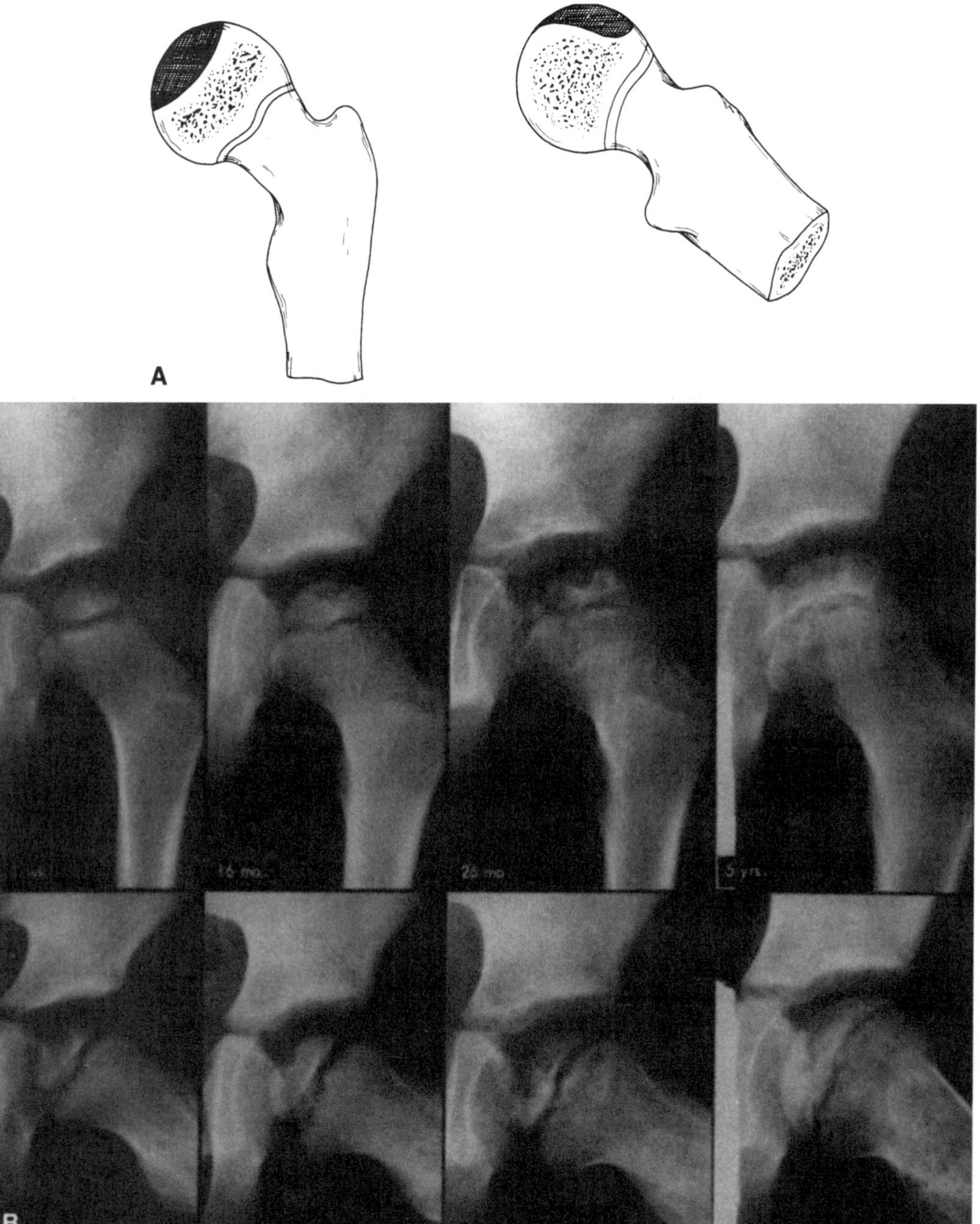

Figure 11-17 ▪ Catterall classification (anteroposterior and frogged radiographs). (**A**) Type I with evidence of anterior femoral head involvement. (continued)

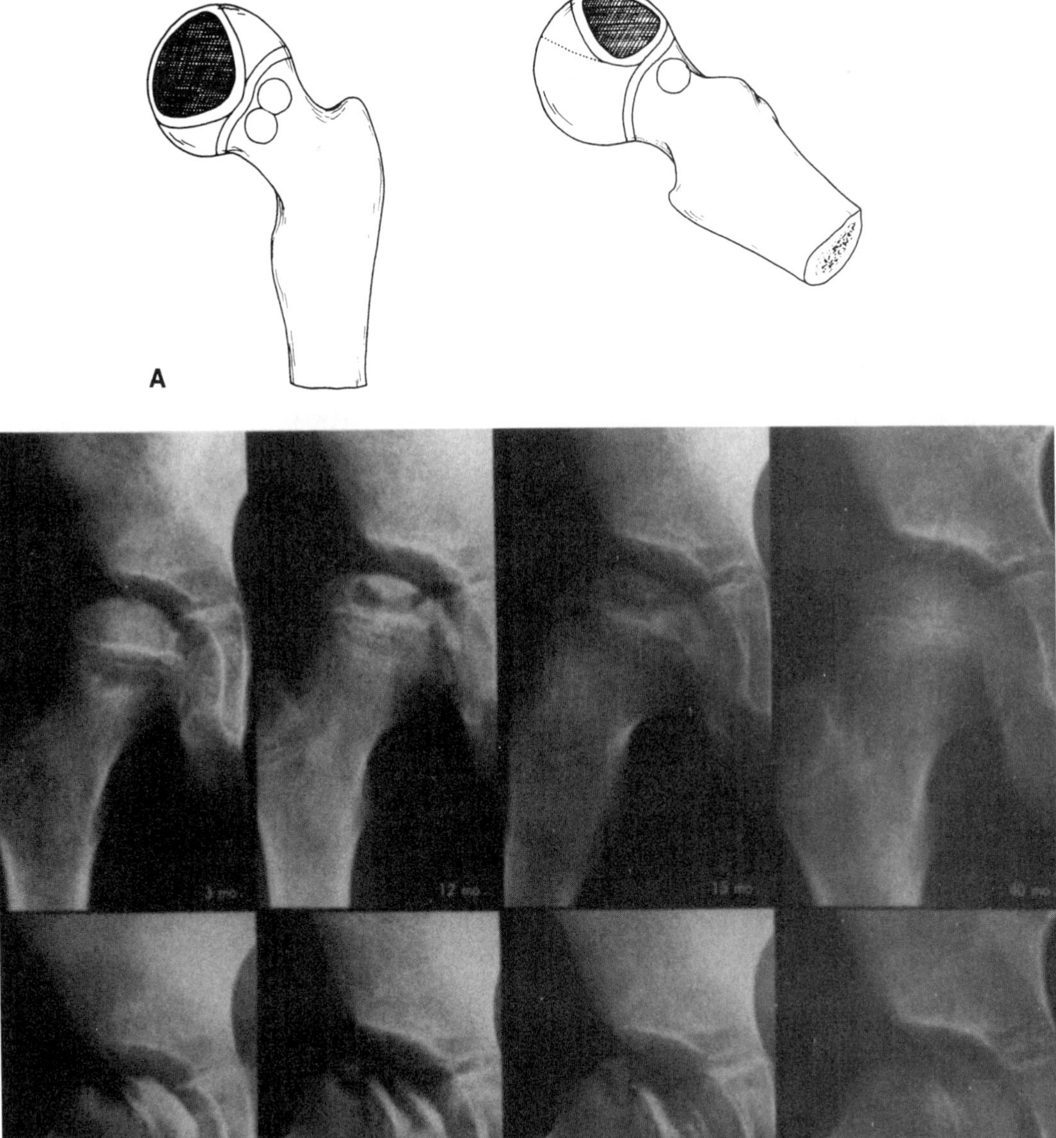

Figure 11-17 (Continued) ▪ (**B**) Type II anteriolateral involvement of femoral head ans sequestrum or differention between the involved and uninvolved portions of the femoral head. (continued)

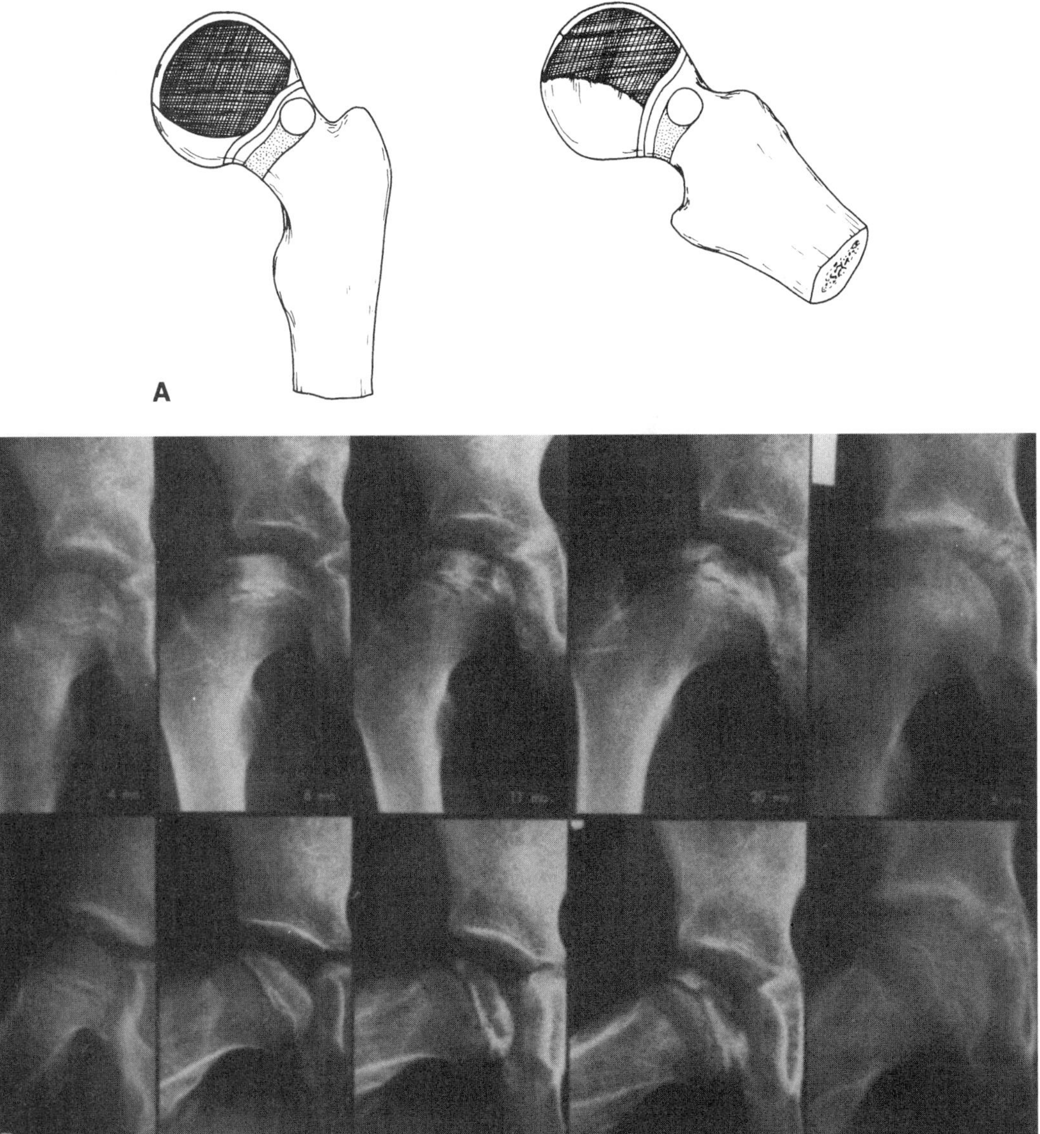

Figure 11-17 (Continued) ▪ (**C**) Type III, large portion of femoral head is involved with sequestrum and collapse of the involved portion. (continued)

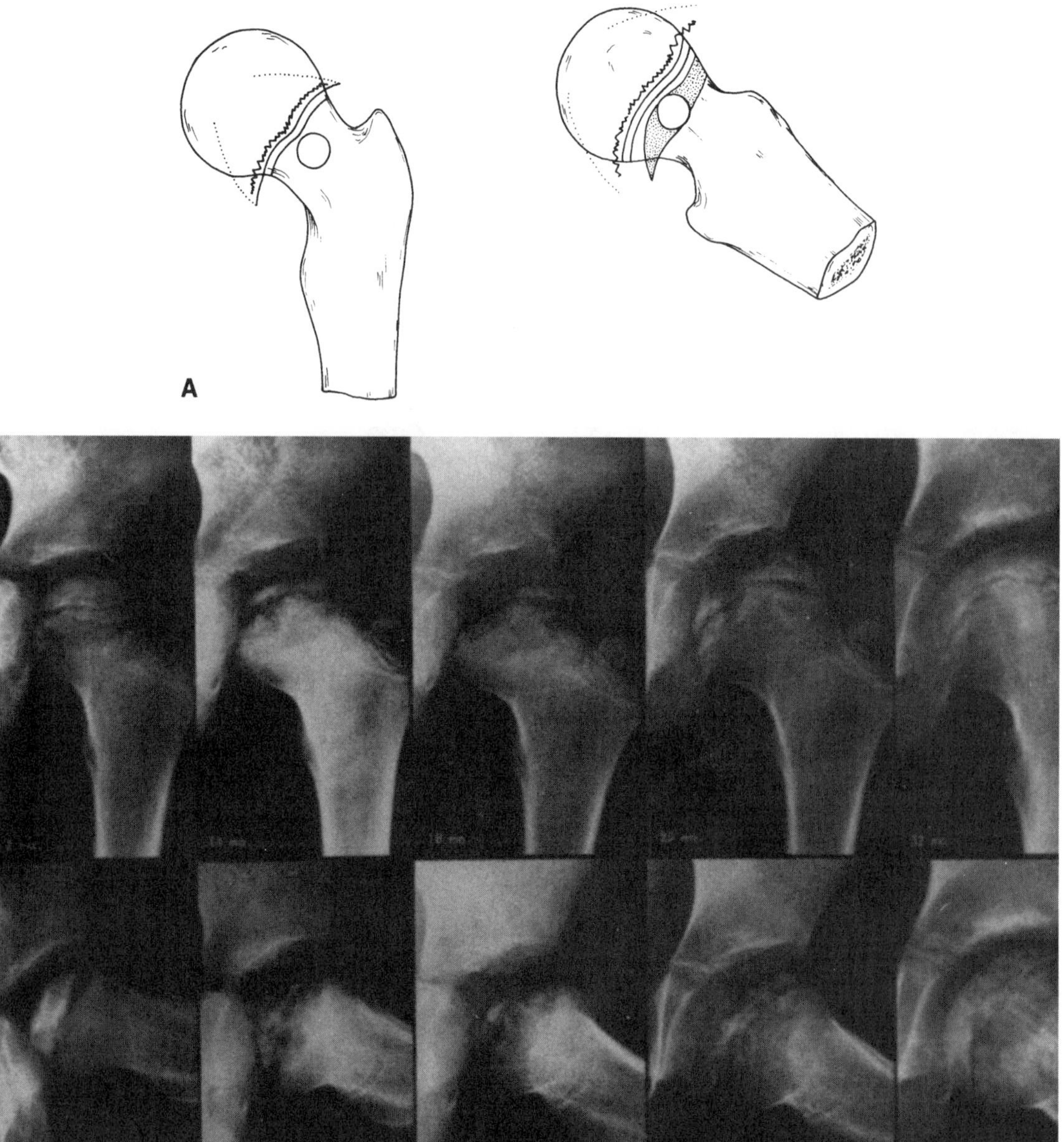

Figure 11-17 (Continued) ■ (**D**) Type IV, involvement of entire femoral head and metaphyseal lesion.

Petrie cast or Scottish-Rite Orthosis, or surgical procedures such as a varus osteotomy (Figs. 11-18 and 11-19).[79]

There remains much debate in the literature over the treatment methods that obtain the best outcome, and further research is needed before definitive treatment protocols can be outlined. Generally, those children with a poorer prognosis for full recovery are girls, children over the age of 8 or 9 years, and the extent of involvement of the femoral head.[78] Children with Catterall Type I generally do not benefit from any form of treatment; they have a good outcome with or without treatment. A long-term multicenter proceptive study is presently being conduted to compare the results of various treatment interventions. Very preliminary results support that the theory treatment for children less than 6 years of age should focus on alleviating symptoms of pain. Children ages 6, 7, or 8 years of age with a bone age of less than 6 years may benefit from containment methods of treatment. Children over the age of 9 years will usually not accept an orthotic device and often are candidates for surgical containment of the femoral head.[79]

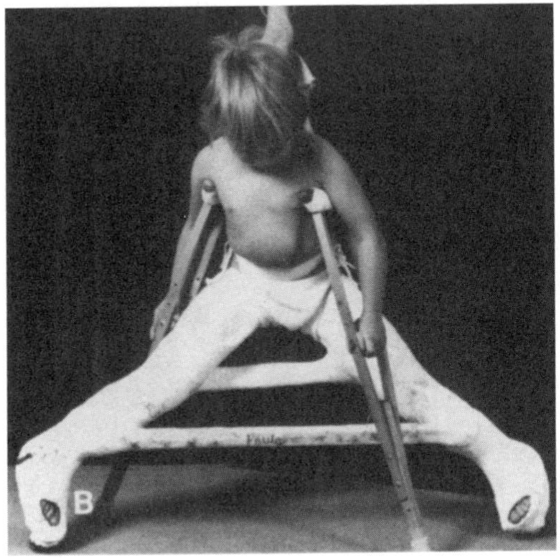

Figure 11-18 ▪ Petrie cast.

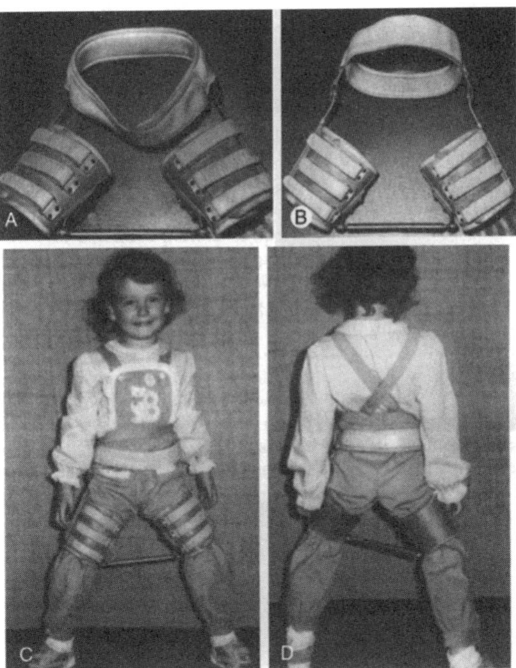

Figure 11-19 ▪ Scottish-Rite orthosis. The abduction bar contains a swivel joint that allows reciprocal motion of the legs.

If an orthotic device has been used as the method of femoral head containment, it may need to be used for a prolonged period of time, up to 1 to 2 years. While wearing the orthosis and after healing, physical therapy is often warranted to address ROM limitations and strength deficits. After removal of the orthotic device, children may continue to walk with a Trendelenburg-type gait because of weakness of their hip extensors and hip abductors. Physical therapy after surgical intervention focuses on gait training and restoration of hip ROM and strength.

Slipped Capital Femoral Epiphysis

Slipped capital femoral epiphysis (SCFE) occurs when the femoral head slips, or is displaced, from its normal alignment with the femoral neck. Excessive stresses on the growth plate are thought to contribute to the displacement of the femoral head. Stresses may include mechanical problems such as excessive weight, torsional forces secondary to trauma, or weakness of the growth plate secondary to sudden growth. The incidence of SCFE varies according to age, sex, and race. The incidence is higher in males and the African-American population, and is often associated with the onset of puberty.[53,80,81] Bilateral occurrence is present in 22% of young adolescents.

SCFE is classified by both duration of symptoms and radiographic findings. Acute SCFE is defined as a sudden onset of painful symptoms of less than 3 weeks' duration, whereas chronic SCFE is characterized by a gradual onset of symptoms for greater than 3 weeks. The third type is acute-on-chronic SCFE with a history of mild pain for greater than 3 weeks and a recent sudden exacerbation of symptoms.[80] Classification according to the severity of the displacement of the femoral head is defined as Grade I, displacement of the femoral head up to 1/3 of the width of the femoral neck; Grade II, more than 1/3 but less than 1/2 displacement; Grade III, displacement is greater than 1/2 (Fig. 11-20).[22,72]

Clinical presentation of young adolescents with SCFE includes pain in the groin, medial thigh, or knee; limping; external rotation of the leg; and limited hip ROM, especially flexion, abduction, and internal rotation.[53,72] External rotation is noted with attempts to flex the affected hip. With an acute onset, pain is often severe and the adolescent is unable to bear weight on the affected lower extremity. History may include a traumatic or gradual onset. If an undiagnosed young adolescent presents to physical therapy with the preceding symptoms, he or she should be immediately referred to a pediatric orthopedist for further work-up.

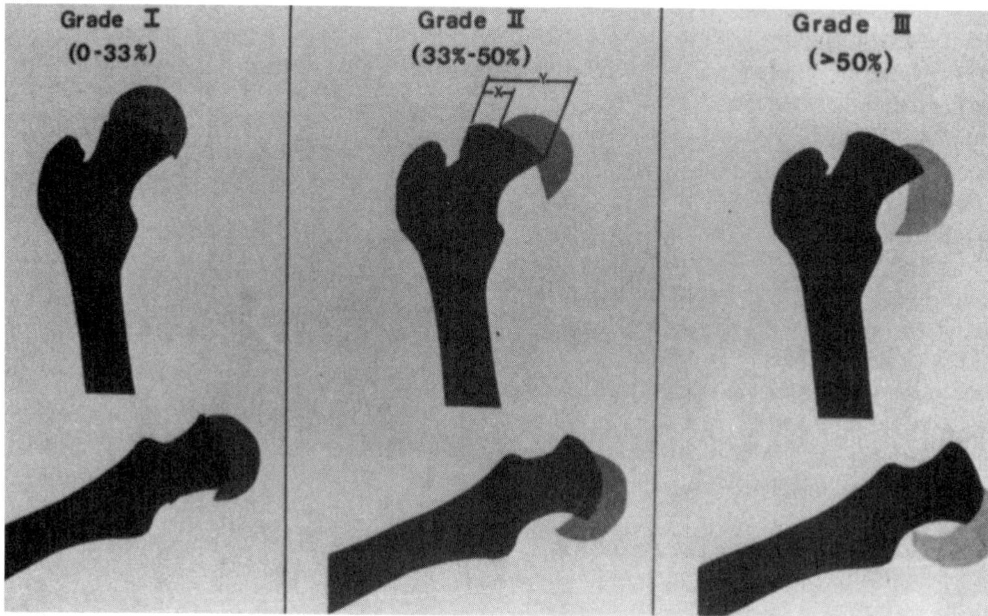

Figure 11-20 ■ Classification of the three grades of slipped capital femoral epiphysis.

MANAGEMENT

The goals of treatment include stabilization of the growth plate to prevent further displacement and prevention of complications, including avascular necrosis, chondrolysis, and early osteoarthritis.[22,82] Stabilization is achieved through surgical pin fixation. Nonsurgical treatment, including bedrest, traction, and casting, have not been successful with long-term outcomes of limited hip ROM, pain, and surgical procedures necessitated by early osteoarthritis. Physical therapy includes gait training with an assistive device postsurgically; weight-bearing status is usually NWB during the acute recovery period.

Tibia Vara (Blount's Disease)

Tibia vara, or Blount's disease, is a growth disorder of the medial aspect of the proximal tibia, including the epiphysis, epiphyseal plate, and the metaphysis.[22] Tibia vara is classified as three types, depending on the age of onset: (1) infantile, less than 3 years of age; (2) juvenile, between 4 and 10 years; and (3) adolescent, 11 years of age or older.[83] Diagnostic radiographic changes include sharp varus angulation in the metaphysis, beaking of the medial tibial metaphysis, wedging of the medial epiphysis, widening of the growth plate, and the presence of cartilage islands in or near the metaphyseal beak (Fig. 11-21).[84] This growth disturbance is thought to be the result of aymmetric excessive compressive and shear forces across the proximial tibial growth plate.[22,85]

Clinically, the child with tibia vara presents with a bow-legged stance. Infantile tibia vara must be distinguished from normal physiologic genu varum and medial tibial torsion. Physiologic genu varum gradually decreases until a genu valgus alignment is present between 2½ and 3 years of age. Toddlers with tibia vara are often obese, early walkers, and may exhibit a lateral thrust of the knee during stance.[22,86] Tibia vara increases in severity, whereas physiologic genu varum decreases as the child grows and develops. Other diagnoses that must be ruled out include various skeletal dysplasias, rickets or vitamin D deficiency, or a fracture that involved the growth plate of the proximal medial tibia. Juvenile or adolescent tibia vara may result from infection or trauma that disrupted growth of the proximal medial tibia.

MANAGEMENT

Treatment is dependent on the age of the child and the stage of the disease. Langenskiöld differentiated tibia vara into six stages with guidelines for prognosis and intervention.[87] Stage I occurs between 18 months and 3 years of age, and is characterized by breaking of the medial metaphysis and delay in growth of the medial epiphysis of the tibia. The stages progress in severity until Stage VI. Stage VI is seen between 10 and 13 years of age and is characterized by fusion of the medial aspect of the epiphyseal plate while growth continues laterally.[22,84,87]

Treatment options include orthotic devices or surgical procedures. Orthotic intervention is recommended for children under 2 to 3 years of age with radiographic findings consistent with Stage I or II. An HKAFO is recommended to be worn 23 hours a day.[84,86] Valgus correction of the orthosis is increased every 2 months. Physical therapy intervention may include family instruction in donning and doffing the orthosis, developing a wearing schedule, and instruction in skin inspection while the orthosis is used. Gait training with or without an assistive device may also be warranted.

After the age of 4 years, surgical options produce better outcomes than orthotic devices.[84] Tibial osteotomy is indicated for children under 5 years of age and for those toddlers who present with more advanced stages of tibia vara. After age 5 years, additional surgical procedures other than a tibial osteotomy are often indicated. The disease has often progressed to the more advanced stages and surgical options, such

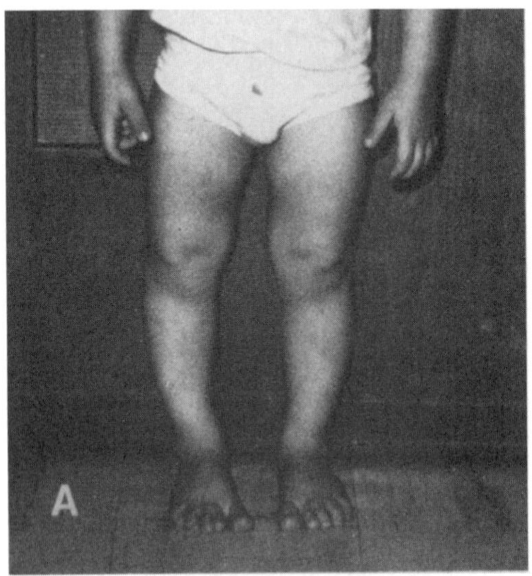

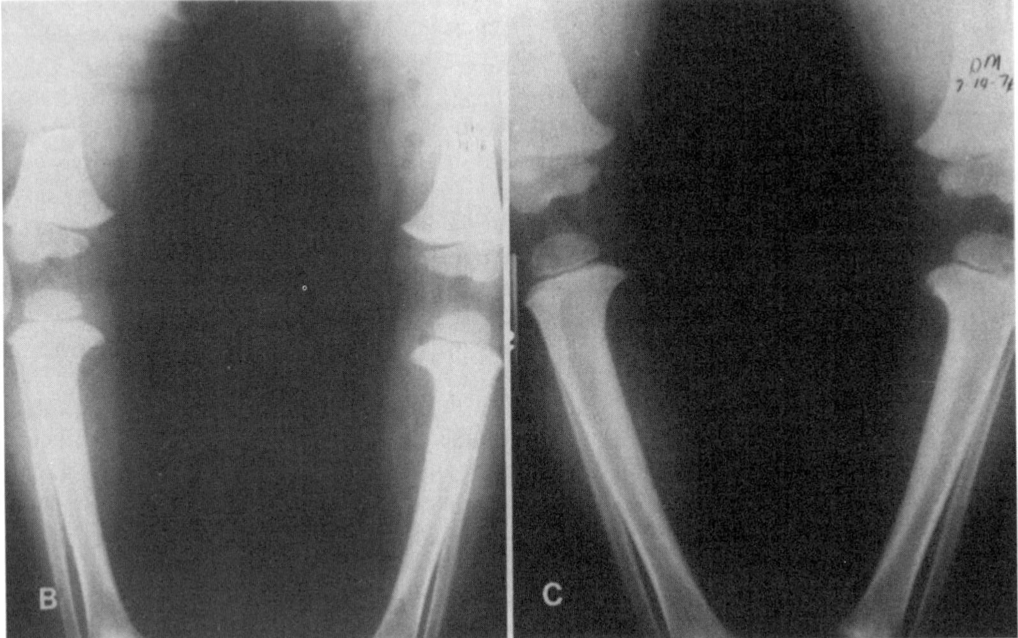

Figure 11-21 ■ (**A**) A 2-year-old child with varus on weight bearing. (**B**) A radiograph of the same child at 2 years of age showing early Blount's disease. (**C**) Same child at $2\frac{1}{2}$ years of age and progression of the Blount's disease; note the varus angulation and beaking of the medial tibial metaphysis.

as a lateral epiphysiodesis or removal of a medial bony bridge, may be necessary.[86]

Limb Length Discrepancy

A limb length discrepancy may be caused by shortening or overgrowth of one or more bones of the leg. Inequality of leg lengths may result from congenit conditions such as limb deficiencies or hemihypertrophy, infections or fractures that injure the physis, neuromuscular disorders, tumors, or trauma that results in overgrowth and disease processes. Injuries to the physes are often asymmetric and result in angular deformities in addition to the shortening of the affected limb. Leg length differences range from 1 to 10 cm or greater.

Measurements must be taken when a leg length difference is suspected. Clinical measurements can be taken by placing blocks of known height under the shorter leg or by measuring from the medial malleolus to the anterior superior iliac spine. The pelvis must be level prior to recording of measurements. More precise measurements are needed to predict the leg length discrepancy that will be present at maturity, evaluate treatment options, and predict the timing of surgical intervention if necessary. To assist with prediction of future growth and treatment options, the orthopedist uses radiographic methods to obtain accurate measurements and determine bone age, and uses growth charts to predict future skeletal growth of the child.

Intervention is generally not indicated for leg length differences of less than 2 cm.[22,34] A lift inside the shoe may be used for differences of 1 to 2 cm. Significant leg length discrepancies are a cosmetic issue as well as functional. Gait is less efficient and awkward, and postural compensations of the pelvis and spine often develop. Postural compensations may not lead to a structural deformity, but they may cause discomfort in adulthood.

MANAGEMENT

Treatment is dependent on the age of the child and growth remaining, severity of the leg length difference, and preference of the family and child. Surgical treatment options involve either shortening of the longer limb or lengthening of the shorter limb. Limb shortening is commonly achieved through epiphysiodesis. The predetermined physis(es) are surgically destroyed by the physician to arrest growth in the longer leg. Epiphysiodesis is indicated for leg length discrepancies of 2 to 5 cm.[22,34,53] Most physicians opt for lengthening the shorter limb when the discrepancy is greater than 5 cm.

If the adolescent has reached skeletal maturity and epiphysiodesis is not an option, shortening of the longer limb can be accomplished through osteotomy. A portion of the bone is removed to equalize leg lengths; 5 to 6 cm is the maximum for removal in the femur and 2 to 4 cm is the maximum for the tibia.[34] The disadvantages of shortening by osteotomy are the reduction in overall height of the individual, body proportions may be cosmetically unappealing, the amount of equalization is limited, and the uninvolved leg has undergone surgery.[34]

In the past 15 to 20 years, limb lengthening procedures have been used more frequently and effectively. Limb lengthening techniques are directed at the involved leg and allow for equalization of greater discrepancies. Limb lengthening may be indicated for discrepancies greater than 5 cm.[22] Limb lengthening techniques involve either metaphyseal or diaphyseal distraction and are based on the principles of fixation of the fragments to allow vascular ingrowth; the distraction rate correlates to the osteogenic activity and goals of minimal disruption of intramedullary vessels and the periosteum.[22,53] The Wagner and the Ilizarov methods are two lengthening techniques used in pediatrics.

The Wagner technique utilizes the principle of diaphyseal lengthening. An osteotomy is performed followed by rapid distraction of the bone that is stabilized through an external device. When the desired length is achieved, the external device is removed and internal fixation and bone grafting are performed to support the gap in the bone. When the gap is filled through new bone growth, the internal fixation is removed. The Wagner method is relatively quick, depending on the length to be achieved and the number of external pins is minimal. However, the entire process involves three operative procedures and cannot be used to correct angular or rotational deformities.

The Ilizarov method utilizes metaphyseal lengthening and involves a corticotomy rather than an osteotomy. Circular rings are placed above and below the level of the corticotomy and are attached to the bone through multiple pins existing the skin. The rings are connected by telescoping rods with a dial (Fig. 11-22). The dial is turned to provide a slow distraction force that keeps pace with the body's ability to lay down new bone. Postoperatively, the distraction rate is 1 mm/day performed in increments of .25 mm four times a day.[53] After the desired length is achieved, the external fixator device is kept in place until bone consolidation is complete. The pins are then removed without the need for an additional operative procedure. The Ilizarov method is used to correct angular and rotational components of limb leg discrepancies. The disadvantages of the Ilizarov method are the multiple pin sites, bulkiness of the apparatus, and the length of time required to achieved the desired length.

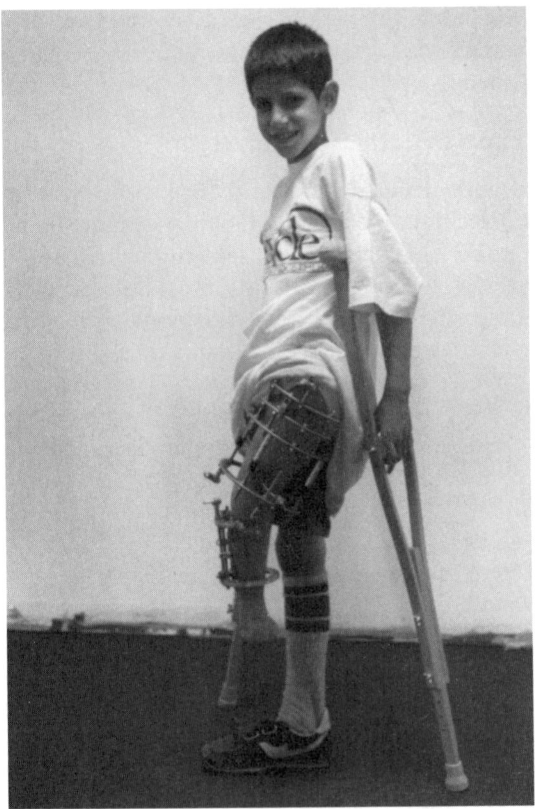

Figure 11-22 ▪ A 9-year-old boy with a diagnosis of proximal femoral focal deficiency who is presently undergoing an Ilizarov lengthening. The lengthening will provide a longer level arm when wearing his prosthesis and bring the height of his knees closer together.

Limb lengthening procedures bring their own set of problems to the child, family, and the professionals involved in the care of the child. Families must be able to make multiple appointments over a period of time, perform daily pin care, and carry out exercise programs. Problems that may be encountered during the course of a lengthening procedure include infection at the pinsites, joint stiffness, subluxation or dislocation (especially of the proximal tibia), nonunion, and fractures. The rate of distraction with the Ilizarov method is meant to keep pace with bone growth and therefore minimize the complications of nonunion and fracture. With both techniques, ROM limitations occur secondary to shortening of the soft tissues and the rate of soft tissue growth compared with that of bone.

PHYSICAL THERAPY

Immediately after surgery, the physical therapist is involved for gait training activities and promoting early weight bearing for most children who have undergone the Ilizarov procedure. Instruction in pin care must also begin immediately postoperatively. Joint ROM limitations occur but should be minimized. Ankle dorsiflexion ROM is often difficult to maintain. Preventive splinting should be implemented early on to maintain the ankle in a plantigrade position. Knee flexion and extension ROM can also become limited. Again, splinting can be implemented to maintain a prolonged stretch on the soft tissues. Muscle weakness is also usually present as the muscles lengthen to accommodate the new limb length. Strengthening exercises should begin early on and continue throughout the duration of the lengthening procedure.

Scoliosis (Idiopathic)

Scoliosis is a lateral curvature of the spine. Idiopathic denotes that the scoliosis is of unknown origin and is the most common form of scoliosis. Idiopathic scoliosis can be further delineated by age of onset: infantile occurs in children from birth to 3 years of age, juvenile occurs between the ages of 3 and 10 years, and adolescent develops after 10 years of age.[22] This section will focus on adolescent idiopathic scoliosis. The prevalence of idiopathic scoliosis in North America is 2 to 3% for curves 10 degrees or less and decreases to 0.2% to 0.3% for curves of 20 degrees or greater.[22,88]

Scoliosis is defined as either structural or nonstructural. Structural curves are fixed and do not correct with lateral trunk bending or traction. Structural curves have a rotary component that is visible when the trunk is flexed forward. Nonstructural curves correct on lateral trunk bending and often have as their etiology a pelvic obliquity, limb length discrepancy, or medical factors such as a tumor or muscle spasm. Structural scoliosis is further identified by the location and direction of the apex of the curve. For example, a curve with the apex in the thoracic region and convexity toward the right would be labeled as a right thoracic curve. Most curves have a primary curve and a compensatory curve. The compensatory curve is the body's attempt to keep the head and trunk aligned vertically. In the preceding example of the right thoracic curve, there may be smaller compensatory curves in the cervical or lumbar regions with their convexity toward the left (Fig. 11-23).

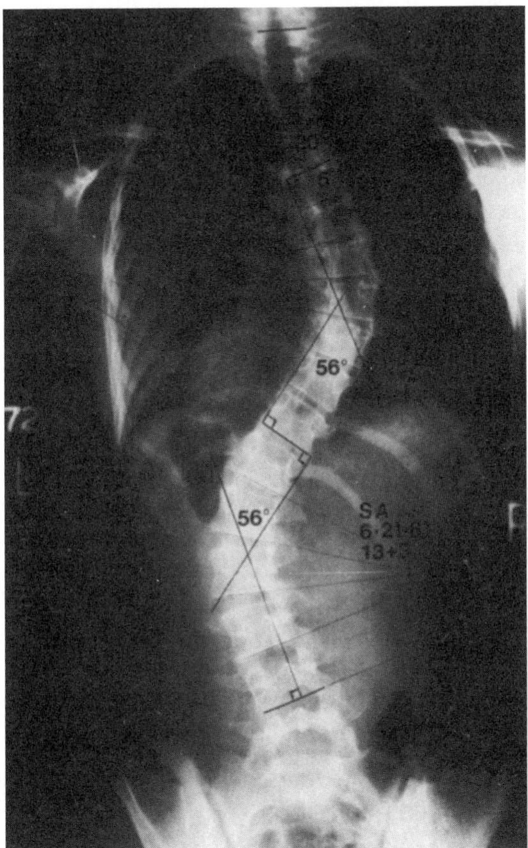

Figure 11-23 ■ A right thoracic, left lumbar scoliosis. The degree of curvature is measured using the Cobb method. The end vertebrae, or the vertebrae that tilts toward the concavity the most, are identified. Lines are drawn extending the end plate of the top and bottom vertebra for each curve. Perpendicular lines to the end plate lines are then drawn. The degree of curvature is defined as the angle of the intersection of the end plate and perpendicular lines.

Multiple structural changes occur with scoliosis, and their severity is related to the severity of the curve.[22] Changes occur in the growing spine in response to compression and distraction forces that are altered in the presence of a curvature. The vertebrae become wedge shaped and higher on the convex side, and compressed on the concave side, and muscles on the concave side become shortened. The vertebral body rotates toward the convex side so that the spinous process is rotated toward the concave side. Because the ribs are attached to the thoracic vertebrae, they also rotate. The rotation of the ribs produces a rib hump posteriorly, which is noted on the forward bend test.

SCREENING

Screenings for scoliosis occur in many schools and target the early adolescent population between 10 and 15 years of age.[89] The goal of school screenings is early detection to limit progression of the curvature. A screening should include anterior and posterior views of the trunk with the shirt removed and a forward bend test (Fig 11-24). On the anterior and posterior views, the examiner is looking for asymmetries in shoulder, nipple, scapular, or pelvic heights, asymmetric folds of the trunk, and curvature of the spine. The adolescent is then asked to bend over, keeping the knees extended and allowing the arms to dangle toward the floor. During the forward bend test, the examiner is looking for asymmetries in the contour of the back indicating a rotary component to the curvature.

When a scoliosis is detected, the adolescent should be referred to an orthopedist. Accurate measurement of the curve is performed through a variety of methods. A common method of measurement is a radiograph and the Cobb measure. To limit radiographic exposure, other measurement methods include Moire topography and

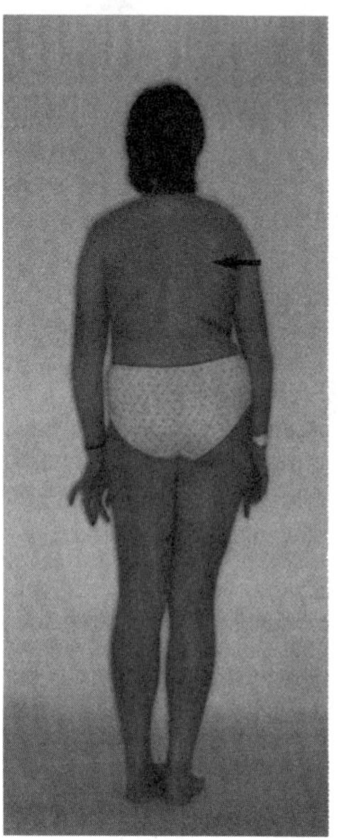

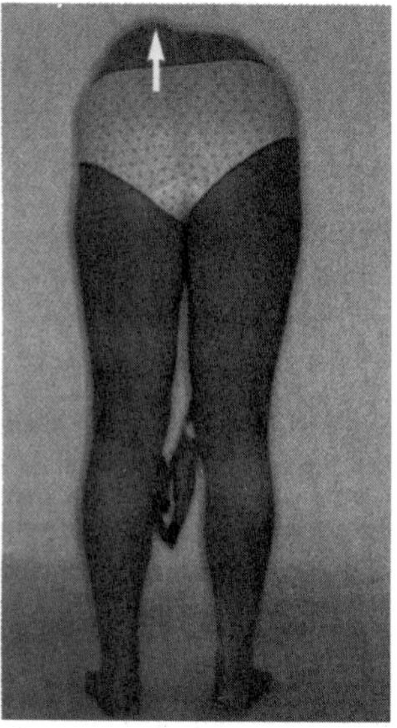

Figure 11-24 ■ Forward bend test. Rib hump is visible on bending forward.

Integrated Shape Investigation System (ISIS).[90] Moire topography is a photogrammetric technique that visually depicts shadow patterns that assess asymmetries. ISIS utilizes computer images in the transverse, frontal, and sagittal planes to develop contours of the adolescent's trunk. The goal of measurement is to determine a baseline and monitor progression of the curve.

MANAGEMENT

Treatment intervention is based on the sex, age, and skeletal maturity of the adolescent and the severity of the curvature.[22,58,91] Young adolescents who are prepuberty are almost certain to exhibit progression of their curvature. Females with a bone age of 15.5 years and males with a bone age of 17.5 years generally do not require treatment. Curves less than 25 degrees can be observed on a regular basis to monitor progression of the curve. Curves between 25 and 40 degrees should be treated with nonsurgical methods. Adolescents with curves greater than 40 degrees are candidates for surgical intervention.

NONOPERATIVE MANAGEMENT. The goal of nonoperative intervention is to maintain the curvature, not to correct the curvature. Nonoperative intervention methods have included exercise, electrical stimulation, and orthoses. Exercise or physical therapy has not been proven beneficial in reducing or altering the progression of a curvature. Exercise is indicated to maintain strength of muscles when an orthotic device is used. Electrical stimulation was attempted as a means of strengthening the

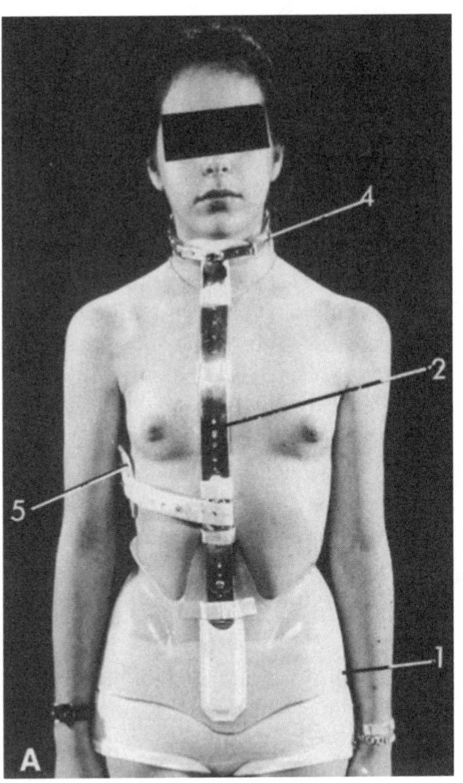

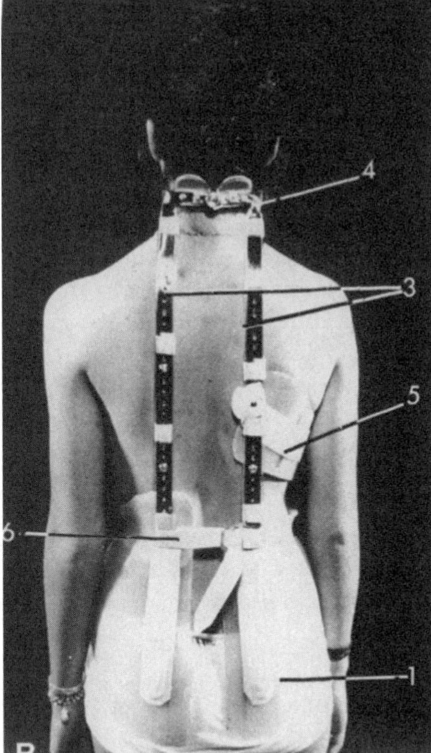

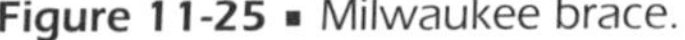
Figure 11-25 ▪ Milwaukee brace.

paraspinal muscles on the convex side of the curve but has been shown to be ineffective.[92]

Orthotic devices have been used in the treatment of scoliosis for many years. Most orthotic devices operate on the principle of three-point pressure against the apex of the curve and may also incorporate a traction component. The Milwaukee brace was one of the first orthotic devices developed for scoliosis. The orthosis consists of a collar that supports the chin and occiput and a pelvic component connected by metal uprights. Lateral pads are present in the pelvic component to provide pressure against the lumbar component of the curve and a thoracic pad is attached to a metal upright to provide pressure against the thoracic component of the curve (Fig 11-25).

Many orthoses presently incorporate a lower profile system that eliminates the chin and occiput component of the Milwaukee brace and are often referred to as a thoraco-lumbar-sacral orthosis (TLSO) (Fig 11-26). The pelvic stabilization and lateral pressure pads are present in a TLSO. Adolescents are generally instructed to wear the orthosis between 18 and 23 hours a day until skeletal maturity or unless the curve continues to progress and surgery is indicated.

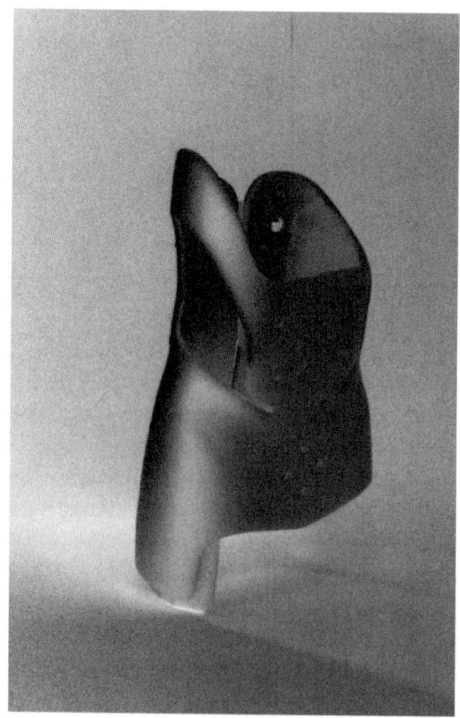

Figure 11-26 ▪ Boston Brace (thoraco-lumbar-scral-orthosis; TLSO).

Instruction in donning and doffing the orthosis, developing a wearing schedule, skin care, and an exercise program to maintain ROM and strength while wearing the orthosis are provided by a physical therapist. Exercise should be focused on maintaining flexibility and muscle strength. Hip flexion contractures can develop with use of the orthosis; routine stretching of the hip flexors should be instituted when orthosis wearing is initiated. Muscle strength must be maintained while wearing the orthosis so that the trunk muscles are strong when the use of the orthosis is discontinued. Exercise should include strengthening for abdominals, gluteal muscles, and paraspinal musculature.

Operative Management. Surgical intervention is warranted if the curve is greater than 40 degrees, the curve is progressing with conservative management, or there is decompensation of the spine or thoracic cavity.[22] The goal of surgery is to obtain as much correction as possible and to stabilize the spine and maintain the correction over time.

There are many types of instrumentation available but the main principles of instrumentation are distraction and compression of the curve appropriately, correction, or minimization of the rotary component, and stabilization of the spine to maintain the correction. Harrington rods, both a compression and a distraction rod, were the standard instrumentation for many years. Alterations have been made to the Harrington rods, and many other types of instrumentation have been introduced. Much of the newer instrumentation aims to maintain the normal lordotic and kyphotic curves of the spine, control the rotary component of the curve, and provide additional stability to the spine.

PHYSICAL THERAPY. Ideally physical therapy has been involved preoperatively with ROM and trunk strengthening exercises. Instruction in deep breathing and coughing exercises should be initiated preoperatively and adhered to immediately postoperatively. Depending on the instrumentation used, the adolescent is encouraged to begin early mobilization, including transfers and gait training. Time frames for ambulation depend on the instrumentation, surgeon's preference, and whether or not a supportive orthosis is needed.

Summary

The growth and development of a child's musculoskeletal system were discussed in this chapter. The immature musculoskeletal system of a child is susceptible to abnormal forces and stresses. Physical therapists must be alert to those forces and the consequences they may have on an immature musculoskeletal system. Many orthopedic diagnoses were discussed in this chapter as examples of the effect of abnormal forces on the developing child and how those forces can at times be beneficial in treatment. However, the principles that were discussed and the assessment procedures that were outlined can be applied to any child seen by a physical therapist, not just those children with a diagnosis of orthopedic origin. Identifying potentially deforming forces and developing treatment protocol based on your findings is the challenging but very rewarding aspect of pediatric physical therapy.

REFERENCES

1. Crelin ES. Development of the musculoskeletal system. *Clin Symp.* 1981;33:2–36.
2. Walker JM. Musculoskeletal development: a review. *Phys Ther.* 1991;71:878–889.
3. Arkin AM, Katz JF. The effects of pressure on epiphyseal growth. *J Bone Joint Surg (Am).* 1956;38:1056–1076.
4. Storey E. Growth and remodeling of bone and bones. *Dent Clin North Am.* 1975;19:443–454.
5. LeVeau BF, Bernhardt DB. Developmental biomechanics: Effect of forces on the growth, development and maintenance of the human body. *Phys Ther.* 1984;64:1874–1882.
6. Dunne KB, Clarren SK. The origin of prenatal and postnatal deformities. *Pediatr Clin North Am.* 1986;33:1277–1297.
7. Haley SM, Tada WL, Carmichael EM. Spinal mobility in young children: A normative study. *Phys Ther.* 1986;66:1697–1703.
8. Florence JM, Pandya S, King WM, et al. Clinical trials in Duchenne dystrophy: Standardization and reliability of evaluation procedures. *Phys Ther.* 1984;64:41–45.
9. Pandya S, Florence JM, King WM, et al. Reliability of goniometric measurements in patients with Duchenne muscular dystrophy. *Phys Ther.* 1985;65:1339–1342.
10. Stuberg WA, Metcalf WK. Reliability of quantitative muscle testing in healthy children and in children with Duchenne muscular dystrophy using a handheld dynamometer. *Phys Ther.* 1988;68:977–982.
11. Bleck EE. *Orthopedic Management in Cerebral Palsy.* Philadelphia: JB Lippincott; 1987.
12. Donovan BM, Munson SH, Richtel A. Correlational analysis between goniometric values obtained from straight leg raise testing and a passive knee extension test for measurement of hamstring length. Unpublished Masters Thesis, Philadelphia College of Pharmacy & Science, February 1998.
13. Kendall FP, McCreary EK. Muscles: Testing and function. Baltimore: Williams & Wilkins; 1993.
14. Hinderer KA, Hinderer SR. Muscle strength development and assessment in children and adolescents. *Int Persp Phys Ther.* 1993;8:93–140.
15. Beasley WC. Quantitative muscle testing: Principles and applications to research and clinical services. *Arch Phys Med Rehabil.* 1961;42:398–425.
16. Bohannon RW. Manual muscle test scores and dynamometer test scores of knee extension strength. *Arch Phys Med Rehabil.* 1986;67:390–392.
17. Effgen SK, Brown DA. Long-term stability of hand-held dynamometric measurements in children who have myelomeningocele. *Phys Ther.* 1992;72:458–465.
18. Hinderer K, Gutierrez T. Myometry measurements of children using isometric and eccentric methods of muscle testing (Abstract). *Phys Ther.* 1988;68:817.

19. Stuberg WA, Koehler A, Wichita M, et al. Comparison of femoral torsion assessment using goniometry and computerized tomography. *Pediatr Phys.* 1989;1:115–118.
20. Staheli LT, Corbett M, Wyss C, et al. Lower-extremity rotational problems in children. *J Bone Joint Surg.* 1985;67A:39–47.
21. Cusick BD, Stuberg WA. Assessment of lower-extremity alignment in the transverse plane: Implications for management of children with neuromotor dysfunction. *Phys Ther.* 1992;72:3–15.
22. Tachdjian MO. *Pediatric Orthopedics,* 2nd Ed. Philadelphia: WB Saunders Co.; 1990.
23. National Institutes of Health. *Research plan for the national center for medical rehabilitation research.* Publication 93-3509. Bethesda, MD: National Institutes of Health, 1993.
24. Palisano RJ, Campbell SK, Harris SR. Clinical decision-making in pediatric physical therapy. In Campbell SK (Ed): *Pediatric Physical Therapy.* Philadelphia: W.B. Saunders, 1994, pp. 183–204.
25. Spranger J, Benirschke JG, Hall W, et al. Errors of morphogenesis: Concepts and terms. *J Pediatr.* 1982;100:160–165.
26. Day HJB. The ISO/ISPO classification of congenital limb deficiency. *Prosth Orthot Int.* 1991;15: 67–69.
27. Wright PE, Jobe MT. Congenital anomalies of the hand. In Canlae ST, Beaty JH (Eds): Operative Pediatric Orthopedics. Philadelphia: Mosby–Year Book; 1991, pp. 253–330.
28. Swanson AB, Barsky AJ, Entin MA. Classification of limb malformations on the basis of embryological failures. *Surg Clin North Am.* 1968;48: 1169–1179.
29. Heikel HVA. Aplasia and hypoplasia of the radius. *Acta Orthop Scand (Suppl).* 1959;39:1.
30. Aitken GT. Proximal femoral focal deficiency: Definition, classification and management. In *Proximal Femoral Focal Deficiency: A Congenital Anomaly.* 1969; Washington DC: National Academy of Sciences, pp. 1–22.
31. Epps CH. Current concepts review proximal femoral focal deficiency. *J Bone Joint Surg (Am).* 1983;65:867–870.
32. Shurr DG, Cook TM. *Prosthetics and Orthotics.* East Norwalk, CT: Appleton & Lange, 1990; pp. 183–193.
33. Bayne LG, Klug MS. Long-term review of the surgical treatment of radial deficiencies. *J Hand Surg (Am).* 1987;12:169–179.
34. Herzenberg JE. Congenital limb deficiency and limb length discrepancy. In Canale ST, Beaty JH (Eds): *Operative Pediatric Orthopedics.* Philadelphia: Mosby–Year Book; 1991, pp. 187–252.
35. Kruger LM. Lower-limb deficiencies: Surgical management. In Bowker JH, Michael JW (Eds): *Atlas of Limb Prosthetics: Surgical, Prosthetic, and Rehabilitation Principles.* Philadelphia: Mosby–Year Book; 1981, pp. 795–834.
36. Gillespie R. Principles of amputation surgery in children with longitudinal limb deficiencies of the femur. *Clin Orthop Rel Res.* 1990;256:29–38.
37. DeVito D. *Lengthening and Shortening Solutions of Lower Extremity Deficiencies.* Presentation and handout at APTA Combined Sections Meeting, 1996.
38. Gover AM, McIvor J. Upper limb deficiencies in infants and young children. *Infants Young Child.* 1992;5:58–72.
39. Setoguchi Y, Rosenfelder R. *The Limb-Deficient Child.* Springfield, IL: Charles C Thomas; 1982.
40. Coventry MD, Harris LE. Congenital muscular torticollis of infancy. *J Bone Joint Surg (Am).* 1959;41:815–822.
41. Suzuki S, Yamamura T, Fujita A. Aetiological relationship between congenital torticollis and obstetrical paralysis. *Int Orthop.* 1984;8:175–181.
42. Binder H, Eng GD, Gaiser JF, et al. Congenital muscular torticollis: Results of conservative management with long-term follow-up in 85 cases. *Arch Phys Med Rehabil.* 1987;68:222–225.
43. Morrison DL, MacEwen GD. Congenital muscular torticollis: Observations regarding clinical findings, associated conditions and results of treatment. *J Pediatr Orthop.* 1982;2:500–505.
44. Emery C. The determinants of treatment duration for congenital muscular torticollis. *Phys Ther.* 1994; 74:921–929.
45. Tom LWC, Rossiter JL, Sutton LN, et al. Torticollis in children. *Otolarynogol-Head Neck Surg.* 1991; 105:1–5.
46. Emery C. Conservative management of congenital muscular torticollis: A literature review. *Phys Occup Ther Pediatr.* 1997;17:13–20.
47. Canale ST, Griffin DW, Hubbard CN. Congenital muscular torticollis: A long-term follow-up. *J Bone Joint Surg (Am).* 1982;64:810–816.
48. Bredenkamp JK, Hoover LA, Berke GS, et al. Congenital muscular torticollis. *Arch Otolaryngol, Head Neck Surg.* 1990;116:212–216.
49. Hensinger RN, Jones ET. Developmental orthopedics: the lower limb. *Dev Med Child Neurol.* 1982; 24:95–116.
50. Dunn PM. Congenital postural deformities. *Br Med Bull.* 1976;32:71–76.
51. Bleck EE. Metatarsus adductus: Classification and relationship to outcomes of treatment. *J Pediatr Orthop.* 1983;3:2–9.

52. Beaty JH. Congenital anomalies of the lower and upper extremities. In Canale ST, Beaty JH (Eds): *Operative Pediatric Orthopedics.* Philadelphia: Mosby–Year Book; 1991, pp. 73–186.
53. Staheli LT. *Fundamentals of Pediatric Orthopedics.* Philadelphia: Lippincott-Raven; 1992.
54. Irani RN, Sherman MS. The pathological anatomy of idiopathic clubfoot. *Clin Orthop Rel Res.* 1972; 84:14–20.
55. Lovell WW, Hancock CI. Treatment of congenital talipes equinovarus. *Clin Orthop Rel Res.* 1970; 70:79.
56. Hensinger RN. Congenital dislocation of the hip, treatment in infancy to walking age. *Orthop Clin North Am.* 1987;18:597–616.
57. Mubarak MD, Garfin S, Vance R, et al. Pitfalls in the use of the Pavlik harness for treatment of congenital dysplasia, subluxation, and dislocation of the hip. *J Bone Joint Surg (Am).* 1981;63:1239–1247.
58. Leach J. Orthopedic Conditions. In Campbell SK (Ed): *Physical Therapy for Children.* Philadelphia: WB Saunders Co.; 1994, pp. 353–382.
59. Goodman RM, Gorlin RJ. Arthrogryposis. In Goodman RM, Gorlin RJ (Eds): *The Malformed Infant and Child.* New York: Oxford University Press; 1983, pp. 42–44.
60. Thompson GH, Bilenker RM. Comprehensive management of arthrogryposis multiplex congenita. *Clin Orthop Rel Res.* 1985;194:6–14.
61. Banker BQ. Neuropathic aspects of arthrogryposis multiplex congenita. *Clin Orthop Rel Res.* 1985; 194:30–43.
62. Williams P. The management of arthrogryposis. *Orthop Clin North Am.* 1978;9:67–88.
63. Staheli LT. Torsional deformity. *Pediatr Clin North Am.* 1977;24:799–811.
64. Knittel G, Staheli LT. The effectiveness of shoe modifications for intoeing. *Orthop Clin North Am.* 1976;7:1019–1024.
65. Marini JC. Osteogenesis imperfecta: Comprehensive management. *Adv Pediatr.* 1988;35:391–426.
66. Binder H, Hawks L, Graybill G, et al. Osteogenesis imperfecta: Rehabilitation approach with infants and young children. *Adv Pediatr.* 1984;65:537–541.
67. Binder H, Conway A, Gerber LH. Rehabilitation approaches to children with osteogenesis imperfecta: A ten-year experience. *Arch Phys Med Rehabil.* 1993;74:386–390.
68. Sillence D. Osteogenesis imperfecta: An expanding panorama of variants. *Clin Orthop Rel Res.* 1981; 159:11–25.
69. Riggs BL. Treatment of osteoporosis with sodium flouride: An appraisal. *Bone Min Res.* 1983;2: 366–370.
70. Gerber LH, Binder H, Weintrob J, et al. Rehabilitation of children and infants with osteogenesis imperfecta. *Clinical Orthop Rel Res.* 1990;251: 254–262.
71. Bleck EE. Nonoperative treatment of osteogenesis imperfecta: Orthotic and mobility management. *Clin Orthop Rel Res.* 1981;159:111–122.
72. Canale ST. Fractures and dislocations. In Canale ST, Beaty JH (Eds): *Operative Pediatric Orthopedics.* Philadelphia: Mosby–Year Book; 1991, pp. 837–1032.
73. Tooms RE. The amputee. In Lovell WW, Winter RB (Eds): *Pediatric Orthopedics,* 2nd Ed. Philadelphia: JB Lippincott; 1985, pp. 999–1053.
74. Kruger, LM. Recent advances in surgery of lower limb deficiencies. *Clin Orthop Rel Res.* 1980;148: 97–105.
75. Canale TS. Osteochondroses. In Canale TS, Beaty JH (Eds): *Operative Pediatric Orthopedics.* Philadelphia: Mosby–Year Book; 1991, pp. 743–775.
76. Thompson GH, Salter RB. Legg-Calvé-Perthes disease: Current concepts and controversies. *Orthop Clin North Am.* 1987;18:617–634.
77. Wenger DR, Ward WT, Herring JA. Current concepts review: Legg-Calvé-Perthes disease. *J Bone Joint Surg (Am).* 1991;73:778–788.
78. Catterall A. The natural history of Perthes disease. *J Bone Joint Surg (Br).* 1971;53:37–53.
79. Herring JA. Current concepts review: The treatment of Legg-Calvé-Perthes disease. *J Bone Joint Surg (Am).* 1994;76:448–458.
80. Aaronson DD, Loder RT. Treatment of the unstable (acute) slipped capital femoral epiphysis. *Clin Orthop Rel Res.* 1996;322:99–110.
81. Loder RT. The demographics of slipped capital femoral epiphysis: An international multicenter study. *Clin Orthop Rel Res.* 1996;322:8–27.
82. Ordenberg G, Hansson IL, Sandstrom S. Slipped capital femoral epiphysis in southern Sweden: Long-term result with closed reduction and hip plaster spica. *Clin Orthop Rel Res.* 1987;220: 148–154.
83. Thompson GH, Carter JR. Late-onset tibia vara (Blount's disease). *Clin Orthop Rel Res.* 1990;255: 24–35.
84. Schoenecker PL, Meade WC, Pierron RL, et al. Blount's disease: A retrospective review and recommendations for treatment. *J Pediatr Orthop.* 1985; 5:181–186.
85. Carter JR, Leeson MC, Thompson GH, et al. Late-onset tibia vara: A histopathologic analysis, a comparative evaluation with infantile tibia vara and slipped capital femoral epiphysis. *J Pediatr Orthop.* 1988;8:187.
86. Johnston CE. Infantile tibia vara. *Clin Orthop Rel Res.* 1990;255:13–23.

87. Langenskiöld A. Tibia vara: Osteochondrosis deformans tibiae: A survey of 23 cases. *Acta Chir Scand.* 1952;103:1–8.
88. Rogala EJ, Drummond DS, Gurr J. Scoliosis: Incidence and natural history, a prospective epidemiological study. *J Bone Joint Surg (Am).* 1978;60:173–177.
89. Lonstein JE. Natural history and school screening for scoliosis. *Orthop Clin North Am.* 1988;19:227–237.
90. Cassella MC, Hall JE. Current treatment approaches in the nonoperative and operative management of adolescent idiopathic scoliosis. *Phys Ther.* 1991;71:897–909.
91. Hall JE. Nonoperative and operative management of adolescent idiopathic scoliosis. Presented at APTA Combined Sections Meeting, February 1998.
92. Sullivan JA, Davidson R, Renshaw TS. Further evaluation of the scolitron treatment of idiopathic adolescent scoliosis. *Spine.* 1986;11:903–906.

Juvenile Rheumatoid Arthritis

Susan E. Klepper and Shirley A. Scull

Rheumatic diseases are characterized by inflammation of connective tissue. Between 160,000 and 290,000 children in the United States are reported to have some type of rheumatic disease.[1] Juvenile rheumatoid arthritis (JRA) is the most common rheumatic disease of childhood, and a significant cause of disability. Prevalence data for JRA are inconsistent because of wide variations in data collection methods.[2] A study by the Mayo Clinic reported a prevalence of 113.4 per 100,000 in the general population of children at risk in Rochester, MN.[3] A recent survey found that children with JRA accounted for 28% of patients seen in pediatric rheumatology clinics in the United States over a 3-year period.[4] Age at onset and gender distribution vary in the different types of JRA, although there is a predominance of females in most types.[5] Several studies suggest the majority of children with JRA are Caucasian, with less frequent occurrence among children of African-American, Chinese-American, and Native-American ancestry.[6]

Other rheumatic diseases seen in children include psoriatic arthritis, juvenile ankylosing spondylitis, scleroderma, systemic lupus erythematosus, and dermatomyositis. In recent years, clinics have seen an increase in the number of children with Lyme disease, and regional or diffuse musculoskeletal pain syndromes.

Criteria for Diagnosis and Classification of JRA

Display 12-1 shows the two sets of criteria currently used for the diagnosis and classification of conditions causing chronic arthritis in children: the American College of Rheumatology (ACR) criteria for JRA,[7] used primarily in North America, and the criteria proposed by the European League Against Rheumatism (EULAR) to define and classify juvenile chronic arthritis (JCA).[8] Investigators continue to study these classification systems to develop more sensitive and specific criteria that reflect the heterogeneity of these conditions.[9–11]

The ACR criteria define JRA as persistent arthritis in one or more joints, lasting 6 weeks or longer, in a child younger than 16 years of age, when all other causes of childhood arthritis have been excluded. There is currently no definitive test for JRA, although laboratory tests and radiographs may support a preliminary diagnosis. The erythrocyte sedimentation rate (ESR) is often elevated and may be useful in guiding treatment. Radiographs early in the disease are not usually diagnostic but serve as a

DISPLAY 12-1

Criteria for Diagnosis and Classification of Childhood Arthritis

ACR* Criteria for Juvenile Rheumatoid Arthritis (JRA)

1. Onset <16
2. Arthritis of at least 6 weeks
3. Onset subtype defined by manifestations during the first 6 months:
   Pauciarticular: arthritis affecting ≤4 joints
   Polyarticular: arthritis affecting ≥5 joints
   Systemic: JRA with intermittent fever, with or without rheumatoid rash
4. Exclusion of other conditions listed, including other rheumatic diseases, infectious arthritis, inflammatory bowel disease, and nonrheumatic conditions of bones and joints

EULAR+ Criteria for Juvenile Chronic Arthritis (JCA)

1. Onset <16 years
2. Arthritis for at least 3 months
3. Subgroups:
   Juvenile ankylosing spondylitis
   Seropositive juvenile rheumatoid arthritis
   Seronegative chronic arthritis—defined by onset into:
      Systemic—requires intermittent fever
      Pauciarticular—arthritis in four of fewer joints during the first 3 months
      Polyarticular—arthritis in five or more joints during the first 3 months
   Psoriatic arthritis
   Arthropathy associated with inflammatory bowel disease

*ACR, American College of Rheumatology; +EULAR, European League Against Arthritis.

baseline measure of joint and bone integrity. Early confirmation of the diagnosis is vital to rule out other illnesses and to initiate adequate treatment before joint damage occurs.

Table 12-1 lists the criteria for classification of the three major onset subtypes of JRA, and variations within the subtypes based on the presence or absence of the rheumatoid factor (RF) and antinuclear antibody (ANA), clinical course, and outcome. *Systemic onset disease* occurs in about 10% of children with JRA.[5] Onset can occur at any age, and there is an equal male to female ratio. The disease is marked by high spiking fevers of 39°C once or twice a day, with normal or subnormal temperatures between spikes. The fever is often accompanied by arthralgia and myalgia, and a migratory, salmon colored rash on the trunk or limbs.

Laboratory findings include negative tests for both the RF and ANA. In about one-third of these children, arthritis may be absent early, but severe polyarthritis may develop several weeks or months after the systemic symptoms.[5,10] Visceral signs include pleuritis, pericarditis, hepatosplenomegaly, lymphadenopathy, and myocarditis. Systemic symptoms may subside after several months to a few years, although some children experience recurring episodes or persistent systemic disease.[5] About 25% demonstrate severe systemic disease and unremitting arthritis.[5]

Polyarticular disease occurs in approximately 40% of children with JRA, and affects mostly girls.[13] These children present with arthritis in five or more joints during the first 6 months. Onset is usually insidious, with a progressive increase in joint involvement. Arthritis is symmetric, involving both large and small joints. The temporomandibular joints and cervical spine are often involved. Systemic symptoms, if present, are usually milder and less persistent than in systemic onset JRA.

Two subgroups of polyarticular JRA have been identified, based on the presence or absence of the RF. The majority of children with RF+ polyarticular JRA are female, with onset after the age of 8 years.[10] About half of these children develop rapid, severe arthritis resembling adult rheumatoid arthritis (RA), with joint erosions seen as early as 6 months after onset.[10] Listlessness, fever, and anorexia are common symptoms. Subcutaneous nodules may be found at the elbow, tibial crest, or fingers.[5] A +ANA test is found in 50% to 70%.[13]

Onset of RF– polyarticular JRA can occur at any time before the age of 16 years. About half of this group is younger than 6 years of age at onset, with another peak seen in the preadolescent age group.[10] Arthritis is symmetric, involving both large and small joints, with a tendency for ankylosis of the carpal and tarsal joints. Joint contractures, juxta-articular osteoporosis, muscle atrophy, weakness, and local and generalized growth disturbances are common. Nodules are rarely seen. Severe, persistent arthritis occurs in about 25%. There is a fairly high incidence of a +ANA, and about 10% develop chronic uveitis.[10]

Pauciarticular onset disease occurs in approximately 50 to 55% of children with JRA, and affects fewer than five joints.[5,13] When only one joint is involved, the physician must be careful to rule out infection or trauma as the cause.[5] Three subgroups have been identified, divided by age, gender, and clinical presentation. One group includes predominantly females, with onset before 6 years of age. Joint involvement is usually asymmetric, and arthritis may present initially in one knee, elbow, wrist, or ankle, but rarely the hip. These children generally have a good clinical outcome, but 15% to 20% experience unremitting disease and subsequent polyarthritis. The inflammation leads frequently to accelerated growth in the affected limb and eventual leg length discrepancy. Most are RF–, but 50% test positive for the ANA. Ocular damage may result from chronic uveitis or iridocyclitis, and 10% may actually lose their sight.[5,13] Frequent eye exams are recommended for children at risk. Topical corticosteroids are used to control the inflammation.

TABLE 12-1
Subtypes of JRA

		Polyarticular Onset (25–40%)		Pauciarticular Onset (50%–55%)		
Variable	**Systemic Onset**	**RF-**	**RF+**	**Type I**	**Type II**	**Type III**
Frequency	10–20%					
Number of joints	Variable	>5	>5	<5 Knee, ankle, elbow rarely hip	<5 Lower limb subsequent sacroillitis	<5 Large and small joints
Onset age (years)	Any age <16	<16	>8	<6	>10	<16
Sex predominance	Equal	Girls	Girls	Girls	Boys	Girls
Systemic manifestations	Prominent	Growth abnormalities	Nodules vasculitis			
Laboratory	(–) RF, (–) ANA	25% (+) ANA	50%–70% (+) ANA	50% (+) ANA	(–) ANA 60% (+) HLA-B27	17–50% (=) ANA 40% (+) HLA-B27
Occurrence of uveitis	Rare		5%	Chronic uveitis, iritis 10% blindness	10–20% have acute iritis	10–20% have chronic iritis
Prognosis	25% have severe disease	25% have severe disease	50% have severe disease	15–20% have subsequent polyarthritis	40% have subsequent JAS	Subsequent psoriasis

A second group of children with pauciarticular JRA includes mostly boys with disease onset in late childhood, usually 10 years of age or older. Laboratory findings show a +HLA–B27, and –ANA. These boys often experience arthritis in the hip, and sacroiliac joints, and 40% are eventually diagnosed with juvenile ankylosing spondylitis (JAS).[13] The third subgroup includes mostly females, with disease onset anytime before age 16 years. Both large and small joints may be involved. Laboratory findings include a +ANA (17% to 50%), and a +HLA–B27 (40%). Chronic iritis occurs in 10% to 20%, and many experience subsequent psoriasis.[5,13]

Etiology and Pathogenesis

The cause of JRA is unknown, although there is evidence of an immunoinflammatory pathogenesis, activated by contact with an external agent, such as trauma or systemic infection, in a child with a specific genetic predisposition.[5,14] The group of conditions now called JRA may actually be several separate diseases, linked by the presence of arthritis. Alternately, a single pathogenic vector may manifest itself differently, based on the specific reaction of each host.[10,15]

There is usually no family history of rheumatoid arthritis, and multiple cases of JRA within the same family are rare.[14] However, recent immunologic studies provide strong support for the role of genetics as a predisposing factor in JRA. For example, children with JAS often have the human leukocyte antigen HLA–B27. Specific genetic markers have also been found in children with pauciarticular and polyarticular onset JRA.[5]

Although the term JRA implies the disease is similar to adult RA, there are distinct differences.[5] Unlike adults, most children with JRA have a negative test for the RF, and many do not experience the serious systemic manifestations commonly found in adults with RA. However, a small group (10%) of children with JRA are older at disease onset, are RF+ and experience aggressive disease.[16]

Prognosis

Most children with JRA are able to lead independent and productive lives with proper and timely medical and therapeutic management. The greater thickness and potential for growth and repair of articular cartilage in children may provide some protection against joint erosions.[17] However, persistent synovitis increases the risk for joint damage and deformity.[17] A review of several long-term outcome studies indicated that 10 years after disease onset, 31% to 55% of children with all types of JRA had persistent synovitis, 55% to 59% had radiographic evidence of joint erosions,[18,19] and between one-third and one-half entered adulthood with active arthritis.[17] Ten years after disease onset, synovitis persists in 22% to 71% of children with pauciarticular JRA, 40% to 50% of those with polyarticular disease, and 25% to 58% of those with systemic disease.[17] Children with pauciarticular JRA appear to have the best prognosis for joint function and mobility.

Musculoskeletal problems, including contractures, joint deformities, postural deviations, and growth abnormalities, may persist long after disease remission, and may contribute to significant pain and disability. Joint erosions, malalignment, and instability also increase the child's risk for further injury and joint degeneration. Joint replacement surgery may be necessary during adolescence when skeletal maturity is nearing completion.

Pathology

The inflammatory process affects the tissues within and surrounding synovial joints. Changes include villous hypertrophy, hyperplasia of the vascular endothelium, and increased production of synovial fluid with swelling and distention of the joint capsule. Synovial cells multiply, forming a massive overgrowth called a pannus, which spreads over the articular cartilage, causing it to soften and weaken. Degradative enzymes are released from the cartilage matrix into the synovial fluid. These enzymes further disrupt the normal cartilage fiber network.[20] Intra-articular adhesions and osteophytes occur later. Fibrosis of periarticular tendons and ligaments results in joint contractures.

Articular surfaces become irregular, and joint congruency, alignment, and stability are compromised as erosions occur in articular cartilage and subchondral bone. Subluxation may occur at the wrist and small joints of the hands and feet. Posterior subluxation of the tibia on the femur may occur in the presence of longstanding knee flexion contractures. The problem is exacerbated by weak quadriceps and an immobile patella.[5]

Early radiographic changes include soft tissue swelling, widening of the joint space owing to effusions, juxta-articular osteopenia, and periosteal new bone, especially noted in the phalanges, metacarpals, and metatarsals.[5] With persistent disease, radiographs often show joint space narrowing, marginal erosions, and osteophytes owing to thinning and loss of articular cartilage. In advanced disease, fibrous or bony ankylosis may be seen in the carpal or tarsal joints or in the cervical spine.[21] Instability of C1 on C2 may occur in some children, although this is found less often in children with JRA than in adults with RA.[21]

Muscles surrounding joints may atrophy as a result of reflex inhibition and disuse. Inflammatory and morphologic changes in muscle tissue, and atrophy of type II muscle fibers, with loss of muscle strength, have been documented in adults with RA.[22] Although this has not been confirmed in children with JRA,[23] there is evidence of protein-energy malnutrition, resulting in a reduction of lean body mass.[24] Additionally, systemic use of glucocorticoids results in muscle atrophy.[25] Soft tissue shortens when the joints are held in flexed positions to accommodate effusions and reduce pain. The result is a loss of joint stability and compliance during loading under motion, increasing the risk for degenerative changes.

Abnormalities in skeletal maturation, with both local and generalized growth disturbances, are common in children with JRA. Increased blood flow to the joint during active disease leads to bony overgrowth, seen most often in the humeral head and radial head of the upper extremities, and the femoral head, medial femoral condyle, and proximal tibia in the lower extremities. Protrusion of the femoral head into the acetabulum may occur in older children with persistent disease.[5] Active disease may also result in premature epiphyseal closure in the bones of the hands and feet.

Juxta-articular osteopenia observed early in the JRA may result from the inflammatory process in rheumatoid synovium. The more generalized demineralization seen later appears to be related to continued disease activity, and is associated with an increased risk of fracture in the vertebrae and long bones.[26] Possible nutritional deficiencies, low body weight, and decreased physical activity may contribute to low bone density.[27] These problems are exaggerated by long-term use of systemic corticosteroids.[28]

Goals of Management

The *goals of management in JRA* are to (1) quickly control the joint inflammation, using the safest and most effective drug therapy; (2) preserve joint integrity, mobility, and function; (3) promote independence in necessary and desired activities; and (4) provide education and support so the child and family can lead normal, healthy lives. This complex agenda requires a multidisciplinary team of health professionals, including a pediatric rheumatologist, nurse, nutritionist, social worker, and physical and occupational therapists, with periodic consultation and intervention by ophthalmologists, orthotists, and orthopedic surgeons. Routine care between rheumatology clinic visits is carried out by the child and family, family physician, school nurse, and community therapists.

Guidelines for physical therapy practice for children with arthritis are available from the Children's Arthritis Centers of New England.[29] The role of the therapist varies depending on the setting. In the rheumatology clinic, the therapist participates in evaluating the child and developing a therapy plan, educates the child and family about the effects of arthritis on the musculoskeletal system and the benefits of exercise, and serves as a liaison to the school and community therapists. Daily therapy may be provided in an acute care setting during an exacerbation or following surgery. More often, therapy is provided on a limited basis in an outpatient clinic, the child's school, or home. Physical and occupational therapists often serve as consultants, designing and teaching home treatment programs to the child and family, making splints, or ordering adaptive equipment.

Pharmacologic Management

There is currently no cure for JRA, but a variety of drugs are used to suppress the chronic synovitis, relieve pain and stiffness, and control dangerous systemic complications (Table 12-2). A wide range of *non-steroidal anti-inflammatory drugs (NSAIDs)* are the first agents used to control the child's arthritis.[30] These medications are considered safe and effective in most patients, although the use of aspirin has declined because of concerns about its association with Reye's syndrome during influenza or varicella infection.[30] The analgesic effects of NSAIDS are rapid, and may lessen pain and stiffness, allowing a child to exercise. Anti-inflammatory effects are achieved within 1 to 3 months in children who respond favorably to NSAID therapy.[30]

Approximately two-thirds of children with JRA do not respond to an NSAID along,[30] and the addition of a second-line drug may be considered. These slow-acting anti-rheumatic drugs (SAARDs) are more toxic than NSAIDs and take longer to produce beneficial effects. However, many rheumatologists now believe earlier aggressive treatment is necessary to prevent the irreversible damage to cartilage, joint surface, and periarticular tissues caused by uncontrolled inflammation.[31] Methotrexate, a folic acid analogue, has been shown to be an effective anti-inflammatory agent relatively early after institution and is currently the second-line drug of choice in many clinics.[30,32] Methotrexate appears to be relatively safe for several years of treatment.[33]

Glucocorticosteroids are effective anti-inflammatory drugs, but the adverse effects of oral steroids are numerous, including general growth retardation, osteoporosis, hypertension, and Cushing's syndrome. Oral steroids are usually reserved for treating severe unremitting arthritis or life-threatening systemic complications.[30] Corticosteroid drops are prescribed for iritis. Intra-articular steroid injections are used to treat severe inflammation in large joints. Recent studies show prolonged remission of active disease for periods up to 12 months in injected knee joints.[34]

Studies of drug efficacy in JRA have led to a decrease in the use of oral gold, injectable gold salts, D-penicillamine, and hydroxychloroquine in many clinics.[30] The future of drug therapy for children with arthritis may include using current drugs in new combinations, new drugs directed at modifying the immune responses producing inflammation, and gene therapy.[30]

The therapist must be aware of the child's medication regimen because therapy may be enhanced by appropriate timing within the medication program. Because joints are more vulnerable to damage during active inflammation,

TABLE 12-2
Drug Therapy for JRA

Medication	Dose	Indication	Toxicity
Aspirin	75–90 mg/kg/d	Control of pain, stiffness, and inflammation	Salicylism (lethargy, hyperpnea, tinnitus), gastrointestinal irritation, bleeding, hepatitis
Nonsteroidal anti-inflammatory agents	Varies with drug	Control of pain, stiffness, and inflammation	Gastrointestinal irritation, hepatitis, decreased renal function
Hydroxychloroquine	7 mg/kg/d	Selective use for arthritis	Dermatitis, keratopathy, retinopathy
Gold salt	0.75 mg/kg/mo	Polyarthritis unresponsive to nonsteroidal anti-inflammatory agents	Dermatitis, nephritis, stomatitis, bone marrow suppression
D-Penicillamine	10 mg/kg/d	Polyarthritis unresponsive to other regimens	Dermatitis, nephritis, lupus-like syndrome
Sulftasalazine	40–60 mg/kg/d	Polyarthritis unresponsive to other regimens	Bone marrow suppression dermatitis, gastrointestinal irritation
Corticosteriod drugs			
systemic	Prednisone, 1mg/kg/d (as low a dose as possible)	Life-threatening systemic disease, chronic uveitis	Growth retardation infection, Cushing's syndrome
Ophthalmic	4 drops/d	Chronic uveitis	Cataracts, glaucoma
intra-articular	30 mg prednisolone—TBA	Selective use for arthritis	Infection
Immunosuppressive	Varies with drug	Life-threatening systemic disease	Infection, bone marrow suppression, sterility

From Cassidy JT, Petty RE. *Textbook of Rheumatology*. 2nd ed. New York: Churchill Livingstone; 1990, with permission.

aggressive therapy should be avoided when the child is acutely ill or when arthritis is not well controlled. A child beginning NSAID therapy or taking less than a therapeutic dose may experience pain relief, even though active synovitis persists. Therapy should be guided by objective signs of arthritis, such as joint effusion and tenderness, as well as pain.

Physical Therapy Assessment

Many of the same outcome measures are used in both adult and childhood arthritis. These include the active joint count (JC), range of motion (ROM), muscle strength, and timed walk. Other measures have been developed to reflect the specific needs of children with arthritis, and focus on the child's ability to perform necessary and preferred activities within the home, school, and community. These instruments are self-report in nature, and assess physical or psychosocial function, pain, and overall status.

This section will address the components of *physical therapy assessment* of the child with JRA (Display 12-2). The musculoskeletal impairments, secondary conditions resulting from these impairments, motor skills, and functional status of the child are assessed. This information provides the basis for setting appropriate treatment goals and developing a management plan. A thorough assessment may require several

DISPLAY 12-2

Components of the Physical Therapy Assessment in JRA

- Observation
- History
- Musculoskeletal assessment
  - Active joint count
  - Range of motion
  - Muscle strength
  - Muscle endurance
- Aerobic endurance
- Postural assessment
- Gait assessment
- Pain assessment
- Functional assessment

clinic visits. The time demands and stress on the family may be reduced when physical and occupational therapists combine their assessments.

Observation and History

The assessment begins with *observation* of the patient's movements to detect gross abnormalities, such as muscle atrophy, joint swelling or malalignment or postural deviations. Observing the child perform tasks, such as walking, picking up toys from the floor, or climbing steps, provides initial information about the child's mobility and gait pattern.

A *history* is taken from the parent, although an older child or adolescent can provide information. Asking the parent or child to describe a typical day provides information about disease symptoms and their effect on the child's function. Questions focus on the duration of morning stiffness, pain or fatigue during the day, current use of splints or adaptive equipment, and ability to perform daily activities at home and school. The therapist may also learn about coping strategies used by the child and family, including current therapy, the effects of any home remedies tried, and the time and resources available for the family to carry out a home treatment program. One of the functional assessment tests discussed in a later section can be administered at this time.

Active Joint Count

The extent of disease activity is assessed by the active joint count. Active inflammation is defined as the presence of any one of the following signs: joint effusion, tenderness, or stress pain. Limited joint motion alone, although a result of the arthritis, does not indicate active disease in the absence of these other signs of inflammation. The wrist and ankle are each considered individual joints. The hips and neck are not included in this scheme, owing to the difficulty of evaluating inflammation in these areas.[35] The active joints are recorded on a visual format, such as a stick figure, showing all major joints (Fig. 12-1).

Joint effusion is verified by demonstrating fluctuation of synovial fluid from one area of the joint to another. Figure 12-2, (right) illustrates one method, using two fingers, one pressing downward, and the other sensing the upward movement of fluid or bulge. In the knee joint, a bulge sign will detect a small effusion. The synovial pouch medial to the patella is emptied by stroking upward, and refilled by stroking upward or downward on the lateral side. Figure 12-2 (left) illustrates the four-finger method, used in the joints of the fingers or toes. Because the collateral ligaments prevent bulging of synovial fluid, the sensor fingers should be placed dorsal to these ligaments and proximal to the base of the middle phalanx.[35] The joint is scored as normal if there is not a clear indication of effusion.

Articular tenderness is assessed by applying firm pressure directly over the joint line. In an active joint, tenderness felt by pressure over the joint line should be greater than that elicited by pressure on the bone adjacent to the joint.[35] *Stress pain* is assessed by moving the limb to the end of the available range and applying pressure to move the limb a little further. Pain during

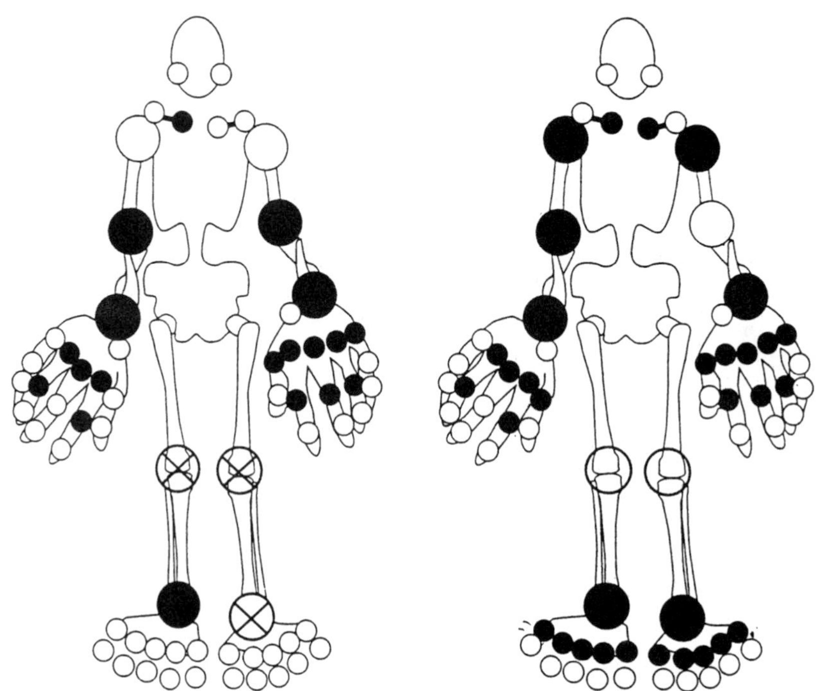

Figure 12-1 ■ Example of the visual format used to record active joint count in a child with polyarticular disease. The left figure shows joints with an effusion (solid circle) or soft tissue swelling (X). The right figure shows joints with stress pain or tenderness (solid circle). (From Wright V, Smith E. Physical therapy management of the child and adolescent with arthritis. In Walker J, Helewa A, eds. *Physical Therapy in Arthritis.* Philadelphia: W.B. Saunders; 1996: 211–244, with permission.)

the arc of motion is usually owing to friction of bone rubbing bone as a result of cartilage damage, and does not necessarily indicate active inflammation. The pressure applied should be about 20% less than that required to elicit tenderness by squeezing the triceps or lower calf muscles.[35]

Range of Motion

A screening examination, asking the child to perform a series of movements to elicit full range of motion, can help to identify gross limitations. A game of "Simon Says" may be useful in young children to gain their cooperation with the examination. Standard goniometric technique is used to document *passive range of motion* (PROM). The child should be completely relaxed to reduce any restrictions owing to action of antigravity muscles. The therapist should be aware that in some children with JRA, who exhibit ligamental laxity and joint hypermobility, a mild contracture may not be obvious. The therapist should make bilateral comparisons when measuring PROM and check for general signs of hypermobility.[36] Joint motion is recorded in degrees, using the anatomic position as the starting point. Using consistent methods of measuring and recording ROM pre-

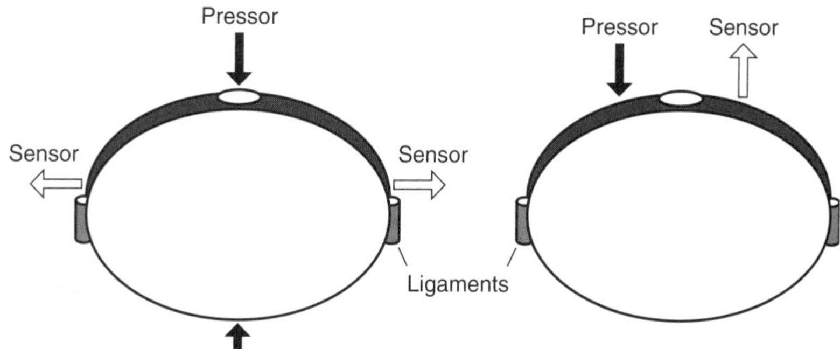

Figure 12-2 ▪ Two ways of detecting joint effusions. (From Smythe H, Helewa A. Assessment of joint disease. In Walker J, Helewa A, eds. *Physical Therapy in Arthritis.* Philadelphia: W.B. Saunders; 1996: 129–148, with permission from H. Smythe, M.D., FRC[C].)

vent confusion when consecutive measurements are done by more than one person.

Although each child responds differently to the disease, common patterns of joint restriction occur in children with JRA. Awareness of these patterns allows the therapist to anticipate potential problems and adjust the therapy plan accordingly. *Lower extremity restrictions* include loss of hip extension, abduction, and rotation, knee flexion contractures, loss of motion in the ankle and subtalor motion, and excessive forefoot pronation or supination. The Ober test is used to assess tightness of the iliotibial band, which contributes to valgus deformity at the knee. Foot deformities in arthritis include hallux valgus, hammertoes, overlapping toes, loss of extension at the metatarsal phalangeal joints, and subluxation of the metatarsal heads. In the child with polyarticular disease, restrictions often occur in glenohumeral abduction, flexion, and rotation, forearm supination, elbow and wrist extension, and finger flexion and extension.

The *cervical spine* is examined using active motion only. The therapist should stabilize the shoulder girdle whereas the child performs the six cardinal motions of the cervical spine. The first signs of cervical spine involvement are decreased extension and rotation. Later changes include loss of the normal cervical lordosis, and fusion of the apophyseal joints. In some children, instability and subluxation of C1 or C2 may occur.[5]

Involvement of the *lumbar spine* is unusual in JRA,[37] but spasm of the spinal extensor muscles or hip flexion contractures may limit mobility of the lumbar spine. The Schober test is used to measure lumbar flexion. Involvement of the *temporomandibular joints* may result in pain and difficulty chewing and opening the mouth. Undergrowth of the mandible may cause malocclusion. Jaw motion is assessed by having the child open the mouth and insert three fingers held vertically.

Loss of motion may be the first sign of joint damage. Joint play motions are examined for stiffness, as well as instability. Angular deformities, such as valgus or posterior subluxation at the knee, are noted. Bony crepitus, from loss of articular cartilage, may cause sudden pain often felt away from the joint line during motion.[35] A review of radiographs provides additional evidence of damage, such as joint space narrowing and erosions. Joint damage can be recorded on a stick figure diagram, similar to that used to record active disease.

Muscle Strength and Endurance

Several recent studies have documented deficits in muscular fitness in children with arthritis. Giannini and Protas, using an isokinetic dynamometer, found significantly lower peak isometric quadriceps strength in 30 children with JRA compared with controls.[38] Vostrejs et al. found differences of more than 10% in peak isometric torque, between the quadriceps, in children with monarticular JRA and knee involvement.[39] Children with polyarticular JRA also scored lower than controls on a timed sit-up test of abdominal muscle strength and endurance.[40] Finally, Oberg et al., using surface electromyography (EMG) in 10 children with JRA and controls, reported reduced EMG responses to fatigue in the patient group, which normalized after training.[23]

Traditionally, therapists have assessed *muscle strength in children with JRA* using break testing of isometric contractions, because many children are not able to tolerate resistance through the full range. Muscle strength is scored on a 0 to 5 scale on a manual muscle test (MMT). Good intra- and interrater reliability has been reported for MMT scores in boys with Duchenne's muscular dystrophy (DMD), when the examiners were highly skilled in evaluating muscle strength in this patient population and strict standards were followed for limb position and testing procedures.[41] However, the usefulness of MMT in adults with RA has been questioned because of the variability in grades above 3 (Fair) and the difficulty in standardizing limb position when contractures, pain, or deformities limit motion.[35] Instrumented measures of muscle strength, using handheld dynamometers, may provide more reliable and discrete data.[42] Smythe and Helewa suggest using the manometer method in patients with arthritis.[35] The rolled cuff is placed distally as far as possible on the limb, without crossing a painful joint. The tester applies pressure to the cuff with a flat hand. The patient pushes against the cuff, while the tester increases pressure gradually for 5 seconds. The highest pressure sustained by the patient is recorded (Fig. 12-3).[35] Reliability and sensitivity to change has not been demonstrated for any of these measures of strength in children with JRA. The method used is often determined by the individual therapist's experience and availability of equipment. Regardless of the method used, it is important that consistent procedures be followed and, reliability be established among testers within the clinic.

Dynamic muscle strength can be assessed in children with inactive disease and no pain on motion by measuring the child's repetition maximum (RM).[43] The RM refers to the maximal amount of weight the child can lift for a specified number of repetitions, maintaining proper form throughout the range. With greater resistance, fewer repetitions are possible, so that a 1-RM resistance is greater than a 6-RM resistance. For children, a measure of a 6 to

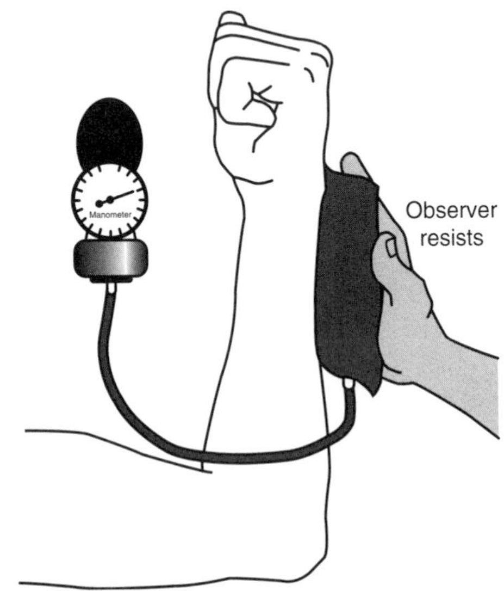

Figure 12-3 ▪ Use of modified blood pressure cuff to measure isometric triceps strength. (From Walker J, Helewa A, eds. *Physical Therapy in Arthritis.* Philadelphia: W.B. Saunders; 1996: 129–148, with permission from H. Smythe, M.D., FRC[C].)

10 RM is sufficient to establish baseline levels of strength, determine the amount of resistance to be used during exercise, and evaluate progress during the training program.[43] Dynamic muscle testing should not be done if a child is not able to tolerate resistance through the range or has any pain on joint motion. A safe alternative might be isometric testing at multiple angles, which can provide an estimation of the child's dynamic strength and reveal specific points of weakness within the ROM. Local muscular endurance can be assessed by having the child perform as many repetitions as possible at a specified percentage (60% to 80%) of the 6-RM resistance.

A warm-up period should precede all muscle testing. Strength and endurance testing should not be done during the same session, because fatigue may affect performance.[43] Muscles are usually tested in functional groups to identify patterns of atrophy and weakness. Special attention is paid to antigravity muscles, such as the hip extensors, abductors, knee extensors, and plantar flexors. The deltoids, elbow flexors and extensors, and wrist extensors are often weak. Grip and pinch strength measurements are used to assess hand strength. Bilateral girth measurements help to quantify asymmetry in muscle bulk. Functional strength in a child too young to cooperate in specific tests can be done by observing the child perform age-appropriate motor tasks.

Aerobic Endurance

Recent research indicates children with JRA often have reduced aerobic capacity (VO_2max) and poor endurance. Giannini and Protas reported significantly lower VO_2max, lower peak heart rate, and shorter exercise time in 30 children with JRA compared to healthy controls.[44] Klepper et al. reported children with polyarticular JRA scored significantly lower than matched controls on a 9-minute run-walk test of aerobic endurance.[40] Poor exercise tolerance and fatigue after moderate physical activity limit a child's ability to keep pace with peers and participate in age-appropriate activities.

Aerobic fitness should be assessed prior to the child's participation in an aerobic conditioning program. Laboratory assessment of VO_2max should be performed in any child with cardiac or respiratory complications. Assessment of submaximal oxygen consumption can provide an estimate of aerobic fitness in children without systemic symptoms. These tests compare the workload achieved and the heart rate response to exercise during a standardized protocol on a treadmill or cycle ergometer. Simple, inexpensive field tests, such as a walk-run test, measure either the time required to travel a specified distance, or the distance traveled over a specified time.[45] Results are compared to normative data or health standards, based on age and gender. Test results can be used to evaluate the effectiveness of the exercise program.

Postural Assessment

Postural alignment is assessed in sitting and standing. The child is observed from the front, back, and lateral positions. Common postural deviations in children with JRA include forward head, kyphosis, excessive lumbar lordosis, hip and knee flexion contractures, genu valgus, and various ankle and foot deformities. The child is examined for leg length discrepancies in both supine and standing, measuring from the anterior superior iliac spine to the medial malleolus. In the presence of a knee flexion contracture, the femur and tibia are measured individually to determine leg length. Pelvic obliquity and scoliosis may result from leg length differences. The standing–bend over test is a good screening tool for scoliosis, because asymmetry of the trunk is easily detected owing to vertebral rotation. Foot deformities, such as subtalor valgus or varus, and excessive forefoot pronation or supination may also contribute to postural deviations.

Gait Assessment

Gait deviations are often observed in children with JRA. Two studies, using computerized motion analysis, reported decreased gait velocity, cadence, step and stride length in children with JRA compared to controls or normative data.[46] These studies also found increased anterior pelvic tilt throughout the gait cycle, decreased hip extension at terminal stance, and decreased plantar flexion force at push-off in the patient groups. Gait deviations may result directly from weakness and decreased range of motion in the lower extremities. Shortened step length is possibly related to decreased hip extension and ankle plantar flexion at the end of stance.[46] Foot problems, including synovitis, loss of ankle and subtalor motion, excessive forefoot pronation or supination, hallux valgus, and a variety of other toe deformities, are common in children with JRA,[47] and probably contribute to many of the changes observed in foot pressures during stance and decreased push-off.

Gait assessment is often done by simple visual inspection, since laboratory gait analysis is expensive and not universally available. Ideally, the child should be observed walking with and without shoes, although some children may experience pain walking barefoot. The child's gait pattern should be observed for symmetry, step and stride length, as well as alignment of the lower limb at heelstrike, midstance, roll over, and swing. A timed walk can be used to determine gait velocity. The assessment should include walking on level surfaces, inclines, stairs, and curbs, and while running. Use of any assistive devices (cane, walker, orthotic devices, wheelchair) for mobility should be noted.

Footprint analysis, using pressure sensitive paper, is a relatively inexpensive alternative to computerized analysis and yields objective and reliable data on step length, width, foot angle, and velocity.[48] A combination of footprint analysis and videography provides a permanent record of the child's performance.

Pain Assessment

Early studies reported children with JRA experienced less pain than adults with RA.[49] However, these studies failed to consider the differences in the way children and adults conceptualize and report pain. Subsequent studies, using assessments more sensitive to the cognitive developmental stages of children, found that pain is often a prominent feature of JRA and a major factor in the child's adjustment to the disease.[50,51]

The *Pediatric Pain Questionnaire (PPQ)* is a comprehensive assessment, modeled on the McGill Pain Questionnaire for adults,[52] which addresses the sensory, affective, and qualitative nature of pain, and considers the developmental differences in perception of pain, with separate forms for the child, adolescent, and parent. The PPQ includes three instruments to assess the intensity, location, and quality of pain in children.[51] These are often used separately. A visual analogue scale (VAS) is used to measure present pain or worst pain intensity over the past week. With VAS, a 10-cm line is anchored at either end by a happy or sad face, and words are used to indicate no pain or severe pain. The VAS is a reliable and valid pain assessment in children as young as 5 years of age.[51] To assess the affective quality of pain, the child is supplied with a list of words and asked to circle all that apply to his or her pain. Wilkie et al. demonstrated good test-retest reliability of pain descriptors, as well as concurrent validity between pediatric pain descriptors from a supplied word list and pain intensity scores and number of pain sites.[53] Body outline figures and color-coded rating scales allow the child to indicate the location and relative intensity of pain (Fig. 12-4).[54]

Functional Assessment

Self-care and mobility in the home, school, and community are assessed. The child is observed while performing functional tasks for quality,

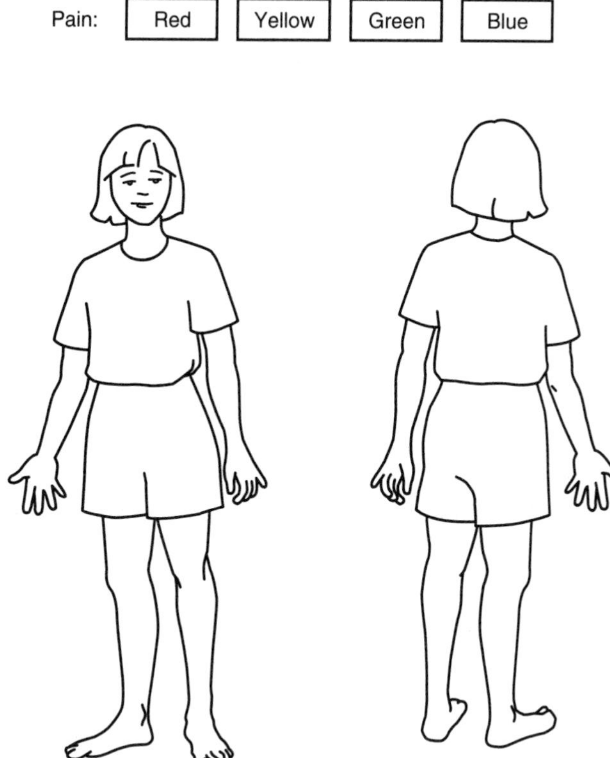

Figure 12-4 ▪ Example of a body outline figure and rating scale used to assess pain intensity and location in children.

speed, and proficiency. The therapist should assess current adaptive equipment, splints, or braces and explore the need for additional equipment. Motor skills and function in a young child can be assessed by using a standardized developmental test. The *Pediatric Evaluation of Disability Inventory (PEDI)* assesses the child's function in self-care, mobility, and social interaction, and can be completed by the parent or caregiver, based on their observation of the child's performance.[55]

Self-report functional assessments developed or adapted specifically for children with arthritis include the Juvenile Arthritis Assessment report for parents or children (JAFAR),[56] Child Health Assessment Questionnaire (CHAQ)[57] (see Display 12-3), the Juvenile Arthritis Functional Status Index (JASI),[58,59] and the Juvenile Arthritis Quality of Life Questionnaire (JAQQ).[60] These measures demonstrate acceptable test-retest reliability when the child is the respondent.[56,57,59] Validity and sensitivity to change are being evaluated. Table 12-3 lists functional assessments currently in use or under development for children with JRA.[60]

Summary of Evaluation

The therapist analyzes the child's current functional limitations, develops hypotheses regarding the relationship between these limitations and the musculoskeletal impairments and secondary conditions, and tries to anticipate the potential risk for future problems. Figure 12-5 illustrates one method of classifying the find-

DISPLAY 12-3

Health Assessment Questionaire*

In this section, we are interested in learning how your child's illness affects his/her ability to function in daily life. Please feel free to add any comments on the back of this page. In the following questions, please check the one response which best describes your child's usual activities (averaged over an entire day) OVER THE PAST WEEK. If your child has difficulty in doing a certain activity or is unable to do it because he/she is too young but NOT because he/she is RESTRICTED BY ARTHRITIS, please mark it as "Not Applicable." ONLY NOTE THOSE DIFFICULTIES OR LIMITATIONS THAT ARE OWING TO ARTHRITIS.

	Without Any Difficulty	With Some Difficulty	With Much Difficulty	Unable To Do	Not Applicable
Dressing and Grooming					
Is your child able to:					
▪ Dress, including tying shoelaces and doing buttons?	______	______	______	______	______
▪ Shampoo his/her hair?	______	______	______	______	______
▪ Remove socks?	______	______	______	______	______
▪ Cut fingernails/toenails?	______	______	______	______	______
Arising					
Is your child able to:					
▪ Stand up from a low chair or floor?	______	______	______	______	______
▪ Get in and out of bed or stand up in crib?	______	______	______	______	______
Eating					
Is your child able to:					
▪ Cut his/her own meat?	______	______	______	______	______
▪ Lift a cup or glass to mouth?	______	______	______	______	______
▪ Open a new cereal box?	______	______	______	______	______
Walking					
Is your child able to:					
▪ Walk outdoors on flat ground?	______	______	______	______	______
▪ Climb up five steps?	______	______	______	______	______

*Please check any AIDS or DEVICES that your child usually uses for any of the above activities:

______ Cane

______ Walker

______ Crutches

______ Wheelchair

______ Devices used for dressing (button hook, zipper pull, long-handled shoe horn, etc.)

______ Built-up pencil or special utensils

______ Special or built-up chair

______ Other (specify: ________________)

*Please check any categories for which your child usually needs help from another person BECAUSE OF ARTHRITIS

______ Dressing and grooming

______ Arising

______ Eating

______ Walking

(continued)

DISPLAY 12-3

Health Assessment Questionaire* (Continued)

	Without Any Difficulty	With Some Difficulty	With Much Difficulty	Unable To Do	Not Applicable
Hygiene					
Is your child able to:					
▪ Wash and dry entire body?	______	______	______	______	______
▪ Take a tub bath (get in and out of tub)?	______	______	______	______	______
▪ Get on and off the toilet or potty chair?	______	______	______	______	______
▪ Brush teeth?	______	______	______	______	______
▪ Comb/brush hair?	______	______	______	______	______
Reach					
Is your child able to:					
▪ Reach and get down a heavy object, such as a large game or books, from just above his/her head?	______	______	______	______	______
▪ Bend down to pick up clothing or a piece of paper from the floor?	______	______	______	______	______
▪ Pull on a sweater over his/her head?	______	______	______	______	______
▪ Turn neck to look back over shoulder?	______	______	______	______	______
Grip					
Is your child able to:					
▪ Write or scribble with a pen or pencil?	______	______	______	______	______
▪ Open car doors?	______	______	______	______	______
▪ Open jars that have been previously opened?	______	______	______	______	______
▪ Turn faucets on and off?	______	______	______	______	______
▪ Push open a door when he/she has to turn a door knob?	______	______	______	______	______
Activities					
Is your child able to:					
▪ Run errands and shop?	______	______	______	______	______
▪ Get in and out of car or toy car or school bus?	______	______	______	______	______
▪ Ride bike or tricycle?	______	______	______	______	______

(continued)

DISPLAY 12-3
Health Assessment Questionaire* (Continued)

Activities (Continued)

- Do household chores (e.g., wash dishes, take out trash, vacuum, do yardwork, make bed, clean room)? ________ ________ ________ ________ ________
- Run and play? ________ ________ ________ ________ ________

*Please check any AIDS or DEVICES that your child usually uses for any of the above activities:

______	Raised toilet seat	______	Bathtub bar
______	Bathtub seat	______	Long-handled appliances for reach
______	Jar opener (for jars previously opened)	______	Long-handled appliances in bathroom

*Please check any categories for which your child usually needs help from another person BECAUSE OF ARTHRITIS

______	Hygiene	______	Gripping and opening things
______	Reaching	______	Errands and chores

Pain

We are also interested in learning whether or not your child has been affected by pain because of his or her illness.

- How much pain do you think your child has had because of his or her illness IN THE PAST WEEK? Place a mark on the line below to indicate the severity of the pain.

No Pain ———————————————— Very Severe Pain
0 ———————————————— 100

Health Status

1. Considering all the ways that arthritis affects your child, rate how your child is doing on the following scale by placing a mark on the line.

0 ———————————————— 100
Very Well ———————————————— Very Poorly

2. Is your child stiff in the morning? ____________ Yes ____________ No
If YES, about how long does the stiffness usually last (in the past week)? Hours/Minutes ________

*Adapted from Singh G, Athreya B, Fries JF, Goldsmith, DP. Measurement of health status in children with juvenile rheumatoid arthritis. Arthritis Rheum 1994; 37:1761–9.

ings, using an adaptation of the model of disability proposed by the National Center for Medical Rehabilitation Research.[61] Based on the child's current status, the therapist, in consultation with the parent, child, and other team members, develops a treatment program directed toward decreasing impairments, improving physical status and function, and preventing disability. Display 12-4 lists general goals of physical therapy for a child with JRA. Short- and long-term objectives are based on the specific needs of the child.

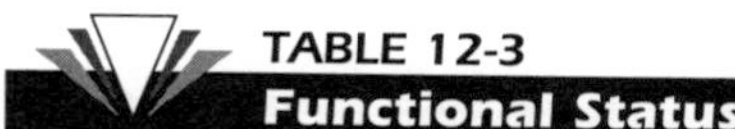

TABLE 12-3
Functional Status Measures in Use in Children with JRA

Instrument	Development	Description	Time to Complete	Dimensions	Reliability and Validity
Childhood Arthritis Impact Measurement Scale	77 children (2–17 yrs) with JRA from 250 clinic attenders	Parent-administered questionnaire for all ages	30–40 min	Physical disability Pain	Pain scale only reliable Poor discriminant validity
Juvenile Arthritis Functional Assessment Scale	71 JRA patients and 63 controls (7–18 yrs)	Trained observer record of 10 tasks in clinic setting	10 min	Physical	Good reliability and validity on initial report only to date
Juvenile Arthritis Functional Assessment Report	72 JRA patients (7–18 yrs) in rheumatology clinic	Child and parent report questionnaire on 23 activities or ADLs	10 min	Physical	Good reliability and validity on initial report only to date
Childhood Health Assessment Questionnaire	72 JRA patients (1–19 yrs)	Parent- or self-administered questionnaire	< 1 h	Physical Pain Vision Global assessment	Good reliability and validity only in initial study
Juvenile Arthritis Quality of Life Questionnaire	40 JRA and spondyloarthropathy patients and parents	Parent-administered questionnaire with 100 items	40–50 min	Fine gross motor, psychosocial, pain, systemic symptoms	Content validity demonstrated
Juvenile Arthritis Self-Report Index	Items generated from 11 children (8–18 yrs), parents, and physicians	Self-report questionaire containing 100 items	30 min	Self-care Domestic Mobility School	Not available
Childhood Arthritis Health Profile	JRA patients	Parent report questionaire containing >200 items	< 1 h	Physical Psyhosocial Pain Treatments	Not available

From Murray KJ, Passo MH. Functional measures in children with rheumatic diseases. *Pediatr Clin North Am.* 1995;42(5):1127–1154.

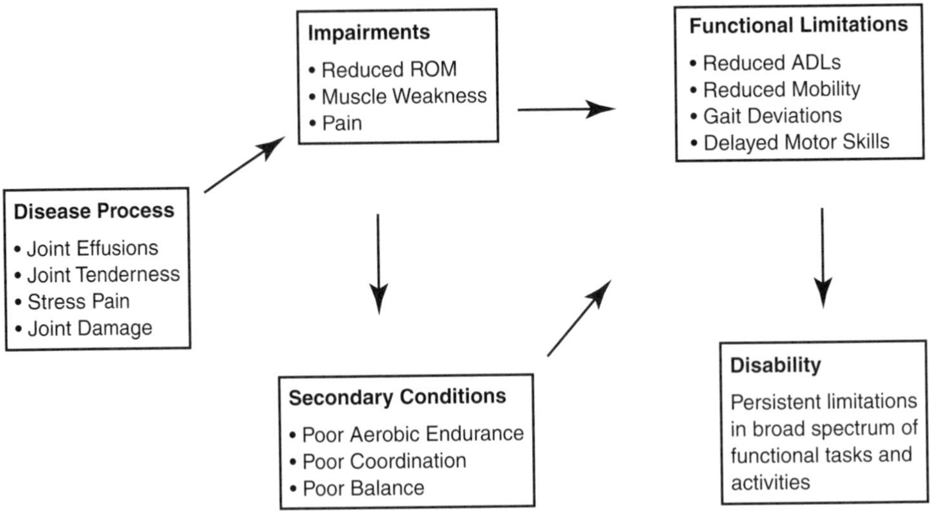

Figure 12-5 ▪ Conceptual model of disablement in JRA.

DISPLAY 12-4

Physical Therapy Goals for Children with JRA

- Reduce impairments
  - Preserve/improve ROM
  - Preserve/improve muscle strength and endurance
  - Preserve/improve aerobic endurance
  - Reduce postural deviations
- Preserve/improve function
  - Preserve/improve stamina for physical activity
  - Preserve/improve pattern and efficiency of gait
  - Preserve/improve ability to perform ADLs
  - Preserve/improve ability to participate in age-appropriate recreational activities
- Provide education and support to child and family
  - Provide information about JRA
  - Provide information about the benefits of exercise
  - Consult with schools/community therapists
  - Asist child/family in setting realistic goals
  - Encourage adherence to the medical and therapeutic regimen
  - Promote responsibility for self-management

Treatment

Several principles guide the physical therapy treatment for children with arthritis. Treatment must be appropriate to the child's cognitive and emotional development to ensure the child's understanding of the procedures and active participation in the therapy program. The intensity, duration, frequency, and type of exercise must be modified according to the child's overall disease status, and to disease activity within individual joints. Treatment and ongoing assessment should be proactive, anticipating future problems, based on the therapist's understanding of common patterns of contracture in JRA. Although developmentally based play therapy can be effective in encouraging younger children to move their joints and increase their physical activity, specific attention must be given to individual joint and muscular impairments to prevent or minimize deformity and subsequent disability.

Pain Management

Pain often has a major impact on the child's ability to cope with the disease and actively participate in therapy.[50] Many drugs used to control inflammation provide some pain relief. Physical measures, such as heat or cold, are also used to reduce stiffness and pain prior to or during exercise. Superficial heat applied for 20 minutes increases blood flow, washes out pain-producing metabolites, increases pain threshold, decreases muscle spasm, and improves extensibility of connective tissue.[62] Local application of cold may also be effective in reducing muscle spasm and pain, although some children prefer heat to cold. Cold is used primarily to treat injured or acutely inflamed joints. In acute injury, cold is combined with rest, compression, and elevation to decrease swelling and prevent further injury.

Exercise in a heated pool allows a child with active inflammation to move with less pain. A warm bath or shower, combined with ROM exercises on arising, will reduce morning stiffness. A sleeping bag or blanket-sleeper pajamas may also be useful in maintaining the body's natural heat and reducing stiffness.[63] Hydrocollator packs may be used to reduce spasm of muscles in the cervical or lumbar spine. Paraffin wax is used occasionally for the wrist and hands, although some children may be fearful of dipping their hands into the wax and prefer to paint the wax on their hands.

Deep heat, such as ultrasound or shortwave diathermy, may be effective in stretching tight fibrotic contractures in the iliotibial band or plantar fascia.[64] However, higher intra-articular temperatures may increase inflammation and activity of collagenolytic enzymes, and is generally not recommended over the immature epiphyseal plate in children.[65] Its use near cemented joints should also be avoided.[66]

Transcutaneous electrical nerve stimulation (TENS) has been used in adults to relieve severe pain, but research showing the effectiveness of TENS in patients with RA is limited.[67] Because the dosage of TENS or other electrotherapy modalities depends on feedback from the patient, their use should be limited to children old enough to understand instructions and report the sensations produced by the modality.

Cognitive-behavioral techniques, such as progressive muscle relaxation (PMR), meditative breathing, hypnosis, guided imagery, EMG biofeedback, and modification in pain behaviors, may prove to be useful in managing the impact of pain on children with JRA. Lavigne et al.[68] reported reduced self-rated pain intensity and expression of pain behaviors in eight children with JRA who participated in a program using PMR and EMG biofeedback biweekly for 3 months. Parents were counseled in behavior techniques to manage their child's pain behaviors. A study by Walco et al.[69] also found short-term reduction in subjective pain in children with JRA, ages 5 to 15 years of age, after 8 weeks of training to use PMR, meditative breathing, and guided imagery to moderate pain. The long-term benefits of cognitive-behavioral measures to modify pain and improve function in children with JRA have not been assessed.

Range of Motion Exercise

Exercise is an essential part of treatment in children with arthritis. The purpose of exercise is to preserve joint mobility and integrity, stretch soft tissue contractures, increase strength and endurance of muscles surrounding joints, preserve or improve aerobic endurance, and maximize function. The exercise prescription (intensity, duration, and frequency) is adjusted, based on disease status. Gentle warm-up and cool-down activities should accompany the exercise program. The child should be taught to distinguish the normal symptoms associated with beginning an exercise program (mild stiffness and soreness) from the objective signs of overuse (heat, swelling, increased joint pain) and to make appropriate changes in the exercise program.

EXERCISE TO PRESERVE OR IMPROVE RANGE OF MOTION

All joints should be moved through the available range of motion three to five repetitions, preferably twice a day to maintain or improve joint mobility and flexibility of the muscle and connective tissue. Because daily exercise is usually done in the home, the child and parents should be taught to recognize the signs of inflammation and adjust the exercise accordingly. During acute joint inflammation, when the joints and soft tissue are more prone to injury from overstretching, only gentle active and active-assistive exercise is used. Daily positioning is used to prevent or reduce flexion contractures in the lower limbs. The child lies prone for at least 20 minutes, with the hips and knees extended and feet over the edge of the bed (Fig. 12-6). With mild hip or knee flexion contractures, positioning time should be increased, with a sandbag or broad strap placed over the buttocks to stabilize the pelvis and prevent the child from rotating sideways.[64]

When the arthritis is under medical control, a *stretching program* is started, targeting those joints with loss of motion. Aggressive passive stretching is avoided because of the risk for damage to epiphyseal areas at the tendon–bone interface. Excessive stretching of the hamstrings, using a long lever arm (pressure placed on the distal tibia) in a child with a longstanding knee flexion contracture may cause posterior subluxation of the tibia.[64]

Brief stretching, with a 60-second hold at the end of the available range, provides a temporary increase in flexibility of the muscle fibers and connective tissue. This stretching method is useful to lengthen tissues prior to placing the limb in a splint. Research indicates a need for repeated static stretching, holding the maximal stretch for several minutes to achieve permanent increases in the length of connective tissue.[70,71] The contract-relax technique may be useful in increasing joint range of motion. The amount of resistance applied to the active muscle contraction should be varied according to the child's tolerance.

It is important to gain the child's cooperation during stretching, and to minimize pain and reflex muscle spasm. Prewarming, using local superficial heat or a warm bath, may

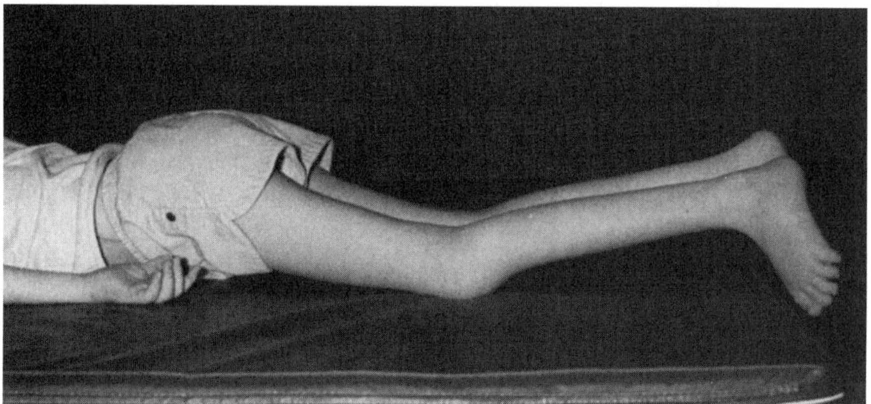

Figure 12-6 ▪ Child with bilateral knee flexion contractures lying in a prone position.

help to facilitate relaxation during stretching. Stretching should be combined with active exercise to strengthen the antagonists and promote use of the joints within the newly acquired range.

Splints and Orthotic Devices

Splints and orthotic devices are important adjuncts to the exercise program for children with JRA. The type of splint selected depends on the therapeutic goal. The three categories of splints include resting splints, corrective splints, and functional splints.[72]

The *resting splint* is used to rest an inflamed joint in a position of function. The splint is often worn during the hours of sleep or as needed during an acute flare of disease activity. It avoids having the patient rest the joint in a position of potential deformity. The wrist and fingers may be placed in a resting splint with the wrist in about 20 degrees of extension (Fig. 12-7). The knee is also commonly splinted in extension at night with a posterior shell. Some children are able to ambulate immediately on arising, because the knee has not become stiff overnight in a flexed position.

Corrective splints, in combination with an appropriate exercise program, are used to improve joint ROM and may include serial splints or casts as well as dynamic splints. The joint is splinted at its maximum range and held in this position for extended periods daily. The splint is adjusted serially as the range of motion improves. Serial casts must be changed frequently, usually every 48 to 72 hours, in order to avoid creating an iatrogenic fusion of the joint. Figure 12-8 shows a dial-lock joint on a knee orthosis, used to adjust the degree of extension as the child gains motion. It may also be used as functional orthosis to control valgus at the knee during gait or to provide external support for weak quadriceps.

Dynamic splints use springs or rubber bands to provide a constant stretching force to reduce a contracture. Commercially available dynamic splints can be ordered and fit to specific joints. The tension at the joint can be controlled by the therapist and set to patient tolerance. Most patients will tolerate a dynamic splint for 1-hour

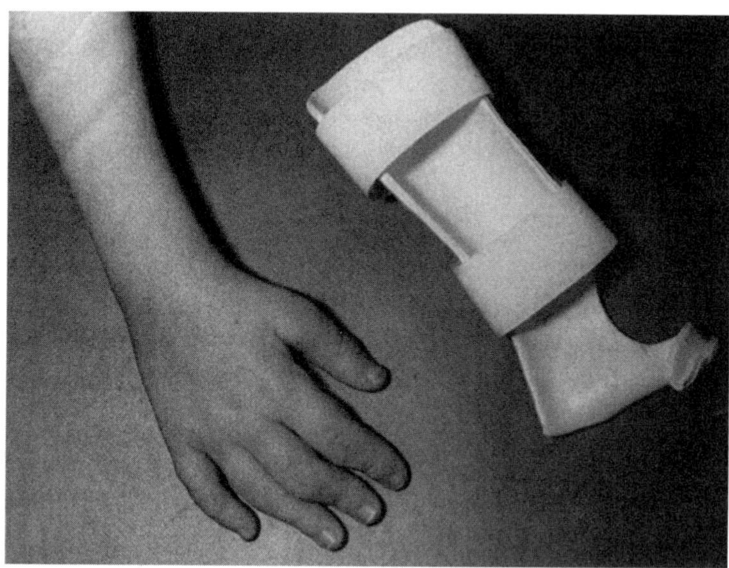

Figure 12-7 ▪ A resting splint that was customized for the child with rheumatoid arthritis.

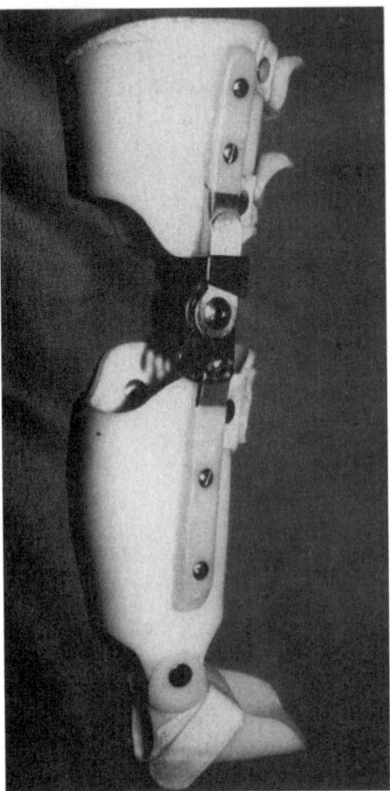

Figure 12-8 ■ Example of a dial-lock knee joint.

periods during the day. If tolerated, they can also be used during sleep.

Functional splints or orthoses are used to support the joint during daily activities. In the upper extremity, a small wrist splint may be used to help during school work or to protect the joint during sports. A lower extremity orthosis such as an ankle-foot orthosis (AFO) may be used to improve stability or reduce pain during weight bearing.

Strengthening and Endurance Exercises

Strengthening exercises are prescribed to address specific muscle deficits. Table 12-4 lists the benefits, precautions, and general guidelines for strengthening exercise. Isometric exercise is usually recommended during active joint disease or when motion against gravity causes joint pain. Although there is evidence of strength gains from isometric exercise in adults with RA,[22] this has not been confirmed in children with JRA.[38] Potential benefits of isometric exercise include an increase in static muscle strength and endurance. A regimen of isometric exercises performed at multiple points within the range of motion may prepare the joint for increased dynamic exercise.[73]

Nonelastic webbing or thick Theraband can be used to provide resistance at the end range during isometric exercise. Maximal or prolonged isometric contractions should be avoided, because they may increase intra-articular contact pressures[74] and constrict blood flow through the exercising muscles, contributing to postexercise soreness.[75] The child can be taught to regulate the intensity of the contraction by first contracting the muscle maximally, and then letting go slightly, producing a submaximal isometric contraction. The child should hold the contraction for no more than 6 seconds, exhaling during the contraction, and inhaling during the relaxation phase. EMG biofeedback may help the child isolate the muscle group and learn to regulate the intensity of the contraction.

Dynamic resistive exercise can be initiated once the disease is under medical control and the child can move the limb against gravity for eight to 10 repetitions without pain.[76] Research shows increased muscle strength and endurance with dynamic resistive exercise in adults with RA.[77] Resistance can be provided by the weight of the body part, light free weights, or elastic bands. Although isokinetic equipment has been used to measure strength in children with JRA, it is not universally available and may not be appropriate for training during periods of active disease.

One possible initial training regimen might include one to two sets of six to 10 RMs for two to three sessions spaced throughout the

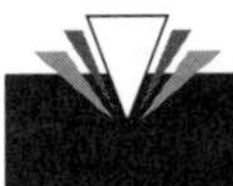

TABLE 12-4

Purpose, Recommendations, and Precautions for Isometric and Dynamic Strengthening Exercises*

Isometric Exercise	Dynamic Exercise
Purpose	
Minimize atrophy Improve tone Maintain/increase static strength and endurance Prepare for dynamic and weight-bearing activity	Maintain/increase dynamic strength and endurance Increase muscle power Improve function Enhance synovial blood flow Promote strength of bone and cartilage
Recommendations	
Perform at functional joint angles Exhale during contraction: avoid valsalva maneuver Intensity: ≤70% one MVC Duration: 6 second contraction Frequency: 5 to 10 repetitions daily	Capable of 8 to 10 repetitions of motion against gravity before additional resistance Progressive resistive regimen Perform in pain-free range Use functional activities/movement patterns Intensity: progress to <70% one RM Duration: progress to 8 to 10 exercises, 8 to 10 repetitions Frequency: two to three times/week on alternate days
Precautions	
Decreased muscle blood flow May increase intra-articular pressure May increase blood pressure	May increase biomechanical stress on unstable or malaligned joints Avoid force on involved hands and wrists

*MVC = maximal voluntary contraction; RM = repetition maximum

(From Minor MA: *Rest and Exercise: Clinical Care in the Rheumatic Diseases.* Atlanta: American College of Rheumatology, 1996;75, with permission.)

week to allow time for recovery and adaptation. The amount of resistance is adjusted, based on reassessment of the child's RM. If elastic bands are used, lighter bands are used first, progressing to more resistive bands as strength increases, provided there is no joint pain or other signs of active disease.[78]

The prescription should include diagrams of all exercises to be performed. A useful resource is the Quick-Fit for Kids (SPRI Products, Inc., Buffalo Grove, IL), a complete kit that includes clear, reproducible diagrams and instructions for resistive exercise. Reasonable goals should be established in collaboration with the child and parent. Goals might include increasing strength, reducing fatigue, and improving specific functional abilities, such as climbing stairs. Functional movement patterns incorporated into the training program may increase the benefits of training. Periodic reassessment, using one of the self-report functional tests, such as the CHAQ or JASI, can provide information about the impact of training on the child's function.

Aerobic Conditioning Exercises

Recent research strongly suggests children with arthritis can improve their aerobic endurance through participation in low impact aerobic training programs. Moncur et al. reported significant gains in maximal aerobic capacity in seven subjects with JRA, who trained on a stationary bicycle, three times a week for twelve weeks.[79] Klepper and colleagues investigated the effects of an 8-week program of low-impact aerobic exercise in 25 children and adolescents with chronic arthritis.[80] Aerobic endurance performance on a 9-minute walk-run test was assessed at study entry, after an 8-week control period, and after the 8-week exercise program. Subjects demonstrated a significant increase in performance from the pre- to postexercise tests. Both studies reported a decrease in disease signs and symptoms after training, suggesting low-impact aerobic training is safe and effective in children with arthritis.

The *aerobic training prescription* is determined by the intensity, duration, and frequency of the exercise. Children who are deconditioned may need to start with short exercise periods once or twice a week. Aerobic exercise for 30 minutes a day, at an intensity of 60% to 75% of the child's maximal heart rate, three to five times a week, appears to be safe for children with arthritis. Duration and frequency can be increased as the child's physical condition improves. Exercise intensity can be monitored by having the child take the radial or carotid pulse or use a modified 0 to 10 version of the BORG Rating of Perceived Exertion Scale.[81]

The *mode of exercise* depends on the child's age, motor skill, disease status, and individual interests. Nonimpact or reduced-impact aerobic activities, such as swimming, walking, stationary cycling, or low-impact aerobic dance, are encouraged, because they utilize large muscle groups while avoiding excessive loading on the joints. Group exercise sessions in the pool or gym may be more fun for the child and increase motivation. Weight-bearing activities should be encouraged to improve bone density. A balanced physical conditioning program should include exercises to improve all components of fitness, including aerobic endurance, muscular strength and endurance, flexibility, and body composition.[82]

Moderation is stressed during any physical conditioning program, because high-intensity exercise or a rapid progression in intensity often results in pain or injury, and poor adherence. Training in proper exercise form at the beginning of the training program and frequent monitoring are essential to ensure safety and effectiveness of the exercise. Pain reports by the child should be assessed for specific cause. Discomfort from delayed onset muscle soreness or overstretching may occur early in the program, and should resolve with time. Overuse of a joint, accompanied by swelling, heat, and pain, should be treated with cold, elevation, and rest, and appropriate modification of the program.

Recreational Activities

The child should be encouraged to participate in a variety of recreational activities in the school and community. Activities should be chosen based on the child's age, physical and emotional development, and status of joint disease. Children with arthritis are encouraged to participate in all activities within their tolerance.[5] However, there are concerns that some children with arthritis may choose inappropriate activities or overexert themselves in an effort to fit in with their friends, whereas others may limit their activity because of their own or their parents' fear of injury. A recent review of sports and exercise in children with arthritis addressed this concern, suggesting sports and other physical activities appropriate for children with JRA, based on each child's abilities and disease activity.[84]

Activities suitable for most children with arthritis include music, arts and crafts, drama, and computer activities. Appropriate aerobic activities include cycling, swimming, walking, and low impact aerobic dance. The height of the bicycle seat should be set so the knee is at an angle of 10 to 15 degrees of flexion when the child's foot is at the apex of the downstroke.[83] Exercise in a heated pool (88 to 92°F) is recommended throughout the year, especially for children who have difficulty walking and exercising on land. Cooler pool temperatures, between 82 and 86°F, are more suitable for aerobic exercise.[83]

Several *exercise videotapes* are available for people with arthritis. "Where Are the Indians"[84] features young children performing range of motion exercises through dances performed to music. Older children and adults can exercise to the "Range of Motion Dance,"[85] "People with Arthritis Can Exercise (PACE),"[86] or "Good Moves for Everybody."[87] Therapists can also help children make their own personal exercise video.

School-age children should be encouraged to participate in physical education class whenever feasible. The therapist can provide the school with guidelines for adapting the program to meet the child's needs and minimize the potential for injury. Activities such as somersaults and headstands should be avoided to prevent injury to the cervical spine. Contact sports and activities requiring weight-bearing on the hands are also discouraged.

Functional Activities

A primary goal for the child with arthritis is to achieve independence in age-appropriate activities of daily living (ADLs) and functional mobility in all environments. Expectations for independence in a toddler or young child will differ significantly from the skills valued in older children or adolescents. In younger children, the emphasis may be on acquiring independence in dressing, bathing, feeding, and motor skills within the home and school. Although these skills remain important throughout life, older children become more interested in participating in sports and other social activities. For the adolescent and young adult, independence may revolve around the ability to drive, socialize with friends, and acquire a job.

The *role of the therapist* is to (1) assess the child's ability to perform necessary and preferred tasks in the home, school, and community; (2) provide interventions to achieve improved mobility and motor skills; (3) suggest appropriate assistive devices, environmental modifications, and adaptive equipment, and train the child in their use; and (4) consult with school personnel and suggest adaptations to the child's educational program.

A child with minimal joint involvement may only need advice about the most efficient method of performing tasks, whereas a child with more severe limitations may need instruction in the use of *adaptive equipment* or advice on environmental modifications to promote greater independence. A dressing stick can be useful for a child with limited range of motion who is having trouble donning pants. A hoop made from a wire coat hanger can help with donning shirts (Fig. 12-9). Zippers, buttons, and snaps can be replaced with Velcro to simplify dressing. Most children are able to use regular eating utensils, but some may need adapted utensils to allow a normal hand-to-mouth pattern. Sufficient shoulder and elbow range of motion is important for self-feeding. When neck extension is limited because of cervical spine involvement, using a straw may help a child drink from a glass without tilting back the head.

The therapist should teach the child and parent the *principles of joint protection* and ways of adapting activities to decrease the physical and mechanical stresses on vulnerable joints. The child should be encouraged to use large joints to perform tasks whenever possible, because they tolerate stress better than the small joints. For example, using a backpack to carry books avoids stress across the wrists and finger joints. Diagrams, demonstration, and practice of joint protection techniques may improve adherence.[88]

Architectural modifications may be necessary, especially for a child who depends on a wheelchair. The child should have easy access to the tub, toilet, and sink with adequate support to ensure safety and privacy. Items that may promote independence include a special tub seat,

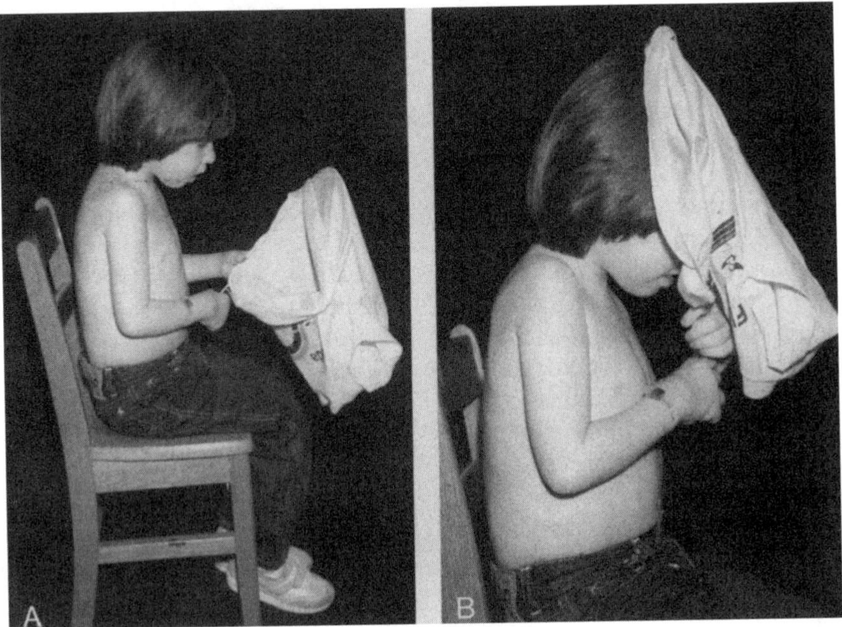

Figure 12-9 ▪ (**A**) and (**B**). A wire hanger may be used to facilitate donning a shirt by a child with limited motion at the shoulder.

support bars, handheld shower hoses, and long-handled sponges. It may also be necessary to widen doors throughout the home, and install a ramp or wheelchair lift.

Functional Mobility

Continued weight-bearing and ambulation are vitally important for the child with JRA to increase bone density, improve muscle strength, and prevent flexion contractures. Treatment and ongoing assessment should anticipate and address potential problems, such as joint contractures, muscle weakness, or pain, that may contribute to difficulties in ambulation. Leg discrepancy should be corrected within a quarter inch to prevent postural compensations, such as knee flexion of the longer limb, pelvic obliquity, or scoliosis. A daily schedule of standing in a supine or prone stander may be helpful for a child with hip and knee contractures.

Custom foot orthoses are sometimes prescribed to reduce pain on weight-bearing and improve gait. Careful assessment of the lower quarter, with emphasis on the foot and ankle, should be done to determine the orthotic prescription. The alignment of the lower extremity is noted for rotation, or valgus/varus deformities, and the presence of a normal longitudinal and transverse arch. Range of motion should be assessed at the ankle mortise, the subtalor joint, the midtarsals and the toes. Ankle swelling can be detected on a figure 8 measurement using a cloth tape and consistent anatomical landmarks. Examination of the skin helps to identify pressure points from weight-bearing or improper alignment. The shoe should also be examined inside and outside for clues to points of pressure or gait deviations. Palpation of the foot can also locate problems such as tenosynovitis or plantar fasciitis.

The weight-bearing foot may look different than the foot in non–weight-bearing. A vertical calcaneus is ideal, with weight-bearing spread across the first and fifth metatarsal heads and the calcaneus. The navicular should remain on a line between the medial malleolus and the head of the first metatarsal. If the patient does not adopt this alignment in standing, the examiner should determine if it can be achieved with manual correction. The child should also be asked to roll onto the forefoot in order to assess pain and foot function during roll over.

The *choice of an orthosis* will vary, based on whether the deformities are fixed or flexible. Flexible deformities may be managed by fabricating the orthosis to hold the joint in correct anatomic alignment. For example, an orthosis with a heel cup molded out of thermoplastic material may help to correct metatarsus adductus. Off-the-shelf orthoses may provide inexpensive alternatives. Fixed deformities require accommodative orthoses. For example, a patient with hallux rigidis, with loss of great toe extension, may need a metatarsal bar added to the sole of the shoe to create a mechanical means of rolling over in gait. Shoes with extra depth are needed to accommodate hammer toes. Fixed hindfoot varus may require posting to achieve comfortable weight-bearing.

The *arthritic foot* without special needs should be properly fitted with a sneaker or similar shoe with a flexible sole and good support for the longitudinal arch. Simple cushioning of the sole may alleviate pain on weight-bearing for many children and can be achieved with a thin liner of cushioning foam. Weight-bearing can sometimes be distributed more comfortably with special pads, for example, a metatarsal dome that can alleviate uncomfortable weight-bearing from the center metatarsals.

When a child begins to have *problems with ambulation,* the cause should be determined and efforts made to keep the child ambulatory. If lower extremity pain has increased, a posterior walker or a regular walker or crutches with platform attachments may be helpful (Fig. 12-10). In a child with unilateral hip pain or weakness, a crane used on the side opposite the involved hip reduces the load on the painful joint. A change in medications or temporary hospital admission for intensive therapy may be needed. An exercise and walking program in the therapy pool will help to improve flexibility and strengthen weakened trunk and lower extremity muscles without causing additional pain to inflamed joints. Activities to improve postural awareness, balance, coordination, and protective responses

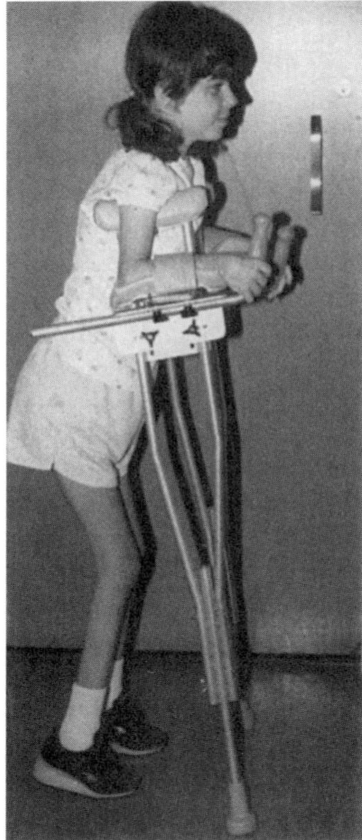

Figure 12-10 ▪ Platform crutches facilitate ambulation by shifting weight bearing of the upper extremities from the hands and wrists to the larger, more proximal joints.

to reduce the risk of falling may be helpful in a child who has not been walking.

Despite these efforts, some children will need to use wheeled mobility to travel long distances to preserve energy and improve function. Powered wheelchairs are generally reserved for children with severe disability. Tricycles or bicycles with training wheels are good alternatives for young children. Older children and adolescents can use a properly fitted lightweight sports wheelchair or powered scooter to move around their school, college campus, or community. The child should be encouraged to get out of the wheelchair often during the day, standing and walking as tolerated to prevent contractures and muscle weakness.

Issues Related to School

Arthritis does not affect cognitive function, but academic problems may occur as a result of frequent absences owing to illness or medical appointments, or decreased attention because of pain, stiffness, and fatigue in school.[89,90] Problems related to school can be assessed with a school check list, such as the one described by Atwood.[91] Using this list, the child indicates problems related to his or her ability to perform necessary tasks in school, the impact of stiffness or pain on various activities, mobility within the school and grounds, and the ability to tolerate the school day.

The therapist can provide information to teachers and other school personnel about specific ways in which arthritis affects the child's school performance, and can suggest possible adaptations to the educational program. Adaptations might include providing a second set of books for home, adapted writing tools or alternatives to writing, such as a word processor or tape recorder, or an easel top desk for a child with cervical spine involvement. Modifications in the schedule may be necessary, including grouping classes in one area of the building to limit travel time, providing the child with a place to rest during the day, and opportunities to stand and move to prevent stiffness from long periods of sitting. Children with lower extremity pain or limitations may need to use the elevators.

Participation in physical education classes is encouraged when the activity is within the child's abilities. The child may also do his or her own exercise routine during gym class. The therapist should recommend appropriate sports activities for the student, and consult with coaches when the child is involved in team sports.

Many schools will provide these and other modifications without a formal process, but a formal evaluation by the school and development of an individual education plan (IEP) may be necessary in some circumstances. The manual "Educational Rights for Children with Arthritis" is available from the American Juvenile Arthritis Organization (AJAO),[92] and it may be very helpful for parents. A thorough discussion of physical therapy in the public schools is provided in Chapter 15.

Surgery and Postoperative Physical Therapy

Children with JRA may require orthopedic surgery when severe contractures or disabling pain fail to respond to conservative treatment, and significantly interfere with function.[93] The decision to perform surgery must be made by an interdisciplinary team, based on an analysis of the risks and benefits. The physical therapist is involved in the preoperative assessment and planning, as well as the postoperative rehabilitation.

Joint contractures that fail to respond to conservative measures are managed in a number of ways, depending on the disease stage and condition of the joint. Intra-articular steroid injection, using triamcinolone hexacetonide, is effective in reducing acute synovitis, plain, and muscle spasm in large joints, such as the hip or knee, when there is no fixed deformity when examined under anesthetic and no evidence of erosion subluxation or ischemic changes on x-ray study.[94] Children 7 years of age or older are usually able to tolerate the procedure with a local anesthetic or mild sedation, although a younger child may require conscious sedation.[5] When joint irritability subsides following injection, hydrotherapy and exercise are initiated. Reported benefits include a reduction in pain and synovial proliferation in injected hip and knee joints lasting 12 months or longer.[5,94] Possible adverse effects include subcutaneous atrophy at the injection site or intra- or periarticular calcification, but these problems are usually mild and without symptoms.[5] There are also some concerns about the long-term effects on articular cartilage in children.

Soft tissue releases are done to manage fixed contractures of the hip flexors, adductors, hamstrings, and heel cords. Reduction in pain, improved ROM, and decompression of the joint often result in improved joint nutrition and healing by fibrocartilage.[95] The postoperative exercise program is aimed at improving range of motion and strength. Immobilization is kept to a minimum to avoid further loss of motion. A continuous passive motion machine (CPM) may be used[96] (Fig. 12-11). Splinting and positioning several times a day and during the night help to preserve motion.

Synovectomy is not usually done in children with JRA, because of problems with postoperative pain and spasm and disappointing long-term results.[97] Synovectomy may be done in combination with soft tissue releases to treat hip flexion contractures.[94] It may also be done arthroscopically for acute synovitis of the knee, when effusion and overgrowth of rheumatoid synovium stimulate the adjacent epiphysis, re-

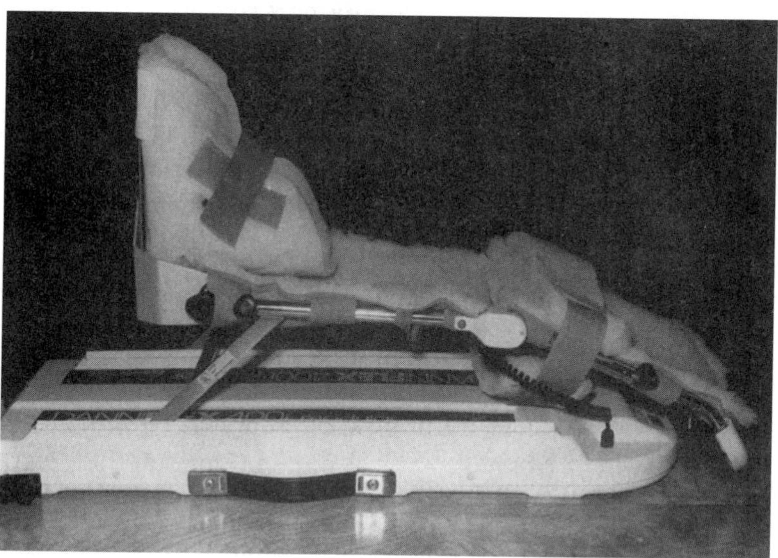

Figure 12-11 ▪ A continuous passive motion machine for use at the knee.

sulting in lengthening of the limb.[95] Tenosynovectomy may be done in a child with seropositive disease to treat synovial proliferation at the metacarpophalangeal joints.[95]

Supracondylar osteotomy, in addition to soft tissue releases, may be required for a severe flexion contracture at the knee or when there is a valgus deformity and evidence of joint damage.[95] An arthrotomy is usually done at the same time if there is a poorly formed or overgrown patella that is fixed to the femoral condyle, limiting joint motion.[95] Postoperatively, the leg is immobilized in a cylindrical cast, with immediate weight-bearing. The case is removed when there is evidence of adequate bone union.

Arthroplasty or arthrodesis are considered when irreversible joint destruction and severe pain significantly limit the child's function. Total or partial joint replacement is done most often for the hip or knee, although prostheses are available for other joints, including the shoulder, elbow, or ankle. Fusion of the wrist or ankle joints may be done to eliminate disabling pain on motion and stabilize the joint in a functional position.

The child's age, disease status, condition of other lower extremity joints, ability to use the upper extremities to assist with weight-bearing after surgery, and the ability of the child and parent to carry out the intensive postoperative rehabilitation program are all considered in the decision to perform a total joint replacement. *Joint replacement surgery* is usually delayed until the epiphyses have fused or there is little chance of further growth of the limb,[94] although children as young as 12 years of age have received hip replacements.[93]

Timing of procedures is extremely important in a child who requires multiple joint replacements. Fusion of a damaged or painful wrist may be necessary first to allow the child to use crutches after hip or knee surgery.[37] When both hips and knees must be replaced, the hip joints are usually done first. When there are severe hip flexion contractures and joint destruction, both hips are replaced at the same time.[37] Preoperative physical therapy includes an exercise program to strengthen the bone, muscles, and soft tissues around the target joints and improve overall endurance. The child is trained to use crutches after surgery and to protect the joint during daily activities.[37]

Custom-designed hip prostheses that are porous are usually used to accommodate the smaller bones in children with JRA and allow for biologic fixation, because cemented prostheses are more susceptible to loosening after several years.[94] The postoperative program for total hip replacement includes range of motion exercise, with precautions to avoid hip flexion past 90 degrees, adduction past neutral, and internal rotation. A foam abduction pillow is used for 6 weeks, alternating with a CPM machine and prone positioning.[98] Isometric exercises of the hip extensors and abductors and quadriceps may be started early. Gait training with an assistive device can begin during the first week. Active exercise in shallow water and ambulation in chest deep water may begin as soon as wound healing is complete.[98]

Total knee arthroplasty is usually done using a cemented prosthesis, and may be accompanied by soft tissue releases to resolve a flexion contracture, release of the lateral retinaculum to prevent further valgus deformity, and resurfacing of the underside of the patella.

ROM exercises are also begun on day 2, and a CPM machine can be used immediately. Prone positioning is also encouraged to preserve knee extension. The goal is 0 to 100 degrees of knee motion. A program to strengthen lower extremity musculature is begun with isometric and straight leg raising exercises. Aquatic exercise and stationary cycling, using a range limiter on the pedal to control the amount of knee flexion, may also be used.[98] Full weight-bearing, using a knee immobilizer, is begun on the second postoperative day.[98,99] Ambulation without assistive devices is allowed when the child demonstrates at least 90 degrees of knee flexion and adequate lower extremity strength and endurance.

The *most common complications* reported with total joint replacement include infection, dislocation, and biologic loosening of the components. One long-term follow-up study of 72 patients with total hip replacements reported that 30% of the patients required revision surgery after 10 years. Hip replacement in children with JRA may be complicated by their smaller bones and osteoporosis, as well as angular deformities in the femur.[94] Soft tissue releases of the hip flexors and adductors may be necessary if hip flexion contracture exist. However, continued advances in customized prosthetic design and surgical procedures should result in improved safety and longevity of total joint replacements.[94]

Management Strategies

Successful management of the physical problems and prevention of disability in the child with JRA depends to a great extent on adherence to the medical and therapeutic regimen. However, the demands placed on the family can be overwhelming. Compliance may be enhanced when the parent and child fully understand the effects of the disease on the body and the benefits of medication, exercise, and other therapeutic procedures to prevent or reduce pain, swelling, contractures, and weakness. Older children, who participate in goal setting and decision making regarding their care, may feel a greater sense of self-efficacy. Because parents and children often have goals related to improving function, rather than reducing impairment, it is important to explain how improvements at the impairment level may help the child to achieve his or her goals.

Educational materials should be appropriate to the child's level of cognitive development and emotional maturity. Several excellent pamphlets, videotapes, and books are available for this purpose from the American Juvenile Arthritis Organization and the Arthritis Foundation. A workbook, *JRA & ME,* uses pictures, games, brief explanations, and puzzles to help school age children understand arthritis and the need for medications and therapy.[100]

Home exercise programs should be individualized to target the child's needs and limited to no more than seven simple exercises, requiring 20 to 30 minutes. The therapist should demonstrate the exercises to the child and parent, periodically reassess the child's performance and progress, and make any necessary changes in the program. With young children, it is best to incorporate the exercises into daily activities, such as bathing, dressing, or play. Positive reinforcement with stickers, small prizes, or special outings can be used to encourage a young child to cooperate in the exercise program. Older children and teens might benefit from a contract, listing their personal goals, the necessary medication and exercise regimen, and the reward or incentive for adherence to the therapeutic program.

Summary

This chapter presented information about the disease process in JRA, the most common physical impairments and functional limitations caused by the disease, and the principles for physical therapy assessment and treatment of the child with JRA. The goal of management is for the child and family to lead as normal a life as possible. An interdisciplinary team (see following Case Study) of professionals is necessary to meet the complex needs of the child with JRA. A total program of care should include medical, and occasionally surgical management, patient and family education, psychosocial support, and physical and occupational therapy.

Case Study—Eric, 15-Year-Old Male with Polyarticular JRA.

Eric is a 15-year-old male with polyarticular JRA of 10 years' duration. Currently, he has limited motion in the cervical spine, both wrists, hips, ankles, and the right knee, and foot deformities. Active disease is evident in the cervical spine, wrists, and the right knee and ankle. Naproxen (375 mg BID), has been prescribed to control the inflammation, and Eric has been given a home exercise program to improve ROM and strength. However, Eric admits to irregular use of the medication and poor adherence to the exercise program. He attends school regularly but is often late because of morning stiffness lasting 1 hour, and complains of fatigue in the afternoon. At this clinic visit, he reports pain in both wrists, neck, low back, and feet. The findings of the assessment are listed in the following.

Active Joint Disease or Joint Damage

Effusions:

1. Both wrists
2. MCP/PIP joints
3. (R) Knee
4. (R) Ankle

Radiographic Signs of Joint Damage

Cervical Spine:

1. Fusion of C2/C3

Impairments

Cervical Spine:

1. Rotation limited by 50%
2. Extension limited to neutral
3. Pain at end range

Wrists and Hands:

1. D-FL: (R) 0–30 (1) 0–25
2. Ulnar deviation
3. Loss of terminal PIP flexion
4. Loss of MCP flexion

Lumbar Spine:

1. Excessive lordosis

Hips:

1. 10-degree flexion contractures

Ankles and Feet:

1. D-FL to neutral
2. Pes cavus
3. Hallux valgus
4. Subluxed metatarsel heads

Knees (right):

1. 10-degrees flexion contracture

Muscle Weakness:

1. Hip extensors
2. Hip abductors
3. Abdominals
4. Quadriceps
5. Plantar flexors

Poor Aerobic Endurance

1. < 40th percentile on 9-minute run-walk test

Functional Limitations

Neck Pain and Fatigue:

1. Riding in car/bus
2. Working at desk

Hand Pain and Fatigue:

1. Pain when writing
2. Difficulty opening jars

Low Back and Foot Pain:

1. Standing
2. Sitting in class
3. Walking for long periods

Gait Deviations:

1. Decreased velocity
2. Short step length
3. Poor push-off
4. Weight borne on lateral side of feet through stance cycle

(continued)

Case Study—Eric, 15-Year-Old Male with Polyarticular JRA. (Continued)

The professional team believed some of Eric's current problems were owing to inadequate disease control and lack of proper exercise, and they thought compliance might improve if he was involved in setting goals and making decisions regarding his care. Eric stated he wanted to participate in afterschool activities, such as intramural sports, have a part-time job, and obtain his driver's license. The team explained how Eric might achieve these goals if his disease was brought under better control by regular use of medication, and his general physical status was improved through daily exercise. Eric agreed to a contract, listing his functional goals, therapy objectives, and a plan of activities aimed at achieving the goals.

Functional Limitation: Decreased Gait Velocity, Step Length

Impairments Contributing to Problem:

1. Bilateral hip flexion contractures
2. Weakness and poor endurance of lower extremity muscles
3. Foot deformities and foot pain

Plan:

1. Daily stretching program for hip flexors, planar fascia
2. Progressive resistive exercises: hip extensors and abductors, quadriceps, and ankle plantarflexors
3. Recommended shoes with cushioned insoles to reduce pain
4. Referral to podiatrist for: custom insoles to accommodate pes cavus deformity; metatarsal bar to allow better roll-off at terminal stance

Functional Limitation: Neck Pain Riding in Car/Doing Deskwork

Impairments Contributing to Functional Limitation:

1. Decreased cervical spine rotation and extension
2. Weakness in the musculature in neck and shoulder girdle

Plan:

1. Daily active ROM exercises for neck and shoulders
2. Isometric exercises for neck muscles
3. Active resistive exercises for upper trunk extensors
4. Recommend semirigid cervical collar when riding in a vehicle
5. Recommend using easel top for desk to decrease neck strain

Functional Limitation: Hand Pain When Writing

Impairments Contributing to the Problem:

1. Active synovitis in joints of the wrist and fingers

Plan:

1. Regular use of night resting hand splints to preserve motion and reduce morning stiffness
2. Active exercise to improve strength
3. Referral to OT to revise functional day splints

The therapist reviewed the exercise program with Eric and arranged to consult with the school physical education (PE) instructor to have Eric do some of his exercises during PE class. Eric agreed to keep a daily log of his medication and exercise. He will be seen in clinic in 3 months.

REFERENCES

1. Newacheck P, Taylor W. Childhood chronic illness: prevalence, severity, and impact. *Am J Pub Health.* 1992;82:364–371.
2. Oen K, Cheang M. Epidemiology of chronic arthritis in childhood. *Semin Arthritis Rheum.* 1996;26(3):575–591.
3. Towner SR, Michet CJ, O'Fallon UM, et al. The epidemiology of juvenile arthritis in Rochester Minnesota. *Arthritis Rheum.* 1983;26:1208.
4. Boyer S, Roettcher P. Pediatric rheumatology clinic populations in the United States: results of a 3 year survey. *J Rheumatol.* 1996;23:1968–1974.
5. Cassidy J, Petty R. Juvenile rheumatoid arthritis. In: Cassidy J, Petty R, eds. *Textook of Pediatric Rheumatology,* 3rd ed. Philadelphia: W.B. Saunders; 1995:133–223.
6. Hanson V, Kornreich H, Berstein B. Three subtypes of juvenile rheumatoid arthritis: correlates of age at onset, sex, and serologic factors. *Arthritis Rheum.* 1977;20(suppl):184–186.
7. Cassidy JT, Levinson JE, Bass JC, et al. A study of the classification criteria for a diagnosis of juvenile rheumatoid arthritis. *Arthritis Rheum.* 1986;29(2): 274–281.
8. European League Against Rheumatism (EULAR). *Nomenclature and classification of arthritis in children,* Bulletin 4. Basel, National Zeitung AG; 1977.
9. Fink C. Proposal for the development of classification criteria for idiopathic arthritides of childhood. *J Rheumatol.* 1995;22(8):1566.
10. Fink CW, Fernandez-Vina M, Stastney P. Clinical and genetic evidence that juvenile arthritis is not a single disease. *Pediatr Clin North Am.* Philadelphia: W.B. Saunders; 1995: 1155–1169.
11. Hochberg M. Classification criteria for childhood arthritic diseases. *J Rheumatol.* 1995;22(8): 1445–1446.
12. Singsen BH. Pediatric rheumatic diseases. *Primer of the Rheumatic Diseases,* 9th ed. Atlanta: Arthritis Foundation; 1988:160–164.
13. White P. Juvenile chronic arthritis. In: Klippel JH, ed. *Rheumatology.* London: Mosby–Year book; 1994.
14. Nepom B. The immunogenics of juvenile rheumatoid arthritis. *Rheumatic Disease Clinics of North America.* 1991;825–842.
15. Lipnick RN, Tsokos GC, Magilavy DB. Immune abnormalities in the pathogenosis of juvenile rheumatoid arthritis. In: Athreya B, ed. *Rheumatic Disease Clinics of North America.* Philadelphia: W.B. Saunders; 1991:843–857.
16. Shore A. Arthritis in childhood. *Med North Am.* 1988;26:4869–4877.
17. Wallace, CA, Levinson JE. Juvenile rheumatoid arthritis: Outcome and treatment for the 1990s. *Rheumatic Disease Clinics of North America.* 1991: 891–905.
18. Ansell BM, Wood PH. Prognosis in juvenile chronic polyarthritis. *Clin Rheum Dis.* 1976;2: 397–412.
19. Rennebohm R, Correll JK. Comprehensive management of juvenile rheumatoid arthritis. *Nurs Clin North Am.* 1984;19:647–662.
20. Smith R. Soluble mediators of articular cartilage degradation in juvenile rheumatoid arthritis. *Clin Orthop Rel Res.* 1990;259:31–37.
21. Ansell BM, Swann M. The management of chronic arthritis of children. *J Bone Joint Surg.* 1983;65B: 536–543.
22. Galloway MT, Joki P. The role of exercise in the treatment of inflammatory arthritis. *Bull Rheum Dis.* 1993;42(1):1–4.
23. Oberg T, Karsznia A, Andersson Gare B, et al. Physical training of children with juvenile chronic arthritis. *Scand J Rheumatol.* 1994;23:92–95.
24. Henderson C, Lovell D. Assessment of protein-energy malnutrition in children and adolescents with juvenile rheumatoid arthritis. *Arthritis Care Res.* 1989;2(4):108–113.
25. Hicks JE. Exercise in patients with inflammatory arthritis and connective tissue disease. *Rheum Dis Clin North Am.* 1990;16:845–870.
26. Elsasser U, Wilkins B, Hesp R, et al. Bone refraction and crush fractures in juvenile chronic arthritis. *Arch Dis Child.* 1982;57:377.
27. Cassidy JT, Langman CB, Allen SH, et al. Bone mineral metabolism in children with juvenile rheumatoid arthritis. In: Miller M, ed. *Pediatr Clin North Am.* 1995;42(5):1017–1033.
28. Varonos S, Ansell BM, Reeve J. Vertebral collapse in juvenile chronic arthritis: its relationship with glucocorticoid therapy. *Calcif Tissue Int.* 1987; 41:75.
29. DeNardo B, Rhodes V, Gibbons B, et al. *Physical Therapy Practice Guidelines for Children with Chronic Arthritis.* The Affiliated Children's Arthritis Centers of New England; 1994.
30. Giannini EH, Cawkell GD. Drug treatment in children with juvenile rheumatoid arthritis. *Pediatr Clin North Am.* 1995:42(5): 1099–1125.
31. Athreya B, Cassidy JT. Current status of the medical treatment of children with juvenile rheumatoid arthritis. *Rheum Dis Clin North Am.* 1991;17(4): 871–889.

32. Giannini EH, Cassidy JT, Brewer EH, et al. Comparative efficacy and safety of advanced drug therapy in children with juvenile rheumatoid arthritis. *Semin Arthritis Rheum.* 1993;23:34–46.
33. Graham LD, Myones BL, Rivas-Chacon RF, et al. Morbidity associated with long-term methotrexate therapy juvenile rheumatoid arthritis. *J Pediatr.* 1992;120:468–473.
34. Allen R, Gross K, Laxer R, et al. Intra-articular triamcinolone hexacetonide in the management of chronic arthritis in children. *Arthritis Rheum.* 1986; 29:997–1001.
35. Smythe H, Helewa A. Assessment of joint disease. In: Walker J, Helewa A, eds. *Physical Therapy in Arthritis.* Philadelphia, PA: W.B. Saunders; 1996: 129–148.
36. Gedalia A, Person DA, Brewer EJ, et al. Hypermobility of the joints in juvenile episodic arthritis/arthralgia. *J Pediatr.* 1985;107(6):873–876.
37. Emery HM, Bowyer SL, Sisung CE. Rehabilitation of the child with a rheumatic disease. *Pediatr Clin North Am.* 1995;42(5): 1263–1285.
38. Giannini MJ, Protas EJ. Comparison of peak isometric knee extensor torque in children with and without juvenile rheumatoid arthritis. *Arthritis Care Res.* 1993;6:82–88.
39. Vostrejs M, Hollister JR, Bowyer S. Quadriceps muscle function after recovery from monoarticular JRA: Follow-up with physical therapy intervention. *Arthritis Care Res.* 1989;2:S16.
40. Klepper S, Darbee J, Effgen S, et al. Physical fitness in children with polyarticular juvenile rheumatoid arthritis. *Arthritis Care Res.* 1992;5(2):93–100.
41. Florence J, Pandya S, King W, et al. Intrarater reliability of manual muscle test (Medical Research Council Scale) grades in Duchenne's muscular dystrophy. *Phys Ther.* 1992;72(2):115–126.
42. Stuberg WA, Metcalf WK. Reliability of quantitative muscle testing in healthy children and in children with Duchenne muscular dystrophy using a hand-held dynamometer. *Phys Ther.* 1988;68: 977–982.
43. Kraemer WJ, Fleck SJ. *Strength Training for Young Athletes.* Champaign, IL: Human Kinetics; 1993.
44. Giannini MJ, Protas EJ. Aerobic capacity in juvenile rheumatoid arthritis patients and healthy children. *Arthritis Care Res.* 1992;4:131–135.
45. McSwegin P, Pemberton C, Petray C, et al. *Physical Best: Instructors Guide.* Reston, VA: American Alliance for Health, Physical Education, Recreation, and Dance; 1989.
46. Lechner D, McCarthy C, Holden M. Gait deviations in patients with juvenile rheumatoid arthritis. *Phys Ther.* 1987;67:1335–1341.
47. Spraul G, Koenning G. A descriptive study of foot problems with juvenile rheumatoid arthritis (JRA). *Arthritis Care Res.* 1994;7(3):144–150.
48. Wright V. Evaluation of gait using footprint analysis: Demonstration of a practical technique for assessment of children with arthritis. Presented at the 31st National Meeting, Association of Rheumatology Health Professionals, Orlando, FL; 1996.
49. Laaksonen AL, Laine V. A comparative study of joint pain in adult and juvenile rheumatoid arthritis. *Ann Rheum Dis.* 1961;20:386–387.
50. Lovell DJ, Walco GA. Pain associated with juvenile rheumatoid arthritis. *Pediatr Clin North Am.* 1989;36(4):1015–1027.
51. Varni JW, Thompson KL, Hanson V. The Varni/Thompson pediatric pain questionnaire: I. Chronic musculoskeletal pain in juvenile rheumatoid arthritis: An empirical model. *Pain.* 1987;28: 27–38.
52. Melzack R. The McGill pain questionnaire: Major properties and scoring methods. *Pain.* 1975;1: 277–299.
53. Wilkie DJ, Holzemer WI, Tesler MD, et al. Measuring pain quality: Validity and reliability of children's and adolescents' pain language. *Pain.* 1990;41:151–159.
54. Savedra MC, Tesler MD, Holzemer WL, et al. Pain location: Validity and reliability of body outline markings by hospitalized children and adolescents. *Res Nurs Health.* 1989;12:307–314.
55. Haley SM, Coster WJ, Fass RM. A content validity study of the Pediatric Evaluation of Disability Inventory. *Pediatric Phys Ther.* 1991;3:177–189.
56. Howe S, Levinson JL, Shear E, et al. Development of a disability tool for juvenile rheumatoid arthritis: The Juvenile Arthritis Functional Assessment Report for children and their parents. *Arthritis Rheum.* 1991;34:873–880.
57. Singh G, Athreya B, Fries J, et al. Measurement of health status in juvenile rheumatoid arthritis. *Arthritis Rheum.* 1994;37:1761–1769.
58. Wright V, Law M, Crombe V, et al. Development of a Self-Report Functional Status Index for juvenile rheumatoid arthritis. *J Rheumatol.* 1994;21: 536–544.
59. Wright V, Longo Kimber J, Law M, et al. The Juvenile Arthritis Functional Status Index (JASI): A validation study. *J Rheumatol.* 1996;23:1066–1079.
60. Murray KJ, Passo MH. Functional measures in children with rheumatic diseases. *Pediatr Clin North Am.* 1995;42(5):1127–1154.
61. National Advisory Board on Medical Rehabilitation Research, *Draft V: Report and Plan for Medical*

Rehabilitation Research. Bethesda, MD: National Institutes of Health; 1992.
62. Michlovitz S. *Thermal Agents in Rehabilitation.* Philadelphia: F.A., Davis; 1986;258–274.
63. Brewer EJ. Reduction of morning stiffness and/or morning pain using a sleeping bag. *Pediatrics.* 1975;56:621.
64. Emery HM, Bowyer SL. Physical modalities of therapy. In: Athreya B, ed. *Rheum Dis Clin North Am.* 1991;17(4):1001–1014.
65. Harris ED, McCroskey PS. The influence of temperature and fibril stability on degradation of cartilage collagen by rheumatoid synovial collagenase. *N Engl J Med.* 1974;290:1–6.
66. Zisken MC, McDiarmid T, Michlovitz S. Therapeutic ultrasound. In: Michlovitz S, ed. *Thermal Agents in Rehabilitation.* 2nd ed. Philadelphia: F.A. Davis; 1990:134–169.
67. Helewa A. Physical therapy management of patients with rheumatoid arthritis and other inflammatory conditions. In: Walker J, Helewa A, eds. *Physical Therapy in Arthritis.* Philadelphia: W.B. Saunders; 1996:245–263.
68. Lavigne JV, Ross CK, Barry SL, et al. Evaluation of a psychological treatment package for treating pain in juvenile rheumatoid arthritis. *Arthritis Care Res.* 1992;5(2):101–110.
69. Walco GA, Varni J, Hartstein G, et al. Cognitive-behavioral interventions for pain in children with juvenile rheumatoid arthritis: A preliminary report. Presented at the Joint Meeting of the Canadian and American Pain Societies, Toronto; 1988.
70. Bohannon RW. Effect of repeated eight-minute muscle loading on the angle of straight leg raising. *Phys Ther.* 1984;64(4):491–497.
71. Godges JJ, MacRae PG, Engelke KA. Effects of exercise on hip range of motion, trunk muscle performance, and gait economy. *Phys Ther.* 1993;73(4): 468–477.
72. Donovan WH. Physical measures in the treatment of juvenile rheumatoid arthritis. *Arthritis Rheum.* 1977;20:533–577.
73. Fleck S, Kraemer W. *Designing Resistance Training Programs.* Champaign, IL: Human Kinetics; 1987.
74. Krebs DE, Elbaum L, O'Riley P, et al. Exercise and gait effects on in vivo hip contact pressures. *Phys Ther.* 1990;71:301–309.
75. James MJ, Cleland LG, Gaffrey RD, et al. Effect of exercise on ^{99m}Tc-STPA clearance from knees with effusions. *J Rheumatol.* 1994;21:501–504.
76. Minor M. *Clinical Care in the Rheumatic Diseases.* Atlanta: American College of Rheumatology; 1996.
77. Ekdahl C, Andersson S, Moritz U, et al. Dynamic versus static training in patients with rheumatoid arthritis. *Scand J Rheumatol.* 1990;19: 17–26.
78. Gordon N. *Arthritis: Your Complete Exercise Guide.* Champaign, IL: Human Kinetics; 1993.
79. Moncur C, Marcus R, Johnson S. Pilot project of aerobic conditioning of subjects with juvenile arthritis. (Abstract). *Arthritis Care Res.* 1990; 3(suppl):S16.
80. Klepper S, Effgen S, Athreya B, et al. Effects of an 8 week physical conditioning program on the signs and symptoms of chronic arthritis in children. *Arthritis Rheum.* 1996;30(9):S1716.
81. Williams J, Eaton R, Stretch C. Use of the rating of perceived exertion to control exercise intensity in children. *Pediatric Exer Sci.* 1991;3:21–27.
82. Klepper S, Giannini MJ. Physical conditioning in children with arthritis: Assessment and guidelines for exercise prescription. *Arthritis Care Res.* 1994; 7(4):226–236.
83. Scull SA, Athreya B. Childhood arthritis. In: Goldberg B, ed. *Sports and Exercise for Children with Chronic Health Conditions.* Champaign, IL: Human Kinetics; 1995:135–148.
84. Carmen D. *Where are the Indians? An Exercise Video for Children.* Dallas: Scottish Rite Hospital for Children; 1991.
85. ROM Institute: *ROM Dance: A Range of Motion Exercise and Relaxation Program.* Madison, WI. ROM Institute New Ventures of Wisconsin, Inc.
86. Arthritis Foundation. *People with Arthritis Can Exercise (PACE).* Atlanta: Arthritis Foundation; 1987.
87. ARTC: *Good Moves for Everybody.* Exercise videotape. Columbia, MO: Arthritis Rehabilitation Research and Training Center.
88. Carmen D, Browne R. Joint protection education for children with arthritis: Can handouts replace professional instruction? *Arthritis Rheum.* 1996; 39(7):S1714.
89. Whitehouse R, Shape J, Sullivan D, et al. Children with juvenile rheumatoid arthritis at school. *Clin Pediatr.* 1989;28:509–514.
90. Stoff E, Bacon M, White P. The effects of fatigue, distractibility, and absenteeism on school achievement in children with rheumatic disease. *Arthritis Care Res.* 1989;2:54–59.
91. Atwood M. Treatment considerations. In: Melvin J, ed. *Rheumatic Disease in Adult and Child: Occupational Therapy and Rehabilitation.* 3rd Ed. Philadelphia: F.A. Davis ; 1989:215–234.
92. Arthritis Foundation. *Educational Rights for Children with Arthritis: A Manual for Parents.* Ameri-

can Juvenile Arthritis Organization. Atlanta: Arthritis Foundation; 1989.

93. Hyman BS, Gregg JR. Arthroplasty of the hip and knee in juvenile rheumatoid arthritis. *Rheum Dis Clin North Am.* 1991;17:971–983.

94. McCullough CJ. Surgical management of the hip in juvenile chronic arthritis. *Br J Rheumatol.* 1991;33:178–183.

95. Swann M. The surgery of juvenile chronic arthritis. *Clin Orthop Rel Res.* 1990;259:70–75.

96. Salter RB. The biologic concept of continuous passive motion of synovial joints: The first 18 years of basic research and its clinical application. *Clin Orthop.* 1989;242:21–25.

97. Jacobson ST, Levinson JE, Crawford AH. Late results of synovectomy in juvenile rheumatoid arthritis. *J Bone Joint Surg.* 1985;85:8–15.

98. Scull S. Juvenile rheumatoid arthritis. In: Campbell S, ed. *Physical Therapy for Children.* Philadelphia: W.B. Saunders; 1994:207–225.

99. Richlerman I, Keenan MA. Surgical interventions. In: Walker J, Helewa A, eds. *Physical Therapy in Arthritis.* Philadelphia: W.B. Saunders; 1996; 95–112.

100. Rocky Mountain Juvenile Arthritis Center. *JRA & Me.* Rocky Mountain Juvenile Arthritis Center at the National Center for Immunology and Respiratory Medicine; 1987.

Rehabilitation of the Child with Burns

Laurie Grigsby de Linde

The purpose of this chapter is to provide a basic description of pediatric burn care and to discuss the role of the therapist in the treatment of the child with burns—from the acute phase through the rehabilitation phase, with emphasis on the latter.

It frequently has been said that children are not small adults. Certainly, the treatment that is appropriate for adults with burn injuries is not necessarily applicable to children with these same injuries and vice versa. Moreover, the treatment for a 9-month-old baby may differ from that for a 3-year-old child, which, in turn, may be different from the approach used for a 10-year-old child. The discussion in this chapter concerning therapy generally is limited to children younger than 12 years of age because children 12 and older are physiologically more similar to adults.

The role of the therapist is broadly addressed. The specific role of the therapist is defined, in part, by the individual setting and also may be dependent on the particular facility's medical and surgical techniques and approach.

Epidemiology, Etiology, and Prognosis

The exact number of burn injuries that occur each year in the United States is not known because there is no comprehensive system for gathering such data. However, estimates are based upon information collected by several voluntary registries and compiled by surveys.

Each year, approximately 1.25 million people in the United States seek medical attention for burns or have at least one-half day of restricted activity because of a burn injury.[1] Approximately 250,000 children aged birth to 17 years were treated for burns.[2] Most burn injuries occur at home and are treated on an outpatient basis.[3] However, 15,000 children are hospitalized each year with burn injuries. About 5500 people die annually as a result of fires and burns, of which one-fifth are children.[2,4]

Preschoolers account for the highest age-specific incidence of burns and for 47% of all deaths in residential fires.[5] The leading cause of accidental death in the home for children ages 1 through 14 years is fires and burns.[6]

Most children, about 200,000, are burned by contact with hot substances and objects, with scalds from spilled food and beverages accounting for about 100,000 of these injuries, and scalds from hot tap water about 5000 of these injuries.[2] Contact with hot objects, such as curling irons, hair curlers, and ranges, comprise about 60,000 injuries.[2] Other frequent sources of burns to children are fireworks (3200), gasoline (1500), and cigarettes and other tobacco products (1500).[2]

According to one source[7] of burn statistics, scald burns are the most frequent type of burn injury for infants and toddlers, accounting for 72% of burns in this age group, whereas flame and contact burns represent 25% of the burn injuries for this group. A water temperature of 140°F can cause a deep partial-thickness to full-thickness burn in 3 seconds, and this same depth of injury can occur within 1 second when water is heated at 156°F.[8] Percolated coffee is 180°F, and hot grease or hot oil is approximately 400°F.[9] One can imagine in terms of pediatric development how scald injuries might easily occur, because children at these ages are learning to reach and grasp and to walk and climb.

The frequency of scald burns is decreased to 54% between 2 and 4 years of age, whereas flame burns are increased to 34%.[7] Most burn injuries in this age group occur as a result of play activities and include children beginning to experiment with matches and lighters.[7] In the 5- to 12-year and 13- to 18-year age groups, flame burns are the most prevalent type of burn injury.[7] In the former age group, children are most often burned by a fire near where they are playing or standing.[7] Adolescents in the latter age group are often burned during a variety of activities, such as lighting fires, riding in or driving vehicles, and during cleaning or repair activities.[7]

A greater number of boys than girls are burned in all age groups.[7] Most burn incidents in very young children occur indoors while at home.[7] As the age of the child increases, burn injuries tend to happen outdoors, both at and away from home.[7] There is an increase in the number of vehicular and work-related burn injuries during adolescence.[7] For all age groups, the kitchen is the most common place for burn injury.[7] In younger children, this is followed by the bathroom, whereas for older children, the yard is the next most likely site of injury.[7]

Persons 5 to 34 years of age have the best survival rates.[7] Older children have a better survival rate than younger children, and the survival rate becomes progressively worse as age decreases.[7] As one might expect, mortality increases with severity (extent and depth) of injury.

Child Abuse and Neglect

Ten percent of all physical child abuse is by burning.[10] Approximately 2% of all pediatric burns are intentional.[11] According to one source, child abuse or flagrant neglect accounts for 20% to 30% of all pediatric burn admissions.[12]

Blakeney and Herndon,[13] citing over a dozen authors or studies, list the following as indicators of child abuse. Although any one indicator should arouse suspicion, the presence of two or more has been found to identify 60% of abusive situations, according to other authors.[14]

- Child is brought for treatment by an unrelated adult
- An unexplained delay of 12 or more hours in seeking treatment
- Inappropriate parental affect: parent(s) appear inattentive to child; lack empathy; may appear to be under the influence of alcohol or drugs
- Attribution of guilt for injury to the patient's sibling or to the patient
- An injury that is inconsistent with the description of the injury
- History of injury that is inconsistent with the developmental capacity of the patient
- Prior history of accidental or nonaccidental injury to the patient or siblings
- Prior history of failure to thrive
- Historical accounts of the injury that differ with each interview
- Injury localized to genitalia, perineum, and buttocks (because of frequency with which injury occurs related to toilet training)
- "Mirror image" injury of extremities (Fig. 13-1)
- Inappropriate affect of child; child appears withdrawn with flattened affect
- Evidence of unrelated injuries, for example, scars, bruises, welts, fractures

All states have laws requiring that certain professionals, including physical therapists and occupational therapists, report suspected cases of child abuse. However, such reporting is often done by another professional, such as a physician or social worker.

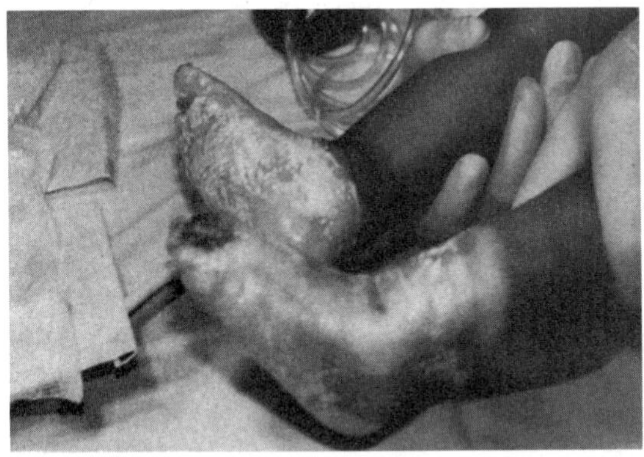

Figure 13-1 ■ Acute, circumferential, mostly full-thickness burns of both feet in a "sock" pattern, sustained by a child younger than 1 year of age. Child abuse was suspected. (Note: To help decrease pain and to limit the time of wound exposure, the topical antimicrobial agent has been applied to gauze instead of directly on the patient, and the dressing to be applied has been prepared before the old bandage is removed.)

Prevention

Because of the high incidence and common pattern of distribution of types of burn injuries among children of various age groups, prevention efforts have been directed toward educating parents, children, and others as to how these injuries occur and how they can be prevented. Several suggestions for preventing pediatric burn injuries include the following:

- Lowering water heater temperature settings to 124°F or lower
- Keeping cords to coffee pots and cups with hot liquids out of reach of young children
- Keeping young children in a safe place during food preparation and serving
- Turning pot handles toward the back of the stove and cooking on rear burners when possible
- Supervising children in the bathtub and testing bathwater with a liquid crystal thermometer before placing the child in the tub

- Keeping young children in a safe place when using appliances such as a clothes iron or curling iron, and allowing these items to cool while out of the reach of children
- Placing safety caps on electrical outlets
- Teaching children that matches are tools, not toys
- Teaching older children and adolescents about the dangers of high-voltage wires and about the dangers of and safe use of gasoline and other flammable liquids
- Teaching children about the dangers of fireworks

Additionally, other prevention efforts have focused on federal regulations mandating the use of flame-retardant fabrics and materials in such articles as children's sleepwear and mattresses to help decrease the number and severity of burns resulting from the ignition of these items. In April 1996, the Consumer Product Safety Commission relaxed the standard for children's sleepwear flammability, which became effective January 1, 1997. The change allows the sale of tight-fitting sleepwear and infant sleepwear for those 9 months and younger even if the clothing does not meet the flammability standard previously applicable.[15] Efforts are focused on the development of a safer child-resistant cigarette lighter design, a "fire-safe" cigarette standard, and eventual laws promoting the sale of such, and there are endeavors in some local communities to support legislation requiring that home water heaters have a maximum temperature setting.

Structure and Functions of the Skin

The skin, like the heart and lungs, is a vital organ of the body. In fact, it is the largest organ of the body, varying in thickness from 0.5 mm in the eyelids to 4 mm in the palms and soles.[16] The skin is composed of the more superficial and thinner (20 to 400 μ) layer, the epidermis, and of the deeper and thicker (440 to 2500 μ[17]) layer, the dermis. In the basal layer of the epidermis are granules of melanin that give skin its color.[16] The dermis is vascular, and the epidermis, although avascular, has its deeper layers nourished by fluid from the dermis (Fig. 13-2).[16] Contained in the skin are sweat glands, hair follicles, sebaceous glands, and on the fingers and toes, nails. Sensory nerves and sympathetic fibers to vessels, to arrector pili muscles, and to sweat glands abound in the skin.[16] The skin helps regulate body temperature, preserves body fluids, protects against infection (by serving as a barrier and also by having certain bactericidal abilities), protects against radiation, and acts as a barrier to help protect vital organs and other body structures against external objects and fluids. Because of nerve endings that sense touch, pain, and temperature, the skin aids in both protective and discriminatory sensation. The skin also assists in vitamin D production. The skin, along with its appendages, can help reveal an individual's race, age, sex, and health. Ridges in the skin on the fingertips give each person a unique set of fingerprints. The skin on the face, with fluctuations in blood flow (e.g., blushing) and with the action of the underlying muscles, can express an individual's emotions.

Whenever the skin is significantly damaged or destroyed, these functions may become impaired. Because the skin is an organ, when the skin is damaged or destroyed, there are not only local but also systemic effects.

Classification of Burns

Burns can be classified by depth, by size (percentage of body surface area [BSA] burned), and by causative agent, or they can be classified as minor, moderate, or major for purposes of triage.

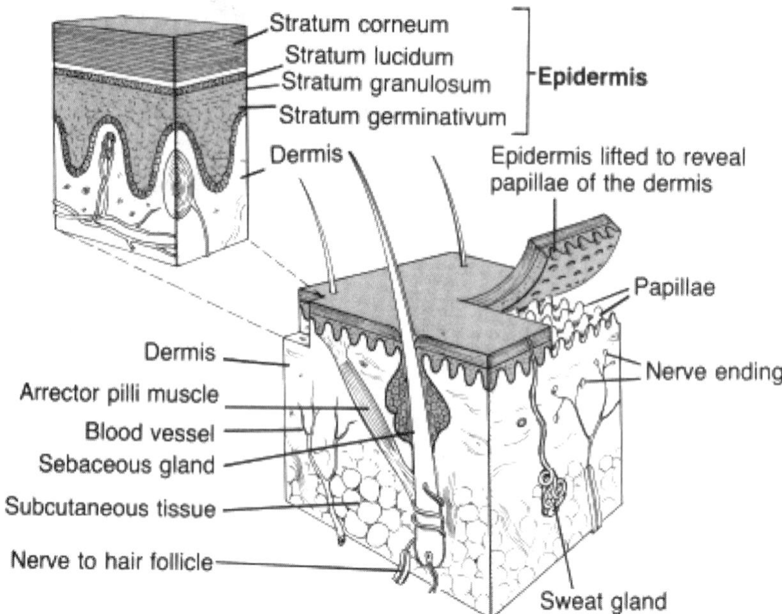

Figure 13-2 ▪ Anatomy of the skin. (From Rosdahl CB. *Textbook of Basic Nursing*. 5th ed. Philadelphia: JB Lippincott; 1991:117.)

Depth

Burns can be classified according to the depth of skin damaged or destroyed (Fig. 13-3). They are variously classified as partial-thickness burns (formerly known as first-degree and second-degree burns) or as full-thickness burns (previously referred to as third-degree burns). Partial-thickness burns can be either superficial or deep. Superficial partial-thickness burns involve the epidermis and the upper portion of the dermal papillae. They are painful, appear red, and

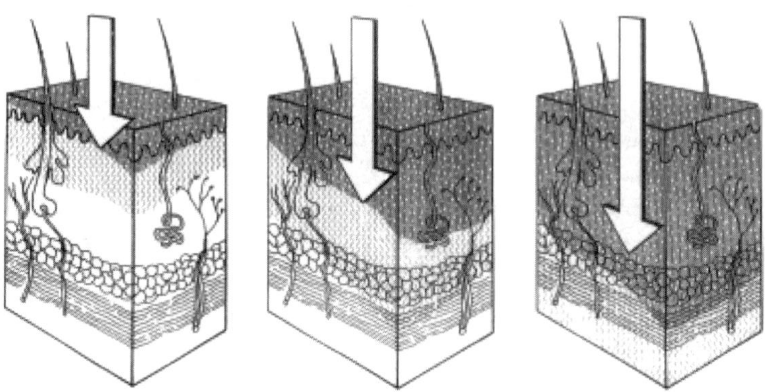

Figure 13-3 ▪ Diagram of depth of burn: partial thickness, superficial (left); partial thickness, deep (center); full thickness (right).

frequently present with blisters. Superficial partial-thickness burns will heal in about 2 weeks or less without scarring.

Deep partial-thickness burns injure the dermis. They are waxy-white in appearance and are pliable. Such burns may be insensitive to light touch but painful to deep pressure. If they become infected, dry out, or have impaired circulation, deep partial-thickness burns can convert to full-thickness wounds. Deep-partial thickness burns will heal spontaneously by epithelial cells from remaining dermal appendages, but the time required for healing may be 3 to 6 weeks or longer, and such burns heal with scar tissue that can hypertrophy and contract. Although deep partial-thickness burns will heal spontaneously without skin grafting, because of the prolonged healing time and frequently poor functional and cosmetic outcome, as well as other reasons listed later, many surgeons elect to excise and graft these wounds when possible and indicated.

Full-thickness burns, by definition, destroy the full thickness of the skin. Such burns can appear as cherry red, white, or brown and leathery; and thrombosed veins may be visible. Hairs can be easily extracted owing to the death of hair follicles. Because the nerves have been destroyed, full-thickness burns are anesthetic to touch. (This does not mean that there is no pain associated with such burns. Activation of the nerves around the periphery of the burn, exposure of the wound to air by removal of dead tissue, or manipulation of the wound can cause extreme pain.[18]) Full-thickness burns will not heal without skin grafting. Even with skin grafting, such burns may result in scar contraction and hypertrophy. Electrical burns often damage muscle, nerve, and bone; histiologically they resemble crush injuries. Treatment of these injuries often varies from that of other burns, and so will not be dealt with in this chapter.

The actual depth of injury may not be accurately or easily determined on the first day, even by the most experienced surgeon. Burn injuries frequently present with varying depths of involvement and usually are not of uniform depth; such factors as how the injury occurred, the thickness of body skin in the area of the burn, and whether or not the individual was wearing clothes have a bearing on the depth of injury. The skin of infants and young children is thinner than that of adults, so, for example, a hot liquid that would cause a superficial, partial-thickness burn in an adult may cause a deeper injury in an infant or toddler. Knowing the depth of the burn is important in determining triage, resuscitation, wound care and closure, and prognosis.

Size

Burns are also classified according to size or total percent of body surface area (TBSA) burned. The TBSA is counted as 100%. The palm of an individual's hand is estimated to be about 1% of the TBSA. Frequently, for adults, the "Rule of Nines" is used to calculate the TBSA burned. According to this rule, in an adult, the head represents 9% of the TBSA, each upper extremity counts as 9%, the trunk represents 36%, each lower extremity represents 18%, and the genitalia is assigned 1%. However, a child's head (especially that of a baby) is larger in proportion to the body than an adult's head is, and a child's lower extremities are smaller in proportion to the body than an adult's lower extremities are to the body. For example, the head of a baby who is younger than 1 year of age is counted as 18%, whereas each lower extremity represents 13.5%. Because of such differences, modified versions of the "Rule of Nines" are used to calculate the TBSA burned in children. One such pediatric burn extent assessment chart has been developed by Lund and Browder.[19] Estimating the TBSA burned is important in determining triage of the patient, figuring fluid resuscitation and nutritional needs, planning wound closure, and predicting prognosis.

Causative Agent

A third way of classifying burns is according to the causative agent or method: scald, contact, flash, flame, chemical, radiation, or electrical. Knowing the causative agent or method can be important in giving appropriate treatment. For example, if an individual sustains a chemical burn, knowing which chemical caused the burn is necessary in order to apply the correct antidote and in determining the need for copious water lavage, which would not necessarily be done for an electrical burn or a flame burn.

Minor, Moderate, and Major Classifications

Burns also can be classified as minor, moderate, or major according to guidelines established by the American Burn Association (ABA) for purposes of triage. For example, a minor burn for an adult might be a partial-thickness burn involving less than 15% of the TBSA; such a patient could be treated as an outpatient. A minor burn for a child might be a partial-thickness burn involving less than 10% of the TBSA, but hospitalization might be considered for such a patient. The ABA recommends that an individual with a major burn be admitted or transferred to a burn center.

BURN CENTER

In 1990, the ABA published guidelines for the development and operation of burn centers,[20] defined as "a service system based in a hospital that has made the institutional commitment to meet the criteria specified in this guide."[20] Although these guidelines were not applied to the hospitals that responded to a survey to be included in the ABA's *Burn Care Resources in North America 1996–1997* directory, the directory lists 135 hospitals in the United States with burn services. Of these, at least 15 are exclusively pediatric facilities.

BURN TEAM

In its guidelines for burn centers, the ABA specifies which personnel should staff the burn center, as well as which specialists and personnel should be on call or available for consultation. (The criteria state that "Both physical and occupational therapy should be represented in the burn center staff.") Within the ABA guidelines, each burn center establishes its own burn team. Personnel who comprise the burn team and their specific roles may vary from institution to institution or according to the individual needs of a given patient or the particular phase of healing, although there generally is a core team. The pediatric burn team frequently includes a surgeon, nurse, occupational therapist, physical therapist, social worker, respiratory therapist, dietitian, child life therapist, hospital chaplain, discharge planner, various specialists (pediatrician, pulmonologist, psychiatrist, plastic surgeon, infection control specialist, etc.), and most importantly, the child and family. Because many children do not have a traditional nuclear family, it is often necessary to determine who, in the child's view, comprises the family.

Scar Hypertrophy and Contraction

As previously mentioned, there are two common, though often avoidable, sequelae of deep partial-thickness and full-thickness burns: scar hypertrophy and scar contraction. Scar hypertrophy and scar contracture can impede both physical and psychological functioning. *Scar hypertrophy* is a raised, thick, usually hard, often knotty-appearing, area of scar tissue (Fig. 13-4; see Figs. 13-5 and 13-9). Scar hypertrophy results from an imbalance of collagen synthesis and collagen lysis. Hypertrophic scars are, at times, also called keloids, although some investigators distinguish between the two. Although debate persists concerning the distinction be-

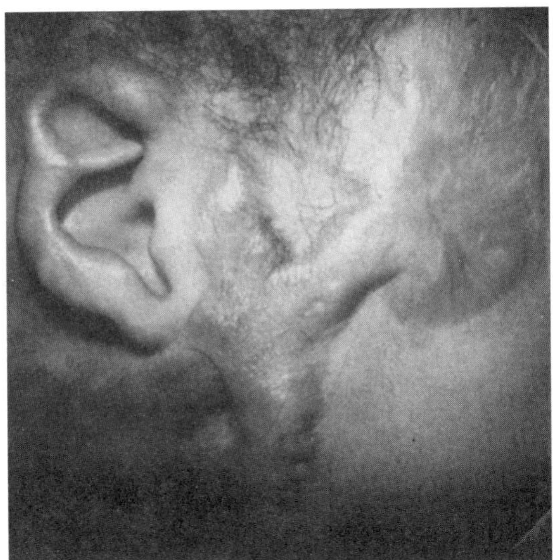

Figure 13-4 ▪ Scar hypertrophy of a healed, ungrafted, deep, partial-thickness burn of the face.

tween hypertrophic scars and keloids. Linares, in a review of the controversy, concluded that keloids are only extreme variants of hypertrophic scars.[21]

To determine which variables might be predictors for the development of hypertrophic scarring, Deitch et al. considered such factors as the race and age of the patient, the location of the burn, and the length of time before the (ungrafted) burn was healed. The investigation concluded that the length of time required to heal the burn was the most important indicator. One-third of the anatomic sites became hypertrophic if the burns healed between 14 and 21 days. If healing occurred after 21 days, hypertrophic scar incidence increased to 78%.[22] African Americans in the study had a greater incidence of hypertrophic scarring than others if the burn took more than 10 to 14 days to heal. The investigators attributed the increased incidence of hypertrophic scars in certain anatomic sites to wound tension. Another investigator[23] has also concurred that increased tension, which promotes collagen deposition and lessens collagen lysis, may contribute to the formation of hypertrophic scars, evidenced by the appearance of hypertrophic scars in areas of motion, such as the joints (Fig. 13-5). The authors of the first-mentioned study, citing other investors,[24] also acknowledge that the depth of the wound is related to the incidence of hypertrophic scarring because burns of the reticulodermis are likely to heal with a hypertrophic scar, whereas more superficial burns involving the papillary dermis do not. However, these authors report that it is more accurate to quantify length of healing time rather than to estimate the depth of the wound subjectively. In the study, the age of the patient was not found to correlate with an increased incidence of hypertrophic scarring. However, others[25,26] have suggested that younger patients may have an increased incidence of hypertrophic scars compared with other age groups, probably because of an increased rate of collagen production.

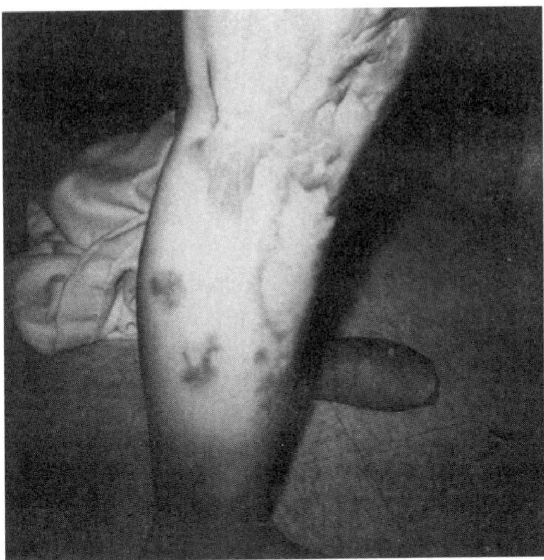

Figure 13-5 ▪ Scar hypertrophy of a healed, ungrafted, deep, partial-thickness burn of the right lower extremity. Note the increased hypertrophic scarring around the knee joint, which may be the result of increased tension-promoting collagen deposition and lessening collagen lysis.

Scar contraction is the pulling or shortening of scar tissue, which can result in the loss of joint motion or skin mobility. Scar contracture is a fixed shortening of the scar tissue that may be amenable only to surgery. Contraction may be attributed to myofibroblasts, cells that have contractile properties, and are found in the healing burn wound. Scar contraction that is not located over a joint can lead to disfigurement, especially if such contraction involves the face. Scar contraction over a joint can lead to loss of joint range of motion (ROM) or posture and gait deviations (Fig. 13-6). Because of the contracting force of scar, which results in loss of skin mobility, a loss of joint ROM also can result from contracting scar tissue that is adjacent to, although not covering, a joint (Fig. 13-7). The scar will contract until it meets an equal or opposing force.[29] What is initially just loss of motion from contracting scar can, if left uncorrected, lead to a gradual shortening of joint capsules, muscles, tendons, and ligaments. A contracting scar in an adult may not cause any loss of motion, whereas that same size scar in a small child may cause a loss of motion.[28]

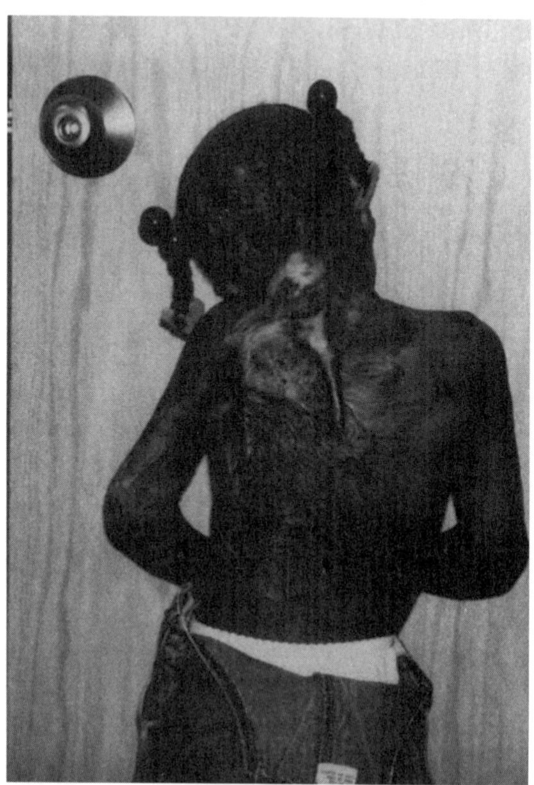

Figure 13-6 ▪ Severe scar contracture and hypertrophy resulting not only in disfigurement and loss of motion, but also affecting posture and ambulation.

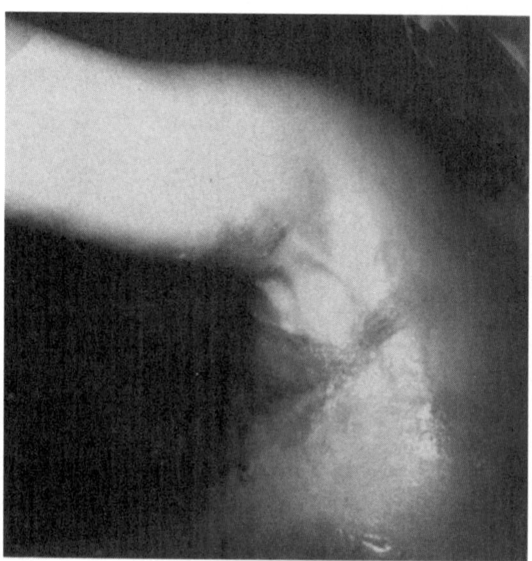

Figure 13-7 ▪ Scar contraction of the axilla in a child who sustained deep partial-thickness and full-thickness burns to the trunk and upper extremity. Sheet-grafting has been performed. Although the axilla itself was spared, contracting scar on both sides of the joint has resulted in a loss of motion.

The processes of scar contracture and hypertrophy begin almost as soon as the burn wound begins healing, although initially they may not be readily visible. Collagen formation begins within 24 hours of the burn injury.[21] There is a high rate of collagen synthesis in the wound,[29] and such activity returns to a normal pace by 6 to 12 months.[30] The scar is initially red because of an increased blood supply, but it usually fades over time. When the scar no longer is actively hypertrophying and contracting, it is said to be mature. The period of scar maturation for most children is approximately 12 to 18 months. For adults, this period may be shorter. While the scar is active, particularly during the first 6 months, the processes of hypertrophy and contraction can be controlled or corrected by nonsurgical approaches, such as pressure, splinting, and ROM exercises, which will be discussed later. As scar maturation progresses, these treatments become less effective in altering scar. After the scar is mature, most nonsurgical treatments are no longer effective, and surgery, if indicated, may afford the only treatment alternative.

Initial Treatment and Medical Management

The initial treatment and medical management of the pediatric burn patient depend, in part, on the depth, size, and location of the burn; the presence of other concomitant injuries, such as smoke inhalation; the age of the child; and the premorbid health of the child. The injury itself will trigger physiologic responses that, in turn, will affect treatment requirements.

Airway and Breathing

Establishing and maintaining an adequate airway and breathing are the first concerns when treating a thermally injured patient. If the patient has inhaled steam or noxious gases, intubation may be necessary because bronchospasm and upper airway edema[31] may develop, possibly resulting in airway obstruction within hours.[32] Oxygen is administered if the patient has inhaled high levels of carbon monoxide. The endotrachial tube may be removed once edema has subsided, usually within a few days.[31] Patients with more extensive airway or lung injuries will require sustained or more involved treatment.

When a patient's respiratory status is evaluated initially, cardiac hemodynamic status is also assessed, and the patient is examined for other injuries[33] such as fractures and lacerations. Prophylactic tetanus toxoid is administered to help prevent infections. A careful past medical history and a history of the burn incident are recorded. The wounds are evaluated, cleaned, and bandaged.

Fluid Resuscitation

Because of the inflammatory process and increased capillary permeability in patients with deep partial-thickness or full-thickness burns, fluid leaves the blood and is dispersed into the interstitial spaces. Patients with burns of less than 10% to 20% of their TBSA, depending on other considerations, may be able to compensate for this fluid shift physiologically through such measures as vasoconstriction and urine retention.[32] Patients with burns involving a greater percentage of TBSA will develop hypovolemic shock and can die if not treated. Replacement of the circulating fluid loss is termed fluid resuscitation. Fluids cannot be administered orally to patients with larger area burns because of ileus (obstruction of the bowel), which occurs secondary to shock. Fluids, with electrolytes similar to serum, and colloid are given intravenously. Patients with smaller burns may be able to take fluids orally. However, children, in particular, may be unwilling to drink and, therefore, may require intravenous fluids. In a few days, with adequate fluid replacement, the fluid in the interstitial spaces returns to the intravascular spaces, and the patient will diurese, signaling successful fluid resuscitation.[32] After fluid resuscitation, the patient may still require the administration of fluids because fluid is also lost through the burn wound and because the patient may be unwilling or unable to take sufficient fluids orally.

A urinary catheter is placed in patients with large burns so as to monitor urine output during resuscitation. Patients with perineal burns may also require catheterization to keep bandages dry or to protect newly placed skin grafts during the skin graft phase.

Escharotomy and Fasciotomy

Full-thickness burned skin is inelastic. Because of the body's response to injury and fluid resuscitation, the patient will become edematous. This is a systemic response that also occurs in the unburned parts of the body. In the case of circumferential burns of the extremities, the combination of inelastic skin and increasing edema can cause a tourniquet effect, resulting in compromised circulation to the distal extremities. If treatment is not initiated, ischemia and tissue damage or necrosis can occur. Monitoring of adequate circulation is usually accomplished by checking capillary refill in the fingers, by assessing the pulses through Doppler flowmetry, or in the case of extremely deep burns, by measuring muscle compartment pressures.[34] Investigators in a study of children who had escharotomies based on elevated compartment pressures found that 92% had intact peripheral pulses at the time of escharotomy. More than 75% of children required extension of the escharotomy to viable tissue or fascia because of continued elevated compartment pressures. The authors concluded that compartment pressure may be the only truly accurate method to determine circulatory compromise.[35]

When circulation is found to be compromised, an *escharotomy* is performed, which involves releasing the constricting inelastic burned skin by surgically incising it longitudinally down to subcutaneous fat on the midmedial and midlateral aspects of the limbs proximally to distally.[36] Escharotomy is usually performed within the first 24 to 48 hours of onset of the burn injury. Escharotomies may need to be performed on the chest to allow for adequate chest expansion and breathing in patients with deep circumferential burns of the trunk. Exercise and activities are permitted following escharotomy. When delayed escharotomy results in compartment syndrome, when deep burns involve muscle (as is often the case with electrical burn injuries), and when burns are accompanied by associated skeletal or soft tissue injury, the fascia will need to be released surgically,[36] a procedure termed a *fasciotomy.*

Nutrition

Initially, oral intake of fluids and food is prohibited in patients with larger burns in order to prevent the development of ileus. A nasogastric tube is inserted to empty the stomach to prevent vomiting and possible aspiration. Once bowel sounds return to normal, the patient can resume oral intake. In response to the burn injury, the patient is in a hypermetabolic state and caloric and nutritional requirements are greatly increased. Adequate nutrition is necessary to prevent wasting and to promote proper wound healing. The pediatric burn patient, because of the injury and a strange environment, may be unwilling to eat. The severity or location of the burns may make it difficult or impossible to eat. A patient with a larger burn may find it hard to consume the volume of food necessary to obtain sufficient calories. Additionally, the patient will be prohibited from eating on days when a surgical procedure is scheduled in the operating room. Because of such factors, the patient may receive a large portion of nutrition through enteral tube feedings or through peripheral vein infusions. Patients with smaller burns who are willing and able to eat may obtain all nutrition orally. When wound healing is complete, or following skin grafting procedures, if the patient is eating and drinking adequately, tube or parenteral feeds may be discontinued. The dietitian often instructs the parent in good nutritional practices before discharge.

Pain Management

A burn injury is one of the most painful events an individual can experience. In addition, the treatments administered, including some administered by the therapist, are themselves painful.

Sheridan et al. stated that poorly controlled pain and anxiety each has adverse psychological and physiologic effects that account for the 30% rate of posttraumatic stress disorder in individuals who suffer severe burns. They also contended that excessive pain and anxiety further fuels the hypermetabolic response by increasing the liberation of stress hormones.[37] Writing about the psychosocial care of the severely burned child, Knudson Cooper and Thomas[18] cite the following research to plead for adequate pain management of burn patients. Studies have shown that medical professionals who treat burn patients underrate the patients' pain when compared with the patients' own estimates of their pain.[38,39] Additionally, the first-mentioned authors state that medical personnel generally believe that babies and children may experience pain differently than do adolescents and adults, although there is no reason for them to believe that babies and children feel less pain.[40,41] In some facilities, children may not receive medication for acute pain![42] The child's pain and anxiety must be considered and treated appropriately throughout all phases of healing.

Pain management is essential for avoiding what would otherwise amount to torture and for enabling the patient to cooperate with treatment and to be involved in self-care. In addition to a variety of pharmacologic agents, relaxation techniques, hypnosis, and other methods of pain management can be employed effectively with children.[43] Besides specific medications and pain management techniques, the facility and each professional should have a treatment approach that has as a goal caring for the burn patient in a way that causes the least amount of pain. Some suggestions for minimizing patients' pain are made throughout the chapter.

Wound Management

The primary goals of wound management are to provide an optimal environment for wound healing, to provide a healthy tissue bed to receive a skin graft, and to protect healing tissue or a recently placed graft. Such goals are accomplished mainly through removing dead tissue, keeping the wound clean and minimizing bacterial invasion, preventing the wound or new skin graft from drying out, and protecting newly healing tissue or recent skin graft(s) from disruptive mechanical abrasion.

Dressing Changes

Many objectives of wound management are achieved through daily wound care and proper application and changing of bandages. Most burn patients will undergo bandage (also called dressing) changes at least daily. In some burn centers, therapists are responsible for or may assist with daily wound care for both inpatients and outpatients. (It may also be the case that the therapist, before or during performance of outpatient therapy, will need to change the patient's bandage.) During a dressing change, the old bandage is removed and the wound may be superficially débrided (nonviable tissue removed). At the same time, the wound is cleaned and examined, ROM is quickly checked (or the patient may be briefly exercised by the therapist), and a topical antimicrobial agent and clean gauze bandages are applied. There are other wound dressings that may be used depending on the extent and depth of injury, the phase of healing, and the protocol of a given burn center. For example, a biologic dressing, such as human cadaver skin (allograft) or pigskin (xenograft), or a biosynthetic dressing, may be placed on the wound. Enzymatic débriding agents, which break down the necrotic tissue without harming the intact tissue, may be placed on the wound.

A review of pediatric burn deaths shows that sepsis is a major contributing factor and that the wound is the primary source of infection.[44] In a burn injury, the protective barrier of the skin is lost, and the burn wound becomes a host for bacteria. Topical antimicrobials play a vital role in helping minimize bacterial colonization of the wound. Several topical antimicrobials may be employed depending on the specific wound and the organisms to be controlled.

Dressings should not excessively inhibit motion. The thumb, for example, should not be wrapped into the palm, nor should bandages restrict chest expansion. However, bandages can be used to help position the patient. For example, during the emergent phase (see later section), bulky bandages can be used in place of splints to support the fingers and wrists in infants and toddlers.

Despite pain medication, the daily dressing change is undoubtedly one of the most painful experiences that the burn patient must endure. There are measures that can minimize the pain and trauma of this event. The patient should be adequately medicated before the dressing change. The patient's response to the dose received should be monitored, and when possible, the physician should adjust the dose or select a different medication accordingly. Bandages that stick to the wound not only cause pain on removal but if they are "ripped off," some of the newly healed tissue may also be removed. When indicated, the bandage can be soaked off, or sterile water (not saline solution, which causes more pain) can be poured over the bandage to loosen it. Even very young children can participate in removing their dressings, which may help minimize pain and offer some sense of control and independence in a situation in which they might otherwise feel helpless. Because some of the pain experienced during a dressing change is caused by exposure of the wound to air, such exposure time should be limited. Limiting the exposure time to air will help prevent the tissue from drying out and will also limit exposure to bacteria. To minimize the time required for a dressing change, bandages should be prepared ahead of time so that they may be quickly applied. Health care professionals who wish to observe the patient's wound should be present at the time of the dressing change so that the patient is not waiting with an undressed wound for them to arrive. Additionally, applying the topical antimicrobial agent to the gauze and then applying the gauze to the wound (instead of applying the topical agent directly to the wound and then applying the gauze) will also help minimize pain during the dressing change.

Other measures may be helpful in minimizing pain and trauma during dressing changes in pediatric patients. Some of these include visualization and relaxation techniques, distraction techniques, and toys and music brought into the treatment room. If the parent desires, and if appropriate, the parent's presence during the dressing change can be beneficial for both the parent and the child. In some cases, however, children may cry more in the presence of a parent because they expect the parent to "rescue" them from the dressing change.

Hydrotherapy

Hydrotherapy is used in some burn centers as a part of wound management. The purpose of hydrotherapy is to help remove the old topical antimicrobial agent, to clean the wound, to help superficially débride the wound (through the effect of the agitator), to increase circulation in order to promote wound healing, and to provide an environment for exercise. The drawbacks of hydrotherapy are that it can spread infection; it can increase the length of time required for a dressing change; it can increase cost (because of the additional personnel required to perform the procedure and clean the equipment); it can increase edema (especially if a limb is placed in a dependent position); and patients, particularly children, may find it to be more traumatic or painful than a dressing change without hydrotherapy, thus making it an unsuitable environment for exercise. Because of the drawbacks of hydrotherapy, some burn centers limit is use to specific wounds or to certain phases of wound healing, or use hand-held showerheads to help clean the wound.

Surgical Management

One of the primary goals of the surgeon is to achieve permanent closure of the wound. Although there have been many advances in wound healing and surgical techniques in the past decade, an autograft is the most widely used method—and is considered to be the preferred permanent method—for wound closure. By definition, an autograft is a skin graft taken from and donated to the same individual. A detailed description of the autografting procedure is provided later in this chapter.

Because a superficial partial-thickness burn will heal in approximately 2 weeks with normal skin, the goals of the surgeon in such cases are to keep the wound free of infection, to provide adequate nutrition and fluids, and to manage pain until the wound is healed. Depending on the size and location of the superficial partial-thickness burn, the age of the patient, and the ability of the parent, many of these burns can be treated on an outpatient basis.

A deep-partial thickness burn can heal without surgical intervention if adequate medical treatment and wound management are provided. However, as discussed earlier, depending on the size of the wound, deep partial-thickness burns may take 3 to 6 weeks or longer to heal spontaneously. The surgeon may elect to graft the deep partial-thickness burn in a procedure called tangential excision and grafting. Such excision and grafting can be done within the first week of the burn injury and is ideally performed 2 to 5 days after the burn injury (termed *early excision and grafting*). Early excision and grafting may also apply to other wounds, particularly full-thickness wounds, which may be excised to fascia. Tangential excision and grafting of deep partial-thickness wounds during the first week shortens the patient's hospital stay, lessens pain, decreases the incidence of infection, improves cosmetic and functional outcome (by minimizing the amount of hypertrophic scar tissue development and scar contraction), and decreases the need for subsequent reconstructive procedures.[45,46]

There are drawbacks associated with early tangential excision and grafting of deep partial-thickness wounds, however, and not all patients are candidates for this procedure. Early excision and grafting of deep partial-thickness burns usually involves significant intraoperative blood loss that may require substantial transfusion; this may not be recommended for medically unstable patients or those with inhalation injury. When a burn involves a significant percentage of TBSA, and particularly when the burn area consists of both deep partial-thickness and full-thickness burns and there is a limited number of donor sites for skin grafts, excision and grafting of deep partial-thickness burns is generally delayed or such wounds are allowed to heal spontaneously. This is because the full-thickness burns have to be grafted first. Deep partial-thickness burns can be grafted after the first 3 to 5 days. However, the later such wounds are grafted, the more likely the wound is to be colonized by bacteria, and some other benefits of early excision may be diminished.

Smaller deep partial-thickness burns that are to be grafted can be treated on an outpatient basis for several days until the patient is admitted to the hospital for grafting or until the surgeon determines that the wound is indeed deep partial-thickness and would be treated best by excision and grafting.

A full-thickness burn, by definition, destroys the full thickness of the skin. Usually, the only way for such burns to heal is for the dead tissue to be removed and a skin graft to be applied. However, full-thickness burns that are small or narrow and are located over certain anatomic surfaces can be excised and closed primarily. ("Fourth-degree" burns, which involve subcutaneous fat, fascia, muscle, or bone, may also require local or regional flaps for definitive coverage.[47])

Skin Graft and Donor Site

A *skin graft* is a piece of skin that is surgically shaved from an unburned part of the patient's body (called the donor site) and placed on the burned area. Obviously, if a full-thickness piece of skin from the unburned donor site were taken and placed on the burned area, the burn would heal, but a wound of similar dimensions to the burn would remain at the donor site. Therefore, only a partial- or split-thickness (approximately 0.008-inch thick[48]) piece of skin is taken. Some areas of the body are preferred donor sites because of the thickness, texture, or color of the skin, because they are areas that will heal well, and also because they are in a region not usually visible. Common preferred donor sites include the lateral thighs and buttocks. However, when these areas are burned, or in an extensively burned individual, almost any skin on the body can be used.

Before the skin graft can be placed, the burned, necrotic skin, called *eschar,* must be removed. This is usually accomplished surgically, but enzymatic débriders may also be used on partial-thickness wounds. Surgical excision usually extends down to a level of viable tissue. Excision can be effected immediately before placing the skin graft, or, depending on the depth and extent of the wound, it may be accomplished earlier, in a separate operation. If a full-thickness wound is not grafted during the same procedure, granulation tissue will develop that will help prepare the site for grafting.

Once the patient has been anesthetized, the skin is shaved from the donor site with an electric knife—known as a dermatome—that has settings to adjust the thickness of skin excised. Removal of the skin that is to be used for grafting is called *harvesting.* The procedure is called a sheet graft when the skin is placed "as is" on the excised burned area (also known as the recipient or graft site) (Figs. 13-8 and 13-9; see Fig. 13-7). Alternatively, the skin may be placed in a skin mesher before its application to the recipient site. The mesher cuts small slits in the graft, after which the graft is stretched or expanded before placement on the recipient site. Such a graft is known as an *expanded mesh graft* (Fig. 13-10). The main purpose of meshing is to allow a skin graft to cover a larger area than

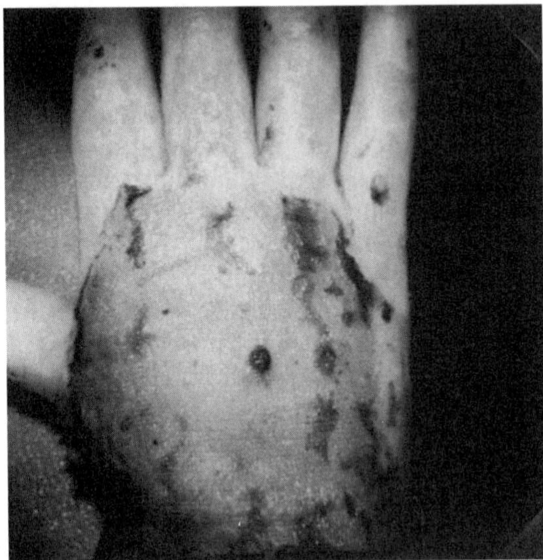

Figure 13-8 ▪ Sheet graft of the dorsum of the hand (wrist to metacarpophalangeal joints) approximately 5 to 7 days after graft application. This patient can now be measured for commercially available, custom-fitting elastic pressure garments, and may be ready for light-pressure dressings worn over bandages.

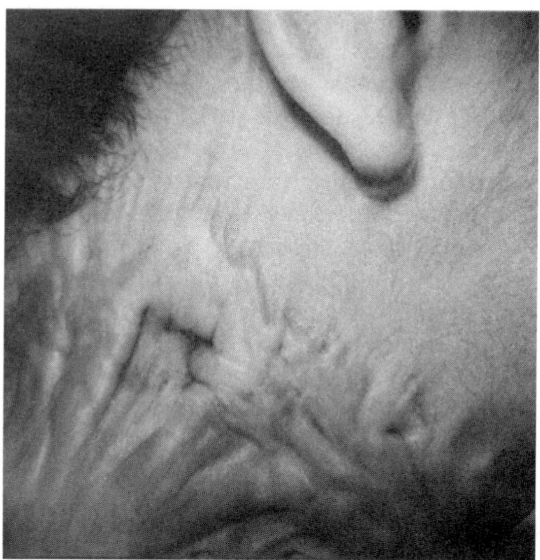

Figure 13-9 ■ Sheet graft of the neck. Note the hypertrophic scarring and contraction of the borders of the graft and of the healed, ungrafted areas. Note also the contraction under the graft.

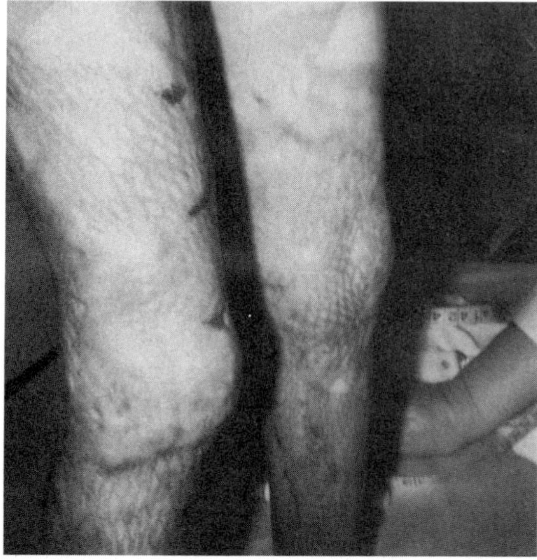

Figure 13-10 ■ Healed meshed grafts of the lower extremities. (Marks are soluble ink used in the measurement of this patient for custom-made pressure garments.)

could otherwise be covered using a sheet graft. The amount of expansion achieved is expressed as a ratio of the expanded to the unexpanded size. For example, an expanded mesh graft that covers one and a half times its original or unmeshed size would be referred to as a 1.5:1 mesh graft. One advantage of a mesh graft is that compared with a sheet graft, there is less likelihood that hematomas or serous fluid will collect under the graft, causing the graft to be nonadherent. A disadvantage of a mesh graft, particularly a large-ratio mesh graft, is that scarring occurs within the interstices or holes and such scarring can hypertrophy and contract. The permanent meshed pattern of the graft may also be cosmetically unattractive. Because sheet grafts provide a better cosmetic outcome with less contraction and hypertrophy, they are the graft of choice in burns involving less than 30% of TBSA that are not excessively colonized by bacteria and other microbes.[49] Sheet grafts should also be used on the face, neck, and hands, and are often preferred, when possible, for other functional areas of the body, such as the feet and the axillae.

The surgeon may secure the graft with surgical staples, stitches, or Steri-strips. The graft usually requires 4 to 7 days to become adherent or to "take." The grafted area is protected during this period by bulky dressings. If the graft site is over a joint, the joint is usually immobilized with a splint during this initial period, and exercise of the joint is discontinued for that same period. Movement or shearing forces can result in graft loss. Other factors that can contribute to graft loss or less-than-optimal graft take are infection, inadequate nutrition, or a poor graft bed or inadequate débridement.

The donor site itself is now a partial-thickness wound and is treated as such. The donor site will usually heal within 10 days to 2 weeks with normal skin, although it may be many months before the skin color appears normal. In some cases, there may be some permanent skin discoloration. Occasionally, a thicker graft is inadvertently taken (remember that the skin of infants and young children is thinner than that of adults), and the donor site, because it is now deeper than a superficial partial-thickness wound, will heal with scar tissue. A donor site that heals with normal skin can be reused, if necessary. Such reuse is called *reharvesting*.

In the case of a burn involving a large percentage of TBSA, even when multiple donor sites are available, the surgeon may elect not to graft the entire burn at once because of the stress of surgery to the patient, particularly if the patient is already medically compromised or unstable. If the grafts do not take, not only is there still a large TBSA burn, but the donor sites are now additional wounds that must be healed, and the donor sites cannot be reused for about 10 days.

FULL-THICKNESS SKIN GRAFT

Although a split-thickness skin graft (STSG) is the most commonly used type of graft to close a burn wound, a full-thickness skin graft (FTSG), if available, can be used or is the preferred graft in some cases to close the wound acutely or during burn reconstructive surgery. Because a FTSG is a full-thickness piece of skin, it usually is harvested from an area, such as the groin, which can be sutured or primarily closed (although a STSG could be used to close the donor site).

The advantages of a FTSG versus a STSG are that a FTSG provides more padding, a better color match, a more nearly normal hair pattern, and less contraction in the recipient site than does a STSG.[1] In addition, the primarily closed donor site of a FTSG usually heals more quickly than that of a STSG and results in a line scar, often in an area not visible, which in some cases, may be more cosmetically acceptable than the donor site of a STSG. The disadvantages of a FTSG are that a FTSG requires near-ideal conditions for survival, and because the donor site is usually primarily closed, the size and number of FTSGs available for use is limited.[50]

Full-thickness skin grafts are recommended for closure of deep palmar burns of the hand.[51,52] Schwanholt et al. reported that young pediatric patients who received FTSGs to close deep palmar burns had better ROM and needed fewer reconstructive procedures than did those who received STSGs.[51] Morris and Saffle reported that patients treated with FTSGs on deep palamar burns needed less therapy and a shorter period of pressure garment use than would be expected if STSGs had been used.[52]

Cultured Autografts and Dermal Substitutes

Several advances in wound healing and surgical techniques during the past decade have improved the outcome and increased survival of burn patients. Among these advances are two that have been shown to increase survival in massively burned individuals who lack sufficient donor sites: cultured autografts and dermal substitutes.

In the 1980s, cultured epithelial autografts (CEAs) or keratinocytes were the newest advancement in wound closure of the severely burned individual. In the case of cultured epithelial autografts, a small piece of unburned skin measuring approximately 1 square inch is taken from the patient and grown in a laboratory. Within several weeks or less, there is enough skin to cover an entire body and this skin can be grafted onto the patient from whom the original sample was taken. However, there are drawbacks and problems with cultured autografted skin. Wound closure must be delayed until the skin is grown, and the rate of graft take, depending on the occurrence of graft site infection varies from 15% to 80%.[53] CEAs, lacking tensile strength, are fragile and easily cut or bruised.[54] Standard therapy regimens, in particular those involving ROM and mobilization, frequently must be altered or their implementation delayed. The cost of the CEA can also be high. Although dermal regeneration occurs below CEAs over 4 to 5 years,[55] the skin lacks hair follicles and sweat glands. Sensory nerves and pigmentation are also absent.[54] Some of the problems associated with the use of CEAs have been mitigated recently by combining a CEA with cadaver skin, that has had the antigenic epidermis removed.

In the mid-1990s, cultured composite autografts (CCAs) were developed. Cultured composite autografts consist of autologous keratinocytes, which form a multilayered epidermal component, and fibroblasts, which form an extracellular dermal matrix. The rate of CCA take is reported to be 80%, and the CCA is durable. Dermal elements, such as hair follicles and sweat glands, are lacking in cultured composite autografted skin. The product is expensive; however, the resulting decreased hospitalization from the use of CCA may offset the high cost.[56]

Several dermal substitutes or dermal analogues are now available for use after decades of research. One such substitute, Integra (Integra LifeSciences Corp., Plainsboro, NJ) is an artificial dermis composed of two layers: a dermal replacement layer of bovine tendon collagen and a substitute epidermal layer of silicone.[57] Integra is placed on the excised wound. The porous dermal replacement layer serves as a matrix for the infiltration of elements from the wound bed that then construct a neodermis. Although the patient's own neodermis is being constructed, the bovine collagen dissolves. During the period of neodermis construction, about 2 weeks, the silicone epidermal layer acts to control moisture loss from the wound. Once neodermis construction is complete or later, the surgeon removes the silicone layer and replaces it with very thin autografts from the patient. One major benefit of Integra is that there is no scar formation associated with its use. Other benefits are that it is immediately available for use; it allows for immediate postexcisional wound coverage, early ambulation and rehabilitation, delayed autografting of the neodermis if necessary, more rapid healing and better cosmetic outcome of donor sites because of ultrathin autograft use, and the ability to save certain donor sites for use on cosmetically sensitive areas.[58] Some disadvantages of Integra are that it lacks hair follicles and sweat glands. However, sensory function returns at the same level and time course as it does following normal STSG autografting.[59] Integra is expensive, but such expense may be justifiable if the use of Integra can decrease morbidity and mortality and improve outcome. The high cost of the product may be offset by the lower costs associated with its use if it can hasten wound closure and decrease the rehabilitation needs and future reconstructive needs of the patient.

Another dermal replacement product that is also available for use is allografted skin, AlloDerm (AlloDerm, LifeCell Corp., The Woodlands, TX), which, once the antigenic epidermis and antigenic cells from the dermis are removed, leaves a dermal matrix that will accept an ultathin STSG. Less scarring and contraction result with the use of AlloDerm and an ultrathin STSG than with an STSG alone, and the use of ultathin grafts with the Alloderm results in quicker healing and less scarring of donor sites.[60] The color of the combined Alloderm and STSG closely matches that of the surrounding skin. As is the case with Integra, the high cost of AlloDerm may be offset by the lower costs of decreased length of stay and fewer rehabilitation needs or future reconstructive surgeries.

Role and Goals of the Therapist

The therapist plays a crucial role in the rehabilitation of the pediatric burn patient. The therapist's goals for the pediatric burn patient are to maintain or increase active and passive range of motion, manage soft tissue contours, maintain or increase strength and endurance, promote normal development and function, and inhibit loss of motion, deformity, hypertrophic scarring, and contraction. The therapist is involved in all phases of the burn injury from the acute through the rehabilitative and the reconstructive. The therapist is a member of the burn team and consults with other team members, including the patient and parents, when planning and executing treatment.

The role and goals of the therapist is discussed for each phase of recovery with emphasis on the rehabilitative phase. Although the primary focus is on the rehabilitative phase, rehabilitation essentially begins when the patient is admitted to the hospital, and the acute therapeutic intervention can affect the type, intensity, length, and outcome of rehabilitation.

The Emergent Phase

The emergent phase generally includes the first 48 to 72 hours after the burn injury. Whether the therapist works in a general hospital or in a burn center, it is advisable to have established a protocol with the surgery department dictating a consult on the patient's admission if the patient has sustained deep or extensive burns. This arrangement ensures that the therapist is available and becomes involved as soon as necessary, and allows the therapist to become familiar with the patient's history and to evaluate, plan, and initiate treatment in a timely fashion.

Patient presentation during the emergent phase will depend on the depth, extent, and location of the burn injury and on any associated injuries, such as smoke inhalation. The patient may have extensive edema, be intubated, have undergone escharotomies, and have multiple bandaged areas, or the patient may have only a bandaged limb or chest with a burn of an as yet determined depth. Both the severity of the injury and the age of the child will affect the therapist's goals and specific treatment during this phase. The goals of the therapist during the emergent phase are to begin evaluation, set goals, and plan treatment. When indicated, the therapist may also be involved in controlling edema, beginning and maintaining motion and mobility, splinting and positioning, training in activities of daily living (ADL), and promoting normal development.

EVALUATION, GOAL SETTING, AND TREATMENT PLANNING

The evaluation process beings with a careful chart review. The physical therapist should next evaluate the patient during a dressing change to examine more closely the location, apparent depth, and extent of the burn wounds.

A generalized evaluation of ROM should be undertaken during the dressing change when bandages will not interfere with motion and when the therapist can see the wounds. The patient may be edematous, which may limit full active and passive ROM. Because of young age, severity of injury, or pain, many children are unable to cooperate with ROM instructions. A goniometer cannot be allowed to touch an open wound, but it can be held about a half inch away from the patient during the evaluation. During the emergent phase, however, it is usually more practical to "eyeball" ROM, which should not be forced by the therapist.

Based on information from the chart and that obtained during a general examination, the therapist can then establish general long- and short-term goals and begin treatment planning and execution. One goal is continued evaluation and monitoring of the patient. Evaluation is an ongoing process, and as changes occur in the patient's status or as the depth of wound or the surgical plan becomes known, the therapist's goals and treatment will be affected.

SPLINTING AND POSITIONING

The purpose of splinting and positioning during this 48- to 72-hour period is to help control edema, provide support for edematous extremities, and inhibit contraction and loss of motion.

It is often not necessary to splint children at this time except in the case of older children and adolescents and those who are extensively burned. The therapist should initiate positioning in bed. If the patient is able to get out of bed, the therapist should provide for proper bedside positioning.

An extremity or part of an extremity may be edematous even if it is not burned. Unlike adults, most children do not have long-term problems with edema. Edematous extremities may be elevated on pillows at heart level. Splints to support the wrist in a neutral position or slight extension and splints to position the ankles in approximately a neutral position may be provided for older children with burns in these areas. If necessary, bulky bandages can be used to provide support for younger children and infants.

There is an axiom that states that the position of comfort—flexion—is the position of contracture for burn patients. Patients are thus splinted or positioned to counteract contracting forces. As mentioned previously, it is often not necessary to splint children during the emergent phase, although the therapist, on a surgeon's order, may elect to begin splinting and positioning children with severe burns or older children and adolescents later in this phase. The neck should be positioned in a neutral position or slight extension. Pillows under the head are prohibited because they promote cervical flexion. A splint can be used to position the neck, but it may be easier during this phase to use a roll under the shoulders. The shoulders should be positioned in approximately 90 degrees of abduction and in slight protraction. Again, during this phase, splints can be used or the position can be achieved using pillows under the arms. The limbs should be positioned in extension, with the ankles and wrists in a neutral position or the wrists in slight extension. To protect the extensor mechanism, as well as to prevent contracture, the proper position for a burned hand is for the metacarpophalangeal joints to be flexed, the interphalangeal joints to be extended, and the thumb to be placed in palmar abduction. (The exception to this is the patient with solely palmar burns, in which case the fingers are positioned in full extension and the thumb is placed in radial abduction.) Smaller joints in the hand may be difficult to position correctly because of edema and should never be forced into the ideal position. Splints or bulky bandages that approximate the desired position can be used to position the hand during the emergent phase if necessary.

If splints are used during this phase, they should be applied over the dressings and secured with Kerlix or Kling* (Johnson & Johnson, New Brunswick, NJ) or similar type bandaging because, with emerging edema, straps on splints could cause a tourniquet effect, and elastic wraps also could compromise circulation. The splint can be worn for 24 hours with removal for exercise or activities as desired. In any case, splints should be removed periodically and checked by the nursing and therapy staff for proper application, and circulation of the distal extremities should be monitored to ensure that the splint is not too tight. Written instructions regarding proper splinting should be provided for the nursing staff.

RANGE OF MOTION

Active ROM exercises during the emergent phase help control edema and initiate early motion. Muscle contraction serves as a pumping mechanism to aid venous and lymphatic return.[61] It is not necessary to move younger children during this time, but the therapist may begin gentle active ROM exercises in older children and adolescents. Active ROM may be limited by edema. As stated previously, ROM exercises should be performed during dressing changes when the bandages do not restrict motion, the therapist can see the limitations in motion resulting from edema, the wound can be viewed, and the patient has received pain medication. Passive ROM should not be performed during this period.

ACTIVITIES OF DAILY LIVING AND DEVELOPMENT

Depending on the age of patient, the severity and location of burn, and the patient's mentation, the therapist may introduce several ADL and developmental activities. When appropriate, the therapist should teach bed mobility and transfers.

The Acute Phase

The acute phase extends from the emergent period until skin grafting or wound closure. The goals of the physical therapist are to maintain ROM, inhibit contraction, and promote function and normal development. Generally during this phase, edema subsides, the depth of the wound becomes evident, and the surgeon plans skin grafting or another course of treatment. The therapist should continue to observe the healing wound at regular intervals.

SPLINTING AND POSITIONING

The purpose of splinting and positioning during the acute phase is to maintain or increase ROM by counteracting the force of contracting tissue. As previously discussed, flexion, the position of comfort, is the position of contracture, so patients are positioned to counteract contracting forces. Patients with burns of the neck are splinted in neutral to slight extension, avoiding lateral flexion and rotation, and pillows are prohibited. (Care also should be taken to position the patient to avoid pressure on burned ears, which can result in chondritis.) Shoulders are positioned in approximately 90 degrees of abduction and slight protraction. Elbows and knees are splinted in extension. In the case of deep dorsal burns of the hand, correct positioning is necessary to prevent boutonnière deformities. A boutonnière deformity (hyperextension of the metacarpophalangeal [MCP] joint, flexion of the proximal interphalangeal [PIP] joint, and hyperextension of the distal interphalangeal [DIP] joint) occurs when the central slip of the extensor tendon to the PIP joint ruptures and the lateral bands slide volarly. To help prevent such a deformity, as well as to inhibit contractures, the hand is positioned with the wrist extended 15 to 20 degrees, the MCP joints are flexed approximately 60 to 70 degrees, the interphalangeal joints are extended, and the thumb is abducted (Fig. 13-11). However, especially with younger children, this precise hand position may not be achieved and should never be forced. The hips should be positioned in extension and abducted 15 degrees, and the ankles should be positioned in neutral. The therapist may also need to splint the mouths of patients with deep facial burns in order to inhibit the development of microstomia.

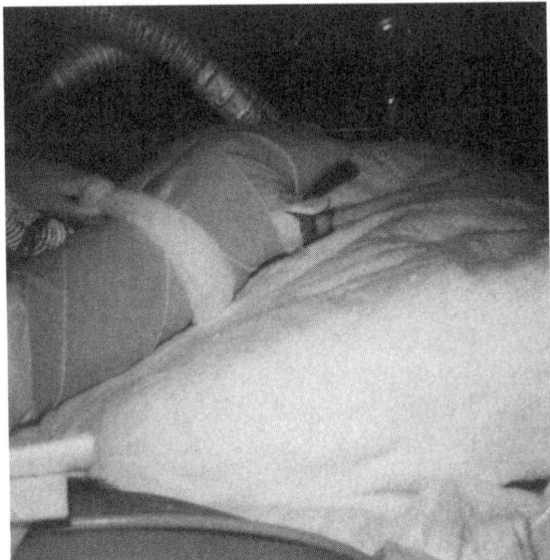

Figure 13-11 ■ A hand splint is used during the acute phase to help maintain range of motion, inhibit contracture, and protect tendons and joints. Elastic bandages are used during this phase to secure splints. Elevation of the extremity may be helpful in decreasing any residual edema.

In general, unburned parts do not need to be splinted or positioned except as they affect the position of burned areas. The therapist should continually monitor ROM, especially in unburned joints in older patients and in patients who are hospitalized for long periods and in whom loss of motion may result from prolonged immobilization. In some cases, it may be necessary to apply foot splints to unburned feet to inhibit footdrop.

If the patient was splinted during the emergent phase, the splint may need to be adjusted in the acute phase to accommodate the changes that result from decreased edema. This process may be less painful to the patient if the therapist adjusts or makes such splints immediately following the dressing change while the patient still has the benefit of recent pain medication. The splint can be applied with elastic bandage wraps during this phase unless significant early edema persists. The splint-wearing schedule will depend on the individual patient. Some patients will wear the splint continually except during dressing changes, during specific activities and exercises, or during periodic evaluation of fit and circulation. Other patients may require splinting only at night. Each patient's schedule may change during the course of the acute phase. One way to determine an adequate splinting schedule is to see how much motion the patient loses when the splint has been off for a specified period.

Although patients must be positioned properly to prevent contractures, their position in bed should be changed periodically over a 24-hour period to help prevent decubiti. The use of special beds or mattresses, designed to decrease pressure over bony prominences and reduce the pressure and shearing forces that might disrupt healing tissue or recent grafts, may be beneficial.

Cardiopulmonary status is also a factor to consider in determining appropriate positioning, particularly in patients who have sustained an inhalation injury or who, because of their injuries, will be at bedrest or hospitalized for a prolonged period. Elevating the head of the bed or placing the patient in a chair at scheduled times may help maximize lung position and chest expansion and maintain or increase endurance. (The therapist should be cautioned, however, that elevating the head of the patient's bed for an extended time can contribute to hip flexion contractures if care is not taken to avoid such contractures through measures such as position changes and ROM exercises.)

Helm[62] raised the concern of preventing peripheral nerve stretch or compression injuries that can be caused by improper positioning of the burn patient. For example, patients with medial thigh burns or a swollen scrotum, or those who are tall, may assume a position of externally rotated hips, flexed knees, and inverted ankles, which can result in footdrop secondary to peroneal nerve palsy.[62]

RANGE OF MOTION

During the acute phase, the purposes of ROM exercises and activities are to maintain or increase ROM by counteracting the contracting forces of healing tissue; to maintain joint motion, tendon gliding, and muscle activity; and to improve circulation. Because edema is resolving, limitations in ROM caused by edema should be decreasing, although during the early part of this phase, some restrictions in motion from edema may persist. During the acute phase, ROM may be limited by inelastic eschar or by contracting tissue. Just as during the emergent phase, ROM exercises should be performed during the dressing change. Once the extent of ROM is known, appropriate exercises can be done at the patient's bedside or incorporated into play activities.

In general, passive ROM exercises should be avoided. However, when children are unable to cooperate because of their injuries or their young age, *gentle* passive ROM, to the limits of resistance by the tissue, can be done. Passive

ROM beyond such resistance can damage healing tissue. When possible, passive ROM exercise can be performed by the therapist in the operating room—while the patient is anesthetized—before any surgical procedure. When performed under these conditions, such ROM exercises are painless, and the therapist is able to ascertain the true limits of motion.

Although maintaining ROM is a primary goal, the author cautions against excessive and aggressive ROM exercise. Overaggressive exercises may damage newly healing tissue and may cause pain that traumatizes the patient and leads to a decreased level of cooperation during the rehabilitation phase. Some infants, toddlers, and younger children who are not extensively burned and who undergo early excision and grafting will be hospitalized only briefly, and may not require daily ROM. Their joints, even if immobilized for several weeks, may not necessarily become stiff, and splinting may help maintain motion. However, the patient's ROM must be closely monitored.

EXPOSED TENDONS AND JOINTS

At some point during the acute or early rehabilitation phase, patients with deep burns may present with exposed tendons or joints. Areas where the tendon or joint is superficial, or where the skin covering them is thin, are common sites for such exposure. Examples of such locations are the dorsum of the hand, particularly over the proximal interphalangeal joints; the posterior elbow; the dorsum of the foot; and the ankle. If the exposed tendon or the exposed joint and periarticular structures appear to be healthy and intact, and depending upon the location of the exposure, the therapist, under the direction of the surgeon, may still perform or ask the patient to perform supervised ROM exercises. (However, in the case of tendon exposure over the PIP joint, full total active ROM of the digit is not permitted.) In cases in which the tendon or joint appears to be fragile or necrotic, or the tendon has ruptured, or the joint and/or periarticular structures are damaged, exercises to the joint must be discontinued, the joint may need to be immobilized, and exercises to the adjacent joints may have to be discontinued or modified or special exercise techniques may need to be employed. The exposed tendons or joints also need to be protected from drying out.

ACTIVITIES OF DAILY LIVING AND DEVELOPMENT

During the acute phase, depending on the age of the child and the severity of the injury, the patient may have difficulty with ADLs or may be dependent on the nursing staff for help with ADLs as a result of treatment. Pain, bulky bandages, and splints may discourage the patient from engaging in such activities. As much as possible, the patient should participate in ADLs and assist with self-care. Splints that inhibit specified ADLs (e.g., self-feeding) should be removed to allow the patient to participate in such activities, after which they can be immediately reapplied. When indicated and appropriate, special ADL equipment (such as built-up handles on eating utensils) can be provided and the patient can be taught necessary techniques, such as transfers.

During the acute phase, patients without lower extremity burns may ambulate. However, because of pain, bandages, or upper extremity splints, such patients may require assistive devices or supervision. Patients with burns of the lower extremity that are not extensive or deep also may ambulate after application of supportive elastic wraps over dressings. However, it may not be necessary to force such early ambulation.

Age-appropriate toys, activities, music, and videos should be supplied according to individual needs, and interaction with other children should be facilitated. Most pediatric facilities have a playroom or employ a child life therapist who interacts with the patient in the unit or at the bedside.

The Skin Graft Phase

The goals of the therapist during the skin graft phase are to help protect the newly grafted area, to maintain motion in the nongrafted joints, and to initiate or finalize discharge planning. The grafted part is usually immobilized for approximately 5 days until the graft is adherent. Depending on the extent of the burn, the patient may undergo several skin grafting procedures.

SPLINTING AND POSITIONING

If the area that has been grafted is over a joint, the joint is usually immobilized with a splint. Besides immobilizing the joint, the splint also maintains the joint in an anticontracture position during this time. If the therapist has not already splinted the joint in an area to be grafted before skin grafting, the therapist now should fabricate a splint that the surgeon can apply in the operating room after the grafting procedure. Alternatively, the surgeon may construct a plaster splint in the operating room. Such construction in the operating room may ensure a more accurate fit over bulky bandages and may be more cost-effective if the splint is to be used only during the skin graft phase. In cases in which the goal of a properly fitted splint cannot be achieved by the means previously described, the therapist may fabricate and apply the splint in the operating room.

RANGE OF MOTION

Although the grafted joint cannot be moved during this period, unburned or burned but nongrafted joints may still be moved. If the unburned or nongrafted area is directly adjacent to a fresh graft, the therapist should seek the surgeon's approval before initiating ROM exercises or other activities that might disrupt the new graft. The patient probably will experience pain or discomfort from the donor site, which may interfere with full active ROM.

DISCHARGE PLANNING

Discharge plans should be finalized by the time of the last skin grafting procedure. However, discharge planning really should begin as soon as the patient has been evaluated and a treatment plan has been proposed. Although each patient should be treated individually and the course for some burn patients is unknown, many such patients follow a predictable course of treatment and have a predictable length of hospital stay. Discharge planning should be a team process, and it is helpful to have a member of the discharge planning department on the burn team.

Ongoing discussion about hospital discharge from the time of admission is encouraging for both the family and the patient, may help them prepare for the patient's eventual return to home, and allows them to be a part of the planning process. Judgment must be exercised during the acute phase in determining what information to share with the family and when.

The therapist should evaluate the patient's needs and the available resources when planning for discharge. Consideration should be given to the type and frequency of therapy necessary and the need for pressure garments or equipment. Additionally, the therapist should consider where the patient lives, the availability of local rehabilitation facilities, whether the local facility and discharging institution will jointly follow the patient and how, what the patient's insurance will cover, the level of family support, and the family's ability to follow through with treatment. Another factor to be considered in discharge planning for school-aged patients is school reentry.[16] If the patient and family have not already met or been given information about burn support groups, this should be done before discharge.

DISCHARGE TEACHING

Just as with discharge planning, discharge teaching should begin as soon as the patient has been evaluated and a treatment plan has been proposed. Of course, the exact information that the family and patient will need cannot be predicted or provided from the outset, but the process of instructing them about therapy and involving them in patient care can begin at admission when appropriate. This approach also allows learning to occur over time and helps the family prepare for eventual discharge. When the patient is ready to be discharged, the topics to be included in the therapist's discharge teaching plan may include skin care, scarring, use and application of pressure garments, ROM, splints, and ADLs or developmental activities.

Teaching methods and instruments can include verbal instructions, demonstrations, written instructions, and/or videos. The family and patient should have ample time and opportunity to review with the therapist the information presented and to practice specific skills, such as applying pressure dressings and garments or splints. The information discussed and the skills demonstrated should be reinforced and expanded on during outpatient visits.

The Rehabilitation Phase

The rehabilitation phase extends from the time of graft adherence—or, for deep partial-thickness burns that are not grafted, from wound closure—until scar maturation. The period of scar maturation for most children is 12 to 18 months after graft adherence or wound closure, with the scar generally being most active during the first 6 months. The goals of the physical therapist during this phase are to achieve mobility and weight-bearing; to maintain or increase ROM; to promote formation of a flat, soft, smooth, pliable scar; to increase strength and endurance; to achieve independence in ADLs; to facilitate normal development and participation in age-appropriate activities; and to facilitate the patient's return to home and school.

Initially, the patient may still have bandages in places to cover small open wounds; these wounds should heal in 1 to 2 weeks, although a few patients have wounds that persist or recur far beyond this period. Some patients have no open wounds but may subsequently develop open areas as a result of scratching or friction in areas of fragile skin. (Wounds, particularly deep wounds or those located over joints, which persist or recur over an extended term may be a sign that the patient has insufficient skin coverage and will require further grafting sooner rather than later.) The donor sites may not be healed during the first week after graft adherence.

WEIGHT-BEARING AND AMBULATION

Patients who have undergone grafting in areas other than the lower extremities can begin weight-bearing on the first postoperative day (if medically stable and with a physician's order). Because the thighs and buttocks are frequently used for donor sites, however, these patients may experience pain or discomfort on weight-bearing, ambulation, or movement. They will frequently stand or ambulate with their trunk, hips, and knees flexed. Because of pain in the donor or graft site, weakness, and their standing posture or gait pattern, these patients may be unsteady and may initially require support or assistive devices. Selecting the appropriate support may be complicated if the grafted site is on the axilla or hand.

Depending on the child's age, medical status, and the size, location, and depth of lower extremity burns, weight-bearing and ambulation or preparation for these activities in the patient with newly grafted lower extremity burns are usually initiated approximately 5 days after grafting. However, on the first day after grafting, the patient can be out of bed in a chair or wheelchair with the legs elevated and the knees and feet properly positioned. A sequence of steps often leads to independent ambulation. Again, depending on the age, medical status, and extent of the injury, the sequence may take from 1 or 2 days to 1 or 2 weeks to complete. Before being placed in a dependent position, the recently grafted lower extremity should be wrapped with elastic bandages or a tubular elastic stocking (e.g., Tubigrip; Seton Products, Ltd., Lancashire, England) should be applied. (However, donor sites on the legs are not usually wrapped.) Such wrapping provides support to prevent blood pooling in the newly adherent graft, which could lead to hemorrhaging of fragile new capillaries and damage to the new graft. Elastic support also helps diminish associated pain, itching, and the dark purple color that results when the lower extremity is placed in a dependent position without elastic support. (Even with adequate support, some of these signs and symptoms may be present to a lesser degree.)

The sequence of steps leading to independent ambulation may begin with leg-dangling. On the fourth to fifth day after graft placement, with elastic support applied, the patient may dangle the legs for brief periods while sitting in bed, in a chair or wheelchair, or on an elevated mat. Next, the patient may attempt weight-bearing with assistance for brief periods, then advance to ambulating with assistance, and finally progress to independent ambulation. Weight-bearing and ambulation often will increase ROM, particularly if the patient has limitations in ankle dorsiflexion. In cases in which a patient has been on prolonged bedrest, a tilt-table may be necessary to initiate the weight-bearing and ambulation process.

SKIN CARE

Daily bathing with a mild soap is recommended to remove dead skin cells and old lotion in order to prevent them from clogging pores. Newly healed tissue or recently adherent grafts are fragile and should be protected from mechanical abrasion. Such areas will become more durable over time. Newly healed tissue and grafts also should be protected from chemicals, such as household cleaners, and from the sun.

Pruritis (Itching). Skin grafts and scar tissue can itch severely during the first year following injury. Such itching can be agonizing and disruptive to the patient's normal activities, particularly sleeping. Scratching can cause open wounds because recently adherent grafts or newly healed tissue is fragile. Itching may be the result of increased histamine, and may be aggravated by dry skin. (Scar tissue and skin grafts do not have the same number of functioning sweat glands[63] and may also lack the number of sebaceous glands that are present in normal skin.) The doctor may prescribe an oral antipruritic. Keeping the skin well lubricated by applying lotions once or more daily can also diminish itching, and cool baths or compresses may also provide relief.[64]

Massage. Massage of scar tissue and skin grafts helps maintain motion by freeing restrictive bands and increasing circulation.[65] Massage may also be helpful in decreasing itching. Initially, only gentle massage should be employed, because the newly healed tissue is often too fragile to tolerate much friction. Many children enjoy massage because it decreases itching, but other children find massage painful or will not sit still for such treatment. Although all patients should have scar tissue and skin grafts lubricated by thoroughly rubbing in lotions—preferably twice each day—the therapist may select particular areas of concern for massage and may also instruct the parent in massage of these areas. Massage should be done before specific ROM exercises, especially passive ROM exercises.

SCAR EVALUATION

There is no universally accepted and practical instrument used to measure scars. However, scar evaluation is important for determining the need for and efficacy of treatment. Several tools or methods that measure one or more aspects of scar have been proposed. Some methods involve the use of tonometry and ultrasonography to measure scar firmness and pliability[66]; the use of tonometry to measure pliability and tension so as to quantify the course of cicatrization and evaluate the efficacy of therapy[67]; the use of laser Doppler flowmetry to study microcirculation in burn scars in order to assess scar maturity[68]; and the use of an elastometer to measure elastic properties of scar so as to objectively document scar response to treatment or scar maturity.[69] The Vancouver Burn Scar Assessment[70] is one instrument that therapists helped develop that appears to be gaining acceptance (Fig. 13-12). This particular method of assessment is a visual scale that rates scar pigmentation, vascularity, pliability, and height. Other than the Vancouver form, the only tools needed are a millimeter rule and a piece of transparent plastic (on which is outlined a 1-inch square box) that is used to depress the scar.

The therapist should periodically document scar changes, particularly as they relate to treatment. Periodic photographs of the scar can also be useful. Besides evaluating scar in healed wounds and grafts, the therapist also should evaluate the donor site for any signs of scarring.

APPLICATION OF PRESSURE

Pressure is used to make or keep scars flat, soft, smooth, and pliable. Although controlled studies are sparse concerning the ability of pressure to prevent or correct scar hypertrophy, and although the exact mechanism of pressure in controlling scar is not known, pressure appears to be clinically effective and is widely used in the United States. Generally, the pressure applied should equal or exceed capillary pressure. For pressure to be therapeutic, it should be applied early, and pressure garments should be worn continuously for the duration of scar maturation. Moreover, the pressure applied should be both conforming and adequate.

Early Application of Pressure Garments. Because the processes of scar hypertrophy and contracture begin almost as soon as the wound begins healing, pressure to control scarring should begin early. Pressure can be applied once grafts are adherent, or when deep partial-thickness wounds are healed so that there are openings no larger than the size of a quarter. Besides controlling scars, pressure in this early stage can provide support to recently adherent grafts or to newly healed tissue. The patient can then be measured for commercially available, custom-made pressure garments. However, because the pressure in such garments and the shearing forces exerted at the time of application are too strong for recently adherent grafts or newly healed scar tissue, the garments cannot be applied for several weeks.

In the interim, lighter pressure can be applied, with gradual progression to stronger pressure over a period of a few weeks. For example, during the first week after graft adherence (about 1 to 2 weeks following graft placement) or during the first week after wound closure, the therapist can use one layer of a tubular elastic stockinette (Fig. 13-13) such as Tubigrip (Seton Products, Ltd., Lancashire, England) or Elastic-net (Beiersdorf-Jobst, Inc., Charlotte, NC), to fashion shirts and shorts to be applied on the extremities and trunk.

Fit. Tubular elastic stockinettes come in various widths ranging from approximately 4 cm to 32 cm. The manufacturer may provide a measuring tape or furnish printed guidelines to help the therapist select the appropriate size; however, the therapist must exercise sound judgment in choosing the best size. Tubular elastic stockinette is too loose if it bags or does not cling to the patient, and it is too tight if it is constrictive, leaves deep indentations on the skin, or restricts circulation. In some cases, one size may be applied on the forearm, whereas a

VANCOUVER GENERAL HOSPITAL
OCCUPATIONAL THERAPY DEPARTMENT

BURN SCAR ASSESSMENT
PATIENT NAME:

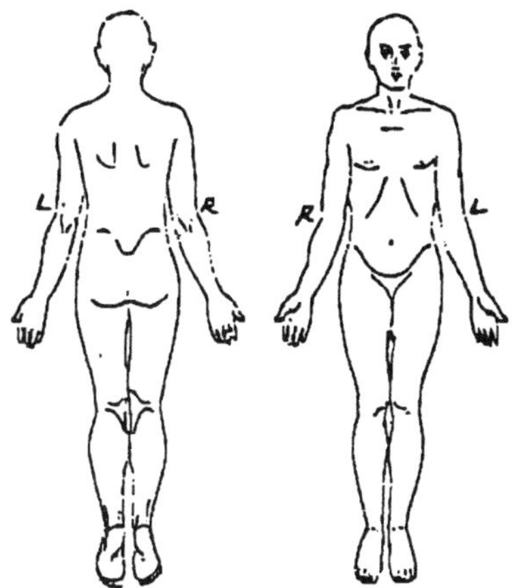

PIGMENTATION (M)

0 normal—color that closely resembles the color over the rest of one's body
1 hypopigmentation
2 hyperpigmentation

VASCULARITY (V)

0 normal—color that closely resembles the color over the rest of one's body
1 pink
2 red
3 purple

PLIABILITY (P)

0 normal
1 supple—flexible with minimal resistance
2 yielding—giving way to pressure
3 firm-inflexible, not easily moved, resistant to manual pressure
4 banding—rope-like tissue that blanches with extension of scar
5 contracture—permanent shortening of scar producing deformity or distortion

HEIGHT

0 normal—flat
1 < 2 mm
2 < 5 mm
3 > 5 mm

Scale in mm

Date	Scar #	Pigmentation	Vascularity	Pliability	Height	Total	OT init

Figure 13-12 ▪ The burn scar assessment form

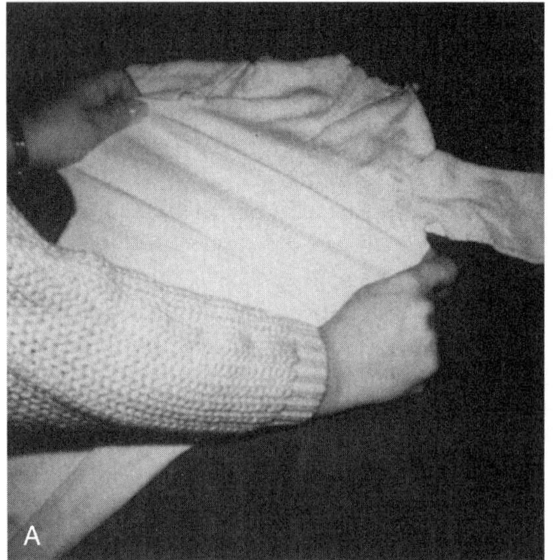

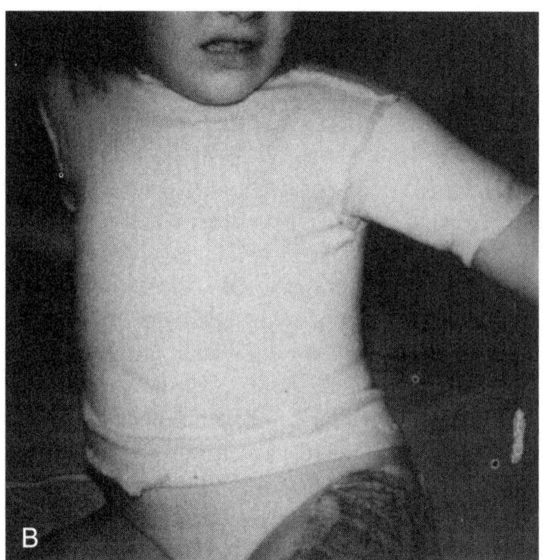

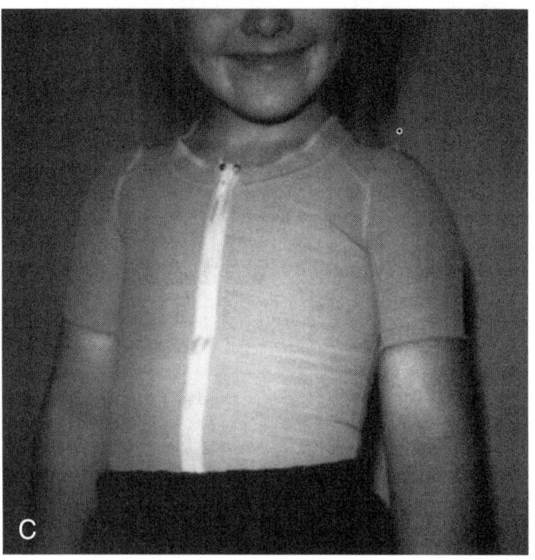

Figure 13-13 ■ (**A**) Shirt constructed of tubular elastic stockinette. (**B**) A child who is approximately 1 week post–skin-graft application to a burned left chest and shoulder. (**C**) The commercially available custom-made pressure garment is worn for 3 to 4 weeks after skin graft placement.

larger size may be needed for the upper arm. In the case of the lower extremity, three different sizes may need to be used.

Application. Before application, any open areas should be covered with a light dressing. Because the friction of application or the shearing forces exerted during movement could cause blisters or even small wounds, fragile-appearing areas also should be dressed with a light bandage. When the tubular elastic stockinette is being applied, it should be lifted over any dressings and gently placed. This technique helps avoid dislodging the dressings, applying friction over open areas or fragile tissue, and causing possible pain. At least one manufacturer of tubular elastic stockinette supplies applicators. The most distal pieces are applied first. For example, in a patient with burns of the buttocks and lower extremity, the piece for the foot would be applied first, followed by the piece for the calf, the piece for the thigh, and finally application of the shorts in that order. Elastic stockinette pieces should also be removed in a precise order, using the reverse pattern. This method of application avoids dislodging of bandages and friction that might lead to blisters, and helps minimize pain. When pieces of various sizes are used on an extremity, each piece should overlap the next by approximately $1\frac{1}{2}$ inches. Such overlap ensures that, during movement, individual pieces will not become separated from other pieces, thereby avoiding both the uncovering of these areas and also swelling of the uncovered areas secondary to increased pressure on each side. Wrinkles and bunching in the tubular elastic stockinette should be smoothed.

By the second week after graft adherence or wound closure, the pressure can be increased by doubling the tubular elastic stockinette and the shirts and shorts made by the therapist. (The elastic stockinette garments provided by the manufacturer should not be doubled.) Several manufacturers of custom-made pressure garments also carry prefabricated, noncustom, pediatric pressure garments that are made of a lighter material and exert a lighter pressure, and these may be able to be introduced at that time.

The temporary or interim pressure garments should be worn about 22 hours per day. They should be removed for dressing changes, bathing, skin care, and specified exercises or activities.

LATER APPLICATION OF COMMERCIALLY AVAILABLE, CUSTOM-MADE ELASTIC PRESSURE GARMENTS. By the third week after graft adherence or wound closure, the patient is usually ready for commercially available, custom-made pressure garments that should have been ordered and received from the manufacturer by that time. At least five or six companies manufacture custom-fitted elastic pressure garments in the United States, including Barton-Carey Medical Products (Perrysburg, OH), Beiersdorf-Jobst (Charlotte, NC), Bio-Concepts (Phoenix, AZ), Gottfried Medical, Inc. (Toledo, OH), and Medical Z (San Antonio, TX). Depending on the company selected, there are a variety of fabric materials and colors, measuring systems, designs, and options available; a span of prices; and a range of services provided (e.g., a company representative who will measure and fit patients instead of the therapist performing the activity).

Fit. Because a garment is custom-made and designed to apply a specific amount of pressure over a given area, it should fit snugly. It is too loose if it can be easily pinched or if it bags or bunches. The garment can be sewn tighter by the therapist, but the patient should be remeasured. The garment is too tight if there is distal swelling, coldness, discoloration, or if the patient is old enough to complain, paresthesias. It is too tight if deep red marks that take longer than 20 minutes to fade are left on the skin from the pressure garment or if there is skin breakdown caused by a seam. The therapist can make small (approximately $\frac{1}{4}$ inch) cuts in the garment to provide a temporary adjustment, but, again, the patient should be remeasured. A second pressure garment should be ordered as soon as the patient is fitted with the first.

Application. There are several methods of application, and the parent and patient will find one that is easiest for them. One method is to apply the garment as is: glove directly on the hand, arm in the sleeve of a shirt, foot into the leotard, and so forth. Another way is to turn the garment inside out and then apply it so that, as it is being donned, it is right side out. Either way, the garment should not be pulled or yanked, because such pulling, if repeated often, can lead to overstretching and can cause a distortion of the garment and lessening of the pressure that the garment is designed to apply. Rather, the garment should be inched on. One technique to ease application of a leotard is to first apply sheer knee-high stockings. The use of such stockings can help decrease the resistance of the skin to application of the leotard and generally does not interfere with the pressure. A similar method can be employed for the upper extremity.

A pressure garment can also be applied over dressings if there are still wounds or if there are wounds that have been created by a patient's scratching. The garment can be lifted over the dressing, or a small piece of elastic stockinette can be used to help hold the dressing in place when applying the pressure garment.

Wearing Schedule. The garment is recommended for wearing approximately 22 hours per day. It should be removed daily for bathing and skin care. Even if the parent does not bathe the child daily, the pressure garment should be removed, the healed area washed, and lotion applied. Patients with wounds also must have dressings changed at least once each day. Depending on the patient, the garment may be removed one or two other times a day for additional lubrication to the scar or graft. The garment also should be removed if there are specified exercises recommended by the therapist, because the garment can impede movement. Moreover, the therapist should be able to observe the part being exercised to determine whether scar is limiting motion and, in the case of passive ROM exercises, to avoid overstretching. Because the pressure garments can impede motion and diminish sensation, children younger than 2 years of age who are wearing pressure garments, such as gloves, may need to have the garment off for brief intervals during the day to experience more normal sensation and movement. Other than the parameters described earlier, children can engage in almost any activity, including swimming, while wearing the pressure garment. Pressure garments should be worn until scar maturation, which, for most children, is within 12 to 18 months.

The patient should have at least two sets of custom-fitting elastic pressure garments so that one set can be washed while the other is being worn. In some cases, three sets are recommended because of the increased wear and tear that certain garments, such as chinstraps and gloves, undergo. Initially, the patient usually receives only one set; the second set is then ordered when it is determined that the first set fits appropriately. At this time, the patient should wear the first set as much as possible, and only wear the temporary pressure garments when the custom-made one is being laundered. Once the patient has two sets of custom-fitting elastic pressure garments, temporary pressure garments should no longer be used. Because the child is growing and because the garments eventually wear out, they should be replaced every 2 to 3 months. Over time, a garment can lose much elasticity, thereby reducing pressure, while appearing to fit well. Because several weeks may elapse between the time the patient is measured and the actual fitting, the therapist should not wait until the garment appears to be too small or too worn before measuring the patient for a new custom-made pressure garment.

Each manufacturer recommends daily laundering of pressure garments. However, washing machines and dryers, heat, and strong detergents can break down the elasticity in the garment, thereby diminishing the pressure provided. Even handwashing the garments contributes to the breakdown of elasticity. Because of this problem and because many young children do not perspire as adults do, this author recommends washing pressure garments only when necessary or just laundering part of the garment (the feet of a leotard, for example). The approach will vary from patient to patient and from garment to garment (e.g., socks may need more frequent laundering than a shirt). Perspiration, petroleum-based lotions, activity, and ozone are other factors that may contribute to the breakdown of elasticity in the garment.

Ensuring Adequate, Conforming Pressure. A child may have received a well-fitting pressure garment (and have worn temporary or interim pressure garments prior to that) and have been compliant with its use, and the therapist still may note scar hypertrophy and contraction a week or more later. Why? Although a garment is designed to apply a specific amount of pressure, the pressure garment itself has no pressure in it. However, once applied, depending on the body surface, material, and fit, as well as other conditions, the garment will generate pressure.

Several factors affect the actual pressure being applied, including characteristics of body surface and movement. Characteristics of body surface that affect pressure are *contour* (concave versus convex surfaces), *resistance* (hard versus soft surfaces), and *surfaces with or without an opposing force*. The therapist should be aware of and anticipate the effects of these characteristics, as well as those of movement.

Contour (Concave Versus Convex Surfaces). Although custom-made pressure garments usually fit well over convex surfaces of the body, such as the forearm or calf, they tend to bridge over concave areas, such as the palm of the hand, between the scapulae, and so on. In the latter case, the garments provide little, if any, pressure over such areas.

Resistance (Hard Versus Soft Surfaces). Pressure is more easily achieved over harder surfaces of the body than over softer ones. Harder surfaces of the body (e.g., muscular or bony surfaces, such as the anterior calf) provide greater resistance than do softer surfaces of the body (such as the stomach or the thigh). For example, one can depress a finger almost an inch into the thigh of a child before significant resistance is met.

Opposing Force. In order for pressure to be applied, there must be an opposing force. For example, a pressure garment over the volar aspect of the forearm helps provide the opposing force for the garment over the dorsal surface of the forearm. Some areas of the body provide little, if any, opposing force when a pressure garment is applied. Examples of such sites include the shoulder and digit web spaces. Additionally, the amount of pressure being applied may tend to diminish distally.

Movement. At any given moment, movement can change the amount of pressure being applied by a garment. Muscle contractions and joint movement can change the contour and hardness of body surface areas and the amount of stretch or laxity in a pressure garment. For example, in one study,[71] a pressure sensor was placed on the dorsum of a hand under a Bio-Concept pressure glove. When the fingers were extended, the sensor gave a reading of 19 mmHg. With the fingers flexed, the sensor demonstrated 45 mmHg.

Inserts. Because of the factors just mentioned, it may be necessary to use inserts to compensate for inadequate pressure provided by pressure garments over certain areas of the body. An *insert* is material that is worn underneath the pressure garment over a specific area and that applies (along with the pressure garment) additional pressure over that area. Many materials can be used as inserts, including Polycushion (Smith Nephew, Inc., Aliplast 4E (molded) (Alimed Inc., Dedham, MA), Otoform K (Dreze, Inc., Unna, Germany), and others, or a combination. The materials used will depend on the specific area of the body and the patient's tolerance, as well as the scar's response to the material, the age of the scar, and when the material is being worn. Otoform K works well over the toes because it molds (forms) into the webbed spaces and contours of the toes. Aliplast 4E (of various thicknesses) molds well over the shoulder, but because Aliplast is semirigid, it may buckle during movement and actually lift pressure off part of the shoulder. Because of this effect, a less rigid (although perhaps not as strong) insert, such as Polycushion, may be used during the day, with Aliplast being used at night.

OTHER METHODS OF APPLYING PRESSURE. Pressure garments are the most common way to apply pressure on scar, but other methods may be as or more effective and have other benefits, such as being easier to apply or less expensive. For example, with a small, localized burn of an extremity, two layers of a snugly fitting tubular elastic stockinette and an insert may be as effective, more comfortable, less costly, and easier to apply than a pressure garment. When a splint is used for a palmar burn, it may be more effective to wear no glove underneath. If the splint is formed well and secured by Coban (3M Medical-Surgical Division, St. Paul, MN), the splint, besides fitting more accurately without the glove, can provide conforming pressure because it is secured with the Coban. However, glove and insert may still be alternated with such a splint to allow for use of the hands.

The transparent plastic facemask was introduced in 1979 by Rivers et al.[72] as an alternative to the elastic facemask to control facial scarring (Fig. 13-14). As its name implies, the transparent facemask is a piece of hard, transparent plastic in the form of a custom-fitting facemask secured to the face by means of straps. The mask is constructed by forming heated plastic over a modified positive mold of the patient's face. The positive mold is made from a negative mold (an impression) of the patient's face. Although an impression may be made of an adult's face when the patient is awake (as described by Rivers et al.), in children, it is advisable to obtain an impression while they are anesthetized. The impression procedure may be scheduled, if possible, when the patient is going to the operating room for débridement and/or grafting of areas other than the face and neck, as long as edema of the head and neck have subsided.

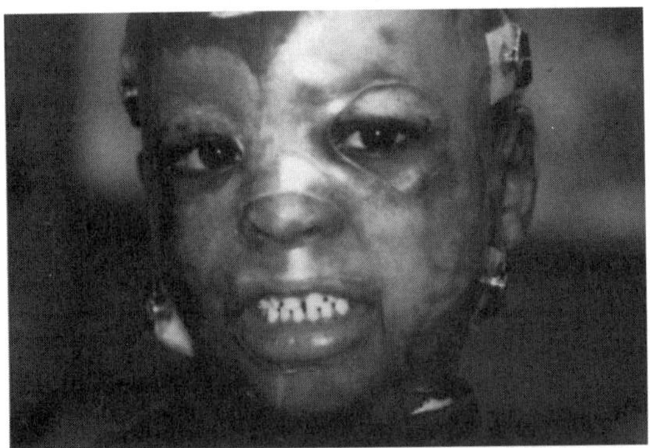

Figure 13-14 ▪ This transparent plastic facemask helps keep scars on the face flat, smooth, and pliable.

The advantages of the transparent facemask versus the elastic facemask are as follows:

- The mask can be constructed and applied to the patient within 24 hours. (There is no waiting for the elastic garment to return from the manufacturer.)
- The therapist can see exactly where pressure is being adequately applied by observing blanching of the scar. The transparent mask can be adjusted accordingly by the therapist to increase or decrease pressure in specific areas.
- The patient's face is visible to other people and is not covered by a "mask."
- The transparent mask usually does not require the construction and exact placement of inserts.
- The transparent facemask may cause fewer problems with head growth and malocclusion than the elastic mask.

There are also several disadvantages of the transparent facemask, including the following:

- The cost of construction (therapist's time and possible operating room costs if the impression is taken under anesthesia and the patient is not undergoing another procedure) for the transparent mask may exceed the cost of an elastic mask.
- Although both types of mask often have to be replaced as the child grows and the mask wears out, the cost of a new transparent mask is probably greater.

- The plastic used to construct the transparent mask is rigid, permits little movement of the facial muscles, and often limits mandible motion.
- The transparent mask may not cover as many areas on the head as the elastic mask. (However, the transparent mask can be used with a chinstrap or alternated with an elastic mask.)
- Perspiration is increased underneath the transparent mask, and plastic may be more uncomfortable than elastic.

Problems With Pressure Garments and Inserts and Some Possible Solutions. Although the application of pressure may be effective in helping to flatten, soften, and smooth scars, potential problems, drawbacks, and difficulties are associated with this approach. The garments are porous, but they can still be uncomfortable, especially in the summer. A small number of children are allergic to the materials in the pressure garment. This may be remedied somewhat by applying a close-fitting garment of another fabric underneath the pressure garment. As discussed earlier, there may also be problems associated with too tight a fit. As also previously discussed, although the patient can engage in most any activity while wearing the garment, the garment can interfere with movement and sensation. Moreover, such garments may interfere with normal ADLs and, in young children, with toilet training, because a leotard or brief is usually too tight for these children to pull down and up without assistance. Also, the elastic chinstrap or facemask may cause snoring or interruptions in normal sleep.

The elastic chinstrap may also cause at least a temporary recession of the mandible,[73] and it, in combination with a neck conformer, may cause increased proclination of maxillary and mandibular incisors.[74] The elastic facemask may impede head growth in very young children[75] and may cause abnormal recession of mandibular growth.[76] Both the elastic facemask and the plastic facemask may affect facial growth.[74] Elastic shirts may cause regressed skeletal growth of the thoracic cage,[76] and elastic gloves may cause narrowing of the palmar arch.[76] However, the burn injury and/or the acute or reconstructive therapy, as well as the grafted skin and scar tissue, may also contribute to these problems.[75–77] When the facemask or elastic chinstrap is used, the child's head growth, facial growth, and dentition should be monitored.

There are several areas of the body where it is difficult to achieve or apply adequate pressure. For example, it is troublesome to apply pressure in the perineum. It is also difficult to apply sufficient pressure over the perineum and the buttocks if the child is in diapers.

Inserts also may cause problems or difficulties. Because most inserts are nonporous, perspiration will be increased in the areas covered by the inserts. Besides causing discomfort, the increased perspiration can lead to a rash or skin maceration, or to skin breakdown because of increased friction. There are several solutions to such problems. One is to remove the insert frequently. Another solution is to apply a layer of stockinette or gauze underneath the insert. If skin breakdown occurs, the area can be bandaged and the pressure garment can still be worn. Occasionally, the insert can still be worn over a bandage.

With normal movement, inserts may slip from their desired location. Children may also intentionally dislodge inserts or remove them.

SPLINTING

The purpose of splinting during the rehabilitation phase is to maintain or increase ROM (Fig. 13-15). This is accomplished by providing an equal and opposing force to that of the contracting scar, by inhibiting contraction, and by maintaining tissue length. If the patient was splinted during the acute phase, the splint may no longer fit because the patient no longer has bulky bandages.

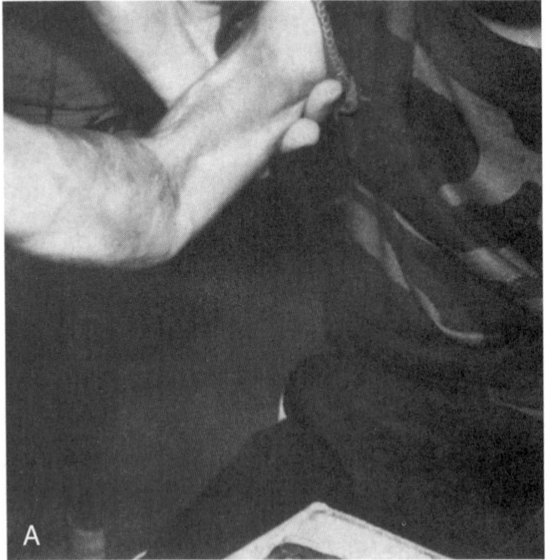

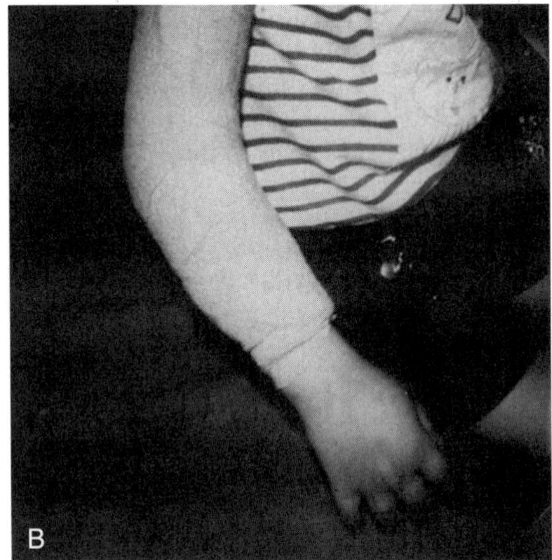

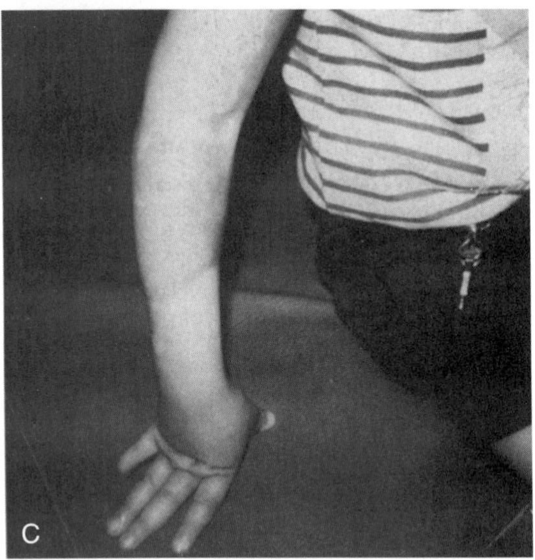

Figure 13-15 ▪ Nonsurgical correction of scar contraction through splinting and pressure. (**A**) Scar contraction causing loss of full elbow extension. (**B**) A splint has been constructed and applied to the anterior surface under a Coban wrap. (**C**) Note the increased joint motion and flatter, smoother scar approximately 24 hours later.

SCHEDULE. The splinting schedule will vary according to the patient's immediate potential for contracture and loss of motion. Such potential should decrease gradually over several months as the scar matures. If a patient loses a significant amount of motion when a splint is off for 2 hours, that patient will, at least initially, require a rigorous splinting schedule. Such a schedule may require the splint to be worn continually except for specified periods (lasting less than 2 hours each) of exercise, activity, and ADLs. Other patients may require splinting only for short periods during the day and then at night, or perhaps just at night. As the scar matures, the active force of the contracting scar should decrease, and the need for the splint should also decrease.

APPLICATION. Splints are worn over pressure garments. Exceptions to this rule occur when a splint both positions and provides pressure, or when a precise fit would be difficult to achieve and maintain in the presence of a pressure garment, as may happen with a small hand. In the former case, the splint would be worn directly against the skin. In the latter case, the splint may be alternated with a glove; alternatively, pressure could be applied to the dorsum by means of a sponge, and both sponge and splint would be secured by a pressure wrap. Elastic bandages are preferable to straps for securing splints in place and helping to maintain splint conformity to the body part. Elastic bandages also provide pressure that can help soften, smooth, and flatten scar; they can also give a slight dynamic quality to a static splint. Coban is very effective in securing pediatric splints and has the additional benefit of being difficult for the child to remove.

During this phase, splints should be custom-made for a child and should fit well. A secure fit helps position the specific joint(s) correctly in addition to providing conforming pressure to the scar.

CASTING. Casting may be used during both the acute and rehabilitation phases to maintain position in pediatric patients when a splint position is difficult to sustain. For example, it may be preferable to immobilize the MCP joints in flexion while allowing active use of the distal joints.[78] Serial casting is effective in correcting contractures in both pediatric and adult burn patients in whom other methods of regaining motion have failed, in noncompliant patients,[79–81] in patients whose splints easily slip or are removed, or in those for whom other methods, such as dynamic splinting, cannot be used.[81] Serial casting can eliminate or delay the need for reconstructive surgery.[81] Once motion is regained through serial casting, it needs to be maintained through continued casting or splinting and ROM exercise. Depending on the particular patient and the phase of healing, casts made of either plaster or synthetic materials may be used. Soft Cast, a synthetic casting material, is particularly useful for children because it sets quickly. In addition, although the child cannot remove it the therapist simply unwraps it rather than using a cast saw, which might frighten the child.

RANGE OF MOTION

The purpose of ROM exercises and activities during the rehabilitation phase is to help maintain or increase ROM by helping maintain scar elasticity and elongation and by opposing the force of contracting scar. ROM exercises and activities during this phase also help maintain muscle balance.

EVALUATION. Pressure garments should be removed for both evaluation of ROM and performance of ROM exercises. The garments can inhibit active and passive ROM, and when the garments are off, the therapist can observe the scar to see if limitations in motion are caused by inelastic scar tissue.

As with other disorders, goniometry is the preferred method of evaluating ROM in children. When evaluating ROM during the rehabilitation phase, the therapist should evaluate active and passive ROM of individual joints, as well as total active and total passive motion across several joints. It is possible, for example, for a child to have full active and passive shoulder flexion with the elbow in flexion but, because of contracting scar, have limitations in shoulder flexion with the elbow in extension. The therapist should also observe the quality of movement and how the motion is performed. For example, a child with burns of the anterior chest will frequently ambulate with protracted shoulders and limited trunk rotation.

ACTIVE RANGE OF MOTION EXERCISES AND ACTIVITIES. Before starting active ROM exercises, it is helpful for the therapist to lubricate and massage the scar tissue over and around the joint or area to be exercised. With younger children especially, it is useful to incorporate enjoyable activities that require the ROM desired. Basketball, for example, is a good activity for achieving shoulder flexion, whereas bicycles or tricycles facilitate hip and knee flexion and extension.

Passive Range of Motion Exercises and Activities. Too often, children with burns have been traumatized by too aggressive or excessive passive ROM exercise. Judgment and experience are required to determine which patients are candidates for passive ROM and to learn how to perform passive ROM exercises for this population. If there is a limitation in passive ROM, before initiating passive ROM exercises, the therapist should attempt to increase motion through changes in the splinting or pressure program. Motion may be lost because the splint was off for too long a period or was incorrectly applied. Also, some joints, particularly the knees and elbows that have limited extension, are amenable to serial splinting. It is difficult for the therapist (and painful for the patient) to stretch hard scar tissue. Softening the scar by increasing the pressure may yield an increase in ROM without the performance of passive ROM exercises. For example, before instituting a passive ROM program to gain shoulder abduction in a child with a burn of the anterior axilla, the therapist should first try to soften the scar in that location by increasing the applied pressure with the addition of an insert. When the scar is softened, the ROM may automatically increase.

It is particularly useful to lubricate and massage scar before performing passive ROM exercises, as dry skin may crack when it is stretched, and massage may soften tissue and facilitate passive ROM. The therapist may stretch the entire band of scar (multijoint), or the scar over a single joint. The therapist may begin by stretching just to the point of slight resistance and maintaining that stretch until resistance is no longer felt. The therapist should stretch the scar until it blanches. If at least slight blanching does not occur, the therapist may not be stretching sufficiently to increase motion. Overstretching, on the other hand, causes unnecessary pain, and the therapist can tear or damage tissue that could then trigger an inflammatory response leading to increased local scarring. Gains in passive ROM should be incorporated into active ROM exercises or functional activities (Fig. 13-16) and maintained through splinting. The splint should be adjusted to accommodate increases in motion.

Passive ROM activities also can be employed, including, for example, placing a child prone or supine over a bolster or ball.

Passive ROM exercises may be contraindicated if there is a substantial wound over a joint, the healing of which may be impeded by stretching. Also, some scars may be too mature to achieve a significant gain in motion from pas-

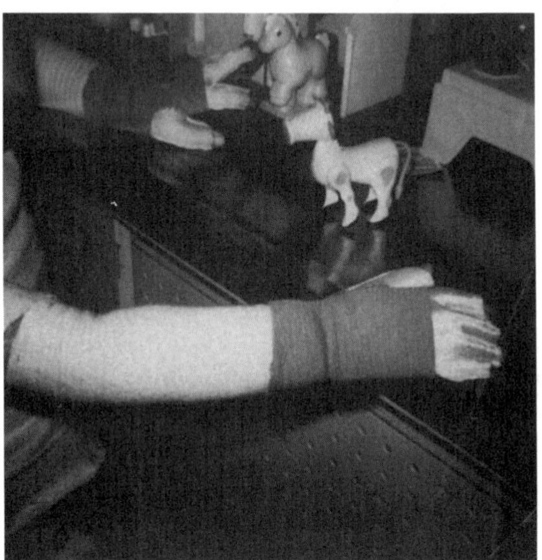

Figure 13-16 ■ Age-appropriate play activities facilitate active range of motion. This child is between 1 and 2 weeks post-graft application and is wearing tubular elastic stockinette and interim pressure gloves constructed of swimsuit lycra.

sive ROM exercises. When increases in range of motion are difficult or impossible to achieve or maintain through any treatment methods previously discussed, the child may simply not have adequate amounts of skin in the area and should be referred for surgical evaluation.

There are several modalities, such as paraffin and continuous passive ROM machines, which can be effective in helping to increase range of motion. These methods are discussed in the section entitled "Therapeutic Modalities."

ACTIVITIES OF DAILY LIVING

Children with small burns often return to age-level functional independence within 1 to 2 weeks of hospital discharge with little or no ADL therapy. Children with more severe burns may have difficulty with ADLs because of the persistence of open wounds, decreased ROM, decreased strength and endurance or interference from pressure garments and splints. ADL problems may also be related to altered or diminished sensation[82] or psychological difficulties. The therapist should provide assistive devices and ADL traning when necessary, while also trying to ameliorate factors that may interfere with functional independence, such as decreased ROM.

STRENGTH AND CARDIOVASCULAR ADAPTATION

Patients who are hospitalized for prolonged periods commonly lose muscle mass and cardiovascular endurance. This loss may be particularly obvious in the burn patient who is in a catabolic state during the acute phase or who has sustained an inhalation injury. Most children with smaller burns appear to have little trouble and take little time resuming preburn activities that require age-level strength and endurance. However, during the early rehabilitation phase, children with larger burns may tire easily. Such patients initially may require strengthening and cardiovascular exercises. These activities must be planned according to the age-appropriate needs of the child, the specific areas burned, and the strengthening and cardiovascular training devices available. Nevertheless, few studies have been done on the pediatric burn patient. One study that involved treadmill stress-testing of pediatric burn patients[83] found that patients who were 1 or more years past the burn injury had an endurance of approximately 3 minutes (one stage) longer than did those patients who were still in the first year after their burn injury. Values for each year after 1 year showed little change. Patients sustaining burns of greater than 40% of their TBSA who underwent fascial excision (instead of tangential excision) or had inhalation injury, or both, showed diminished performance in the first year. After the first year, however, regardless of such complications, all pediatric burn patients tested were able to maximize their recovery, except that the performance of those patients who had sustained inhalation injury never equaled those without inhalation injury.

THERAPEUTIC MODALITIES

Although there has been documented use of some modalities with adults who have been burned, there have been few reports of the use of therapeutic modalities for children with burn injuries. Several modalities that are commonly utilized for burned adults can also be used with certain children.

Paraffin and Sustained Stretch Treatments. Paraffin and sustained stretch treatments may increase collagen extensibility, increase skin pliability, decrease joint discomfort, and increase joint ROM.[84] Because of burn patients' decreased skin tolerance to heat and increased sensitivity to heat, and particularly in the case of children, their fear of hot liquids, the paraffin is cooled before application. (Patients with a particular intolerance for or fear of heat, decreased sensation, or open wounds or fragile skin are not candidates for paraffin and sustained stretch treatments.) The paraffin is combined with mineral oil and the temperature is lowered to 115°F[85] or lower. The joint can be stretched either with the aid of a splint or held manually, and then dipped into the paraffin. The paraffin also can be painted on,[86] or coarse mesh gauze can be dipped into the paraffin and applied to the joint, after which gentle long stretch and active exercises can be performed.[85]

CONTINUOUS PASSIVE MOTION. Continuous passive motion (CPM) machines can be used with burn patients during both the acute and rehabilitation phases.[87] Although their use with burned adults has been studied and documented,[88,89] most machines do not fit small children. Some of the models, however, may be suitable for older children and adolescents. Covey et al. in discussing the use of CPM with patients sustaining hand burns, postulated that the patients who may benefit the most from CPM are those with burns involving multiple kinetic areas (the idea being that the CPM machine could be applied to one limb while the therapist worked on another), comatose patients, and patients who display limited active motion because of pain, anxiety, or edema.[88] Such factors might also apply to the use of CPM with patients who have burns on other areas of the body. Although CPM may provide an additional, useful, therapeutic tool, many of the machines do not take the joint through the full ROM.

OTHER THERAPEUTIC APPROACHES

SILICONE GEL. Topical silicone gel sheets have been used on hypertrophic scars in Europe since the mid-1980s. One controlled study[90] performed in the United States reported significant gains in ROM in patients with elbow contractures who were treated with both silicone gel and exercise compared with those who were treated with exercise alone. In a controlled study[91] by Ahn et al. that used silicone gel sheets to treat hypertrophic scars in adults documented improvement in one or more items of scar texture, color, thickness, durability, pruritus, and (where applicable) ROM assessed during clinical evaluation; and there was an increase in scar elasticity as measured by objective elastometry. In those patients whose scars showed improvement, the silicone gel sheets were worn for at least 12 hours per day for 4 weeks; further improvement was noted after a second 4-week period. The mechanism of action of the silicone gel sheets remains unknown, and the gel sheets appear to work with or without the use of pressure to secure them in place.

Certain problems may be associated with silicone gel sheets, including rashes and skin maceration.[91] A report of the use of silicone gel sheets on scars in pediatric patients[92] revealed another significant problem—poor durability of the gel sheets in active children that, in turn, increased the cost of the treatment.

MYOFASCIAL RELEASE. No studies have been done concerning the use of myofascial release in burn patients. However, therapists trained in myofascial release have begun to employ this technique in burn patients in whom the depth and extent of injury have produced scar problems that may be amenable to myofascial release.

HIPPOTHERAPY. Hippotherapy, or therapeutic horseback riding, has been used with children who have burn injuries. Riding therapy may increase ROM and strength and improve dexterity while providing an exciting activity that may also enhance the burned child's self-esteem and self-confidence.[93]

SWIMMING. Therapeutic swimming can also be useful in the treatment of burned children. The goal of such therapy is to provide a recreational activity designed to increase strength, endurance, and ROM in a medium that may decrease pain.

DEVELOPMENTAL CONSIDERATIONS

The effects of burn injury on child development have received sparse investigation. A recent study[94] of 12 pediatric burn patients who were tested with the Denver Developmental Screening Test revealed delays in six of the subjects. The most severely injured showed the most significant delays. Although most of the delays were in the gross motor sector, delays also were noted in the fine motor-adaptive and personal-social sections of the test for five of the children. None of the subjects showed delays in the language category of the test. These researchers concluded that parents should be apprised of possible developmental delays, and that rehabilitation professionals should include the attainment of developmental goals in their treatment plans. Other than severity of injury, the study did not specifically identify the factors that may have contributed to the delays. A limitation of the study is that it was done early in the child's recovery, so it is not known how long these delays persist.

Other investigators studied a group of children aged 6 months to 6 years. They used the Denver II, Peabody Developmental Motor Scales, the Denver Home Screening Questionnaire, and the Vineland Adaptive Behavior Scales. The results indicated that 43% of children had "suspect" findings overall and 39% had language delays at 6 months after the injury. There were no changes in the Denver II scores, but there were improvements in the Peabody Motor Scales. It is not clear if any of the children had delays prior to the burn injury.[108]

It is not uncommon for hospitalized children to regress developmentally. This is one reason why they should be encouraged to assist with or participate in their own care and ADLs, and should be involved in age-appropriate play and activities when possible. Despite such involvement and activities, to execute necessary treatment, facilitate care, ease the child's pain, and because of the child's injury, certain procedures must be performed that, along with the physical and emotional trauma, separation from family, and relative dependency, contribute to regression. For example, toddlers who have just mastered toilet training may be returned to diapers, and those who had finally been weaned from the bottle may be put back on it. When the child is discharged, the parent may complain that the child has lost mastery of abilities that the parent worked hard to help the child achieve. Such delays appear to be temporary, and earlier skills are usually regained when the child returns home and resumes his or her prior activities.

A developmental evaluation during the acute phase may not yield a true picture of the child's developmental status because of temporary regression or because of pain or a decreased ability to cooperate. The rehabilitation phase may be the preferred time frame for a developmental evaluation and specific remediation. Children who are victims of abuse or neglect may also be developmentally delayed, although it is possible that such delays may have preceded the burn injury.

As previously discussed, treatment during the rehabilitation phase also may interfere with execution of and acquisition of age-level skills. Sensation and movement may be limited by pressure garments. Splints may hinder motion and thus thwart independence in ADLs. Because the child may not be able to don and doff a pressure garment independently, the acquisition of toileting skills may be delayed or the child may require assistance.

RETURNING TO SCHOOL

If the burned child is school-aged, planning for school reentry should begin early during the child's hospitalization. Maintaining contact with the teacher and classmates through cards, phone calls, videos, and when possible, visits, helps the child focus on the goal of returning to school and facilitates reentry. Some hospital settings allow for tutoring. Children who were burned 1 or more years before entering school also may benefit from a school reentry program, particularly if the burns were extensive.

The purpose of the school reentry program is to facilitate the child's physical, social, and emotional return to school by increasing the knowledge and understanding possessed by the teacher, classmates, and other staff and students as to what happened to the burned child. Additional information provided may include reasons for the child's appearance and an explanation of care items, such as pressure garments and splints. The reentry program can also provide increased support for the child (e.g., decreasing both the child's and classmate's fears and increasing self-esteem by describing the child as a hero), practical information for the school staff concerning the patient's splints and pressure garments, and information about he child's ADL needs, such as writing, mobility around the school, and use of the bathroom.

A variety of school reentry programs can be employed, and the physical therapist can play an integral role in a school reentry program. Some of these programs incorporate puppet shows, games, videos, and visits to the school by hospital professionals. Topics that might be included in a reentry program cover:

- What exactly happened to the burned child and information about the hospitalization
- Burn prevention and first-aid
- The noncontagious nature of burns
- The use of pressure garments or splints
- Scars
- The impropriety of teasing and why people stare
- The fact that the burned child is still the same child depsite his or her different appearance
- The ability of the burned child to engage in most or all of preburn activities
- What classmates can do to help

It is usually preferable to have the burned child and family present during the program.

The burn unit's therapist should work in conjunction with the school therapist to determine the patient's needs in school and to confer about the therapy program. The therapist also should provide information to the teacher and the school nurse concerning the application of and schedule for splints or pressure garments, ADL concerns, and handling of potential problems.

BURN CAMP

Just as there are camps for children with various diseases or disabilities (e.g., diabetes camp, spina bifida camp, etc.), there are also about 40 burn camps in North America that offer a variety of programs for children who have sustained burn injuries. Several of these camps are coordinated or staffed by therapists, or therapists are encouraged to attend the camp to help with programs or to assist campers. The purpose of most of the camps is to provide a safe, recreational environment in which children with burns can interact with one another, build self-esteem, learn new skills, and have fun.

COSMETICS

Corrective cosmetics are used on burned adults and may also be of use in certain adolescents and children. Some patients may require hair pieces or prosthetic ears. At least one medical center[95] takes a more comprehensive approach, not only teaching make-up application but also providing instruction in color and fashion analysis and psychosocial skills.

The Reconstructive Phase

Once scars are mature, they usually do not respond to most nonsurgical approaches to correct hypertrophy and contracture, and surgery may offer the only remedy. Burn patients may also require surgery because the type of wound closure accomplished in the acute phase may have resulted in a less-than-optimal cosmetic or functional outcome. A child may be discharged from therapy with full ROM only to develop a contracture later because the scar tissue and grafted skin did not keep pace with growth. Moreover, some reconstructive procedures yield better results when performed at certain times or ages. Children are evaluated regularly as they grow and mature to determine the need for reconstructive surgery.

Reconstructive surgery often is delayed until after scar maturation except in cases in which, for example, a contraction or a contracture resulting in loss of motion cannot be corrected by nonsurgical approaches. After reconstructive surgical procedures, patients may require therapy similar to that described for the rehabilitation phase. In many cases, however, the course of therapy is often shorter and its intensity decreased.

PSYCHOSOCIAL ISSUES

Whether the burn is large or small, it can trigger short- or long-term difficulties for both the child and family. Although many burn injuries are accidental, the parents of the child feel tremendous guilt nonetheless. Often, one parent will blame the other for the incident. Because a parent feels guilty or feels sorry for the child, proper discipline for the burned child may not be maintained once the child is at home. Usually, the entire family will be affected in one way or another by the injury. Siblings of the burned child may feel neglected or resent the "extra attention" the burned child is receiving. The incident may place a burden on the family's finances. Carrying out the necessary daily treatment at home and keeping appointments at the hospital may also be stressful. Certainly, the burned child also has many issues with which to contend. For example, the child may have to endure staring or teasing, and may feel angry about the injury happening and the treatment required. Both the child and family may be angry and grieve over losses such as changes in appearance and function.

The therapist should be aware of these feelings and reactions, and should provide encouragement and support. When indicated, the therapist should involve or alert professionals who can help the patient and family.

There are a number of self-help and support groups for burn survivors and their families that provide a range of services. Among these is The Phoenix Society, Inc. 33 Main St., Suite 403, Nashua, NH 03060; 1–603–889–3000 or 1–800–888–BURN, which will supply a list of local chapters or other self-help organizations on request.

Outcomes

Functions of the Skin

As stated earlier, whenever the skin is significantly damaged or destroyed, the functions of the skin may be impaired. Several functions, such as protection against infection and regulation of body fluids and electrolytes, are primarily disturbed during the acute phase. Other

DISPLAY 13-1
Professional Organizations and Resources

The American Burn Association
625 N. Michigan Ave,
Suite 1530
Chicago, IL 60611
1-800-548-BURN

Periodicals:

Journal of Burn Care & Rehabilitation (official publication of the American Burn Association) St. Louis, MO, Mosby–Year Book, Inc.

Burns (the journal of the International Society for Burn Injuries) Oxford, U.K., Butterworth-Heinemann, Ltd.

functions, such as temperature regulation, can be impaired both during the acute phase and, at times, after healing. Other functions of the skin may be permanently impaired. Normal skin color may be lost. Skin grafts tend to be hyperpigmented, whereas scar tissue often lacks pigment. These color changes are permanent. (However, some partial-thickness burns may heal with skin that is hypopigmented or depigmented, and such pigment changes may be improved by surgery.[96]) No hair will grow in areas where hair follicles are destroyed. Although the cosmetic function of hair can be restored through surgical procedures, such as tissue expansion of the scalp, when sufficient hair remains, there exists no practical answer for major hair losses on the limbs, trunk, and other areas. Nails are frequently damaged or destroyed in deep burns of the hands and feet. Injury or destruction of the sebaceous and sweat glands can lead to dry skin that requires frequent external lubrication. Scar tissue and skin grafts are not as durable as normal skin. A scar at maximum strength may be only 70% as strong as intact skin.[97] Often, the same scrapes and bumps that normal skin can withstand cause tissue breakdown in scarred and grafted skin.

Heat intolerance because of decreased sweating in scarred areas can be a problem in patients with deep partial-thickness and full-thickness burns involving a large percentage of TBSA. A study of sweating in patients with healed burns revealed a decreased number of sweat glands in hypertrophic scar tissue, but the remaining sweat glands in burned areas were more hyperactive than those in normal skin.[63]

Investigations of sensation in grafted skin and healed burns have yielded contradictory results, and there are few studies involving children. One study[98] of sensory loss over grafted areas of burned adults demonstrated diminished or absent sensation, as well as complaints of increased sensitivity to ambient cold, although the decrease in sensation rarely contributed to the subject's long-term impairment rating. The depth of injury appeared to be the best predictor of altered sensation. One researcher[99] concluded that the same graft type can show various degrees of innervation depending on the depth and extent of injury, healing complications, and the amount of scar tissue.

An inquiry[82] of tactile function in burned children found that points or areas tested on the burned side had altered and often diminished sensation when compared with the corresponding unburned side, and that 60% of the subjects had one or more ADL problems related to altered tactile sensation. However, the researchers believed that all of the children appeared to have adjusted well to their tactile skills or problems. One investigator[100] conducted sensory evaluations and histologic studies of the tactile functions in eight adults who had received free full-thickness grafts to the palmar area and digits as infants and who were periodically evaluated over a period of up to 19 years. Nerve endings and fibers were found to be clustered around hair roots, and no encapsulated receptors were found in the grafts, yet with the exception of hyperesthesia, sensation was rated as good. It was concluded that specific sensory organs need not be present for sensation, and that normal sensations can develop after grafting in early childhood before awareness of sensations are firm.

Although scar tissue tends to become more pliable as it matures, it does not have the same elastic properties as normal skin. Thus, some patients with significant facial scarring may actually appear younger than their age because of the increased tautness of scar tissue and grafted skin. However, this same tautness often gives a masklike appearance that does not yield to the normal nuances of facial expression.

Growth and Physiologic Functions

Longitudinal studies[101] of burned children who underwent excisional therapy have revealed that growth delays and nutritional dysfunction, bone growth abnormalities, and physiologic dysfunction, including alterations in cardiopulmonary, renal, audiologic, and immunologic function, can occur. Most of these problems occurred in children with burns over greater than 40% of their TBSA. Some of these deficits were temporary, whereas others appeared to be permanent.

Psychological and Behavioral Adaptation

Most studies on adjustment after burn injury have focused on quite severely injured patients, and not all investigators have been in agreement. As one might expect, children with burn injuries and their families have problems, but research indicates that the long-term adjustment for most of these children is good, suggesting that those with less severe injuries also have positive adjustments.

A study[102] by Blakeney et al. of young adult survivors of severe childhood burn injury revealed that, although some survivors had significant indicators of psychological disturbances, most did not evidence psychopathology more often than did a normal group, and data indicated that they were typical of other people in their age group. A follow-up inquiry[103] concluded that positive psychological adjustment was predicted by increased family cohesion, independence, and increased expressiveness within the family. Intelligence was not a factor, and length of time after injury was a factor only during the first 2 years.

A study[104] of burn-disfigured children of primary-school age who had sustained burns over greater than 80% of their TBSA revealed that all of the children presented with pervasive developmental regression, accompanied by phobias, nightmares, and various other symptoms such as enuresis or encopresis. However, by the fifth year following the injury all of them (except one, who had premorbid deficits) had returned to an average level of progressive personality development. Even the one with premorbid deficits was found to be progressing well within his limitations. The researchers pointed to the parent(s) as being a fundamental factor in facilitating positive self-image in the child and in beginning and preserving the skill of active mastery in the child.

Another study[105] compared perception of body image in children with burns (ages 5 to 15 years) 5 years after the injury with that of a control group of children without burns. No differences between the two groups were noted. Another investigation[106] of body image, self-esteem, and depression among burn-injured adolescents and young adults showed that those who perceived greater social support from family and particularly from friends had a more positive body image, greater self-esteem, and less depression than did those who perceived less support. The study found females to be more depressed than males. Surprisingly, the percentage of TBSA burned, the location of the burn, and the number of years elapsed since the injury were not found to be significant factors in this investigation.

Although the predominantly positive adjustment of those with larger burns would appear to augur well for individuals who have sustained burns involving a smaller percentage of TBSA, the exception to a favorable adjustment for those with smaller TBSA burns may be those with "hidden burns." One paper[107] reported on a group of individuals, predominantly women, who had been burned as children. The burns were primarily small and could be hidden by clothing. This group rarely exposed their scars, most were unmarried, and they expressed unhappiness. As children, they were encouraged to hide their scars to avoid taunting; consequently, they grew up believing that the scars were "bad." The author of the paper recommended that burn care providers educate parents of newly burned children about the possible long-term negative effects of encouraging children to hide their scars. (See Case Studies.)

Case Study 1—Tiffany, 18-Month-Old Female with TBSA Burns

Tiffany is an 18-month-old female who sustained 11% TBSA partial- and full-thickness burns to the face, submental area, neck, chest, right shoulder, and right arm after pulling a bowl of hot soup from the counter. She underwent débridement of the thorax, shoulder, and arm and placement of split-thickness sheet grafting with surgical staples to those sites 4 days after the injury. The buttocks and thighs were donor sites. The physical therapist had seen Tiffany before the grafting and constructed an abduction (airplane)splint for the right shoulder to be applied at the time of grafting. The therapist also discussed treatment goals and provided information to the parents. Tiffany's arm was maintained in the splint for 5 days following surgery, except for dressing changes. During this period, the therapist sewed interim Tubigrip pressure shirts for the trunk and arm and received insurance authorization for commercial custom-made pressure shirts and for outpatient rehabilitation.

On the fifth day after grafting, the surgeon removed the staples and most of the grafts had taken. Small areas of graft loss were present along with open wounds from nongrafted burns. Tiffany had full passive shoulder motion but resisted and cried with attempts to move her arm and did not actively move the arm. She was measured for a custom-made pressure shirt, and a Tubigrip shirt, made by the therapist, was applied over the shoulder following dressing changes. The parents were instructed in proper application of the Tubigrip shirt and shoulder abduction splint (to be worn at night) and in activities to facilitate shoulder motion and use, and passive range of motion exercises to be performed once daily.

Tiffany returned for an outpatient visit 1 week later and still had some scabs and small open wounds. She had full passive range of motion but active abduction limited to 120 degrees with a protracted scapula. The donor site was healed and ambulation was normal. The therapist used the Vancouver Scar Assessment to evaluate the donor site and nongrafted burn areas. The donor site was scar-free but some areas on the chest had changes indicative of scar development. Elastogel (Southwest Technologies) was applied to these areas under the Tubigrip shirt with instructions to remove the material three times each day for 1 hour each. Parents were further instructed to double the Tubigrip shirts and maintain the splint at night. The physical therapist engaged Tiffany in activities to enhance shoulder motion.

One week later, Tiffany returned with active shoulder abduction to 150 degrees, and all wounds closed except for two small (1-cm) sites. The scar under the Elastogel was smooth, soft, and flat, but some adjacent areas were not as good and the Elastogel was replaced with a larger piece to cover the adjacent areas. The custom-made garment was fitted with instructions to alternate its use with the double Tubigrip shirt until the second garment was received and to continue with the splint at night.

At her next visit 2 weeks later, Tiffany had no open wounds and had full active motion, but the scapula still tended toward protraction upon abduction. Scars were all smooth and flat except a small area on the shoulder that was 1 mm thick. The PT molded a $\frac{1}{8}$ inch Aliplast over the shoulder with a $\frac{1}{4}$ inch Polycushion (placed with stockinette over the adhesive side of the Polycushion) over the Aliplast. Two sets of inserts were constructed for the raised area, and splint use at night was continued. The next week saw all scars being flat, smooth, and soft, and full range of active motion had been achieved. Additional inserts were constructed. The parents were instructed to continue use of the pressure garment and inserts but to discontinue the night splint and to call if any changes were noted in the scar or motion.

Monthly visits continued for the PT to reevaluate motion, scars, construct inserts, and periodically remeasure for garments. At 17 months after the injury, the scar was faded, soft, and pliable and Tiffany had full range. At that point, she was discharged from PT with instructions to continue scar lubrication, use sunblock as appropriate, and not hide her scars.

Case Study 2—Robert, 10-Year-Old Boy with BSA Burns

Robert, a 10-year-old male who, while playing with gasoline and matches, sustained 20% BSA burns, partial- and full-thickness, to both lower extremities proximal to the ankles, and his left forearm, sparing the elbow and wrist joints. He was transported to the area burn center about 40 miles from his home. An escharotomy was performed on the deep, circumferential burn to the right calf.

On physical therapy evaluation, Robert's lower extremities and left forearm and hand were edematous. He positioned himself from the left arm abducted to his body with his elbow and wrist in flexion and his forearm pronated. Robert's hips were flexed and abducted, his knees were flexed, and ankles plantar-flexed and supinated. Pain and edema limited active knee motion to 90-degree flexion and −30-degree extension. Robert's ankles dorsiflexed to neutral and there was full active motion in the left arm and hand, both hips, and all toes.

The physical therapist constructed and applied bilateral knee extension splints and a splint that positioned the right foot in neutral. Robert's legs were elevated on pillows, and he was instructed and encouraged to use his left hand for all ADLs and other activities. Active and active-assisted exercises within tissue-limited range were added on the third day after injury.

On day four, Robert received STSG sheet grafts to both calves and posterior left thigh and knee, with the right thigh and back serving as donor sites. Splints were applied at grafting and they kept the graft sites immobilized for the next 5 days except for dressing changes.

Robert's parents had been instructed in treatment goals and techniques, and owing to the distance from home, Robert's rehabilitation was to be provided as an outpatient at a local hospital. The burn center physical therapist was to recommend, monitor, and provide certain services, such as measuring for pressure garments, for the local physical therapist. The burn center physical therapist also contacted the insurance company to justify the need for therapy at both centers and to obtain authorization for pressure garments.

On day five following grafting, the staples were removed and it became obvious that additional grafting was needed for replacement of some lost graft and for an area not previously thought to need grafting on his right lower extremity. Robert was measured for a custom-made leotard with removable socks. Tubigrip was applied over the bandages on Robert's left lower extremity.

Following a second grafting on the next day, Robert was seated in a bedside chair with his legs elevated and bilateral knee extension and foot splints applied. The right splints remained on constantly except during dressing changes, whereas the left splints were also removed for PT that included active and active-assisted and resisted exercise. With elastic bandages applied over the Tubigrip to provide vascular support and support of the new grafts, Robert began to dangle his legs and bear weight on the left lower extremity. At this time, there was full active motion and function of the left upper extremity with many of the wounds closed. Five days after the second grafting (15 days after the injury), staples were removed, Tubigrip was applied to the right lower extremity and doubled on the left lower. Robert was discharged from the burn center the next day after his parents had demonstrated proper treatment skills at that time.

Robert's local outpatient treatment began and was supported by weekly treatments to the burn center for 7 weeks, followed by decreasing frequency to once every 2 months for care primarily regarding pressure garments and inserts. During one such visit, hypertrophic scarring was noted at a donor site on the back necessitating the use of a sleeveless pressure shirt with appropriate inserts.

Robert was initially reluctant to participate in gym class and soccer activities for fear of others seeing the garments and burns on his legs. Therefore, a school reentry and instructional program provided by both PTs was arranged. During the summer following the injury, Robert attended a camp for children with burn injuries.

Acknowledgments

Thanks to God for the privilege of working with children with burns and their families. Thanks to these children and their families for all they have taught me. Thanks to Anne Putnam and Karen Grigsby for all of their practical help and support with this chapter. Thanks to my husband, Jorn, and my children, Andreas Eric and Astrid Karen, for their patience and support during the many hours I spent writing.

REFERENCES

1. Brigham PA. A tour of the burn world—with special reference to children. The 20th Annual Mid-Atlantic Burn Conference; Monmouth, NJ; 1997.
2. National Health Interview Survey, National Hospital Discharge Survey, National Hospital Ambulatory Medical Care Survey, National Electronic Injury Surveillance System. Compiled and provided by PA Brigham, The Burn Foundation, Philadelphia; 1997.
3. Peate, WF. Outpatient management of burns. *Am Fam Phys.* 1992;45:1321.
4. Peter Brigham, Estimates, Burn Foundation of Philadelphia; 1992.
5. McLoughlin E, McGuire A. The causes, cost, and prevention of childhood burn injuries. *Am J Dis Child.* 1990;144:677–683.
6. East MK, Jones CA, Feller I, et al. Epidemiology of burns in children. In Carvajal HF, Parks DH, eds. *Burns in Children: Pediatric Burn Management.* Chicago: Year Book Medical Publishers; 1988: 3–10.
7. Statistics compiled by the now defunct National Burn Information Exchange as reported by East MK, Jones, Feller I, et al. Epidemiology of burns in children. In Carvajal HF, Parks DH, eds. *Burns in Children: Pediatric Burn Management.* Chicago: Year Book Medical Publishers; 1988:3–10.
8. Moritz AR, Henriques FC. Studies of thermal injury. II. The relative importance of time and surface temperature in burns. *Am J Pathol.* 1947;23: 695.
9. Grube BJ, Heimbach DM, Williamson JC. Management of pediatric burns. In Morray JP, ed. *Pediatric Intensive Care.* Norwalk, CT: Appleton & Lange; 1987:471–506.
10. Heath GA, Gayton WF, Hardesty VA. Childhood firesetting. *Can Psychiatr Assoc J.* 1976;21:229–237.
11. Epidemiology of burns in children-who: Victim types, 1964–1984 (n = 18, 764). Ann Arbor, MI: National Burn Information Exchange; 1985.
12. Bailey WC, ed. *Pediatric Burns.* Chicago: Year Book Medical Publishers; 1979:68.
13. Blakeney PE, Herndon DN. Abuse by burning. In Herndon DN, ed. *Total Burn Care.* London: W.B. Saunders; 1996:550–555.
14. Hammond J, Perez-Stable A, Ward C. Predictive value of historical and physical characteristics for the diagnosis of child abuse. *South Med J.* 1991; 84(2):166–168.
15. Cusick JM, Grant EJ, Kucan JO. Children's sleepwear: Relaxation of the Consumer Product Safety Commission's flammability standards. *J Burn Care Rehabil.* 1997;18:469–476.
16. Lockhart RD, Hamilton GF, Fyfe FW. *Anatomy of the Human Body.* Philadelphia: J.B. Lippincott; 1969.
17. Moncrief JA, Grafting. In Artz CP, Moncrief JA, Pruitt BA, eds. *Burns: A Team Approach.* Philadelphia: W.B. Saunders; 1979:275.
18. Knudson Cooper M, Thomas CM. Psychosocial care of the severely burned child. In Carvajal HF, Parks DH, eds. *Burns in Children: Pediatric Burn Management.* Chicago: Year Book Medical Publishers; 1988:345–362.
19. Lund CC, Browder NC. The estimation of areas of burns. *Surg Gynecol Obstet.* 1944;79:352.
20. American Burn Association. Hospital and prehospital resources for optimal care of patients with burn injury: Guidelines for development and operation of burn centers. *J Burn Care Rehabil.* 1990;11: 98–104.
21. Linares HA. Pathophysiology of the burn scar. In Herndon DN ed. *Total Burn Care.* London: W.B. Saunders; 1996:383–397.
22. Deitch EA, Wheelahan TM, Rose MP, et al. Hypertrophic burn scars: Analysis of variables. *J Trauma.* 1983;23:895–898.
23. Hunt TK. *Fundamentals of Wound Management in Surgery—Wound Healing: Disorders of Repair.* South Plainfield, NJ: Chirurgecom; 1976.
24. Parks DH, Evans EB, Larson DL. Prevention and correction of deformity after severe burns. *Surg Clin North Am.* 1978;58:1279–1289.
25. Ketchum LD. Hypertrophic scars and keloids. *Clin Plast Surg.* 1977;4:301–310.
26. Peacock EE, Madden JW, Trier WC. Biological basis for the treatment of keloids and hypertrophic scars. *So Med J.* 1970;63:7–55.

27. Larson D, Huang T, Linares H, et al. Prevention and treatment of scar contracture. In Artz CP, Moncrief JA, Pruitt BA, eds. *Burns: A Team Approach.* Philadelphia: W.B. Saunders; 1979:467–468.
28. Hulnick SJ, former Burn Center Director and Chief of Plastic Surgery, St. Christopher's Hospital for Children, Philadelphia, personal communication, 1988.
29. Diegelmann RF, Rothkopf LC, Cohen LK. Measurement of collagen biosynthesis during wound healing. *J Surg Res.* 1975;19:239–243.
30. Barnes MJ, Morton LF, Bennett RC, et al. Studies on collagen synthesis in the mature dermal scar in the guinea pig. *Biochem Soc Symp.* 1975;3: 917–920.
31. Phillips AW, Cope O. The revelation of respiratory tract damage as a principal killer of the burned patient. *Ann Surg.* 1962;155:1.
32. Jones CA, Feller I, Richards KE. Nursing care of the burned child. In Bailey WC, ed. *Pediatric Burns.* Chicago: Year Book Medical Publishers; 1979:67–106.
33. Carvajal HF. Resuscitation of the burned child. In Carvajal HF, Parks DH, eds. *Burns in Children: Pediatric Burn Management.* Chicago: Year Book Medical Publishers; 1988:78.
34. Robson MC, Burns BF, Smith DJ. Acute management of the burned patient. *Plast Rec Surg.* 1992; 89:1158.
35. Waldbillig A, et al. The adequacy of escharotomy in the pediatric burn patient (abstract). American Burn Association Meeting: New Orleans; 1989.
36. Zuker RM. Initial management of the burn wound. In Carvajal HF, Parks DH, eds. *Burns in Children: Pediatric Burn Management.* Chicago: Year Book Medical Publishers; 1988:99–105.
37. Sheridan RL, Hinson M, Nackel A. Development of a Pediatric Burn Pain and Anxiety Scale. *J Burn Care Rehabil.* 1997;18:455–459.
38. Heidrich G, Perry S, Armand R. Nursing staff attitudes about burn pain. *J Burn Care Rehabil.* 1981; 2:259–261.
39. Perry S, Heidrich G, Ramos E. Assessment of pain by burn patients. *J Burn Care Rehabil.* 1981;2: 322–326.
40. Eland JM, Anderson JE. The experience of pain in children. In Jacox A, ed. *A Source Book for Nurses and Other Health Professionals.* Boston: Little, Brown; 1977:453–473.
41. Wagner M. Pain and nursing care associated with burns. In Jacox A, ed. *Pain: A Source Book for Nurses and Other Health Professionals.* Boston: Little Brown; 1977:391–403.
42. Perry S, Heidrich G. Management of pain during débridement: A survey of US burn units. *Pain.* 1982;13:267–280.
43. Marvin JA, Miller MJ, Blakeney PE, et al. Pain response and pain control. In: Herndon DN, ed. *Total Burn Care.* London: W.B. Saunders; 1996:529–541.
44. Linares HA. Autopsy findings in burned children. In Carvajal HF, Parks DH, eds. *Burns in Children: Pediatric Burn Management.* Chicago: Year Book Medical Publishers; 1988:288–289.
45. Engrav LH, Heimbach DM, Reus JL, et al. Early excision and grafting vs nonoperative treatment of burns of indeterminant depth: A randomized prospective study. *J Trauma.* 1983;23:1001–1004.
46. Heimbach DM. Early burn excision and grafting. *Surg Clin North Am.* 1987;67:93–107.
47. Carvajal HF. Burn injuries. In Behrman RE, ed. *Nelson Textbook of Pediatrics.* Philadelphia: W.B. Saunders, Hartcourt Brace Jovanovich; 1992:233.
48. Parks DH, Wainwright DJ. The surgical management of burns. In Carvajal HF, Parks DH, eds. *Burns in Children: Pediatric Burn Management.* Chicago: Year Book Medical Publishers; 1988: 158,166.
49. Tompkins RG, Burke JF. Alternative wound coverings. In Herndon DN, ed. *Total Burn Care.* London: W.B. Saunders; 1996:164–168.
50. Robson MC. Overview of burn reconstruction. In Herndon DN, ed. *Total Burn Care.* London: W.B. Saunders; 1996:485–491.
51. Schwanholt C, Greenhalgh DG, Warden GD. A comparison of full-thickness versus split-thickness autografts for the coverage of deep palm burns in the very young pediatric burn patient. *J Burn Care Rehabil.* 1993;14;29–33.
52. Morris SE, Saffle JR. Utilization of full-thickness skin-grafting in the treatment of hand burns (abstract). American Burn Association Meeting, Baltimore, 1991.
53. Interview with Heimbach DM. Early excision and grafting: clinical implications. *Boots Burn Manage Rept.* 1992;1:8.
54. Egan M. Cultured skin grafts: preserving lives, challenging therapists. *OT Week.* 1992;6:14.
55. Compton CC. Current concepts in pediatric burn care: The biology of cultured epithelial autografts: An eight-year study in pediatric burn patients. *Eur J Pediatr Surg.* 1992;2:216–222.
56. Lifeskin the next generation in burn care. Culture Technology, Inc.; 1994.
57. Integra training manual. Plainsboro, NJ: Integra LifeSciences Corp.; 1996.
58. Medical economics of Integra artificial skin. Plainsboro, NJ: Integra LifeSciences Corp.; 1996.

59. Burk JF. Observations on the development and clinical use of artificial skin: An attempt to employ regeneration rather than scar formation in wound healing. *Jpn J Surg.* 1987;17:431–438.
60. Wainwright DJ. Use of an acellular allograft dermal matrix (AlloDerm) in the management of full-thickness burns. *Burns.* 1995;21:243–248.
61. Beasley RW. Secondary repair of burned hands. *Clin Plastic Surg.* 1981;8:141.
62. Helm PA. Neuromuscular considerations. In Fisher SV, Helm PA, eds. *Comprehenisve Rehabilitation of Burns.* Baltimore: Williams & Wilkins; 1984:235–241.
63. Cadwallader C, Helm P. Sweat gland distribution in healed severe burns: Quantitative topical distribution and qualitative function (abstract). American Burn Association Meeting, San Francisco, 1984.
64. Bell L, McAdams T, Morgan R, et al. Pruritis in burns: A descriptive study. *J Burn Care Rehabil.* 1988;9:306.
65. Cyriax JH. Clinical application of massage. In Licht S, ed. *Massage, Manipulation, and Traction.* New Haven, CT: Elizabeth Licht Publisher; 1960.
66. Katz SM, Frank DH, Leopold GG, et al. Objective measurement of hypertrophic burn scar: A preliminary study of tonometry and ultrasonography. *Ann Plast Surg.* 1985;14:121–127.
67. Esposito G, Ziccardi P, Scioli M, et al. The use of a modified tonometer in burn scar therapy. *J Burn Care Rehabil.* 1990;11:86–90.
68. Leung KS, Sher A, Clark JA, et al. Microcirculation in hypertrophic scars after burn injury. *J Burn Care Rehabil.* 1989;10:436–444.
69. Bartell TH, Monafo WW, Mustoe TA. A new instrument for serial measurements of elasticity in hypertrophic scar. *J Burn Care Rehabil.* 1988;9:657–660.
70. Sullivan T, Smith J, Kermode J, et al. Rating the burn scar. *J Burn Care Rehabil.* 1990;11:256–260.
71. Reichenbacher F, President of Bio-Concepts, Inc., Phoenix: Personal communication; 1988.
72. Rivers EA, Strate RG, Solem LD. The transparent facemask. *Am J Occup Ther.* 1979;33:109–113.
73. Parks DH, Shriners Burns Institute, Galveston, TX: Personal communication; 1982.
74. Fricke N, Dutcher K, Omnell L, et al. Effects of pressure garment wear on facial and dental development (abstract). American Burn Association Meeting: Salt Lake City, UT; 1992.
75. Grigsby L. The use of the facemask with children. Fifth Annual Meeting of the Mid-Atlantic Association of Burn Care Facilities: Philadelphia; 1982.
76. Leung KS, Cheng JCY, Ma GFY, et al. Complications of pressure therapy for post-burn hypertrophic scars. *Burns.* 1984;10:434–438.
77. McCauley RL, Fairleigh JF, Robson MC, et al. Effects of facial burns on facial growth in children: Preliminary report (abstract). American Burn Association Meeting: Baltimore; 1991.
78. Flesch P. Casting the young and the restless (abstract). American Burn Association Meeting: Orlando, FL; 1985.
79. Jordan MH, Lewis MS, Wiegand LT, et al. Dynamic plaster casting for burn scar contracture—an alternative to surgery (abstract). American Burn Association Meeting: San Francisco; 1984.
80. Bennett GB, Helm P, Purdue GF, et al. Serial casting: A method for treating burn contractures. *J Burn Care Rehabil.* 1989;10:543–545.
81. Ridgway CL, Daugherty MB, Warden GD. Serial casting as a technique to correct burn scar contractures: A case report. *J Burn Care Rehabil.* 1991;12:67–72.
82. Stap L, Brock R, Zissermann L. The tactile functions of burned children. *J Burn Care Rehabil.* 1983;4:291–302.
83. McElroy K. Alvarado MI, Rutan R, et al. Cardiovascular adaptation: Exercise stress-testing the pediatric burn patient, a continuation (abstract). American Burn Association Meeting: Salt Lake City; 1992.
84. Head M, Helm P. Paraffin and sustained stretching in the treatment of burn contractures. *Burns.* 1977;4:136.
85. Gross J, Stafford S. Modified method for application of paraffin wax for treatment of burn scar. *J Burn Care Rehabil.* 1984;5:394.
86. Johnson CL. Physical therapists as scar modifiers. *Phys Ther.* 1984;64:1383.
87. Covey MH. Application of CPM devices with burn patients. *J Burn Care Rehabil.* 1988;9:496–497.
88. Covey MH, Dutcher K, Marvin JA, Heimbach DM. Efficacy of continuous passive motion (CPM) devices with hand burns. *J Burn Care Rehabil.* 1988;9:397–400.
89. McAllister LP, Salazar CA. Case report on the use of CPM on an electrical burn. *J Burn Care Rehabil.* 1988;9:401.
90. Wessling N, Ehleben CM, Chapman V, et al. Evidence that a silicone wound dressing increases range of motion of limbs after contractures (abstract). American Burn Association Meeting: Orlando, FL; 1985.
91. Ahn ST, Monafo WW, Mustoe TA. Topical silicone gel: A new treatment for hypertrophic scars. *Surgery.* 1989;106:781–787.

92. Gibbons M, Zuker R, Brown M, et al. Experience with Silastic gel sheeting in pediatric scarring. *J Burn Care Rehabil.* 1994;15:69–73.
93. Tatum C, Executive Director, Pegasus Riding Academy, Inc., Philadelphia; Personal correspondence, 1989.
94. Moore M, Alvarado MI, Rutan R, et al. Developmental screening: A measure of functional ability (abstract). American Burn Association Meeting: Salt Lake City; 1992.
95. Kammerer-Quayle, B. Personal Image Center at Rancho Los Amigos Medical Center: Downey, CA.
96. Kahn AM, Cohen MJ, Kaplan L. Treatment of depigmentation resulting from burn injuries. *J Burn Care Rehabil.* 1991;12:468–473.
97. Levenson SM, Geever EG, Crawley LV, et al. The healing of rat skin wounds. *Ann Surg.* 1965;161: 293–308.
98. Ward RS, Saffle JR, Schnebly A, et al. Sensory loss over grafted areas in patients with burns. *J Burn Care Rehabil.* 1989;10:536–538.
99. Ponten B. Grafted skin: Observations on innervation and other qualities. *Acta Chir Scand (suppl).* 1960;257.
100. Matev IB. Tactile gnosis in free skin grafts in the hand. *Br J Plast Surg.* 1980;33:434–439.
101. Individual studies with multiple and often different investigators, done at Shriners Burns Institute, University of Texas Medical Branch, Galveston. Reviewed by Robson MC: Burn injuries involving the "whole person." Rehabilitation and reconstruction of the burn patient (symposium), American Burn Association Meeting: Salt Lake City; 1992.
102. Blakeney P, Herndon DN, Desai MH, et al. Long-term psychosocial adjustment following burn injury. *J Burn Care Rehabil.* 1988;9:661–665.
103. Blakeney P, Portman S, Rutan R. Familial values as factors influencing long-term psychological adjustment of children after severe burn injury. *J Burn Care Rehabil.* 1990;11:472–475.
104. Beard SA, Herndon DN, Desai M. Adaptation of self-image in burn-disfigured children. *J Burn Care Rehabil.* 1989;10:550–554.
105. Jessee PO, Strickland MP, Leeper JD, et al. Perception of body image in children with burns, five years after burn injury. *J Burn Care Rehabil.* 1992;13:33–38.
106. Orr DA, Reznikoff M, Smith GM. Body image, self-esteem, and depression in burn-injured adolescents and young adults. *J Burn Care Rehabil.* 1989;10:454–461.
107. Breslau AJ. What can be learned from long-term follow-up of burn patients (unpublished paper). Psychosocial Interest Group. American Burn Association Meeting: Baltimore; 1991.
108. Johnson J, Gorga D, Bentley A, et al. The physical, development, and functional progression of young children (6 months–6 years old) from 1–6 months post-burn (abstract). 29th Annual Meeting of the American Burn Association, New York; 1997.

Pulmonary Disorders in Infants and Children and Their Physical Therapy Management

Jan Stephen Tecklin

Health professionals have the general misconception that respiratory disorders and chronic pulmonary diseases are mainly adult problems. Nonetheless, statistics show that respiratory disease in infants and children is a major problem that accounts for a large share of childhood mortality and morbidity. Mortality statistics show that approximately 30% of all deaths in term infants and 50% to 75% of deaths in premature infants in the United States are either caused by or are closely related to respiratory disease.[1] The morbidity statistics are staggering. Asthma alone is responsible for 10.1 million additional days missed from school when compared with days missed by children without asthma. Children with asthma are about nine times more likely to be unable to conduct their major activities of living when compared with all children without asthma.[2] Acute respiratory infections in children from 1 to 14 years of age are responsible for three to eight illnesses per year per child in both developed and developing nations.[1] Asthma resulted in 12.9 million contacts with physicians and 200,000 hospitalizations in 1988.[2] In the United States, 10% to 20% of children younger than 17 years of age have been reported to have a chronic respiratory problem.[3] Recent data from the Centers for Disease Control and Prevention indicate a 7% incidence of asthma in children.[4] These statistics may seem surprising but not to the health professional who spends a great deal of time treating children with primary pulmonary diseases or respiratory problems secondary to other conditions.

Initially, this chapter provides background information that will enable readers to understand more completely the fragility of the neonatal and pediatric respiratory system, the process of development of that system, and the need for aggressive treatment of disorders of the system. These introductory topics include characteristics of children's lungs, growth and development of the respiratory tract, and predisposition to acute respiratory failure in children and infants. An overview of assessment and treatment by the physical therapist of pulmonary disorders in infants and children is then given. Medical information and a discussion of the physical therapy evaluation and management of four major respiratory problems of children—atelectasis, respiratory muscle weakness, asthma, and cystic fibrosis (CF)—are then presented, followed by questions about future research.

Characteristics of Children's Lungs

Waring[5] described seven unique characteristics of children's lungs that have an impact on the development of lung disease:

1. *Single Cause.* In children, unlike adults, most respiratory signs and symptoms can be explained by a single cause.
2. *Obligatory Miniaturization.* Airflow is related to the cross-sectional area of the airway. The cross section is related geometrically to the airway diameter. As the diameter decreases, the cross section decreases geometrically rather than linearly. As a result, a small obstruction will cause a massive reduction in the cross-sectional area of the lumen in a child's airway. Croup and bronchiolitis, which affect the subglottic trachea and bronchioles, respectively, are caused by edema resulting from infection within those airways. These diseases, which involve severe obstruction of the airways, are seldom, if ever, seen in older children or adults.

   In addition to the ease of airway obstruction, the small size of the child's airway results in different physiologic requirements. Infants and small children, whose distal bronchiolar diameter is 1 mm, have a small cross-sectional area that causes a high resistance to airflow. The result of this high resistance, although normal, is greater work of breathing for the child.[6] When the increased likelihood of an obstruction is combined with the increased work of breathing, it becomes obvious why a child's small airways predispose him or her to severe illness.
3. *Interrelationship of Disease and Growth.* The 25 million pulmonary alveoli that are normally present at birth increase until the child is approximately 10 years of age, at which time the adult complement of 300 million alveoli should be present. Diseases that either interfere with the development of the lungs or destroy existing alveoli will decrease the potential number of alveoli in an adult.[7] The deficit in alveolar development reduces the pulmonary reserve and may predispose the child to lung disease during adulthood.
4. *Immunologic Innocence.* Once the transplacentally supplied antibodies from the mother

are exhausted at 3 to 4 months of age, the infant is defenseless against many infectious microorganisms. The infant's antibodies are developed through periodic exposure to, or infection with, microorganisms.[8]

5. *High Genetic Impact.* Several of the childhood diseases with a major pulmonary component are transmitted genetically. The inheritance pattern may be recessive or dominant. CF is a primary example of a disease with clearly identified genetic factors that ultimately affect the lungs. Asthma has some genetic components, but they are ill-defined, and environment may play an important role in asthma.[9]
6. *Indiscreet Host Curiosity.* Small children explore their environment by placing objects in their mouths. This behavior may cause aspiration of foreign objects into the airway or aspiration of toxic chemicals (e.g., furniture polish, turpentine, and kerosene).
7. *Diagnostic Imperviousness.* Three factors make the diagnosis of childhood pulmonary conditions difficult. A child younger than 5 years of age usually cannot perform pulmonary function tests. Second, because of the small size of their airway, the diagnostic tools commonly used in adults are too large for use in infants. Finally, many people have a psychological or emotional barrier to inflicting pain on children, even when the pain of a blood test or a lung biopsy could yield important information for diagnosing or curing a severe disease.

Growth and Development of the Lungs

A brief review of the major periods of lung development is useful in discussing obligatory miniaturization and the interrelationship between disease and growth, and it will provide insight into some unique aspects of the growth (in number) of pulmonary alveoli.

The earliest sign of lung development occurs during the embryologic period, 24 to 26 days after conception. Endodermal tissue of the primitive foregut expands into an anterior lung pouch when the embryo is 4 mm long. During this separation of the trachea and esophagus, aberrations in development may lead to one of several configurations of tracheoesophageal fistulae. Four days later, the lung pouch differentiates into right and left sides. Mesenchymal cellular tissue surrounding the developing lung buds will later differentiate to become muscle, connective tissue, and cartilage within the bronchial walls. Noncellular tissue will provide the elastic and collagen fibers that support the lung structures.[10]

The lung buds continue to grow and subdivide into smaller airways during the 5th to 16th week of gestation (i.e., the pseudoglandular period). Bronchial epithelium lines the primitive airways, and there is a burst of growth between the 10th and 14th week. Mucus-secreting glands and supportive cartilage appear late in the pseudoglandular period and continue their growth through the canalicular period. Branching and subdivision produces 8 to 32 bronchial generations, with the greatest number of divisions occurring in those lung areas that are most distant from the hilum, or root of the lungs.[10] The bronchial tree is complete from the glottis to the terminal bronchioles by the beginning of the canalicular period.

The major events that mark the 16th to 24th week (i.e., the canalicular period) are thinning and flattening of the bronchial epithelium and the appearance of capillaries. The capillaries, which protrude into the epithelium, provide close proximity of the blood supply to the airways. Thinning of the epithelium and capillarization provides the apparatus—the air–blood interface—for respiration. Gas exchange can take place by the end of the canalicular period.[10]

At approximately 25 weeks, the energy of the developing lung begins to form outpouchings of the terminal bronchioles to produce the pulmonary alveoli. This "terminal sac" or "alveolar" period continues until 8 to 10 years of age. A terminal bronchiole will branch into many alveolar pockets or ducts. These ducts are in continued proximity to the tiny capillaries formed during the canalicular period. Once sufficient numbers of alveolar/capillary units are present, life may be sustained, provided that the biochemical substance surfactant is present within the alveoli.[10]

Surfactant is a phospholipid material secreted by Type II cells that line the pulmonary alveoli. Surfactant reduces surface tension within the alveolus, thus allowing inflation of the alveolus with smaller pressures and less work by the infant than would be needed to inflate a surfactant-deficient alveolus. Surfactant appears at its mature chemical level at approximately 34 weeks of gestation and indicates maturity of the lung by allowing the maintenance of continuous respiration.[11]

After birth, there is a continued subdivision of the alveolar ducts to form alveolar sacs (i.e., the true alveoli). The vasculature continues to parallel the growth in alveoli by branching and multiplying until alveolar growth ceases. From the 25 million alveoli present at birth, there is a 12-fold increase by 8 to 10 years, at which time the adult complement of approximately 300 million is achieved. Destructive processes within the period of alveolar multiplication may limit the potential for development of the adult number of pulmonary alveoli.[12]

Predisposition to Respiratory Failure

The following information is presented to describe more fully several mechanisms of acute respiratory failure and its rapid development in children and infants. Although acute respiratory failure is not a disease, it is often the final common pathway for many diseases that damage the developing respiratory system.

From the mortality data previously cited, it should be obvious that respiratory failure in infants and children is not uncommon. Several structural and metabolic factors in the pediatric population, although entirely normal, predispose them to acute respiratory failure. Respiratory failure can be defined as a condition in which impairment of gas exchange within the lungs poses an immediate threat to life. Downes and associates state that clinical signs and arterial blood gas determinations should be used to monitor infants and children for the development of acute respiratory failure.[13] The arterial blood gas levels compatible with respiratory failure are 75 mmHg of carbon dioxide and 100 mmHg of oxygen when the patient is receiving an inspired oxygen concentration of 100%. Respiratory failure exists when either of these arterial levels is reached in the presence of any of the following clinical signs—decreased or absent inspiratory breaths sounds, severe inspiratory retractions with accessory muscle use, cyanosis with inspiration of 40% oxygen, depressed consciousness and response to pain, and poor skeletal muscle tone.[13]

The most important general factor predisposing infants and children to acute respiratory failure is their high incidence of respiratory tract infections. During the first several years of life, when immunologic defenses are developing, the child is at risk for infections. This risk, which increases as the environment of the toddler expands, probably peaks in the early school years when the child is bombarded with various infectious agents transmitted by classmates, teachers, and other personnel.[14] A recent study by Haskins and Lotch indicates that children in day care centers have an increased incidence of acute respiratory illnesses.[15] As the number of children in day care programs increases, we can expect an increase in the incidence of respiratory infections in the preschool age group.

Two major structural factors—airway size and poor mechanical advantage for the respiratory muscles—contribute to respiratory failure in a young child. The diameter of the tracheal lumen in a 1-year-old child is smaller than the diameter of a lead pencil. More than 85% of the child's peripheral bronchioles are smaller than 1 mm in diameter. A small amount of mucus, bronchospasm, or edema can effectively occlude not only the peripheral airways but may also obstruct the larger, more proximal bronchi. With sufficient airway blockage, respiratory failure may quickly ensue.

The second major structural issue predisposing children to respiratory failure involves five items that cumulatively cause poor mechanical advantage to the respiratory bellows of the child's thorax:

1. Type I fatigue-resistant muscle fibers are not present in adult proportions in the diaphragm or other ventilatory muscles of the infant until 8 months of age.[16] This lack of fatigue-resistant fibers allows the infant's respiratory muscles to tire quickly, causing alveolar hypoventilation that may lead to respiratory failure.
2. Poor development of the abdominal muscles, used for coughing, renders the infant's airway susceptible to obstruction by mucus.
3. Horizontal alignment of the infant's rib cage and the round (rather than oval) configuration of the chest provide poor mechanical advantage to the intercostal and accessory muscles of respiration. These muscles lift the ribs and sternum to increase thoracic diameter and lung volume.
4. Increased chest wall compliance during infancy can result in sternal retractions associated with increased inspiratory effort during times of illness. The relative lack of stiffness in the infant thorax can simulate a flail chest. Intense inspiratory efforts may paradoxically decrease thoracic volume at a time when just the opposite response is necessary and ventilation is further compromised with the potential for hypoventilation. Developmental changes in the chest wall during the second year of life result in chest wall compliance similar to that of adults.[17]
5. The baby's position may affect diaphragmatic excursion. The infant who is in a supine position works harder to ventilate because the abdominal viscera may impede full descent of the diaphragm.

A third important issue for the physical therapist is respiratory metabolism. The high metabolic rate of the child causes increased consumption of oxygen, increased heat loss, and increased water loss secondary to a faster respiratory rate. The range of normal respiratory rates for children is shown in Table 14-1.

In addition to having muscle fibers that are susceptible to early fatigue, the young child or infant has a poor muscle fuel supply. Glycogen supply in the muscle tissue is small in the infant, and is depleted quickly when muscular activity is increased, which occurs during respiratory distress.[18]

The aforementioned general, structural, and metabolic factors, although developmentally and chronologically normal and appropriate, may combine to render the young respiratory tract fragile and prone to failure during periods

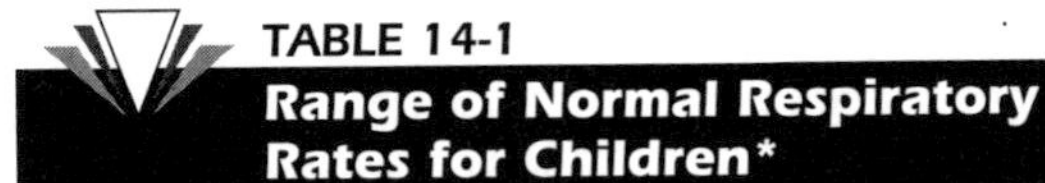

TABLE 14-1
Range of Normal Respiratory Rates for Children*

Age(Yrs)	Mean Respiratory Rate (Range)
1	28(18–40)
2	25(19–35)
3	23(18–32)
4	22(18–29)
5	21(17–27)
6	20(17–25)
8	19(15–23)
10	18(15–22)
12	18(14–21)
14	17(13–21)
16	17(12–20)

*Adapted from Waring WW. The history and physical examination. In: Kendig EL, Chernick V, eds: *Disorders of the Respiratory Tract in Children,* Philadelphia: W.B. Saunders; 1977;83.

of stress, which are commonly seen in respiratory diseases.

Physical Therapy Assessment of Children With Respiratory Disorders

Chart Review

A review of the medical chart and chest roentgenograms, if available, should be the first aspects of the physical therapy assessment of a child. A chart review should provide information regarding the child's medical history; the clinical course of the child's current illness, including signs and symptoms and their precipitating factors; any previous treatment for the illness; and a referral for physical therapy. In addition to the written information found in the chart, physicians and nurses can often provide invaluable and immediate information regarding the child's current state. The chest roentgenograms are useful in identifying specific areas of the lung or thorax that may be affected by the illness. A complete roentgenographic interpretation is beyond the scope of physical therapy practice.

Physical Examination

Careful examination of the infant or child with respiratory distress can offer useful information. The younger the patient, the more the therapist may need to rely on careful observation, because the neonate cannot participate actively in a chest assessment. An age-appropriate description of the activities that the therapist will be performing should precede the actual physical examination.

GENERAL APPEARANCE

The therapist should note the state of consciousness of the child and the level to which the child can cooperate with simple commands. Obvious skeletal abnormalities, peripheral edema, wounds, scars, and abnormal postures should all be considered. The therapist should also note the various pieces of apparatus that are being used (e.g., mechanical ventilator, oxygen hood or mask, intravenous or arterial lines).

HEAD AND NECK

There are several common signs of respiratory distress in the infant or young child. *Nasal flaring* is probably a reflex used to attempt to widen the nasal airway, thus decreasing resistance to airflow during periods of distress. *Head bobbing* that coincides with the respiratory cycle may be the result of attempts to use the accessory muscles of inspiration by an infant who has inadequate strength to fix the head and neck. *Audible expiratory grunting* is thought to be an effort by the infant and young child to maintain airway patency and prevent airway collapse during expiration. Grunting is most commonly heard during lower respiratory tract disorders. Cyanosis and pallor are other common signs of respiratory distress, although they are less specific signs than the several previously noted.

EVALUATION OF THE UNMOVING CHEST

In this portion of the physical examination, the shape and symmetry of the thorax are noted, as are any unusual characteristics of the skin, including rashes, scars, and incisions. The thorax of the infant is more rounded in configuration than the thorax of an adult. The anteroposterior diameter of the thorax in the infant is likely to be equal to its transverse diameter, whereas in the adult's thorax, there is usually a much greater transverse diameter. Congenital defects that may be seen include pectus excavatum (or funnel chest); pectus carinatum (or pigeon-breast); barrel-chest, which is usually associated with hyperinflation of the lungs; and the thoracic deformity that is associated with scoliosis. Muscle development of the thorax should also be examined for symmetry and for the presence of hypertrophy of the accessory muscles, which suggests chronic dyspnea.

EVALUATION OF THE MOVING CHEST

Determination of the respiratory rate is the first item assessed when evaluating the moving chest. Counting of respirations should be done inconspicuously, often when counting the pulse rate. As previously noted in Table 14-1, the younger the patient, the greater the normal resting respiratory rate. Regularity of breathing is a major item for evaluation, particularly in the neonate and in children with neuromuscular disorders. Short periods of apnea are not particularly unusual and may be referred to as periodic breathing in the neonate. True apnea exists when apneic periods exceed 20 seconds. Apnea can be associated with respiratory distress, sepsis, and central nervous system (CNS) hemorrhage. In addition to the rate and regularity, the ratio of inspiration to expiration (I:E) should be determined. This I:E ratio is usually approximately 1:2. Infants and children with obstructive airway disease, such as asthma and bronchiolitis, may have a marked increase in expiratory time; as a result, their I:E ratio may become 1:4 or 1:5. Synchronous motion of the abdomen and thorax should be observed. On inspiration, both thoracic expansion and abdominal bulging should be noted. When this synchrony is lost, a "seesaw" motion of thoracic expansion with abdominal in-drawing occurs on inspiration, with the opposite movements being noted on expiration. The presence of retractions of the chest wall should be noted. Retractions, or in-drawing, may occur in suprasternal, substernal, subcostal, or intercostal areas. Retractions, seen more frequently in pediatric patients, occur as a result of the compliant thorax of the infant and young child. During respiratory distress, the muscles of either inspiration or expiration, or both, place sufficient pull on the thorax to cause an in-drawing in several areas. When retractions are severe, they may reduce effective inspiration.

EVALUATION OF COUGHING AND SNEEZING

Infants probably use sneezing more than coughing as both a protective and a clearance mechanism for the airway. Older infants and children must be able to cough effectively to clear secretions or other debris from their airway. It is important to determine the ability to cough in a child with neuromuscular disease who may be at risk for retention of secretion and aspiration of feedings.

Auscultation

Auscultation—listening to the lungs with a stethoscope—is a useful method of assessment. The stethoscope used for auscultation of the infant and young child is a smaller version of that used for adults (Fig. 14-1). The therapist should warm the stethoscope before using it, and depending on the age of the child, the therapist may show how it is used by demonstrating on a child's doll or on a puppet. Because of the proximity to the thoracic surface of the child's

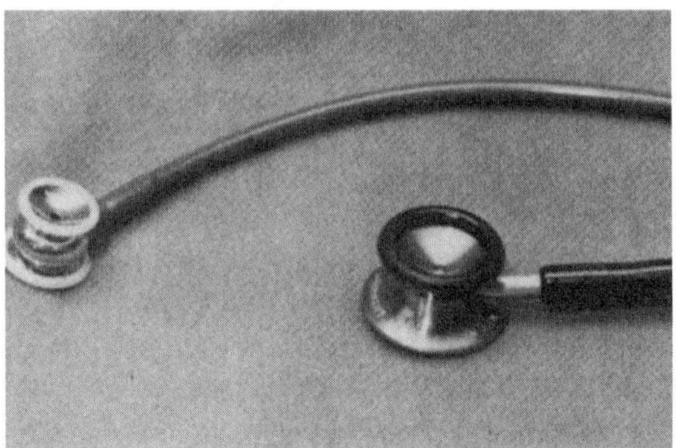

Figure 14-1 ■ Two sizes of pediatric stethoscopes. (Reproduced by permission from Irwin S, Tecklin JS. *Cardiopulmonary Physical Therapy*. St. Louis: CV Mosby; 1985).

airways, as well as the thin chest wall in the young child and infant, sounds are easily transmitted and anatomic specificity may be reduced. A particular sound, therefore, although heard in one area of the thorax, may not correspond to the lung segment directly below the area in which the sound is heard. As a result, auscultation, particularly in the neonate or premature neonate, may not be as precise as in the older child or adult. Nonetheless, the therapist should attempt to ascertain the presence of normal and abnormal breath sounds throughout the lung fields. The therapist should also try to identify adventitious sounds, such as wheezes, crackles, rhonchi, rubs, and crunches. Stridor, a crowing sound associated with upper airway obstruction, and expiratory grunting, associated with airway collapse in the infant, are often audible without auscultation. Because of the ease of transmission of sound through the infant's thorax, the therapist should attempt to correlate auscultatory findings with roentgenographic changes and other physical findings before instituting treatment.

Palpation

Palpation of the thorax in the infant or child is usually limited to examination of the trachea, which will indicate the position of the mediastinum. Palpation to identify subcutaneous emphysema and other gross findings, such as edema, may also be useful. As the child grows, the therapist may palpate to examine chest expansion and its symmetry, as well as the presence of bony lesions, such as rib fractures.

Other Assessments

Although this chapter deals with disorders of the pulmonary system, the therapist must consider all systems when assessing a child. Development assessment is often necessary for a child who has experienced periodic or chronic episodes of hypoxemia, as often occur with pulmonary disorders. Inadequate oxygenation for a period of time may cause minor or major CNS deficit, resulting in a developmental delay. (Normal development and tests of development are discussed in Chapters 1 and 2 of this text.) Various postural abnormalities can be the result of, or can cause, respiratory disorders. Scoliosis with a primary curvature of greater than 60 degrees will usually result in thoracic restriction and a decrease in lung volumes, as will severe pectus excavatum. Some chronic lung diseases, such as severe asthma and CF, lead to hyperinflated, barreled chest with abducted and protracted scapulae. These possibilities must be considered in the assessment of the child with pulmonary disorders. Common orthopedic disorders, some of which have respiratory complications, are discussed in Chapter 11. Finally, an assessment of the family's knowledge and ability to participate in the child's care are important when planning discharge from the hospital, because many pediatric pulmonary disorders are chronic, and will require continuing and effective care at home.

Physical Therapy of Children With Respiratory Disorders

Physical therapy for the infant or child with a pulmonary disorder can be categorized into three general areas:

1. Removal of secretions, either by traditional bronchial hygiene methods or contemporary techniques
2. Breathing exercises and retraining
3. Physical reconditioning

Of course, the degree to which these three areas are used will depend not only on the disease process(es), but also on the age of the child and his or her level of ability and cooperation. Neonates and infants will be treated almost exclusively with traditional bronchial hygiene procedures. Some breathing games and activities can be incorporated into the regimen when the child becomes a toddler. As the child grows older, exercises for breathing retraining, physical reconditioning, and postural exercises become possible. Also, measures for airway clearance that depend on breathing control, such as autogenic drainage and positive expiratory pressure masks, become more applicable as the older child can coordinate the necessary breathing maneuvers.

Removal of Secretions

Removal of secretions from the child's airway is the main goal of bronchial hygiene. Of all types of physical therapy treatment for patients with respiratory problems, bronchial hygiene has been most extensively studied and its efficacy is widely accepted. Bronchial hygiene includes both traditional methods—positioning for gravity-assisted drainage of the airways, manual techniques for loosening secretions, and removal of secretions by coughing and suctioning of the airway—and contemporary techniques, involving huffing, forced expiratory technique, positive expiratory pressure, flutter valve, and high-frequency chest compression.

TRADITIONAL BRONCHIAL HYGIENE

POSITIONING FOR GRAVITY-ASSISTED DRAINAGE. Using a working knowledge of bronchopulmonary segment anatomy, the therapist can position the infant or child to drain areas of the lung in which secretions are found during the assessment. The positions place the segment or lobe of lung to be drained uppermost, with the bronchus supplying that lung area in as close to an inverted position as possible. In adults and older children, specific positioning for segmental drainage often involves the use of treatment tables or tilting beds. In infants and young children, the therapist's lap and shoulder serve as the "treatment table." The baby can be held and comforted while in each of the 10 drainage positions (Fig. 14-2). When the child reaches 2 or 3 years of age, the transition may be made from lap to treatment table, but many therapists and parents will continue to use the lap for children up to 4 or 5 years of age. Because most families do not have a hospital bed or tilt-table at home, other methods can be used for proper positioning (Fig. 14-3).

MANUAL TECHNIQUES OF PERCUSSION AND VIBRATIONS. The manual techniques of percussion and vibration are used to loosen or dislodge secretions from the bronchial wall, thus allowing easier removal when the child coughs, sneezes, or undergoes airway aspiration with a suction catheter. Although some major differences exist, the techniques used are similar to those performed on adults. One of the major differences is the amount of force used for either percussion or vibration. Common sense should dictate that minimal amounts of force should be used on the thorax of a premature infant who weighs 1 to 2 kg or less. Increased amounts of percussion and vibration force can be safely applied as the infant grows and as the bones and muscles of the thorax become stronger.

As with adults, the percussion and vibration should be applied to the area of thorax that corresponds to the lung and airways in which secretions are present. Another difference in the pediatric group is that a therapist's percussing or vibrating hand often covers the entire thorax. Other implements have been suggested for percussion and vibration in the infant as a result of this discrepancy in size. Several items used for percussion are shown in Figure 14-4, and different hand configurations for percussion of the infant are shown in Figures 14-5 to 14-9. Crane has identified the following contraindications for chest percussion in the neonate: a significant drop in transcutaneous (or arterial) oxygen level during percussion, rib fracture or other thoracic trauma, and hemoptysis.[19] Crane also identified various conditions in which percussion should

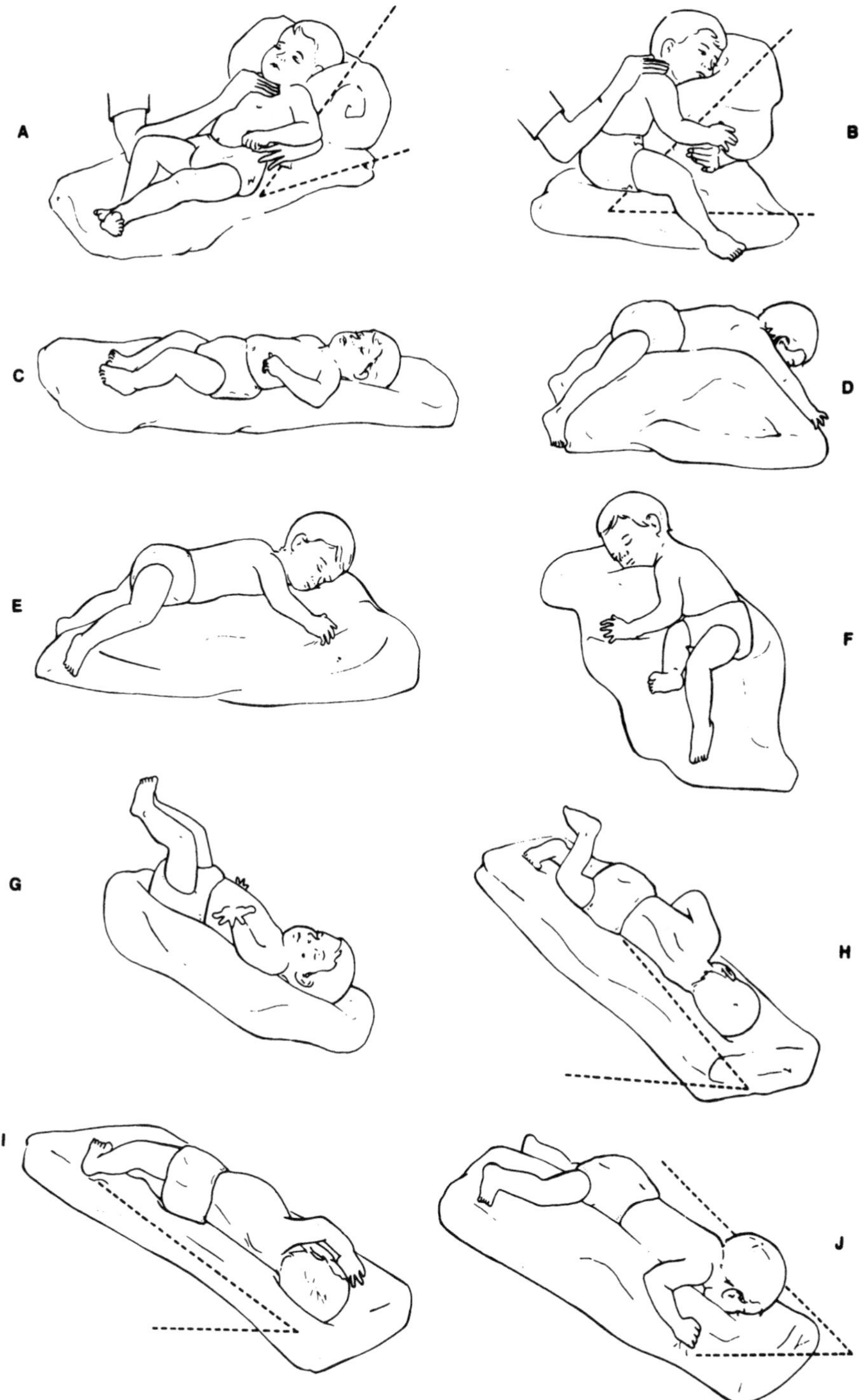

Figure 14-2 ▪ Ten positions for postural drainage (H and I demonstrate lying on the right and left sides). (Reproduced by permission from Irwin S, Tecklin JS. *Cardiopulmonary Physical Therapy*. St. Louis: CV Mosby; 1985.)

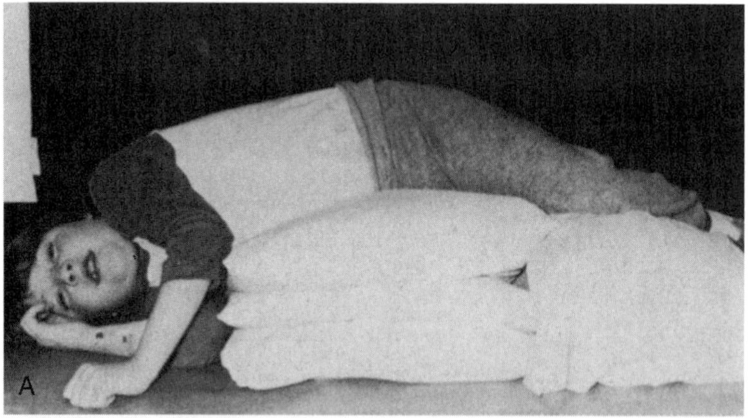

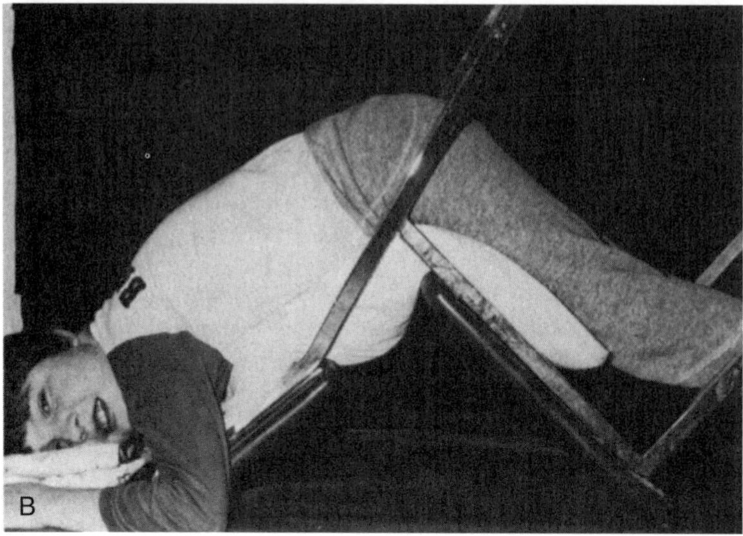

Figure 14-3 ▪ Positioning methods for bronchial drainage at home using bed pillows (**A**); a desk chair (**B**); a stack of magazines with a bed pillow (**C**); and a bean-bag chair (**D**). (Reproduced by permission from Irwin S, Tecklin JS. *Cardiopulmonary Physical Therapy*. St. Louis: CV Mosby; 1985.)

be used carefully in a child, including poor condition of the infant's skin, coagulopathy, osteoporosis or rickets, cardiac arrhythmias, apnea and bradycardia, increased irritability during treatment, subcutaneous emphysema, and subependymal or intraventricular hemorrhage.[19] Vibration, which may be used in addition to or in place of percussion, is a less vigorous technique than percussion. There are few true contraindications to vibration with the exception of hemoptysis and reduced oxygenation during treatment. Because vibration is usually done during the expiratory phase of breathing, and because the infant with respiratory disease often has a rate of 40 or more breaths per minute, it is difficult to coordinate manual vibration with the expiratory phase of breathing. Some persons use various battery-powered vibrators that can be held against the infant's thorax during expiration and then quickly removed during inspiration. The modifications and precautions for both percussion and vibration become fewer as the infant grows, and treatment begins to parallel more closely that used for an adult.

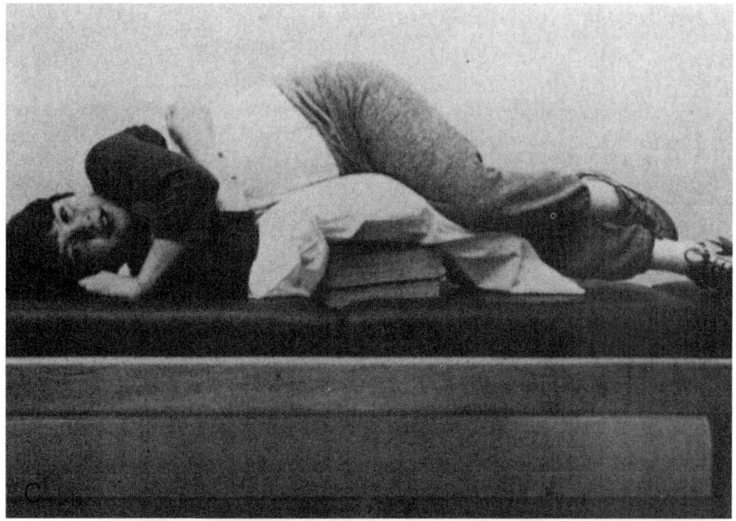

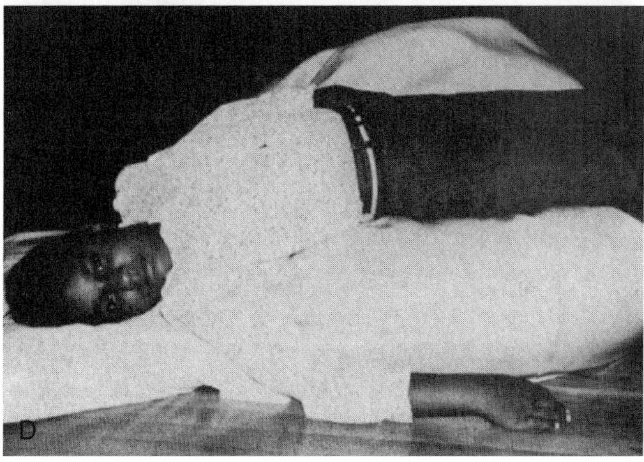

Figure 14-3 ▪ (Continued)

Coughing and Suctioning. Infants and young children will seldom cough on request. Toddlers and school-aged children have the language skills to understand the request for coughing but will often choose not to cough. Imaginative means, including storytelling, coloring games, and nursery rhymes, have been suggested to entice young children to cooperate.[20] In addition, the author has found that by prompting these young children either to laugh or cry (preferably the former), a useful and productive cough can often be elicited. External stimulation of the trachea ("tracheal tickling") using a circular or vibratory motion of the fingers against the trachea as it courses below the sternal notch may be another useful technique for removing loosened secretions (Fig. 14-10). However, given the relative small size and fragility of the structures involved with this technique, great care must be employed to avoid injury. Coughing is particularly difficult for the child who has undergone thoracic surgery. Splinting the incision with the hands or with a doll or stuffed animal pressed close to the

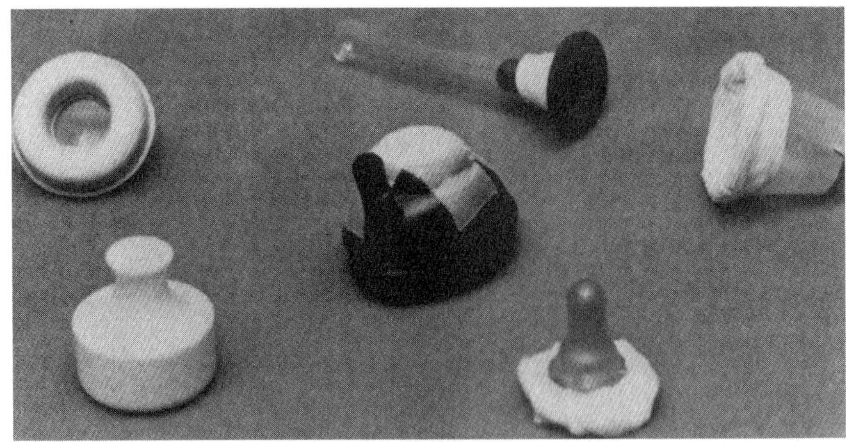

Figure 14-4 ▪ Commercially available and adaptable devices for percussion. (Reproduced by permission from Irwin S, Tecklin JS. *Cardiopulmonary Physical Therapy.* St. Louis: CV Mosby; 1985.)

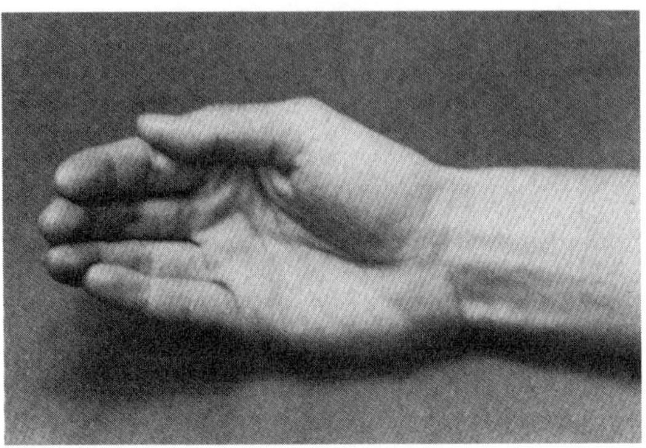

Figure 14-5 ▪ Fully cupped hand for percussion. (Reproduced by permission from Irwin S, Tecklin JS. *Cardiopulmonary Physical Therapy.* St. Louis: CV Mosby; 1985.)

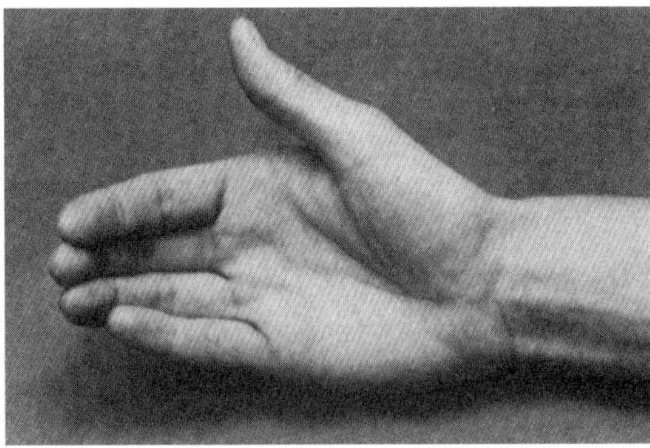

Figure 14-6 ▪ Four fingers cupped for percussion. (Reproduced by permission from Irwin S, Tecklin JS: *Cardiopulmonary Physical Therapy.* St. Louis: CV Mosby; 1985).

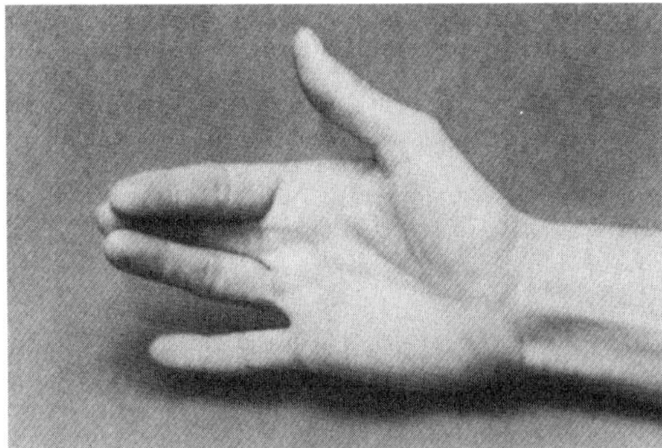

Figure 14-7 ▪ Three fingers cupped for percussion with the middle finger "tented" (anterior view). (Reproduced by permission from Irwin S, Tecklin JS. *Cardiopulmonary Physical Therapy.* St. Louis: CV Mosby; 1985.)

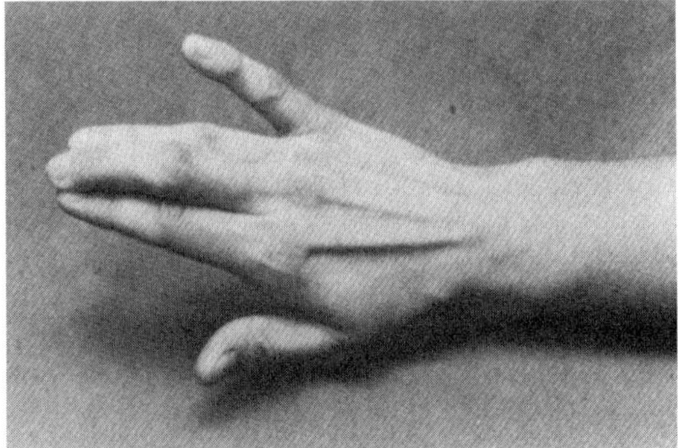

Figure 14-8 ▪ Three fingers cupped for percussion with the middle finger "tented" (posterior view). (Reproduced by permission from Irwin S, Tecklin JS. *Cardiopulmonary Physical Therapy.* St. Louis: CV Mosby; 1985.)

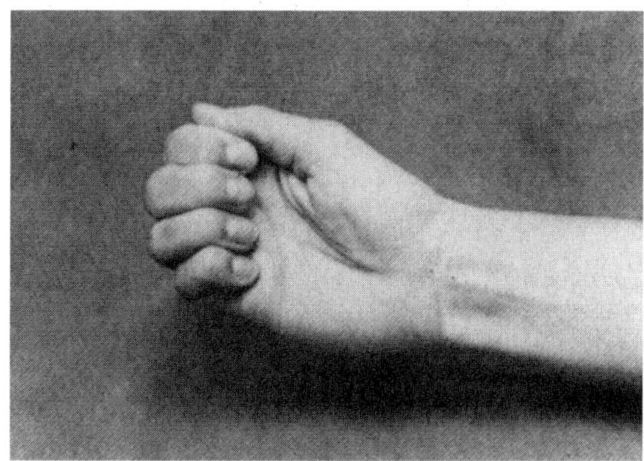

Figure 14-9 ▪ Thenar and hypothenar surfaces for percussion. (Reproduced by permission from Irwin S, Tecklin JS. *Cardiopulmonary Physical Therapy.* St. Louis: CV Mosby; 1985.)

child's chest promotes the development of an effective cough (Fig. 14-11).

Airway aspiration by suctioning is often needed, particularly in the neonate, to remove secretions. Suctioning must always be done carefully because it has significant risks, even when performed under the best circumstances. Crane has detailed a protocol for endotracheal aspiration.[19]

CONTEMPORARY APPROACHES TO BRONCHIAL HYGIENE

During the 1980s, several new approaches to bronchial hygiene were developed. Various breathing maneuvers used to loosen and transport mucus were the common feature of these approaches. In addition, these new techniques were all designed to eliminate the need for an individual other than the patient to perform traditional manual techniques of percussion and vibration. These approaches were developed primarily for children and young adults with CF, although they are appropriate for all individuals with chronic lung disease that produces copious sputum.

Autogenic Drainage. This approach was introduced by Dab and Alexander, who describe autogenic drainage as follows[21,22]:

1. The child sits in an upright, or sitting position.
2. The child takes deep breaths at a "normal or relatively slow" rhythm.
3. Secretions move upward as a result of the breathing.
4. When secretions reach the trachea, they are expelled with either a gentle cough or slightly forced expiration.

The authors recommend that slightly forced expiration be used because of their belief that the high transmural pressures that develop during coughing effectively cause airway collapse, thereby rendering the coughing effort ineffective.[21,22]

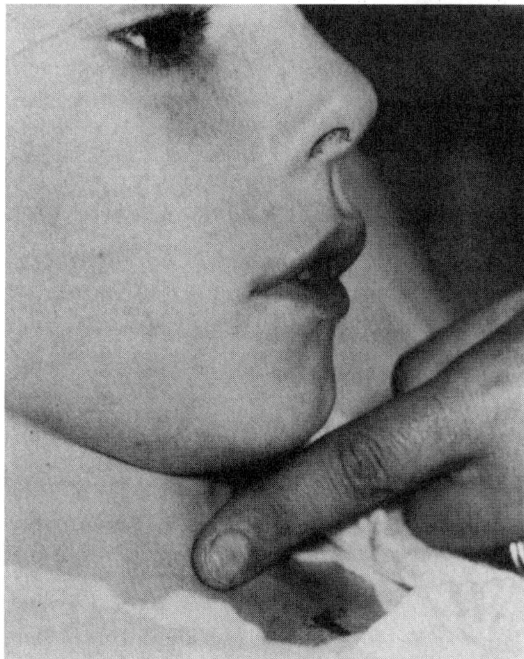

Figure 14-10 ▪ Placement of the finger for the tracheal "tickle" maneuver. (Reproduced by permission from Irwin S, Tecklin JS. *Cardiopulmonary Physical Therapy.* St. Louis: CV Mosby; 1985.)

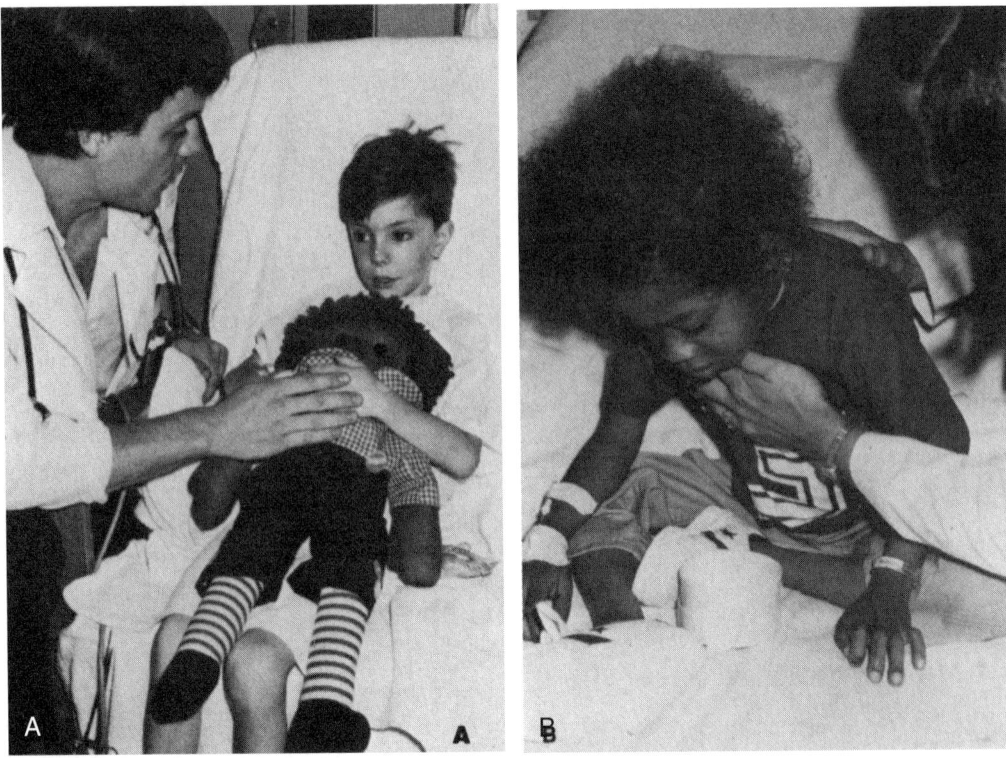

Figure 14-11 ■ (**A**) Incisional splinting during coughing using a favorite stuffed toy. (**B**) Manual compression over the midsternum to facilitate expectoration of sputum. (Reproduced by permission from Irwin S, Tecklin JS. *Cardiopulmonary Physical Therapy*. St. Louis: CV Mosby; 1985.)

Current usage of autogenic drainage recommends not deep breathing but tidal breathing at different lung volumes. That is, the child will breathe at a normal volume but will begin this controlled breathing at a very low lung volume (with most of the resting lung volume previously expelled). After several breaths at low lung volume, the child moves the tidal breathing to a mid-lung volume and then, following several additional breaths, to a higher lung volume. The movement of air through the smaller to the larger airways is thought to loosen secretions and move them proximally. The child should be taught to suppress active coughing until a mere huff cough can clear the secretions from the respiratory system. Although controlled research is minimal, the author has worked with many patients in whom this technique has been successful in clearing the airways. This is a somewhat difficult technique to teach and is most commonly used for patients who are highly motivated and old enough to control their breathing well.[23]

Forced Expiratory Technique. The forced expiratory technique (FET) was developed in New Zealand, but was popularized in the late 1970s and into the 1980s by Pryor, Webber, Hodson, and Batten, all from Brompton Hospital in London.[24] As with autogenic drainage, the primary benefit derived from FET is that it can be performed without an assistant. Because the Brompton group has expressed great concern about what they believed to be misinterpretations of their original description,[25] their description of FET is provided here in a direct quotation from their original article.

> The forced expiratory technique (FET) consists of one or two huffs (forced expirations), from mid-lung volume to low lung volume, followed by a period of relaxed, controlled diaphragmatic breathing. Bronchial secretions mobilized to the upper airways are then expectorated and the process is repeated until minimal bronchial clearance is obtained. The patient can reinforce the forced expiration by self compression of the chest wall using a brisk adduction movement of the upper arm.[24]

In a subsequent article that attempts to clarify the various components of FET, the authors place particular emphasis on huffing to low lung volumes in an effort to clear peripheral secretions. In addition, the phrase "from mid-lung volume" has been clarified to mean taking a medium-sized breath before initiating the huffing. The authors recommend that patients use FET while in gravity-assisted positions, and further suggest that pauses for breathing control and periods of relaxation are part of the overall technique.[25]

The FET has been reconstituted by the Brompton group into a series of approaches called active cycle of breathing technique (ACBT). The ACBT employs a number of individual skills including controlled breathing, FET, huff coughing, and thoracic expansion exercises. As was the case for the FET, there have been little or no attempts at controlled research for the ACBT.

Positive Expiratory Pressure (PEP) Breathing. PEP breathing was developed in Denmark in an attempt to maintain airway patency and employ channels of collateral ventilation to provide airflow distal to accumulated secretions. The airflow in the distal portions of the airway is presumed to dislodge and move secretions proximally toward larger airways. In addition, PEP provides expiratory resistance that appears to stabilize smaller airways, thereby preventing their early collapse during expiration and huff coughing. This technique is thought to be effective in both reducing air-trapping and enhancing secretion removal. The original technique relied upon breathing through an anesthesia face mask but more recent devices use mouthpieces.

When using PEP, the therapist attempts to have patients breathe with a level of expiratory pressure of approximately 15 cm H_2O. Devices to provide PEP usually offer varied resistance and have some type of indicator to identify when the 15 cm of pressure has been achieved. The child attempts to maintain that level of pressure throughout the expiratory phase of breathing for 10 to 15 breaths followed by huff coughing (controlled coughing with an open glottis) to clear the secretions. Some recommend using PEP breathing while the child assumes each of the several bronchial drainage positions.[26] Figure 14-12 shows commercially available PEP devices. (DHD Healthcare, Canastota, NY).

Flutter. The Flutter is a small, hand-held pipelike device that produces an oscillating sistance during expiration. The oscillations are created by a small ball within the device that is moved out of its seat during expiration but then rapidly moves back into its seat through the effects of gravity. The ball is then moved out of the seat again by the continuing force of the expiratory airflow. This repeated movement of the ball rapidly opens and occludes the orifice of the device that results in the rapid oscillations or vibrations transmitted into the airway. These rapid oscillations are thought to loosen the secretions for ease of removal. As with PEP breathing, airway collapse is reduced by the PEP generated by the device. Use of the Flutter is followed by attempts to clear secretions by

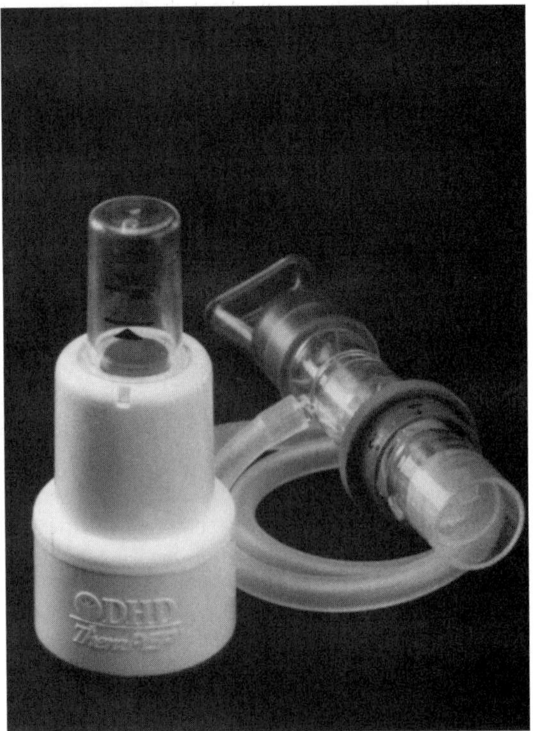

Figure 14-12a ▪ An example of a positive expiratory pressure device TheraPEP (DHD Healthcare, Canastota, NY)

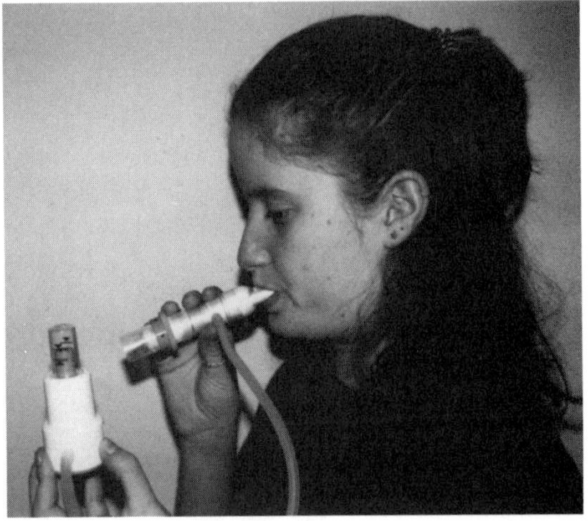

Figure 14-12b ▪ TheraPEP device in use (compliments of A. Tecklin).

huff coughing. Figure 14-13 shows the Flutter device (Vario Raw SA; distributed by Scandipharm, Inc., Birmingham, AL).

HIGH FREQUENCY CHEST COMPRESSION (HFCC). This technique of treatment uses an inflatable vest and an air-pump system that produces pulsations of variable speed and force to the external chest wall. The child simply applies the vest, turns on the pump and treatment begins. The pulsations are thought to have several effects on the respiratory tract. First, the shear forces developed help dislodge secretions from the airway wall. There may also be physical alteration of secretion in that the mucupolysaccharide chemical bonds are altered to render the secretions more fluid. The ciliary escalator may also be enhanced by increasing the amplitude of ciliary beating and improving ciliary smooth muscle function.[27] Figure 14-14 demonstrates a ThAIRapy® Vest (American Biosystems, St. Paul, MN).

Breathing Exercises and Retraining

Because many of the commonly used breathing exercises require voluntary participation by the child, the classic methods for teaching improved diaphragmatic descent, increased thoracic expansion, and pursed-lip breathing may not be useful in the infant or young child. DeCesare suggests using neurophysiologic techniques, such as applying a quick stretch to the thorax to facilitate contraction of the diaphragm and intercostal muscles, to increase inspiration for the baby or young child.[20]

The toddler can participate in games that require deep breathing and control of breathing. Asking the child to breathe in time to music or to the beat of a metronome can present the skill of paced breathing. Blowing bubbles from a bubble wand or blowing a pinwheel will help emphasize increased control and prolonged expiration, which may be useful for the child with obstruc-

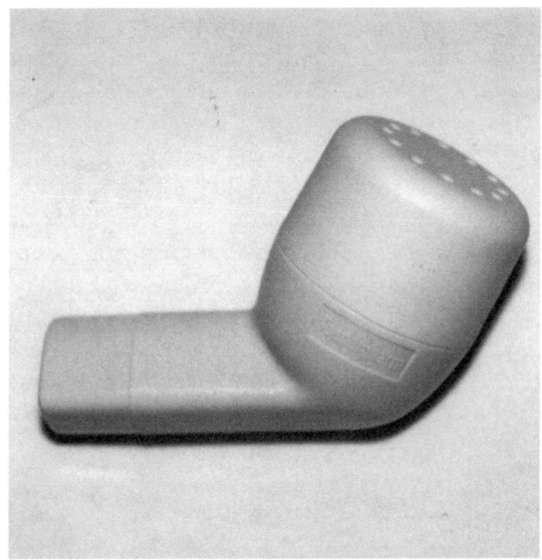

Figure 14-13A ▪ Flutter device (VarioRaw SA; distributed by Scandipharm, Inc., Birmingham, AL).

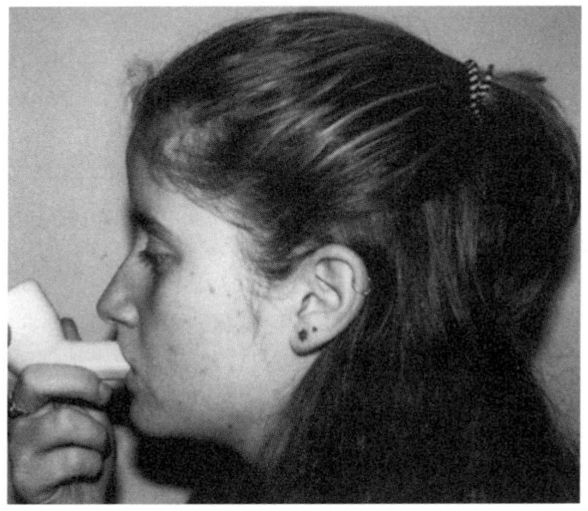

Figure 14-13B ▪ Flutter device in use (compliments of A. Tecklin).

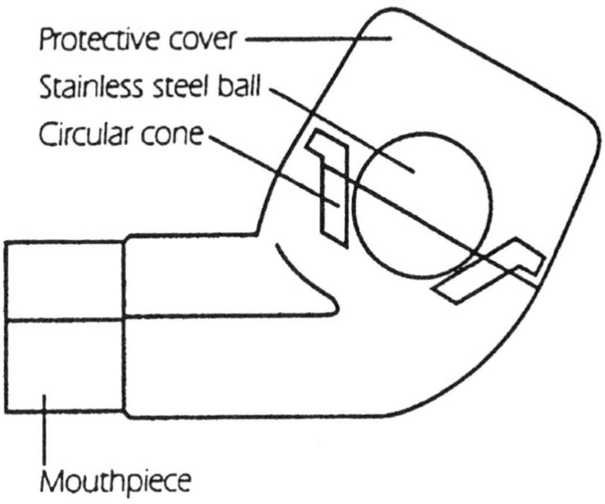

Figure 14-13C ▪ Cross-section of Flutter device.

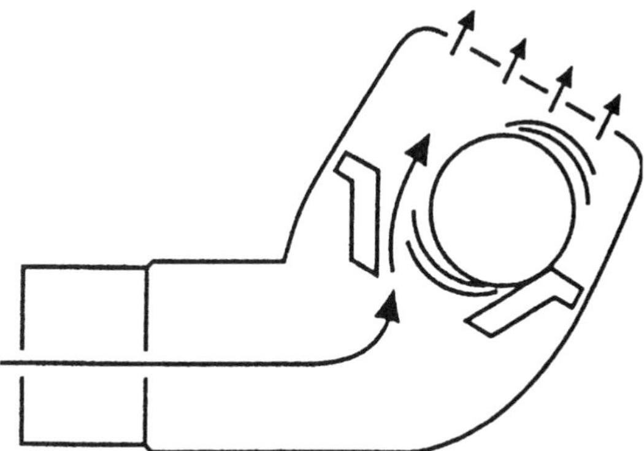

Figure 14-13D ▪ Cross-section of Flutter device with representation of oscillating ball.

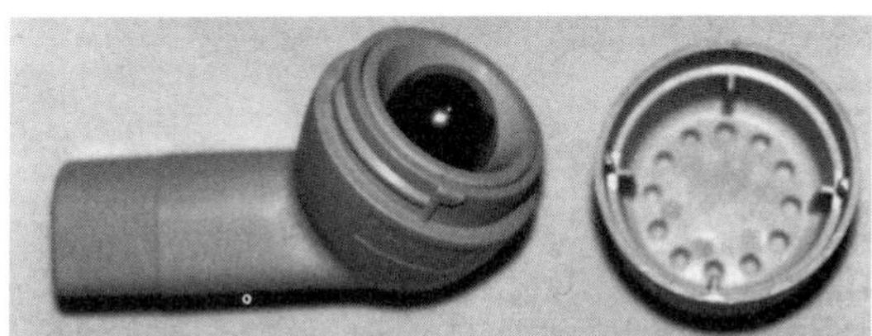

Figure 14-13E ▪ Flutter device with oscillating ball

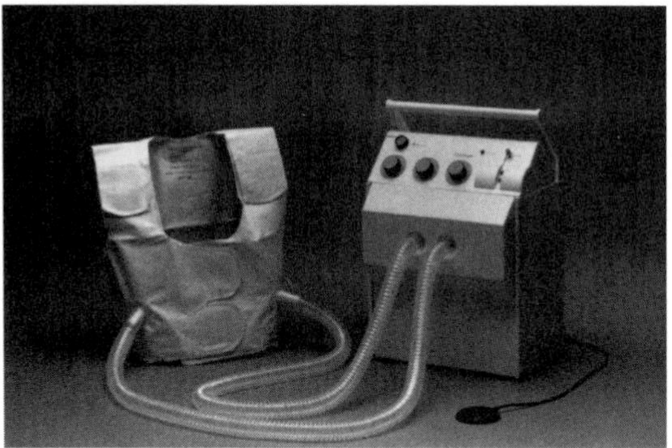

Figure 14-14 ▪ ThAIRapy Vest (American Biosystems, St. Paul, MN).

tive disease. Blow bottles may be useful as a means of strengthening the respiratory muscles. The bottles can be set up for inspiration or expiration, and various target levels of water transfer can be set for the child. Numerous types of incentive spirometers are also useful for enhancing deep inspiration after either medical or surgical diseases. Incentive spirometry has been studied extensively and is generally considered to be a useful adjunct to postoperative pulmonary care and a means of strengthening respiratory muscles.[28,29] Improving ventilation to the lower lobes by using diaphragmatic breathing and lateral costal expansion also helps reduce postoperative pulmonary complications.[28]

Participation in breathing exercises usually improves as the child grows older. When appropriate, the therapist may use manual contact to teach diaphragmatic breathing, lateral costal expansion, and segmental expansion. Depending on the findings from the assessment of the moving chest, the therapist will choose one or more of these types of breathing exercises. The older child with severe, perennial asthma and the child with CF will often exhibit many of the same characteristics as adults with chronic obstructive pulmonary disease (COPD). Paced diaphragmatic breathing may be very useful for these children and young adults. Reduced expenditure of energy is one of the major benefits of diaphragmatic breathing. Because exercise intolerance becomes a problem for children with asthma and CF, diaphragmatic breathing may improve the child's ability to walk, climb stairs, and perform other vigorous physical activities. Pursed-lip breathing may also be useful for breath control in the child with chronic lung disease. Relaxation exercise for the child with asthma is often suggested as a means of reducing breathlessness. Although there is no scientific evidence of any change in the pulmonary function of these children with relaxation exercise, there is strong anecdotal evidence of a reduction in the anxiety associated with dyspnea.

Physical Development

Activities to improve physical function in the infant or child with a pulmonary disorder may begin in the neonatal nursery. When possible, physical therapy treatments should be done with the infant removed from the isolette or warming bed. The handling and tactile stimulation provided by the bronchial hygiene session may be helpful adjuncts to the sensorimotor development of the infant, who may spend great amounts of time in a supine position. Of course, this type of movement is not always possible, particularly for the critically ill baby. As the pulmonary condition improves, the infant should begin to receive, in addition to respiratory physical therapy, appropriate intervention to assess and, if necessary, to treat delays in motor development. Chapter 3, devoted to the high-risk infant, describes an approach to this type of child.

PHYSICAL TRAINING

Children with asthma and CF and those with respiratory disease secondary to neuromuscular or musculoskeletal problems represent two distinct groups for whom physical training is important. A case example of each group follows in this chapter. Programs of physical training usually include exercises to improve strength and range of motion (ROM), posture, and endurance.

Strength training is helpful in both groups of children. Children with severe asthma and moderately advanced CF are often limited in strength owing to inactivity and chronic or periodic hypoxemia. Darbee and Cerny advocate a strengthening program involving isotonic resistive exercise performed at a high number of repetitions rather than high levels of resistance.[30] They also believe that exercise should stress the shoulder girdle and thoracic musculature as a means of facilitating the respiratory pump.[30] Although data are sparse, one must assume that improving strength in these children will decrease their physical inactivity and disability. The group of children with neuromuscular disease, such as myopathy or spinal muscle atrophy, and musculoskeletal disease, such as juvenile rheumatoid arthritis, will have weakness that prohibits their full participation in normal childhood activities. A carefully planned, judiciously administered strengthening program should help both groups.

Decreased ROM is more commonly a problem for those with neuromuscular/musculoskeletal problems than for those with asthma and CF. When thoracic motion is considered as a part of ROM, however, then the children with asthma and CF have been found to have decreases similar to those occurring in children who have undergone recent thoracic surgery. This surgical group will have reduced thoracic motion after surgery and are at risk for both loss of shoulder motion and development of scoliosis. Exercises for deep breathing, thoracic expansion, segmental expansion, and upper extremity function can help either prevent loss of motion or regain motion that has been lost.

Strengthening of respiratory musculature has been scrutinized in recent years. Just as other skeletal muscles respond to training for both endurance and strength, the muscles of inspiration and expiration will respond similarly. Studies of groups of children with chronic obstructive disease and groups with specific respiratory muscle weakness have shown that significant improvement in respiratory muscle function accompanies breathing activities aimed at either endurance or strength, or both.[31] Inspiratory muscle training and strengthening have resulted in improvement in numerous physiologic indices; however, the clinical or functional benefits have been defined less completely. Nonetheless, inspiratory muscle strengthening and endurance training should be considered if weakness is suspected in the vital respiratory pump. Expiratory muscle strengthening may benefit exercise tolerance and surely should enhance the force of expiratory maneuvers, including coughing. As with inspiratory muscle training, expiratory muscle training lacks completely persuasive clinical study. These exercises are described in the following discussion regarding respiratory muscle weakness.

The child with chronic lung disease will benefit from participation in a program of cardiovascular training or conditioning. Because of the tendency for running to precipitate exercise-induced bronchospasm in children with asthma, this group of young patients seems to respond much better to swimming programs. Children and young adults with CF participate throughout the United States in organized walking or jogging groups. The popularity of these groups can be traced to Dr. David Orenstein and colleagues who first popularized jogging for children with CF and who then studied the benefits for those children.[32] Darbee and Cerny provide an exceptionally complete description of exercise testing and training for children with lung dysfunction.[30]

Regardless of the specific exercise or physical reconditioning program, and regardless of the pediatric pulmonary problem, there is a major role for the physical therapist in treating children with lung disease.

The next section of this chapter describes four common disorders of the respiratory tract in children and their physical therapy evaluation and treatment.

Atelectasis

Atelectasis, or incomplete expansion of a lung or a portion thereof, was first described by Laennec in 1819.[33] Primary atelectasis occurs in the neonate as a result of pulmonary immaturity, and also can occur at any age as a result of inadequate respiratory effort. Secondary atelectasis occurs when gas in a lung segment is reabsorbed without subsequent refilling of that segment. The most common causes of secondary atelectasis include bronchial obstruction, abnormal pressure on the lung tissue, and removal of pulmonary surfactant by disease or trauma.[34]

Primary atelectasis in small areas of the newborn lung is a common finding during the first few days of life. The sick neonate with poor respiratory effort and generalized weakness may not fully expand all areas of the lung for several weeks. Major areas of secondary atelectasis may be the result of abnormal thoracic content causing external compression of the lung tissue or the airways. Among the most common causes of lung compression in young children are an enlarged heart or great vessels, congenital or acquired lung cysts, diaphragmatic hernia, and congenital lobar emphysema. The most common type of atelectasis seen by the physical therapist is caused by airway obstruction secondary to secretion of mucus or other debris, including meconium, amniotic content, foreign bodies, and aspirated gastrointestinal contents. In critical care units, a misplaced endotracheal tube often causes a large area of atelectasis.

Medical Information

Signs and symptoms of atelectasis depend on the degree of involvement of the lungs. Common findings include decreased chest wall excursion of the affected hemithorax, tachypnea, and inspiratory retractions, as well as cyanosis if the atelectasis is large. The trachea will deviate toward the involved lung because of volume loss, and a dull percussion note, which indicates an airless lung, will be present. By auscultation, breath sounds will be reduced or absent. The roentgenogram will often demonstrate a sharply demarcated area of consolidation, although patchy areas of atelectasis are not uncommon in acute respiratory tract infection.

Medical management of obstructive atelectasis is directed toward the removal of the obstructing material or structure. When the atelectasis is associated with an acute infection, therapy that cures the infection will often eradicate the atelectasis. Good hydration will decrease the viscosity of the mucus. Postural drainage with chest percussion, vibration, and coughing, followed by deep inhalations, will help remove mucus, and a bronchodilator may widen the bronchus, thus allowing air past the obstruction. When an obstruction is caused by a neoplasm or other structure that occludes the airway or exerts pressure over the lung parenchyma, surgical removal of the item may be indicated. Endobronchial aspiration using a suction catheter may help remove airway debris, and repositioning of a poorly placed endotracheal tube may correct atelectasis. If none of these more conservative measures is successful, bronchoscopy, using either a rigid or a flexible bronchoscope with administration of general or local anesthesia, is indicated to remove the intraluminal mucus or debris.[35]

Prognosis is usually good if the underlying disease process is not life-threatening and if the duration of the atelectasis has not been prolonged. Permanent damage to the bronchial architecture can occur with delayed or incomplete resolution of atelectasis. Pulmonary fibrosis and bronchiectasis are the most common sequelae of obstructive atelectasis.[35]

Physical Therapy Evaluation

A thorough review of the patient's chart is necessary to understand fully the pathophysiology of the condition and to identify the type of atelectasis (primary or secondary). The treatment for each type will include similar efforts to increase respiratory effort, but only secondary atelectasis requires bronchial hygiene procedures.

Review of the roentgenographic findings will identify the position of the atelectasis. The therapist should use the roentgenogram as a clinical tool when treating a patient with atelectasis. Lateral and posteroanterior exposures provide a three-dimensional view of the lung fields. The patient's chest and breathing should be noted. A large atelectasis narrows the rib interspaces and decreases excursion of the involved hemithorax. The muscular pattern of respiration should be noted—diaphragmatic versus accessory—and the patient's respiratory rate should be determined.

Palpation may indicate a shift of the trachea toward the atelectasis owing to volume loss in the lung. The airless lung has a dull percussion note that helps the therapist locate the atelectasis. Auscultatory findings will vary. The most frequent change is a diminution of breath sounds in the involved area. Complete obstruction of a large or main bronchus may result in complete absence of breath sounds. With patchy or incomplete atelectasis, crackles may be heard for the first of several deep breaths; however, with subsequent deep breaths, the alveoli may open and the crackles may decrease.

Other considerations in evaluating the child include the following:

- Mobility—Has the child been at bedrest for an extended time?
- Pain—Can the child take a deep breath and cough effectively?
- Cough—Can the child cough, and does he or she have sufficient strength or neurologic competence?

Physical Therapy Management

Several studies strongly support physical therapy procedures for the prevention of postoperative atelectasis in adult surgical patients. Therapeutic methods used in these studies included bronchial drainage, percussion, vibration, deep breathing,[36,37] maximal inspiratory efforts,[38] and electrical stimulation of the thorax with direct current.[39] The success of each treatment regimen was unequivocal. (The difference between adults and children in terms of airway cross section and strength of coughing has been previously discussed.)

Finer and associates found a significant decrease in the incidence of postextubation atelectasis in infants who were treated with bronchial drainage, vibration, and oral suctioning when compared with a similar control group treated only with bronchial drainage.[40] Atelectasis after extubation occurs commonly in infants, and is presumably caused by excessive bronchial secretions.

These studies have not evaluated the treatment of atelectasis; however, they have evaluated its prevention, which is the best treatment. Burrington and Cotton have reported the successful use of bronchial drainage, percussion, and coughing, preceded by inhalation of a bronchodilator, in 28 children who had aspirated a foreign body.[41] Of this group, 24 children coughed out the object after physical therapy. Although atelectasis is not always present with a foreign body in the airway, it is a common radiologic finding. When atelectasis is caused by aspirated material, physical methods can remove the material and relieve the atelectasis.[41]

Controlled studies of physical therapy for the treatment of atelectasis have not been published. The development of a rational approach to treatment should be based on the type and cause of the atelectasis. The methods used in the aforementioned studies are often included in the treatment of a child with atelectasis.

Postoperative atelectasis is a combination of primary and secondary atelectasis. Secretions are more abundant owing to irritation of the airway by the anesthetic gases and tube manipulations. With incisional pain, and with the generalized weakness that accompanies thoracic or abdominal surgery, the child has a less effective cough and the volume of inspirations is decreased. Deep breathing to achieve maximal inspiration will often be sufficient to resolve small areas of atelectasis. These efforts should be initiated early in the postoperative period—in the recovery room if possible—to prevent atelectasis. Coaching the child to breathe deeply, splinting the incision to reduce pain, and using proprioceptive techniques to facilitate the inspiratory musculature can help the child increase the depth of respiration. Positioning the patient to drain the major lung fields and percussion/vibration followed by attempts to cough will aid in the prevention of pulmonary complications. Incentive spirometers, used as a breathing game, will stimulate deeper inhalations. Percussion and coughing become critical components of the treatment if the patient develops atelectasis despite preventive measures. Aggressive percussion of the chest over the atelectasis and splinted coughing will work to mechanically dislodge and clear the obstructing mucus. Treatment often includes endotracheal suctioning to remove accumulated mucus and to further stimulate coughing. Early ambulation of the patient after surgery and the resultant stress on the respiratory system helps mobilize secretions by causing the patient to breathe deeply.

Children with medical chest conditions develop atelectasis as a result of retained secretions. These children will find coughing and maximal inspirations easier to do because there is no incisional pain. Liberal and more aggressive use of chest percussion in these nonsurgical patients is helpful. Bronchial drainage with localized percussion will often dislodge the obstructing secretions, and coughing will clear the airway. Many physicians suggest aerosol inhalation, both to moisten the secretions and to deliver a bronchodilator. The rationale for these procedures of inhalation is that moist secretions will drain more easily from a bronchus that is maximally dilated. Data exist to support both of these methods as an adjunct to physical therapy.[42]

The use of autogenic drainage, FET, and PEP should be considered for obstructive atelectosis.

Primary atelectasis caused by respiratory muscle weakness can be resolved by deep breathing and strengthening of the respiratory muscles.

Respiratory Muscle Weakness

Respiratory muscle weakness in children, as in adults, may be the result of a disorder affecting any link in the chain of neuromuscular events that produce a contraction of the respiratory muscles. Weakness or paresis of the respiratory muscles may be either mild and transient or severe and irreversible. The underlying pathologic process is the primary determinant of the duration and severity of the weakness. The physical therapist should develop a therapeutic regimen to treat the muscle weakness and to prevent or treat the resultant pulmonary symptoms within the limitations imposed by the disorder.

In the past decade, a growing population of ventilator-dependent children has arisen as a result of improved technology and care for acute and chronic ventilatory failure. These children, too, require physical therapy for problems associated with respiratory pump failure and for the delay in motor skill development caused by reliance on the mechanical ventilator.

Medical Information

Diffuse pathology of the CNS (e.g., viral encephalitis or barbiturate intoxication) may lead to respiratory failure by paralyzing the voluntary and involuntary portions of the respiratory muscles. Abnormal neural control mechanisms and reflexes may ablate or reduce the physiologic response to chemical and mechanical stimuli. These stimuli may occur within the lungs, the brain stem, the blood, and cerebrospinal fluid (CSF). Examples of childhood disorders that result in a reduced response to respiratory stimuli are familial dysautonomia, sleep apnea, and obesity-hypoventilation syndrome. Lesions affecting the medullary centers that generate the inspiratory drive may cause marked changes in ventilatory patterns.

Spinal cord lesions above the C-4 level may result in total ventilatory paralysis. Because the phrenic nerve, which innervates the diaphragm, leaves the spinal cord at the C-4 level, a lesion above that level will affect all muscles of respiration. Injury to the high-thoracic or low-cervical cord often results in decreased lung volume and reduced chest wall compliance. Coughing will be inadequate if the abdominal muscles are paralyzed. These factors may cause respiratory insufficiency that may progress to respiratory failure. Acute respiratory care and long-term rehabilitation are essential components of a treatment plan for the child with a spinal cord lesion or injury.

Diseases affecting the efferent portion of the neuromuscular system are not uncommon in children. The progressive loss of anterior horn cells seen in Werdnig-Hoffmann syndrome leads to paralysis and early death secondary to respiratory failure. The result of acute polyneuritis (Guillain-Barré syndrome) is often respiratory paralysis. When this syndrome is fatal, it is usually attributable to respiratory failure. Because recovery from Guillain-Barré syndrome is often complete, the respiratory weakness must be treated aggressively and should include acute and long-term rehabilitation measures.

Degenerative diseases of the muscle (e.g., Duchenne myopathy) are characterized by progressive deterioration of pulmonary function. Adequate arterial oxygen and carbon dioxide values are maintained only through active efforts. Death is usually the direct result of respiratory failure, which often follows the development of pneumonia.

The thoracic cage normally provides for adequate function of the respiratory musculature. Abnormalities of the thorax, such as idiopathic scoliosis, scoliosis secondary to neuromuscular disease, and other specific congenital abnormalities, may result in a loss of mechanical advantage of the respiratory muscles.

The examples just mentioned can cause respiratory muscle weakness or mechanical disadvantage. They may also lead to the requirement for long-term management by mechanical ventilation. Mallory and Stilwell identify the physical therapist as a member of the typical team of caregivers for these technology-dependent children.[43] In addition, of the seven rehabilitation goals they have identified for the ventilator-dependent child, six are directly related to physical therapy knowledge, skills, and scope of practice. These seven goals follow:

1. Increase in muscle strength
2. Increase in attention and cognition
3. Decrease in spasticity
4. Increase in chest wall movement
5. Accessory muscle breathing while upright
6. Diaphragmatic breathing
7. Assisted cough

All goals, with the possible exception of the second one, are direct benefits derived from physical therapy.[43]

Physical Therapy Evaluation

The parameters assessed in a comprehensive physical therapy evaluation for a child with respiratory muscle weakness are breathing pattern, respiratory muscle strength, chest and shoulder mobility, and airway clearance (see Case Study, H. E., and Table 14-2). In addition, when appropriate, the therapist should evaluate sensorimotor development.

Case Study—H.E., 14-year-old Caucasian Male with History of Duchenne Muscular Dystrophy

H.E., a 14-year-old Caucasian male with a history of Duchenne muscular dystrophy diagnosed at 4 years of age, was referred for pulmonary physical therapy evaluation. At the time of his referral, a functional evaluation revealed that H.E. could ambulate 25 feet in 20 seconds, could roll from a prone to a supine position and back to a prone position, and had adequate sitting balance. He was unable to run, ascend or descend stairs, rise from the floor or from a chair, sit up from a supine position, or assume a posture on all fours. A modified manual muscle examination indicated strength that was graded from "poor" to "absent" for all isolated muscle groups, with the exception of wrist extensors, which were graded as "fair" to "good." H.E. could function from an electric wheelchair, and he could ambulate slowly using a walker with supervision.

Pulmonary physical therapy evaluation included an assessment of H.E.'s breathing pattern, respiratory muscle strength, chest wall mobility, coughing ability, and oral motor functions. The result of these assessments are presented in Table 14-2.

In addition to the therapeutic regimen outlined in Table14-2, H.E.'s parents were instructed in the techniques of bronchial drainage, chest percussion, vibration, and shaking. Although retention of secretions had not been a problem, the potentially severe effects of a respiratory tract infection were explained. The parents were instructed to begin bronchial hygiene procedures at the first sign of an infection of the respiratory tract.

Determining the breathing pattern is a major part of the evaluation. Minute ventilation—the product of the respiratory rate and the tidal volume—determines the arterial $PaCO_2$. The respiratory rate can be counted for 30 seconds or 1 minute, remembering that the child's normal respiratory rate at rest varies with age (a younger child will have a higher rate).[44] Tidal volume can be easily measured with a spirometer or a Wright respirometer used at the bedside. As with respiratory rate, tidal volume varies depending on the child's height. A taller child has a larger predicted tidal volume.[44] The pattern and symmetry of muscular effort must be ascertained. Is the child using primarily the diaphragm, intercostal muscles, accessory muscles, or glossopharyngeal muscles? Is the muscular pattern similar for each hemithorax?

The therapist has several methods available for evaluating respiratory muscle strength, including measurement of lung volumes, maximal static inspiratory and expiratory pressures, and electromyography. The first two methods are simple and inexpensive, but require the child's full cooperation. With normal lung tissue and without loss of elastic recoil, decreased inspiratory capacity or expiratory reserve volume suggest weakness of the inspiratory or expiratory musculature, respectively.[45] Respiratory failure may be imminent when the vital capacity declines to approximately 30% of predicted values. Maximal inspiratory and expiratory pressures are another good index of respiratory muscles. These pressures can be measured with appropriate pressure manometers, and measurements can be repeated as often as necessary.[46]

Evaluation of the mobility of the chest wall includes determining expansion of the chest wall in anteroposterior, transverse, and vertical directions during inspiration. Thoracic dimensions are determined during inspiration and expiration to document chest motion. ROM in the spine and the shoulder girdle should be examined, including glenohumeral, acromioclavicular, and sternoclavicular joints. Decreased motion at any one of these joints may result in reduced thoracic expansion.

Auscultation of the lungs of a child with respiratory weakness will serve several functions. Decreased breath sounds will help identify areas that are poorly ventilated. Lung areas with decreased or absent sounds may correlate with de-

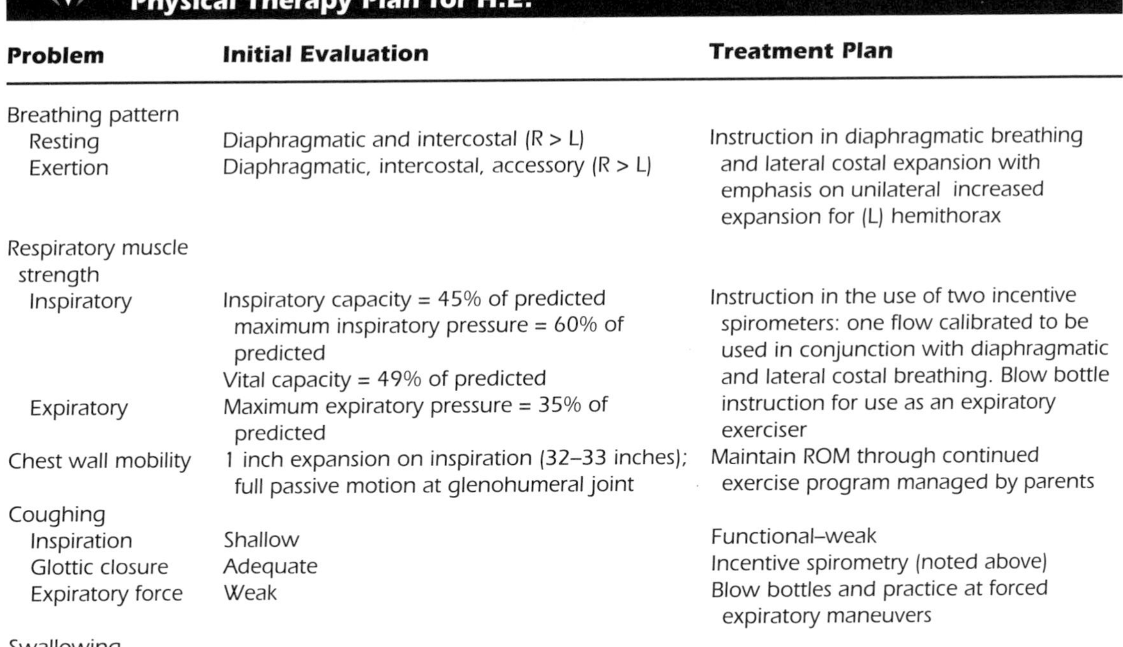

TABLE 14-2
Physical Therapy Plan for H.E.

Problem	Initial Evaluation	Treatment Plan
Breathing pattern		
Resting	Diaphragmatic and intercostal (R > L)	Instruction in diaphragmatic breathing and lateral costal expansion with emphasis on unilateral increased expansion for (L) hemithorax
Exertion	Diaphragmatic, intercostal, accessory (R > L)	
Respiratory muscle strength		
Inspiratory	Inspiratory capacity = 45% of predicted maximum inspiratory pressure = 60% of predicted Vital capacity = 49% of predicted	Instruction in the use of two incentive spirometers: one flow calibrated to be used in conjunction with diaphragmatic and lateral costal breathing. Blow bottle instruction for use as an expiratory exerciser
Expiratory	Maximum expiratory pressure = 35% of predicted	
Chest wall mobility	1 inch expansion on inspiration (32–33 inches); full passive motion at glenohumeral joint	Maintain ROM through continued exercise program managed by parents
Coughing		
Inspiration	Shallow	Functional–weak
Glottic closure	Adequate	Incentive spirometry (noted above)
Expiratory force	Weak	Blow bottles and practice at forced expiratory maneuvers
Swallowing		
Solids	Adequate	
Semisolids	Adequate	

creased chest motion or muscular effort. Breath sounds are the most reliable clinical tool for ensuring good ventilation. Breath sounds can help the therapist evaluate the need for bronchial hygiene. If rhonchi and wheezes are heard, bronchial drainage and removal of secretions are probably necessary. Breath sounds may indicate the resolution or progression of pulmonary complications, such as pneumonia or atelectasis, and the therapist may choose to modify treatment accordingly.

The therapist should evaluate the child's cough. Integral components of a cough are sufficient active inspiration and coordinated closure of the glottis, followed by sudden contraction of the abdominal muscles to markedly increase intrathoracic pressure. With neuromuscular dysfunction, the child may lack any or all cough-related skills. Evaluation of inspiratory effort, glottis closure, and abdominal muscle strength is important in assessing coughing. The child must also coordinate the three components into an effective, sputum-producing effort.

Overall strength, mobility, and coordination, as well as the developmental level of the child, must be evaluated to plan a realistic rehabilitation program. A child who can actively locomote in some manner is less likely to suffer pulmonary complications and may improve pulmonary function as a byproduct of the rehabilitative effort. An aggressive therapeutic regimen is necessary, both to provide early mobility and to strengthen the respiratory musculature, thus improving ventilatory function.[47]

Evaluation of oral motor function—swallowing and feeding—often requires an interdisciplinary effort by physicians, physical therapists, occupational therapists, speech pathologists, other therapists, and nurses. Swallowing must be evaluated for two reasons: eating is the best way for a child to thrive nutritionally, and aspiration of feedings is a major cause of respiratory problems in developmentally delayed and neurologically impaired children.[48] A discussion of aspiration and swallowing function is beyond the scope of this chapter, but a good general overview can be found in Farber's text.[49]

Physical Therapy Management

Physical rehabilitation for the child with neurologic impairment should include an exercise program to improve or maintain respiratory function. The exercises should strengthen inspiratory and expiratory muscles, especially the abdominal muscles that are necessary for effective coughing. A traditional method of "strengthening" the diaphragm by using abdominal weights has not withstood rigorous scientific evaluation.[50] More physiologically appropriate methods of improving inspiratory muscle strength and endurance may include resistive breathing,[51] use of incentive spirometers,[52] and maximal sustainable ventilatory capacity.[53]

Respiratory muscle training has become a recognized approach to reduce the progressive decline in respiratory function in children with Duchenne myopathy. A battery of breathing exercises has improved spirometric values in children with Duchenne myopathy.[54] Specific inspiratory muscle resistive training has been used to improve respiratory muscle strength and endurance in children with Duchenne myopathy. Studies have shown continuing improvement over a 6-month period of training, with much of the improvement sustained at a point as long as 6 months following the cessation of the formal exercise regimen.[55,56] In addition, active and resistive exercises for the neck will strengthen the accessory muscles of inspiration (i.e., the sternocleidomastoid muscles and scalene muscles). Although accessory muscle use increases the energy cost of breathing, the accessory muscles may provide increased inspiratory volume to prevent respiratory insufficiency in the child with neuromuscular disease. Active and resistive exercises for strengthening of the abdomen, which may help develop a strong, effective cough, are well known by physical therapists. Many clinical aspects of respiratory muscle training have been discussed by Watts, Adkins, and Warren.[57–59]

Improving the pattern of breathing of a child with neuromuscular disease may provide two major benefits. First, in improved ratio of alveolar ventilation to dead space ventilation occurs when a slower, deeper pattern of breathing replaces a fast and shallow mode. The therapist may have the child attempt a slower and deeper pattern of breathing using various clinical cues, including counting, a metronome, or a spirogram. Care must be taken to avoid a deep breath, which, owing to increased elastic resistance of the lung parenchyma at high volumes, may increase the work of breathing and negate the presumed improvement. Avoiding inefficient or counterproductive muscular effort is the second major benefit of changing the pattern of breathing. A child with respiratory distress may appropriately use the accessory muscles to aid inspiration and may use the abdominal muscles to enhance full expiration. This muscular pattern, however, can become habitual. If the diaphragm provides adequate ventilation, unnecessary muscular effort is exerted if the child continues to use the accessory muscles. Various training methods have been suggested, including relaxation exercises and neurosensory techniques, but no scientific data support these endeavors, nor do they suggest that short-term changes in muscular patterns during the therapeutic session have a residual effect or replace the inefficient patterns.

Although the importance of maintaining or improving mobility of the thorax in children has been identified and related treatment plans have been outlined,[57–59] no controlled studies of the techniques have been conducted. Active breathing exercises to improve thoracic mobility have been suggested for localized areas or for the entire chest. Manual stretching of the chest wall has been advocated but has not been tested. It is known that adults with decreased thoracic mobility have increased lung compliance and improved oxygenation for several hours after the use of incentive spirometers and positive pressure breathing.[60] It seems logical that a child whose chest wall is normally more compliant than that of an adult, should also benefit from these two methods. Active or passive exercise to improve shoulder girdle mobility in children with paralysis may also improve thoracic excursion. Clinical studies must be undertaken to justify the time-consuming procedures used in the name of respiratory exercises.

Skill at coughing is important because of the smaller airway cross section in children and the predisposition to airway obstruction. Children with muscular weakness often lack an effective cough. Efforts to improve the cough usually involve strengthening of the abdominal muscles. Using sit-ups and straight leg raising has been discouraged because these activities primarily involve the rectus abdominus rather than the strong compressors of the abdominal wall (i.e., the transversalis and oblique muscles).[57] The use of expulsive maneuvers, such as blow-bottles or forced expiratory trials, seems to offer more kinesiologically approximate means of strengthening the cough musculature. Other traditional methods of instruction in coughing rely on a "double cough," "huffing" on expiration, and external stimulation (irritation) of the trachea to elicit a cough.

Because many children with respiratory weakness and general inactivity accumulate secretions, bronchial drainage techniques are an important part of the home treatment program. If the parent suspects an increase in secretions as a result of a respiratory tract infection, the use of positioning for gravity drainage and chest vibration or percussion may prevent the development of pneumonia or atelectasis. Oral or nasal suctioning may be necessary to maintain a clear airway if a child cannot cough well and if secretions are voluminous. Parents should be trained in aspiration techniques and should have proper suctioning equipment in the home.

Despite many articles and textbooks that describe detailed physical therapy programs for patients with neuromuscular weakness of the chest, there is a dearth of well-substantiated clinical research to support many of the suggested treatment procedures.

Asthma

There are many definitions of asthma, all with some features in common, but none is agreed on universally. A panel of the National Heart Lung and Blood Institute proposed the following definition: "Asthma is a lung disease with the following characteristics: (1) airway obstruction that is reversible (but not completely so in some patients) either spontaneously or with treatment; (2) airway inflammation; and (3) increased airway responsiveness to a variety of stimuli."[61] The chronic inflammatory changes in the airway are responsible for bronchoconstriction, edema within the airways, secretion of mucus, and the chronic nature of the disorder.[62]

Medical Information

Asthma is among the most prevalent chronic conditions in the United States affecting approximately 14 million people and 7 percent of children. Asthma is also an expensive disease whose total cost was estimated in 1990 at more than $6 billion in the United States.[63] Importantly, there has been a notable and troublesome increase in asthma mortality since 1977, with the increase seen most significantly in inner cities and among the poor and minority groups, particularly African Americans.[64] There is enormous morbidity associated with the condition, as denoted by days lost from school, hospitalizations, and health care costs. Asthma in children is characterized by several factors. Boys seem to predominate over girls by as much as a 2:1 ratio, although this number is not firm. Exercise-induced asthma is common in children, with a reported prevalence of more than 90%.[65] Children with asthma are often allergic, with the inhaled allergen triggering a type 1 immunoglobin E (IgE)–mediated response. Symptoms may also be provoked by viral infections and emotional problems. Finally, the increasing mortality and continuing high morbidity associated with childhood asthma are attributable, in part, to a growing problem with asthma in the inner city populations.[66]

The physiologic changes responsible for the signs and symptoms of asthma are thought to be initiated by the release of one or more chemical mediators from the mast cells and eosinophils within the airways. These inflammatory mediators—histamine, prostaglandin D_2, leukotriene C_4, and others—stimulate a response that increases bronchial smooth muscle contraction, causes mucous secretions from the goblet cells of the bronchial epithelium, and may result in edema of the bronchial wall. The result of all three processes is often an obstruction of the airways. As airway obstruction progresses, expiratory airflow decreases, lung volumes and airway resistance increase, airway conductance decreases, and ventilation/perfusion inequality leads to arterial hypoxemia. The various pathophysiologic aspects of asthma appear to have a major hereditary component. However, asthma seems to have a complex genetic model without any clear pattern of inheritance.[62]

A fascinating aspect of asthma in children is the exercise-induced component. With strenuous exercise for a period of time, usually for more than 5 minutes, a child can develop many manifestations of asthma (e.g., dyspnea, wheezing, and airway obstruction) that may reverse spontaneously or with treatment. This exercise component is important to the physical therapist who is developing a conditioning program to increase exercise tolerance in the child with asthma. The response can be controlled by having the child using appropriate oral or inhalation medications before the exercise bout.

Medical Management

Medical management of the child with asthma is commonly divided into treatment of the acute attack and control of chronic asthma. Treatment mainstays for the acute attack include inhaled β_2 agonists such as albuterol or isoetharine. Supplemental oxygen is used to maintain an O_2 saturation of approximately 95%. Intravenous aminophylline, and systemic corticosteroids are additional medications for acute asthma. In severe attacks that appear to be unremitting, subcutaneous epinephrine may be employed.[62,67]

The long-term medical management of asthma has several components: pharmacologic, environmental, and immunologic. The pharmacologic agents used may include sympathomimetic agents delivered orally or by aerosol; oral preparations of theophylline (methylxanthines); anti-inflammatory agents, including inhaled and oral corticosteroids; and cromolyn sodium, delivered by inhalation. Control of environmental factors plays a major role in asthma therapy. A dust-free environment for the child is imperative, and special air-filtration units may be required for the child's room. Removal of pets from the home, avoidance of tobacco smoke, and careful selection of foods to which the child is not sensitive are also major aspects of environmental control. If the youngster chooses to be active in athletics, care must be taken either to avoid levels of activity that may provoke bronchospasm or to use appropriate medication before engaging in asthma-inducing levels of physical exertion.

Another method of long-term therapy for allergic asthma is immunotherapy (allergy shots). Once allergens are identified by skin testing, extracts of these allergens are given in gradually increasing strengths by way of periodic injections. The rationale is that the child's immunologic system will respond to the minute doses of allergen by producing circulating antibodies. Once sufficient levels of antibodies are developed, environmental exposure to the allergen (e.g., pollen or food) will result in no symptoms of asthma because the acquired antibodies will alleviate the allergic response of the child. There has been a recent review of the many aspects of immunotherapy.[68]

Physical Therapy Evaluation

As with medical care, physical therapy evaluation and management of children with asthma is largely based on the clinical situation at the time (i.e., whether the child is in an acute, subacute, or chronic stage of the disease). The child with status asthmaticus will generally not tolerate well any maneuvers aimed at either bronchial hygiene or physical training. A notable exception is when the patient is intubated and mechanically ventilated.

The physical therapist's evaluation of a child on a ventilator should include auscultation in an effort to identify secretions and poorly inflated areas of lung. Evaluation of the child's position in bed and initial assessment of shoulder ROM are appropriate. An evaluation of the asthmatic patient in the subacute phases (i.e., when the severe bronchospasm has responded to medication) should include several parameters. The therapist must identify, through auscultation, where bronchial secretions have accumulated and if areas of the lungs are poorly ventilated. The pattern of ventilation and use of accessory muscles should be noted. Measurements of the thorax, including thoracic index, should be made during inspiration and expiration to determine chest mobility. Shoulder-girdle ROM should also be measured. Several or all of these evaluated items will be abnormal. The therapist must reevaluate these items with each treatment until the ROM, thoracic index, breath sounds, and pattern of breathing are normal.

A long-term rehabilitation plan for the child with asthma must also examine exercise tolerance, strength, and posture. Exercise tolerance may be evaluated by semiquantitative measures in the physical therapy department or by sophisticated testing in an exercise laboratory. Heart rate during a particular workload and time of recovery to resting heart rate are useful and simple indices of fitness or exercise tolerance.[69] Quantitative strength measurement of major muscle groups can be made with equipment that is readily available in the physical therapy department. Posture can be evaluated using a grid system.[70]

Physical Therapy Management

There is little, if any, rationale for physical therapy in the child with status asthmaticus, or intractable acute asthma. Status asthmaticus renders a child too dyspneic, anxious, scared, and physically unable to cooperate with the therapist for bronchial hygiene, breathing retraining, posture and ROM evaluation, or any rehabilitative endeavors. Bronchial drainage with chest percussion, vibration, and coughing should be used when the status asthmaticus begins to abate and the patient can tolerate these physical maneuvers. An exception to this approach is when the child is intubated for mechanical ventilation, in which case the child should undergo bronchial drainage, percussion, vibration, and suctioning if secretions are problematic.

When the severe bronchospasm begins to wane, accumulated secretions are often encountered in the previously narrowed airways. Aggressive bronchial hygiene is imperative during this subacute stage. Secretions that are not removed quickly predispose the patient to atelectasis and bronchial infection. Bronchial drainage with chest percussion and vibration is indicated within the limits of the youngster's tolerance and endurance. Secretion volume, color, consistency, and the child's vital signs before, during, and after treatment should be recorded.

In the long-term care of asthmatic children, intermittent bronchial hygiene treatments may be useful, but they are not used routinely as in other conditions, such as CF. Parents must know the drainage positions and manual techniques in order to treat the child at home. Parents should use bronchial drainage at the first sign of a respiratory infection or increased mucous production. The only reported study of the effects of drainage and percussion in children with asthma involved 21 outpatients. These children, who had mild to moderate asthma, were divided into a treatment group and a control group. The mean FEV_1 for the treatment group increased by 10.5% 30 minutes after therapy. The control group had a slight decrease in mean FEV_1 during the same period. The difference in mean FEV_1 values was significant at the 0.05 level.[71] Breathing training combined with relaxation techniques has been suggested for improvement of respiratory patterns in children with asthma. Several rationales for the use of slow, deep diaphragmatic breathing have been given. The work of breathing can be decreased by slowing the respiratory rate and by decreasing the ratio of dead space ventilation to minute ventilation. Increased diaphragmatic excursion also improves regional ventilation to the lower lobes in persons with architecturally normal lungs.[28] Because many small areas of atelectasis are present in the lower lobes, diaphragmatic breathing to improve lower lobe ventilation may be beneficial in asthma.

As a result of greatly increased residual volume and decreased expiratory reserve volume, the child with asthma often develops a shallow, rapid respiratory pattern that uses the accessory muscle of inspiration. Expiratory obstruction may cause expiration, which is usually passive, to become active through abdominal muscle and internal intercostal contraction. The therapist should teach the child to decrease use of the accessory muscles once the residual volume diminishes and expiratory flow improves. Continued use of this abnormal pattern of breathing is energy-depleting and inappropriate when an improvement in symptoms occurs. Jacobson's relaxation techniques have been used to decrease accessory and abdominal muscle use while increasing diaphragmatic excursion.[72] Relaxation techniques have also been advocated to reduce the anxiety and physical stress associated with an episode of asthma. Many anecdotal and verbal reports lend subjective support to the benefits of relaxation techniques in patients with asthma, but controlled studies are lacking. The effects of deep inspiratory and expiratory efforts in asthmatic patients was reported by Gayrard and associates, who found that deep, slow inspiration from functional residual capacity to total lung capacity yielded an immediate increase of 71% in airway resistance.[73] A similar but weaker response occurred with deep expiration. The patient's efforts toward deep, slow breathing must, therefore, be initiated carefully because a maximal effort can result in decreased airway function.[73] Nasal breathing, which warms and humidifies inspired air, has been advocated for patients with asthma who have exercise-induced bronchospasm.[74] Based on the role of heat exchange within the airways, warmed humidified air may provide an easy, cost-free method of reducing the bronchospasm that follows stressful exercise in children with asthma.[75]

Physical rehabilitation to improve endurance, work capacity, and strength are major goals in the long-term management of asthmatic children. Children with chronic asthma are often less physically fit than their normal peers. Exercise-induced bronchospasm may preclude a child with asthma from participating in vigorous exercise and the child may, therefore, be unable to respond to physical demands.[76] Appropriate medication before vigorous exercise may attenuate the bronchospastic response, and the child can derive both the enjoyment and benefits of exercise. A formal physical training program should be preceded by qualitative or, preferably, quantitative evaluation of the child's response to strenuous exercise. The initial evaluation determines the level of exercise needed to improve strength and endurance and is a baseline against which the results of subsequent studies can be compared to determine improvement or deterioration. Among the more commonly used methods of training are free running, treadmill running, bicycle ergometry, and swimming.

Two controlled studies of swimming training in children with asthma showed similar results. Sly and associates assigned children to either a treatment group or a control group.[77] The treatment group participated in a swimming program for 2 hours three times a week for 13 weeks. Although no changes were recorded in pulmonary function or basic personality traits, a marked decrease in wheezing days was noted in the treatment group. The mean number of days of wheezing for the treatment group was 31.3 during the 13 weeks before the training program; this figure declined to 5.7 days of wheezing during the swimming program. A similar control group of asthmatic children had a mean of 10.1 and 13.2 days wheezing, respectively, before and during the 3-week control period.[77]

Fitch and associates conducted a study of the results obtained with a 5-month swimming program in 46 asthmatic children compared with a control group of 10 children.[78] Included in the testing parameters were asthma score (based on wheeze, cough, and sputum), physical work capacity at a heart rate of 170, drug score (based on the amount of medication), FEV_1 levels, and response to an exercise challenge on a treadmill. A marked improvement in asthma score, drug score, and physical work capacity followed the training period. A concomitant improvement in posture was noted. No change was reported in FEV_1 or the severity of exercise-induced asthma. The authors concluded that swimming is an eminently effective method of physical training in asthmatic children.[78] Other aspects of physical therapy management for asthmatic children in terms of posture improvement and shoulder girdle and chest wall mobility exercises have been well described.[57,59,70]

Cochrane and Clarke recently reported the results of a 3-month medically supervised indoor training study of 36 patients with asthma, aged 16 to 40 years.[79] Although the age range largely exceeds childhood, the results are worth discussing. Training included an optimal duration and frequency of 30 minutes three times per week, with the target heart rate at 75% predicted maximum. The training sessions were varied to include cycling, jogging, and aerobics. Each session was preceded by a warm-up and followed by a cool-down, including light calisthenics and stretching. Changes in physiologic parameters were compared with those in a nontraining control group of patients with asthma. There were numerous improvements noted in cardiovascular, respiratory, and metabolic function in the training group but not in the control group. Breathlessness was reduced during work levels corresponding to many activities of daily living (ADLs). There was no change in disease severity between the groups. Although exercise-induced asthma cannot be prevented by physical exercise, there can be little doubt of the potential for physical training in individuals with asthma, but strong motivation and good adherence are important factors for the success of an exercise program for children with asthma.[79,80]

In addition to generalized physical training, a recent double-blind study showed that specific inspiratory muscle training over a 6-month period improved inspiratory muscle strength and decreased asthma symptoms, related hospitalizations, emergency room contacts, absence from school, and medication consumption.[81]

Cystic Fibrosis

Medical Information

CF is the most common lethal genetic disorder affecting Caucasians. It is estimated to occur in 1 of every 1600 to 2000 births, and has a carrier rate of approximately 1 in 20 persons. CF is a generalized disorder of the exocrine glands, which, in its fully manifested state, produces high sweat electrolyte concentrations, pancreatic enzyme deficiency, and chronic suppurative pulmonary disease. The clinical presentation of CF varies, but usually includes combinations of productive cough, abnormally frequent and large stools, failure to thrive, recurrent pneumonias, rectal prolapse, nasal polyposis, and clubbing of the digits. Because of its variable presentation, CF is often misdiagnosed as asthma, allergy, celiac disease, and chronic diarrhea. The well-informed health professional should consider CF when any of these symptoms are encountered.

The gene for CF, the cystic fibrosis transmembrane conductance regulator (CFTR), was identified on the long arm of chromosome 7.[82,83] Formal identification occurred in 1990 when the secretory defect caused by this gene was corrected in vitro.[84] Although one mutation is responsible for approximately ⅔ of all cases of CF, there are more than 600 mutations of the gene recognized.[84,85] The major hypothesis of CFTR dysfunction states that the product of the abnormal gene is responsible for a decrease in chloride and water secretion by airway epithelial cells, thereby resulting in dehydrated mucus. However, the diversity of organ system involvement in CF suggests that other mechanisms are also associated with the CFTR. Regardless of the specific mechanisms, it is agreed that all exocrine glands are impaired to some degree and the variable dysfunction results in a wide spectrum of symptoms and complications for CF.[84]

When two carriers have a child, there is a 25% chance that the child will have CF, a 50% chance that the child is a carrier of the gene, and a 25% chance that the child will be completely free from the CF gene. Testing for the carrier or heterozygous state is now possible, as is prenatal testing.

The incidence in Caucasians has been mentioned. Although CF is much less common in the black population, it occurs in 1 in 17,000 births among African Americans.[1] CF is rare in the Asian population. The course of the disease, like its presentation, is variable. Although severe lung and gastrointestinal disease can be fatal for children with CF, survival rates have improved steadily over the last 25 years. For example, approximately 40% of individuals with CF survive to an age of 30 years and beyond.[1] Reports of large numbers of adults with CF have been published in several journals.[86–88]

The pulmonary disease associated with CF causes the greatest mortality. Pulmonary involvement in CF begins with the production and retention of thick, viscid secretions within the bronchioles. These secretions provide a medium in which bacterial pathogens flourish. The resultant infections produce more secretions and additional obstruction, and a vicious cycle is begun. The earliest pathologic changes may be reversed with aggressive treatment. With continued reinfection, bronchiolitis and bronchitis progress to bronchiolectasis and bronchiectasis. The latter two processes, which are irreversible, destroy elements within the walls of the airways.

In addition to these destructive processes, hyperplasia of mucus-secreting glands and cells occur within the lungs. Large quantities of thick, purulent mucus are produced, causing the airway obstruction that is common in CF. If the obstruction is partial, a ball-valve process may result in hyperaeration of the lung distal to the obstruction. Complete airway obstruction results in absorption atelectasis distal to the obstruction. Small areas of hyperaeration and atelectasis often exist in adjacent areas, and present a honeycomb pattern on a chest roentgenogram. The rapidity of pulmonary progression and success of treatment play major roles in determining the survival of a child with CF.

Pulmonary complications often include lobar atelectasis, bronchiectasis, pneumothorax, hemoptysis, pulmonary hypertension, and cor pulmonale. These problems have been discussed at length by others.[89–91]

Medical Management

Management of CF is directed toward decreasing airway obstruction and pulmonary infection, replacing pancreatic enzymes to help reverse the nutritional deficiency, and providing appropriate psychosocial and emotional support to the child and family. Control of pulmonary infection is the major therapeutic objective. Sputum culture and sensitivity tests to identify pathogens and determine appropriate antimicrobial drugs enable the physician to plan a rational course of medications. The most common bacteria-causing infections in patients with CF are *Staphylococcus aureus* and *Pseudomonas aeruginosa*. Antimicrobial agents may be given orally or parenterally. There is no oral preparation available to combat the Pseudomonas species, so intravenous administration of the anti-pseudomonas drugs is necessary.

In the past decade, the bacterium *Burkholderia cepacia* has become recognized as contributing to infection in people with CF. *B. cepacia* is largely antibiotic-resistant and may be transmitted in epidemic-like fashion. It has been associated in many patients with rapid progression of lung disease, ending in death within several months. It must be noted, however, that not all *B. cepacia* infections react in this manner. The CF Foundation (CFF) and Centers for Disease Control and Prevention have recommended isolating individuals with this infection in order to prevent epidemic outbreaks.[84]

Reduction of airway obstruction is the most time-consuming aspect of comprehensive treatment for CF. Reduction of sputum viscosity by aerosolized or oral medications is thought to enhance physical efforts to loosen and drain mucus from the airways. Physical therapy is a major part of the care.

Two newer approaches to treatment include lung transplantation and gene therapy. Lung transplantation for those with end-stage disease has been successful. Unfortunately, there are major problems with transplantation, including a median waiting time for donor organs of greater than 12 months and the development of obliterative bronchiolitis following transplantation. The waiting period has resulted in approximately 40 percent of patients awaiting an organ dying before receiving the transplant. Bronchiolitis obliterans occurs in about one-half of patients about 2 years after transplantation and follows a steady downhill course. Gene therapy attempts to introduce into the airways normal versions of the CFTR. To date, results have been limited.[84]

Replacement of pancreatic enzymes is essential for the 85% of patients with pancreatic dysfunction. Traditionally the recommended diet for patients with CF has included high-protein, high-carbohydrate, and low-fat foods. With more effective pancreatic preparations, many children have liberalized their intake of fat. Despite apparent control of pancreatic insufficiency with enzymes, patients with CF may need up to 50% more calories than their age- and weight-matched peers. Continually underweight children, or those who experience weight loss with a progression of disease, may benefit from commercial dietary supplements. Supplements must be chosen carefully and added to the diet. A nutritionist's counseling is necessary.

Psychosocial and emotional support for patients with CF and their families is the responsibility of all professionals who work with this population. Issues that must be confronted include chronic life-shortening illness, genetic disease, cost of drugs and care, time-consuming treatments, death of a child, denial, and guilt. Other issues emerge as patients reach adulthood: marriage, occupations, and dependence on others for treatment. A counselor or social worker plays a major role on the CF team, and several publications have addressed the psychosocial aspects of the management of CF.[92–93]

A nationwide network of centers is dedicated to the treatment of CF. These centers are sponsored by the CFF and can reach almost every population center in the United States. The CFF sponsors research projects, fellowships, conferences, fund raising, and other activities in its mandated task of providing the best care for children and adults with CF.

Physical Therapy Evaluation

Physical therapy evaluation for the child with CF is similar to the evaluation for the other disorders discussed in this chapter. Emphasis in CF must be placed on the obstruction by bronchial secretion that causes the numerous pulmonary problems and complications.

Auscultation for secretions must be done with the expectation of finding many areas with sonorous wheezes, harsh breath sounds, and crackles (all abnormal breath sounds). The sounds may not change for several days in a patient with advanced disease, and auscultation on an intermittent, rather than daily, basis may be helpful.

A determination of the child's ability to cough and raise secretions is crucial. An acutely ill child with CF who cannot cough effectively risks further deterioration in airway function. The roentgenogram is useful in identifying specific pockets or patches of advanced destruction of the lung. Many therapists believe that the three-dimensional view of the lungs afforded by posteroanterior and lateral chest films provides specific information to help direct treatment.

Qualitative and quantitative evaluation of exercise tolerance provides a basis for planning an exercise reconditioning program at a level appropriate to the child's tolerance. An evaluation of the child's muscular pattern of breathing may be accomplished by observation or by palpation.

Mobility of the chest wall should be determined for several reasons. A noncompliant thorax increases the work of breathing. Children with CF often have hyperinflated lungs, and so the chest wall may appear barrelled and fixed. If chest wall changes occur, the child may have difficulty developing the necessary pressures and flow rates to cough effectively or to increase ventilation during physical stress. Thoracic index, thoracic girth, and rib motion should be determined during full inspiration and full expiration.

Evaluation of the child's posture is essential to identify early changes caused by the hyperaeration and chronic coughing that accompany CF (Fig. 14-15). The thorax assumes a barrel-shape, with an increase in the normal thoracic kyphosis. Scapular protraction also becomes evident. With the anatomic changes in the upper thorax that accompany hyperaeration, range of motion of the shoulder girdle must be measured. A comprehensive evaluation should include those postural items that may affect both function and cosmesis.

Physical Therapy Management

CONVENTIONAL PHYSICAL THERAPY

The major role of physical therapy for the child with CF is in the aggressive use of bronchial drainage, chest percussion, vibration, and suctioning (if necessary). Treatment should be generalized because mucus is produced in most areas of the lungs. If specific segments have more advanced disease or exhibit increased production of mucus, emphasis for treatment should center on these segments. Early studies of conventional bronchial drainage, percussion, and vibration in CF have helped document their efficacy. Lorin and Denning, for instance, have demonstrated that twice the amount of sputum per cough and per treatment was obtained when a combined treatment regimen of gravity drainage, percussion, and vibration was

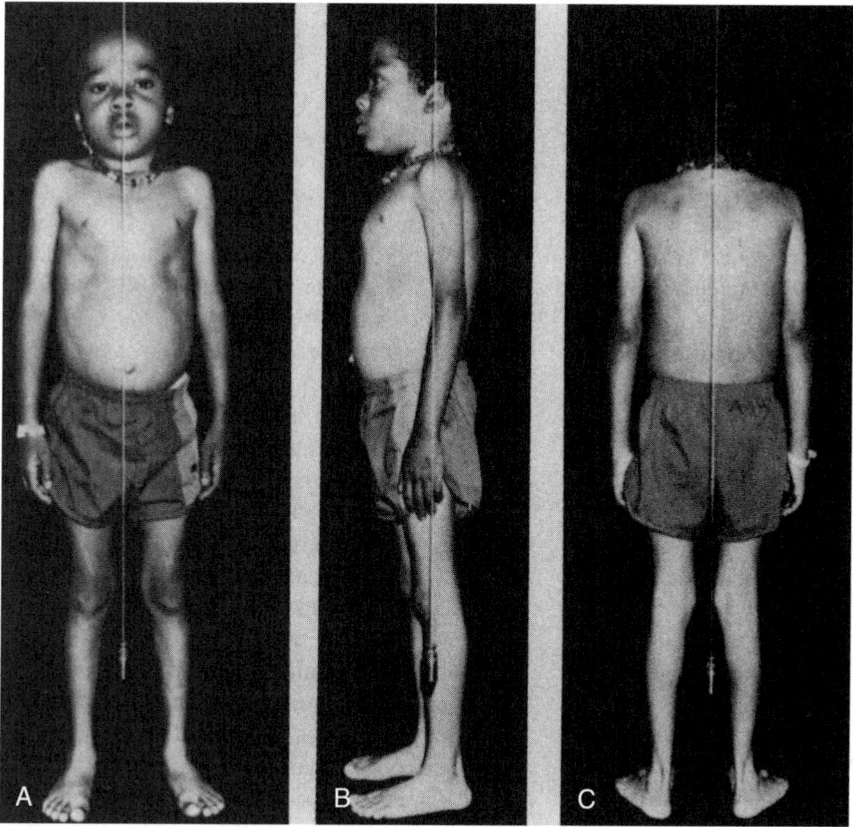

Figure 14-15 ▪ Postural abnormalities in a child with cystic fibrosis. (**A**) Anterior view. Notice that the shoulders are held high, especially on the right. This posture appears to offer better mechanical advantage to the accessory muscles for breathing. The lower ribs are flared, and the thorax appears barreled and elongated because of the hyperinflation of the lungs. A full postural evaluation might reveal other, less obvious abnormalities. (**B**) Lateral view. The thoracic kyphosis and barreled chest seen here are common findings in children with obstructive pulmonary disease and hyperinflation of the lungs. (**C**) Posterior view. The shoulders appear high, with a protraction of the scapulae. Notice the enlargement of the thorax in relation to the rest of this patient's body. Pronated feet are also noticeable. (Reproduced by permission from Irwin S, Tecklin JS. *Cardiopulmonary Physical Therapy*. St. Louis: CV Mosby; 1985.)

compared with cough alone.[94] Tecklin and Holsclaw have documented improvement in forced vital capacity and peak expiratory flow rate after bronchial drainage, percussion, and vibration in 26 children with CF.[95] Weller and colleagues have also reported increased peak expiratory flow rates after conventional treatment.[96] Feldman and associates have demonstrated remarkable improvement in flow rates at low lung volumes 45 minutes after treatment in nine patients with CF.[97] In Feldman's study, the isovolume flow rate near 25% of forced vital capacity increased from baseline by 70% 45 minutes after treatment.[97] These changes in small airway flow rates are consistent with the results of Motoyama.[98]

Desmond and coworkers employed a crossover design to determine whether pulmonary function decreased over a 3-week period during which physical therapy was withheld. There was a statistically significant decrease in flow rates that was reflective of small airway function, forced expiratory flow ($FEF_{25-75\%}$) and Vmax60 (total lung capacity [TLC]), each of which declined by 20% after 3 weeks of no therapy. These values returned to their prior levels shortly after resumption of physical therapy.[99]

ALTERNATIVE AIRWAY CLEARANCE TECHNIQUES

As individuals with CF have grown older to the point where the median age of survival is now more than 30 years, the importance of independent treatment has grown, with the following approaches being those used most universally to either substitute for or serve as an adjunct to conventional physical therapy. A recent and exhaustive review by Williams of the world's literature on various physical therapy methods demonstrated that the most effective form of treatment has yet to be established.[100] Although there are methodological flaws in the many studies reported, it appears clear that the alternative techniques offer benefits and are particularly useful in that several provide total independence in self-care without the need for an assistant to provide the manual techniques.

Autogenic Drainage. Autogenic drainage has been shown to improve pulmonary function and result in increased secretion removal when compared with PEP breathing and conventional physical therapy.[101,102] Other studies that compared autogenic drainage with the active cycle of breathing[103] and with conventional therapy[104] were able to demonstrate improved airway function and secretion clearance. One of the drawbacks with autogenic drainage is that it requires intense individual training by the physical therapist, and some individuals have difficulty learning and performing the technique. Those who are able to participate report good acceptance and use of the procedure and independence in its use.

Forced Expiratory Technique/Active Cycle of Breathing. A number of studies that compared the FET with conventional physical therapy were performed by the physical therapists from Brompton Hospital in London, where the FET was popularized. Although the results of these studies appear to support the FET, the weak or absent statistical analyses, the small numbers of subjects, and other opportunities for experimental bias raises questions about the objectivity and validity of the work.[105–108] Verboon et al. found no difference in pulmonary function in eight subjects who received either FET and postural drainage or FET alone. However, when one deletes one of eight subjects who produced minimal amounts of sputum, the 24-hour sputum collection in Verboon's study actually favors conventional physical therapy over FET.[109]

The Brompton group updated the FET by adding breath control techniques, huffing, and thoracic expansion exercises in various sequences. This newer approach is called active cycle of breathing,[23] but as with the FET, there is little research to support its use in lieu of conventional physical therapy.

Positive Expiratory Pressure Mask. The PEP mask, described earlier in the chapter, may hold the greatest promise in terms of independent removal of excess secretions in children with CF. Several studies have found that the efficacy of the PEP mask, when used in conjunction with FET, was superior to, or at least equal to, that of conventional bronchial hygiene measures, including positioning, manual techniques, and coughing.[110–113] One study found conventional treatment to be superior, but that study used statistical analysis only for within-group changes rather than between-group changes.[114]

Two recent long-term studies of PEP breathing have been reported. McIlwaine et al. compared two groups of subjects with CF who were assigned randomly to a PEP group or a conventional therapy group. At the end of 12 months, the PEP group had small improvements in pulmonary function (FVC, FEV_1, and FEF_{25-75}), whereas the conventional group showed small declines in those values.[115] The second study showed no difference in the rate of decline of pulmonary functions during two 12-month periods in which conventional physical therapy was used for the first period and PEP mask breathing was used for the second period.[116]

FLUTTER. The Flutter is another attempt to offer a measure of independence to young adults with CF. The Flutter was compared with voluntary coughing alone and postural drainage during 15-minute treatment sessions in 17 subjects with CF of varied severity. The Flutter appeared far superior in its ability to help subjects raise secretions. However, few would agree that a 15-minute postural drainage session, using up to 10 positions, represents a treatment comparable to those performed and recommended by most physical therapists.[117] Several subsequent studies of the Flutter found no difference between the device and other modalities of airway clearance. It appears that the Flutter is well accepted by some patients and is equivalent to the effects on sputum clearance and pulmonary function of other types of airway clearance.[118–120]

HIGH FREQUENCY CHEST COMPRESSION. HFCC is most commonly provided by use of the American Biosystems thAIRapy vest. The vest has gained acceptance throughout many CF centers in the United States. Warwick and Hansen examined the efficacy of HFCC in a long-term study of 16 subjects with CF. All but one of the those subjects showed improvement in their respiratory impairment during the trial.[121] Subsequent evaluations of HFCC demonstrated that the technique was at least as beneficial to subjects with CF as conventional physical therapy and PEP breathing.[122,123] The "vest," as HFCC is called, has provided a useful, independent means for older children and adults with CF to continue treatments without an assistant to provide manual techniques. The only drawback to the vest is its cost, which is approximately $16,000 at this writing, but many insurance carriers will provide excellent levels of support for this tool.

In summary, the use of gravity-assisted bronchial drainage with manual techniques as the "gold standard" for children with CF is no longer the case, although a recent report noted that fully 89% of respondents to a questionnaire continued to use these time-honored techniques. This figure was greater than for any of the other techniques noted.[124] Nonetheless, when working with children with CF, the therapist must consider alternative techniques for secretion removal. The choice of procedures should fall largely on the patient and family members who are ultimately responsible for this time-consuming daily procedure.

DIRECTED COUGHING. At least three studies have examined the efficacy of directed coughing for secretion removal in CF. Each study compared coughing alone with conventional therapy and found that the benefits derived did not differ among the approaches.[125–127] The study by De-Boeck and Zinman, however, found that flows at low lung volume, which are usually indicative of small airway function, were significantly improved with conventional physical therapy.[125]

MODIFICATIONS OF BRONCHIAL HYGIENE PROCEDURES

Modifications of usual treatment procedures are often necessary for acutely ill children or for those with certain complications. In a patient with major hemoptysis, chest percussion and vibration should be discontinued temporarily because the physical maneuvers may dislodge a blood clot and prolong the bleeding. FET and PEP may be useful. If the area of hemoptysis can be identified, the child should be positioned to drain the accumulated blood. Percussion and vibration may be reinstituted gradually within 24 to 48 hours if the bleeding abates.

Pneumothorax is often a complication of CF and is commonly treated with an intrapleural chest tube with suction. Gravity drainage is appropriate, although percussion and vibration at the site of tube insertion are contraindicated. FET, PEP, and directed coughing may enable the continued treatment of excessive secretion. Bronchial hygiene treatment for the noninvolved thorax should be continued.[128]

With far advanced destruction of the lung, the child at the final stage of disease will not tolerate drainage positions. These patients may be treated in any position of comfort, with vibration for all areas of the lungs, and this can then be followed by FET or PEP. Vibration during coughing and manual support of the chest will enhance the expulsive coughing effort in the terminal stage of CF. Improvement of diaphragmatic excursion, decreased use of accessory muscles, and relaxation are often advocated for children with CF. The rationale for using these measures in patients with CF is similar to that for those with asthma: decreased work of breathing, decreased dead space ventilation, and reduced anxiety. The efficacy of these treatments has not, however, been tested by appropriate clinical trials.

PHYSICAL EXERCISE

Formal and informal methods of exercise testing and physical conditioning have been recommended for children with CF.[129] Cropp and associates showed that in children with CF, with the exception of those with advanced lung disease, the *cardiovascular* response to exercise was normal during incremental testing on a cycle ergometer.[130] However, the *ventilatory* response to exercise was abnormal because those with CF who had decreased pulmonary function increased their ventilation more than did normal controls at all levels of stress. The authors stated that the relative increase in minute ventilation in subjects with CF was necessary to overcome the airway obstructive element of the disease. Children with advanced disease often had carbon dioxide retention indicative of the inability to increase ventilation sufficiently. These children with advanced disease were also very likely to have arterial oxygen desaturation during exercise.[130] Muscle fatigue as an additional limiting factor in physical exercise was recently identified by Moorcraft et al. Seventy-eight of 104 subjects with CF reported that muscular fatigue was a significant limiting factor during peak exercise testing. Therefore muscle endurance and fatigue should be considered during exercise testing and training.[131]

The relevance of these findings is that physical training and reconditioning, in a formal or informal program, is safe and beneficial in all patients except those with severe lung disease. Even those with severe disease have been shown to benefit from an exercise program if supplemental oxygen is provided. Marcus and colleagues demonstrated that patients with advanced CF who exercised with an FIO_2 of 30% worked longer, had higher maximal oxygen consumption, and experienced less oxygen desaturation than while exercising at room air.[132] Treadmill walking or running, cycle ergometer training, free running or walking, and strengthening exercises are useful methods of increasing cardiovascular fitness, endurance, and general muscular strength. Although several investigators have examined the immediate effects of exercise on children with CF, the effects of a long-term training program have yet to be evaluated.

Keens and associates attempted to improve ventilatory muscle endurance, as measured by the maximal sustainable ventilatory capacity

(MSVC).[31] This study documented an improvement of more than 50% in MSVC after specific ventilatory muscle training in children with CF. Additionally, a group of seven children at a summer camp who underwent a general physical activity program also showed more than a 50% improvement in MSVC. Once the ventilatory exercise or physical activity ceased, a decrease in MSVC was noted. Physical conditioning and training programs will, therefore, affect specific ventilatory muscle endurance.[31]

Summary

This chapter has attempted to provide a summary of unique characteristics of lung disease in children, growth and development of the respiratory system, and the reasons why children and infants are predisposed to acute respiratory failure. Assessment of the child with pulmonary disease and treatments aimed at reducing the severity of pulmonary disease in infants and children have been reviewed. Four major respiratory disorders have been described, along with a discussion of appropriate physical therapy assessment and management. Published evidence for the physical therapy methods has been reviewed. Physical therapy for children with lung disease has been shown to be efficacious, depending on the treatment employed and the problems addressed.

REFERENCES

1. Lemen RJ, Parcel GS, Loughlin G, et al. Pediatric lung diseases. *Chest.* 1992;102(suppl):232S–242S.
2. Taylor WP, Newacheck PW. Impact of childhood asthma on health. *Pediatrics.* 1992;90:657–662.
3. *Vital Statistics of the United States, 1970.* Vol. 2. Mortality, Part A. Rockville, MD: National Center for Health Statistics; 1974.
4. Centers for Disease Control and Prevention. Asthma mortality and hospitalization among children and young adults—United States, 1980–1993. *MMWR Morb Mortal Wkly Rep.* 1996;45:350–353.
5. Waring WW. Respiratory diseases in children: An overview. *Respir Care.* 1978;20:1138–1145.
6. Avery ME. Normal and abnormal respiration in children. Presented at the 37th Ross Conference on Pediatric Research; 1961.
7. Dunhill MS. Quantitative observations on the anatomy of chronic non-specific lung disease. *Med Thorac.* 1965;22:261.
8. Holsclaw DS. Pediatric pulmonary disease: An overview. *Pediatr Ann.* 1977;6:438–443.
9. Woolcock AJ. Asthma—what are the important experiments? *Am Rev Respir Dis.* 1988;138:730–744.
10. Charnock EL, Doershuk CF. Developmental aspects of the human lung. *Pediatr Clin North Am.* 1973;20:275–292.
11. Avery ME. Hyaline membrane disease. *Am Rev Respir Dis.* 1975;111:657–688.
12. Polgar G, Weng TR. The functional development of the respiratory system. *Am Rev Respir Dis.* 1979;120:625–695.
13. Downes JJ, Fulgencio T, Raphaely RC. Acute respiratory failure in infants and children. *Pediatr Clin North Am.* 1972;19:423–445.
14. Holsclaw DS. Early recognition of acute respiratory failure in children. *Pediatry Ann.* 1977;6:467–475.
15. Haskins R, Lotch J. Day care and illness: Evidence, costs, and public policy. *Pediatrics.* 1986;77(suppl):951–956.
16. Keens TG, Ianuzzo CO. Development of fatigue-resistant muscle fibers in human ventilatory muscles. *Am Rev Respir Dis.* 1979;119:139–141.
17. Papastamelos C, Panitch HB, England SE, et al. Developmental changes in chest wall compliance in infancy and early childhood. *J Appl Physiol.* 1995;78:179–184.
18. Pagliara AS, Karl IE, Haymond M, et al. Hypoglycemia in infancy and childhood. *J Pediatr.* 1973;82:365–379.
19. Crane L. Physical therapy for the neonate with respiratory disease. In: Irwin S, Tecklin JS, eds. *Cardiopulmonary Physical Therapy,* 3rd ed. St. Louis: CV Mosby; 1995.
20. DeCesare J. Physical therapy for the child with respiratory dysfunction. In: Irwin S, Tecklin JS, eds. *Cardiopulmonary Physical Therapy,* 3rd ed. St. Louis: CV Mosby; 1995.
21. Dab I, Alexander F. Evaluation of a particular bronchial drainage procedure called autogenic drainage. In: Baran D, Van Bogaert E, eds. *Chest Physical Therapy in Cystic Fibrosis and Chronic Obstructive Pulmonary Disease.* Ghent, Belgium: European Press; 1977;185–187.

22. Dab I, Alexander F. The mechanism of autogenic drainage studied with flow volume curves. *Monogr Paediat.* 1979;10:50–53.
23. Lindsay KL. *Airway Clearance and Breathing Retraining Techniques.* Philadelphia: Presbyterian Medical Center; 1997.
24. Pryor JA, Webber BA, Hodson ME, et al. Evaluation of the forced expiratory technique as an adjunct to postural drainage in treatment of cystic fibrosis. *Br Med J.* 1979;2:417–418.
25. Partridge C, Pryor J, Webber B. Characteristics of the forced expiratory technique. *Physiotherapy.* 1989;75:193–194.
26. Hofmyer JL, Webber BA, Hodson ME. Evaluation of positive expiratory pressure as an adjunct to chest physiotherapy in the treatment of cystic fibrosis. *Thorax* 1986;41:951–954.
27. Gregory R. High frequency chest compression. Presented at Airway Clearance and Breathing Retraining Techniques. Philadelphia: Presbyterian Medical Center; 1997.
28. Shearer MO, Banks JM, Silva G, et al. Lung ventilation during diaphragmatic breathing. *Phys Ther.* 1972;52:139–147.
29. Wetzel J, Lunsford BR, Peterson MJ, et al. Respiratory rehabilitation of the patient with spinal cord injury. In: Irwin S, Tecklin JS, eds. *Cardiopulmonary Physical Therapy,* 3rd ed. St. Louis: CV Mosby; 1995:590.
30. Darbee J, Cerny F. Exercise testing and exercise conditioning for children with lung dysfunction. In: Irwin S, Tecklin JS, eds. *Cardiopulmonary Physical Therapy.* 3rd ed. St. Louis: CV Mosby; 1990:570.
31. Keens TG, Krastins IRB, Wannamaker EM, et al. Ventilatory muscle endurance training in normal subjects and patients with cystic fibrosis. *Am Rev Respir Dis.* 1977;116:853–860.
32. Orenstein D, Franklin BA, Doershuk CF, et al. Exercise conditioning and cardiopulmonary fitness in cystic fibrosis. *Chest.* 1981;80:392.
33. Laennec RTH; Forbes J, trans. *Diseases of the Chest.* 4th ed. London: 1819.
34. Atelectasis. In: Schaffer AT, Avery ME, eds. *Diseases of the Newborn.* 4th ed. Philadelphia: W.B. Saunders; 1977:122–126.
35. Nemir RL. Atelectasis. In: Kendig EL, Chernick V, eds. *Disorders of the Respiratory Tract in Children.* 3rd ed. Philadelphia: W.B. Saunders; 1977.
36. Thoren L. Postoperative pulmonary complications: Observations on their prevention by means of physiotherapy. *Acta Chir Scand.* 1954;107: 193–205.
37. Stein M, Cassara EL. Preoperative pulmonary evaluation and therapy for surgery patients. *JAMA.* 1970;211:787–790.
38. Bartlett RH, Gazzinga AB, Graghty JR. Respiratory maneuvers to prevent postoperative complications. *JAMA* 1973;224:1017–1021.
39. Hymes AC, Yonehiro EG, Raab DE, et al. Electrical surface stimulation for treatment and prevention of ileus and atelectasis. *Surg Forum.* 1974;25:222–224.
40. Finer MN, Moriartey RR, Boyd J, et al. Postextubation atelectasis. A retrospective review and a prospective controlled study. *J Pediatr.* 1979;94: 110–113.
41. Burrington JD, Cotton EK. Removal of foreign bodies from the tracheobronchial tree. *J Pediatr Surg.* 1972;7:119–122.
42. Tecklin JS, Holsclaw DS. Bronchial drainage with aerosol medication in cystic fibrosis. *Phys Ther.* 1976;56:999–1003.
43. Mallory GB, Stillwell PC. The ventilator-dependent child: Issues in diagnosis and management. *Arch Phys Med Rehabil.* 1991;72:43–55.
44. Polgar G, Promadhat V. *Pulmonary function Testing in Children.* Philadelphia: W.B. Saunders; 1971.
45. Derenne JP, Macklem PT, Roussos CH. The respiratory muscles: Mechanics, control, and pathophysiology. Part III. *Am Rev Respir Dis.* 1978; 118:581–601.
46. Black LF, Hyatt RE. Maximal respiratory pressures: Normal values and relationship to age and sex. *Am Rev Respir Dis.* 1969;99:696–702.
47. Braun NMT, Rochester DF. Muscular weakness and respiratory failure. *Am Rev Respir Dis.* 1979; 119:123–125.
48. Williams HE. Inhalation pneumonia. *Aust Paediatr J.* 1973;9:279–285.
49. Farber S. *Neurorehabilitation: A Multisensory Approach.* Philadelphia: W.B. Saunders; 1982.
50. Merrick J, Axen K. Inspiratory muscle function following abdominal weight exercises in healthy subject. *Phys Ther.* 1981;61:651–656.
51. Gross D, Riley E, Grassino A, et al. Influence of a resistive training on respiratory muscle strength and endurance in quadriplegia (abstract). *Am Rev Respir Dis.* 1978;117(4):343.
52. Pontoppidan H. Mechanical aids to lung expansion in non-intubated surgical patients. *Am Rev Respir Dis.* 1980;122(5):109–119.
53. Leith DL, Bradley M. Ventilatory muscle strength and endurance training. *J Appl Physiol.* 1976;41: 508–516.

54. Siegel IM. Pulmonary problems in Duchenne muscular dystrophy: Diagnosis, prophylaxis, and treatment. *Phys Ther.* 1975;55:160.
55. Martin AJ, Stern L, Yeates J, et al. Respiratory muscle training in Duchenne muscular dystrophy. *Dev Med Child Neurol.* 1986;28:314–318.
56. Wanke T, Toifl K, Formanek D, et al. Inspiratory muscle training in patients with Duchenne muscular dystrophy. *Chest.* 1994;105:475–482.
57. Watts N. Improvement of breathing patterns. *Phys Ther.* 1968;48:563–576.
58. Adkins H. Improvement of breathing ability in children with respiratory muscle paralysis. *Phys Ther.* 1968;48:577–581.
59. Warren A. Mobilization of the chest wall. *Phys Ther.* 1968;48:582–585.
60. Bergofsky EH. Respiratory failure in disorders of the thoracic cage. *Am Rev Respir Dis.* 1979;119: 643–669.
61. National Heart, Lung and Blood Institute National Asthma Education Program Expert Panel Report. *Guidelines for the Diagnosis and Management of Asthma.* Bethesda: NHLBI; 1991.
62. Lemanske RF, Busse WW. Asthma. *JAMA.* 1997; 278:1855–1873.
63. Blaiss MS. Outcomes analysis in asthma. *JAMA.* 1997;278:1874–1880.
64. Lang DM, Polansky M. Patterns of asthma mortality in Philadelphia from 1969 to 1991. *N Engl J Med.* 1994;331:1542–1546.
65. Godfrey S. Childhood asthma. In: Clark TJH, Godfrey S, eds. *Asthma.* Philadelphia: W.B. Saunders; 1979.
66. Weiss KB, Gergen PJ, Crain EF. Inner-city asthma: The epidemiology of an emerging US public health concern. *Chest.* 1992;101(suppl): 362S–367S.
67. Avery ME, Wohl ME. Obstructive Diseases. In Avery ME, First LR, eds. *Pediatric Medicine,* 2nd ed. Baltimore: Williams & Wilkins; 1994:289–294.
68. Weber RW. Immunotherapy with allergens. *JAMA.* 1997;278:1881–1887.
69. Lunsford BR. Clinical indicators of endurance. *Phys Ther.* 1978;58:704–709.
70. Kendall HO, Boynton DA. *Posture and Pain.* Baltimore: Williams & Wilkins, 1952.
71. Huber AL, Eggleston PA, Morgan J. Effect of chest physiotherapy on asthmatic children (abstract). *J Allergy Clin Immunol.* 1974;53:2.
72. Rathbone JL. *Relaxation.* Philadelphia: Lea & Febiger; 1969.
73. Gayrard P, Orehek J, Grimand C, et al. Bronchoconstrictor effects of a deep inspiration in patients with asthma. *Am Rev Respir Dis.* 1975; 111:433–439.
74. Shturman-Ellison R, Zeballos RJ, Buckley JM, et al. The beneficial effect of nasal breathing on exercise-induced bronchoconstriction. *Am Rev Respir Dis.* 1978;118:65–73.
75. Deal EC, McFadden ER, Ingram RH, et al. Role of respiratory heat exchange in production of exercise-induced asthma. *J Appl Physiol.* 1979;46: 467–475.
76. Cropp GJA. Exercise-induced asthma. In: Middleton E, ed. *Allergy: Principles and Practice.* St. Louis: CV Mosby; 1978.
77. Sly RM, Harper RT, Rosselot I. The effect of physical conditioning upon asthmatic children. *Ann Allerg.* 1972;30:86–94.
78. Fitch KD, Morton AR, Blanksby BA. Effects of swimming training on children with asthma. *Arch Dis Child.* 1976;51:190–194.
79. Cochrane LM, Clarke CJ. Benefits and problems of a physical training programme for asthmatic patients. *Thorax.* 1990;45:345–351.
80. Thio BJ, Nagelkerke AF, Ketel AG, et al. Exercise-induced asthma and cardiovascular fitness in asthmatic children. *Thorax.* 1996;51:207–209.
81. Weiner P, Azgard Y, Ganam R, et al. Inspiratory muscle training in patients with bronchial asthma. *Chest.* 1992;102:1357–1361.
82. Rommens JM, Iannuzzi MC, Kerem B, et al. Identification of the cystic fibrosis gene: Chromosome walking and jumping. *Science.* 1989;245: 1059–1065.
83. Riordan JR, Rommens JM, Kerem B, et al. Identification of the cystic fibrosis gene: Cloning and characterization of complementary DNA. *Science.* 1989;245:1066–1073.
84. Robinson C, Scanlin TF. Cystic fibrosis. In Fishman AP, ed. *Pulmonary Diseases and Disorders.* 4th ed. New York: McGraw-Hill; 1997:803–824.
85. Kerem B, Rommens JM, Buchanan J, et al. Identification of the cystic fibrosis gene: Genetic analysis. *Science.* 1989;245:1073–1080.
86. Shwachman H, Kowalski M, Khaw KT. Cystic fibrosis: A new outlook. *Medicine.* 1977;56: 129–149.
87. Holsclaw DS, Kovatch A. A clinical profile of adults with cystic fibrosis. *CF Club Abstr.* 1977;18:53.
88. diSant' Agnese PA, Davis PB. Cystic fibrosis in adults. *Am J Med.* 1979;66:121–132.
89. Holsclaw DS. Common pulmonary complications of cystic fibrosis. *Clin Pediatr.* 1970;9:346–355.
90. Goldring RM, Fishman AP, Turino GM, et al. Pulmonary hypertension and cor pulmonale in

cystic fibrosis of the pancreas. *J Pediatr.* 1964;65: 501–524.

91. Holsclaw DS, Grand RJ, Shwachman H. Massive hemoptysis in cystic fibrosis. *J Pediatr.* 1973;76: 829–838.
92. Gayton WF, Friedman SB. Psychosocial aspects of cystic fibrosis: A review of the literature. *Am J Dis Child.* 1973;126:856–859.
93. McCollum AT, Gibson LE. Family adaptation to the child with cystic fibrosis. *J Pediatr.* 1970; 77:571–578.
94. Lorin MI, Denning CR. Evaluation of postural drainage by measurement of sputum volume and consistency. *Am J Phys Med.* 1971;50:215–219.
95. Tecklin JS, Holsclaw DS. Evaluation of bronchial drainage in patients with cystic fibrosis. *Phys Ther.* 1975;55:1081–1084.
96. Weller PH, Bush E, Preece MA, et al. The short-term effects of chest physiotherapy on lung function tests in children with cystic fibrosis. *Monogr Paediatr.* 1979;10:58–59.
97. Feldman J, Traver GA, Taussig LM. Maximal expiratory flows after postural drainage. *Am Rev Respir Dis.* 1979;119:239–245.
98. Motoyama EK. Lower airway obstruction. In: Mangos JA, Talamo RD, eds. *Fundamental Problems of Cystic Fibrosis and Related Diseases.* New York: Intercontinental Medical Book Corp; 1973.
99. Desmond KF, Schwenk F, Thomas E, et al. Immediate and long-term effects of chest physiotherapy in patients with cystic fibrosis. *J Pediatr.* 1983;103:538–542.
100. Williams MT. Chest physiotherapy and cystic fibrosis. Why is the most effective form of treatment still unclear? *Chest.* 1994;106:1872–1882.
101. McIlwaine PM, Davidson AGF. Cystic fibrosis, basic and clinical research. Comparison of expiratory pressure and autogenic drainage with conventional percussion and drainage therapy in the treatment of cystic fibrosis (abst.). *Proceedings of the 17th European Cystic Fibrosis Conference, Copenhagen, Denmark.* Amsterdam: Elsevier Science BV; 1991:54.
102. Pfleger A, Theissl B, Oberwalder B, et al. Self-administered chest physiotherapy in cystic fibrosis: A comparative study of high-pressure PEP and autogenic drainage. *Lung.* 1992;170:323–330.
103. Miller S, Hall D, Clayton CB, et al. Chest physiotherapy in cystic fibrosis a comparative study of autogenic drainage and active cycle of breathing technique (formerly called FET). *Pediatr Pulmonol.* 1993;(suppl 9):267.
104. Butler-Simon N, McCool P, Giles D, et al. Efficacy and desirability of autogenic drainage vs. conventional postural drainage and percussion. *Pediatr Pulmonol.* 1995;(suppl 253):(abst 265).
105. Pryor JA, Webber BA. An evaluation of the forced expiratory technique as an adjunct to postural drainage. *Physiotherapy.* 1979;65:304–307.
106. Sutton PP, Parker RA, Webber BA, et al. Assessment of the forced expiratory technique, postural drainage, and directed coughing in chest physiotherapy. *Eur J Respir Dis.* 1983;64:62–68.
107. Webber BA, Hofmyer JR, Morgan MDL, et al. Effects of postural drainage incorporating the FET on pulmonary function in cystic fibrosis. *Br J Dis Chest.* 1986;80:353–359.
108. Partridge C, Pryor J, Webber B. Characteristics of the forced expiration technique. *Physiotherapy.* 1989;75:193–194.
109. Verboon JML, Bakker W, Sterk PJ. The value of forced expiration technique with and without postural drainage in adults with cystic fibrosis. *Eur J Respir Dis.* 1986;69:169–174.
110. Falk M, Kelstrup M, Andersen JB, et al. Improvement in the ketchup bottle method with positive expiratory pressure, PEP, in cystic fibrosis. *Eur J Respir Dis.* 1984;65:424–432.
111. Tyrell JC, Hiller EJ, Martin J. Face mask physiotherapy in cystic fibrosis. *Arch Dis Child.* 1986;61: 598–600.
112. Tonnesen P, Stovring S. Positive expiratory pressure (PEP) as lung physiotherapy in cystic fibrosis: A pilot study. *Eur J Respir Dis.* 1984;65:419–422.
113. Oberwaldner B, Evans JC, Zach MS. Forced expirations against a variable resistance: A new chest physiotherapy method in cystic fibrosis. *Pediatr Pulmonol.* 1986;2:358–367.
114. Van Asperen PP, Jackson L, Hennessey P, et al. Comparison of a positive expiratory pressure (PEP) mask with postural drainage in patients with cystic fibrosis. *Aust Paediatr J.* 1987;23: 283–284.
115. McIlwaine PM, Wong LTK, Peacock D, et al. Long-term comparative trial of conventional postural drainage and percussion versus positive expiratory pressure physiotherapy in the treatment of cystic fibrosis. *Pediatr Pulmonol.* 1995;(suppl 254):(abst 268).
116. Robins R, Townshend J, Lands LC. One-year experience with positive expiratory pressure (PEP) mask in children with cystic fibrosis. *Pediatr Pulmonol.* 1996;(suppl 13):308 (abstract 357).
117. Konstan MW, Stern RC, Doershuk CF. Efficacy of the Flutter device for airway mucus clearance in patients with cystic fibrosis. *J Pediatr.* 1994;124: 689–693.
118. Geouque D, Engelhardt M. Effect of Flutter device on pulmonary function among the pediatric cystic

fibrosis population. *Pediatr Pulmonol.* 1996;(suppl 13):306(abst 350).

119. Gondor M, Nixon PA, Rebovich PF, et al. A comparison of the Flutter device and chest physical therapy in the treatment of cystic fibrosis pulmonary exacerbation. *Pediatr Pulmonol.* 1996; (suppl 13):307(abst 355).
120. Homnick DN, Marks JH. Comparison of the Flutter device to standard chest physiotherapy in hospitalized patients with cystic fibrosis. *Pediatr Pulmonol.* 1996;(suppl 13):308(abst 356).
121. Warwick WJ, Hansen LG. The long-term effect of high frequency chest compression therapy on pulmonary complications of cystic fibrosis. *Pediatr Pulmonol.* 1991;11:265–271.
122. Braggion C, Cappeletti LM, Cornacchia M, et al. Short-term effects of three chest physiotherapy regimens in patients hospitalized for pulmonary exacerbations of cystic fibrosis: A cross-over randomized study. *Pediatr Pulmonol.* 1995;19: 16–22.
123. Kluft J, Beker L, Castagnimo M, et al. A comparison of bronchila drainage treatments in cystic fibrosis. *Pediatr Pulmonol.* 1996;22:271–274.
124. Chiapetta A, Davis S. Airway clearance practices of respiratory care practitioners, physical therapists, and physiotherapists from CF centers. *Pediatr Pulmonol.* 1996;(suppl 13):307(abstract 353).
125. DeBoeck C, Zinman R. Cough versus chest physiotherapy: A comparison of the acute effects on pulmonary function in patients with cystic fibrosis. *Am Rev Respir Dis.* 1984;129:182–184.
126. Rossman CM, Waldes R, Sampson D, et al. Effect of chest physiotherapy on the removal of mucus in patients with cystic fibrosis. *Am Rev Respir Dis.* 1982;126:131–135.
127. Bain J, Bishop J, Olinsky A. Evaluation of directed coughing in cystic fibrosis. *Br J Dis Chest.* 1988; 82:138–148.
128. Tecklin JS, Holsclaw DS. Cystic fibrosis and the role of the physical therapist in its management. *Phys Ther.* 1973;53:386–393.
129. Darbee J, Cerny F. Exercise testing and exercise conditioning for children with lung dysfunction. In: Irwin S, Tecklin JS, eds. *Cardiopulmonary Physical Therapy.* 3rd ed. St. Louis: CV Mosby; 1995:563–578.
130. Cropp GJA, Pullano TP, Cerny FJ, et al. Adaptation to exercise in cystic fibrosis. *CF Club Abstr.* 1979;20:32.
131. Moorcraft AJ, Dodd ME, Howarth C, et al. Muscular fatigue, ventilation, and perception of limitation at peak exercise in adults with cystic fibrosis. *Pediatr Pulmonol.* 1996;(suppl 13):306(abst 349).
132. Marcus CL, Bader D, Stabile MW, et al. Supplemental oxygen and exercise performance in patients with cystic fibrosis with severe pulmonary disease. *Chest.* 1992;101:52–57.

Physical Therapy in the Public Schools

Karen Yundt Lunnen

Public schools are the most common practice setting for physical therapists who work with children.[1] It is a challenging and rewarding environment that requires physical therapists to use the best of their professional abilities within a context very different from the traditional medical environment.

Historic Background

Physical therapists have been practicing in the public school environment in the United States since the 1930s. During those early years, children with physical disabilities were usually segregated in special orthopedic schools or, in smaller communities, in separate classrooms within the school building. The primary diagnoses that physical therapists were involved with were poliomyelitis, tuberculosis of bones and joints, birth anomalies, and cerebral palsy.[2] Children with intellectual impairment or more severe disabilities did not have access to public education.

Often, physical therapists were employed as "special teachers, with the same privileges and responsibilities."[2] They met the same educational requirements as teachers and had, in addition, "a course in physical therapy from an approved school."[2] Many also had a background in physical education. Physical therapy departments were generally fully equipped treatment areas with whirlpools, parallel bars, treatment mats, and so on.

Pratt describes physical therapy in the educational setting at that time as a "rich and happy field" where the physical therapist had the "privilege of seeing the whole child" and where opportunity existed to not only see a child in his or her individual treatment session but to "follow the child in his peer groups."[2] Physical therapists experienced "great satisfaction in having an active part in the physical and social adjustments which are accomplished over a long period."[2]

Physical therapists who were practicing in educational environments were already addressing the benefits of including children with disabilities in activities with "normal" children. Ruth De Young speaks of an orthopedic school housed under the same roof as the high school allowing a "complete curriculum for little cripples."[3] Hutchinson, in 1937, comments that "it is easier for the crippled child to grow normally when he is in association with regular school children."[4] Yet, for approximately 30 more years, segregation for those with physical handicaps and exclusion for those with mental retardation or severe physical disabilities was the prevailing norm.

In the 1960s and 1970s, parents and other advocates became active in the so-called normalization movement and found support from John F. Kennedy's administration. Kennedy, who had a sister with intellectual impairment, created the President's Committee on Mental Retardation. The committee continues to study issues related to mental retardation and provide assistance and advice to the President. Annual reports are available for public review.

Several landmark decisions in the Supreme Court in the early 1970s paved the way for subsequent legislation guaranteeing the rights of those with disabilities. It is essential that physical therapists understand this legislation at both a federal and state level, because it has directed the provision of special education for children and defined the role of the physical therapist in the educational environment.

The first significant civil rights legislation for individuals with disabilities was the Rehabilitation Act of 1973.[5] It mandated that no program receiving federal moneys (including school programs) would discriminate on the basis of handicap. Section 504 of the Rehabilitation Act states that "no otherwise qualified disabled individual would be excluded from the participation in, be denied the benefits of, or be subjected to discrimination under any program or activity receiving federal financial assistance."[5] Section 504 paved the way for subsequent legislation impacting the provision of special education for children with disabilities in the public schools. It is also significant because it ensures that students with disabilities receive appropriate education even if special education is not required. It is an important source of support and funding for children who do not qualify for services under other legislative acts.

In November, 1975, the U.S. Congress passed the Education for All Handicapped Children's Act (Public Law 94-142),[6] which was the template for dramatic changes in the responsibilities of public schools to educate children with disabilities. PL 94-142 provided for a "free appropriate public education" (FAPE) for all children with disabilities from the age of 6 to 21 years (or from 5 years if that is the age in a particular state when children normally begin their participation in public school). FAPE "emphasizes special education and related services designed to meet their unique needs. . . . "[6]

Related services included ". . . transportation and such developmental, corrective, and other supportive services that are required to assist a handicapped child to benefit from special education, and includes speech pathology and audiology, psychological services, physical therapy, occupational therapy, recreation, early identification and assessment of disabilities in children, counseling services, and medical services for diagnostic or evaluation purposes."

Further provisions of PL 94-142 described a number of important new concepts for the public education of children with disabilities.

1. *Zero reject:* Under the new legislation, no child was to be excluded from receiving a free and appropriate education regardless of the type or severity of his or her disability. The law established two priorities to achieve zero reject: to identify those children currently not receiving any special education services; and to improve services for students with severe disabilities who were receiving an inadequate education, thus eliminating any exclusionary practices.[7]

2. *Least restrictive environment:* Education in the least restrictive environment is more commonly referred to as "mainstreaming" or "inclusion." School systems are required to ensure that: "To the maximum extent appropriate, children with disabilities, including children in public or private institutions or other care facilities, are educated with children who are nondisabled; and that special classes, separate schooling or other removal of children with disabilities from regular classes occurs only when the nature or severity of the disability is such that education in the regular classroom with the use of supplementary aids and services cannot be achieved satisfactorily."[6]
3. *Parent participation:* Parents or primary caregivers are essential members of the multidisciplinary team approach to evaluation, planning, and intervention that was mandated by PL 94-142. Legislation formalized participation of the parents by mandating their involvement in program planning; requiring their permission for evaluation; restricting release of information without their consent; giving them access to all educational records relating to their child; allowing them to serve on local and state advisory panels; and ensuring them due process. Parents' involvement in the planning process facilitates focus on meaningful functional goals for the child and family and consideration of the child's unique needs within a broader context. Physical therapists share with other professionals the responsibility of ensuring that parents are aware of their rights and encouraged to be active participants in program planning for their children. Parents can be powerful advocates, and it behooves physical therapists and others to consider parents an integral part of the team and to be aware of parent support and advocacy groups within their region.
4. *Nondiscriminatory evaluation:* Legislation requires that the evaluation of a child is free from racial or cultural bias, that no one test is used as the sole criterion for placement decisions, and that the test is administered in the child's native language. With their focus on motor skills, physical therapists are not affected by this aspect of the legislation as much as some other professionals, but all professionals are encouraged to use standardized tests that have been normed on a diverse population when possible.
5. *Individualized Education Program:* Every child receiving special education must receive an individualized education program (IEP). This is a comprehensive individualized plan developed by a multidisciplinary team in cooperation with the parents outlining the special education and related service needs of the child. Annual goals and short term objectives are developed by an IEP Team and are reviewed and revised on a predetermined basis.

Almost 11 years later (October 8, 1986) the Education of the Handicapped Act Amendments (PL 99-457) were enacted.[8] Part B of the amendments expanded the provisions of PL 94-142 to include preschool children (3 to 5 years old) "who are experiencing developmental delays . . . in one or more areas."[8] As in PL 94-142, physical therapy for preschool children is considered a related service and is provided only to assist in meeting the educational plan. Part H of the amendments provided early intervention services for infants and toddlers who have developmental delay or who "have a diagnosed physical or mental condition which has a high probability of resulting in developmental delay."[8] The actual amount of delay is specified by individual states, so that a young child might be eligible for early intervention or preschool services in one state but not another.

In October 1991, PL 94-142 and PL 99-457 were reauthorized and amended as PL 102-119, the Individuals with Disabilities Education Act Amendments (IDEA).[9] Now included were provisions to include family training, counseling, and home visits; to expand the related services category to include nutrition and assistive technology, among others; to require coordination of services between public and private agencies; and "to the maximum extent possible to provide services in natural environments, including the home and community settings in which children without disabilities participate. . . ." Under Part H, physical therapy was considered an early intervention service to be provided irrespective of the educational goals for the child. For infants and toddlers, the comprehensive multidisciplinary plan became the individualized family service plan (IFSP). The IFSP is comparable to the IEP but, as its title suggests, involves the infant or toddler and family in the multidisciplinary assessment and intervention plan. The family assessment portion is voluntary, and the child may not be excluded from services if the family does not want to participate in the assessment process. Legislation states that "enhancing the capacities of families to meet the special needs of their infants and toddlers with handicaps" is considered an "urgent and substantial need."[9] The IFSP must be evaluated annually and reviewed at least every 6 months. PL 102-119 also mandated that the IEP or IFSP state provisions for a child and family's transition from one level of service to another.

The Technology Related Assistance for Individuals with Disabilities Act (Tech Act)[10] was originally passed in 1988 and reauthorized in 1993. Under this act, public schools are obligated to acquire but not necessarily purchase needed assistive technology. "An assistive technology device means any item, piece of equipment, or product system whether acquired commercially off the shelf, modified, or customized, that is used to increase, maintain, or improve the functional capabilities of children with disabilities. . . ." Assistive technology services refer to "any service that directly assists a child with a disability in the selection, acquisition, or use of an assistive technology device."[10] IDEA adopted the basic terminology and concepts of the Tech Act.

The Medicare Catastrophic Coverage Act (Public Law 100-360)[11] was instituted to allow Medicaid funds to pay for services outlined as needed in an IEP or IFSP. The intent of this act was to improve access to therapy for children by allowing federal resources other than education to contribute to the related service needs of children.

The Americans with Disabilities Act (ADA), PL 101-336,[12] which was enacted in 1990 and became effective in 1992, extended comprehensive civil rights protection to individuals with disabilities. The law's major impact on public education was the provision that all public buildings must be accessible.

IDEA was reauthorized in June 1997 as Public Law 105-17,[13] supporting most of the provisions of earlier legislation with amendments that expanded or modified the provisions of the law in other areas.

Models of Service Delivery and Team Interaction

As a result of federal legislation, children with multiple disabilities and severe intellectual impairment were now in the public schools, and professionals from all disciplines were challenged to meet their needs. Special education took on a new dimension. With a legal mandate to provide physical therapy for children if it was determined necessary, local education agencies (LEAs) scrambled to employ physical therapists. They found that physical therapists who wanted to work in the public school environment were in short supply and high demand. Questions arose about the qualifications a physical therapist should possess to work in the public schools.[14] Did physical therapists with entry-level professional education have the academic foundation and clinical experience to work with children who had multiple disabilities? Efforts were made to define the competencies required to practice in an educational environment[15] and in early intervention,[16] and to identify a process for specialty certification in pediatric physical therapy.[17]

Physical therapists were challenged both individually and collectively to define their role in the educational environment. Part of the adaptation required of physical therapists was to adjust from the traditional medical model to an educational model. In the medical model prevailing in the late 1970s and into the 1990s, children were evaluated and treated by a physical therapist in a clinical setting. Interaction was primarily between the therapist and child and provided in a center isolated from the child's natural environment.

The educational environment required that therapists consider different models of intervention. Unidisciplinary intervention shifted to multidisciplinary team intervention for assessment, planning, and service delivery. In the federal legislation, the teams were described as "multidisciplinary," although the intent of the legislation was closer to what most would define as a transdisciplinary team model. In the transdisciplinary model, team members jointly assess the child, parents are full and active participants; a primary service provider is assigned to implement the plan with the family; information, knowledge, and skills are continuously shared among team members; and there is a commitment to teach, learn, and work together across disciplinary boundaries to implement a unified service plan.[18] The role release that is required for meaningful team function in the transdisciplinary model is still difficult for physical therapists practicing in the school setting. In a survey of physical therapists practicing in educational environments, Effgen and Keppler[19] found that although they recognized the importance of collaborative team interaction, most physical therapists practicing in educational settings perform evaluations independently of team members, report findings separately, conduct evaluations outside the classroom, and provide treatment as a direct service, also outside the classroom. One reason that physical therapists gave for not fully embracing a collaborative team model was concern about legal issues related to standards of professional practice. Rainforth[20] examined the physical therapy practice acts in each state and concluded that "documents that define legal and ethical practice of physical therapy allow for, and even encourage, role release in educational settings."

Various authors use different terminology to describe models of physical therapy service in the educational setting, but categories commonly referred to are (1) direct; (2) indirect (monitoring); and (3) consultation. Although these are described separately, they often occur together as complimentary components of a comprehensive intervention plan for an individual student. Direct service involves hands-on intervention directly from a physical therapist or physical therapist assistant supervised by a physical therapist. It can be offered in an isolated manner (in a physical therapy clinic or treatment area) or integrated (in the child's classroom or "natural" environment). The expected outcome of direct service is improved skill.[21] Scheduling is one of the limitations of the direct service model, because if a child is receiving physical therapy, he or she is not participating in the normal academic curriculum.

Indirect service (monitoring) involves establishing a management program for a student, instructing others to carry it out, and monitoring the process to ensure positive outcomes. Three outcomes are commonly associated with the indirect model: "(1) the student refines a skill; (2) the student maintains function; and (3) the parents and educators learn to implement a procedure."[21] The indirect model requires that physical therapists can effectively teach others and that they can sell their "product" (i.e., the functional importance of the recommended intervention).

Consultation involves a partnership between the physical therapist and the recipient of the information exchange. The expected outcome of consultation is that "the school environment (human and nonhuman) changes in ways that enable a student to succeed at school despite the limitations imposed by a disabling condition."[21] Bundy describes consultation as "extraordinarily powerful" and recommends it as the primary form of service delivery for most students.[21]

Legislation that related services were provided to enable the child to benefit from special education caused physical therapists and others to reshape their thinking about intervention. Was a child with myelodysplasia who could function independently in the school environment in a wheelchair eligible for physical therapy to work on ambulation with a walker? Were soft tissue contractures reason for physical therapy intervention if they did not interfere with function in the educational environment? What was special education for a child with multiple disabilities and severe intellectual impairment? Was physician referral necessary for all children? Any children? What was our professional liability? What documentation was required? Coming from a medical model in which documentation was required with almost every visit and reassessment was required at least monthly, the minimum requirement of an evaluation every 3 years seemed unthinkable.

A variety of factors have impacted the delivery of pediatric physical therapy in the past 20 years that have blured the distinction between the medical and educational models. McEwen and Shelden[22] summarize the major shifts in pediatric physical therapy as "(1) from neuromaturational and reflex-hierarchial models of assessment and intervention to systems models and motor learning principles; (2) from measuring within a neurodevelopmental framework to measuring within a disablement model that focuses on functional activities; and (3) from center-based and child-centered services to family-centered services in natural environments."[22] It is not possible in this chapter to describe these theoretical shifts in more detail, but they lend support to the model of service delivery adopted in educational environments. Additional research is needed to look at outcomes for children receiving physical therapy under various models (Table 15–1).

The majority of the functions and roles assumed by physical therapists in the public school setting that have been described so far have been student related. Physical therapists can also make significant contributions to program-related needs. Physical therapists may assist others in the educational setting to identify architectural barriers and plan for accessibility modifications; establish guidelines and child-specific modifications for the transport of children with disabilities on school-owned vehicles (e.g., buses); promote acceptance of students with disabilities by both educational personnel and students; plan recreational areas for accessibility; and contribute to the development of

TABLE 15-1
Summary of Trends in the Delivery of Physical Therapy Services to the Pediatric Population

Child-centered	to	Family-centered
Center-based	to	Naturalistic environment
Isolated service	to	Integrated service
Unidisciplinary	to	Transdisciplinary
Direct intervention	to	Indirect (monitoring) or consultation

safety procedures for emergency evacuation of students with disabilities. They may work with physical educators to develop "mutually supportive and effective motor programs."[23] Depending on interest and expertise and the needs of the school system, physical therapists may participate with others in the musculoskeletal screening of athletes; prevention and treatment of sports-related injuries; development of conditioning programs; or education programs for coaches, parents, and students. They may be involved with developing and helping conduct (or training other personnel to conduct) various screening programs (e.g., scoliosis or developmental).

Frequently, physical therapists are the liaison between the educational and medical communities. They may provide background information about various conditions, interpret medical records, facilitate communication between educational and medical personnel, and access resources in the medical community. Physical therapists may also be expected to provide educational personnel with information about physical therapy and topics related to intervention with children who have physical disabilities. Hardy and Roberts[24] recommend conducting a survey of educators' interests and needs to structure inservice education programs that are meaningful. Topics of interest identified from the authors' survey of special educators included specific student disabilities, classroom adaptation, referral guidelines, physical therapist roles and responsibilities, and the difference between an occupational therapist and physical therapist.[24]

Eligibility Determination

Determining who is eligible for related services in the educational environment is often a challenging process. It is important to remember that related services support the educational process and not the medical well-being of the child, and that related services are provided to help a child benefit from special education. Under the provisions of IDEA, if a child does not need special education, he or she is not eligible to receive related services. Decisions about educational relevance are made by the team. Eligibility determination varies from state to state. Borkowski and Wessman[25] surveyed representatives from each American state. Only four states used eligibility criteria that were more specific than those specified in IDEA. Faced with financial constraints, shortages of physical therapy personnel, and legal accountability, many states struggle to improve the objectivity of the process for determining eligibility without losing the mandate for individualized program plans. Criteria or guidelines are customarily not mandatory but help structure decisions about prioritizing who receives physical therapy, the type of services, and the frequency and duration of services.

The Waukesha Delivery Model,[26] developed and first implemented in Wisconsin, has been adopted by many states as a means of guiding decisions about related service eligibility. In the model, students are assigned to one of four levels of service based on the rate of change in the student's physical or functional status. Each level defines the purpose of the intervention, the intensity of service, and personnel responsibilities for the delivery of service. Students exhibiting more rapid rates of change receive a greater amount of the therapist's time and direct involvement under the Waukesha model.

Louisiana and some other states incorporate a controversial method of determining eligibility referred to as "cognitive referencing" or "performance discrepancy criteria," that predicts a child's potential for improvement as a direct relationship between intellectual and motor development.[27] The model presumes a positive correlation between cognitive and motor development and an upper limit for development based on a child's cognitive abilities. Children are eligible for physical therapy services only if motor skills are significantly lower than cognitive abilities. Cognitive referencing particularly limits intervention for children with severe intellectual impairment and accompanying physical disabilities.

The use of various tools adds objectivity and consistency to a process that can be difficult. Giangreco cautions, however, that research does not support the use of these tools and that they can contribute to fragmentation if they are unidisciplinary in design.[28] Unless they are used judiciously, they can negate the individualized approach to evaluation and program planning that the law requires. Each child with a disability has unique needs that must be meshed with the contextual differences in the environments in which he or she functions. Giangreco has given the acronym COACH (choosing options and accommodations for children) to 10 interrelated guidelines that provide alternative ways to think about the provision of related services in educational settings:

1. Establish and maintain a collaborative team.
2. Define components of the educational program.
3. Understand the interaction among program placement and service.
4. Use a value system to guide decision-making: "Only as special as necessary."
5. Determine functions of service providers and their interrelatedness.
6. Apply essential criteria when making service recommendations: educational relevance and necessity.
7. Determine who has authority for decision-making: consensus.
8. Match the mode and frequency of service provision to the function served.
9. Determine the least restrictive location and strategies for service provision.
10. Implement and evaluate related services.

Determining whether the student's needs are educationally related is sometimes difficult. Bundy justifies the provision of either occupational therapy or physical therapy for students if any of the following educational goals can be met or improved as an outcome of the intervention: "Expressing what they have learned, assuming a student role, performing self-care tasks or improving posture and mobility."[21] Bundy's guidelines would exclude physical therapy intervention for acute injuries except in a consultation role. In some instances, when physical and/or occupational therapy *is* the specially designed instruction, these services may be provided as a child's special education program rather than as a related service.

Referral

In the educational setting, a child can be referred for physical therapy services by educational personnel, health care providers, or parents. If the child is not already placed in special education, the referral is processed through the school-based committee. An administrative placement committee approves the recommendations of the school-based committee and makes appropriate placement. An IEP must be developed for the student before initiation of physical therapy service. If a student is determined ineligible for special education, a physical therapist may (at the discretion of the LEA) offer limited consultation to the classroom teacher, physical education teacher, or parent. The referral process can be cumbersome, especially for a child who is not already receiving special education services. Physical therapists may screen a child as a preliminary step and help direct the process of subsequent referral in that way. The newly enacted version of IDEA states that the education of children with disabilities can be made more effective by (among other things) "providing incentives for whole-school approaches and prereferral intervention to reduce the need to label children as disabled in order to address their learning needs."[13] This approach has potential to make the referral process less complicated in the future.

If the state practice act for physical therapy requires physician referral for a client to access physical therapy it is necessary to obtain that medical referral in addition to the procedural steps outlined by legislative guidelines. In states with direct access, a physician referral is not necessary unless dictated by a third party payer (e.g., Medicaid). A physician referral is recommended for students with complex medical needs in part to create a framework and formalize a process for needed communication with the referring physician. Children with disabilities are frequently served by a variety of professionals and social agencies. Communication with others involved in providing care for the child outside of the educational environment is crucial regardless of the decision about medical referral.

Assessment/Evaluation

PL 105-17 requires a "full and individualized initial evaluation" to determine whether the child has a disability and the educational needs of the child. An evaluation requires parental consent, although a mediation process is defined that can be followed if parents deny consent. The legislation further specifies that a variety of assessment tools and strategies must be used to "gather relevant functional and developmental information"; that no single procedure be used as the sole criterion for placement decisions; that technically sound instruments be used; and that testing is nondiscriminatory.[13] The requirement that testing be nondiscriminatory and administered in the child and family's native language has gained in importance as the number of minorities in the public schools has increased. The 1997 amendments to IDEA state that the federal government must "be responsive to the growing needs of an increasingly more diverse society" given the rapidly changing racial profile.[13] Findings state that by the year 2000, one of every three people in the United States will be either African American, Hispanic, Asian American, or American Indian. In large-city schools like Miami, Chicago, Baltimore, Houston, and Los Angeles, 80 to 90 percent of the student population consists of minority groups.

A physical therapy evaluation is one part of the evaluative process. The physical therapist's evaluation will include traditional elements plus an evaluation of the student's ability to participate in and benefit from the educational environment. This would include transportation on the school bus; entering and exiting the bathroom and toileting; eating; and negotiating hallways, doors, distances, stairs, and so on. At least one standardized measure is recommended as a basis for comparison over time. Summaries of assessment instruments available to use with children who have developmental delays are available in published materials.[30,31] Instruments in common use are the Bruininks-Oseretsky Test of Motor Proficiency[32] (which includes a screening tool as well as a comprehensive evaluation); the Gross Motor Function Measure[33]; and Mobility Opportunities Via Education (MOVE),[34] a curriculum particularly useful for children with multiple disabilities.

It is especially important in an educational environment that the physical therapist interpret the results of the testing for others. Depending on their background, members of the team may have varying levels of understanding about concepts and terms common to a physical therapist. Documentation of the testing must also be written in language that can be understood by nonmedical personnel. In a study by Linehan et al.,[35] it was found that teachers had higher expectations for students who had an ecological assessment report (student's observed competencies in his or her daily environment) as compared with a developmental assessment report (student's mental and developmental ages).

Program Development/Intervention

The basis for program planning for children with special needs is the IEP for school-aged children and the IFSP for infants and toddlers. The IEP is defined as a written statement for each child with a disability that is developed, reviewed, and revised in accordance with set criteria. The format for documenting the IEP varies from school district to school district.

INDIVIDUALIZED EDUCATION PROGRAM

The IEP must include[13]:

1. A statement of the child's present levels of educational performance (i.e., how the child's disability affects the child's involvement and progress in the general curriculum or, for preschool children, their participation in appropriate activities);
2. A statement of measurable annual goals including benchmarks or short-term instructional objectives;
3. A statement of the special education and related services and supplementary aids and services to be provided to the child or on behalf of the child and program modifications or supports for school personnel that will be provided for the child to advance appropriately toward attaining the annual goals, to be involved and progress in the general curriculum, and to participate in extracurricular and other nonacademic activities;
4. An explanation of the extent, if any, to which the child will not participate with nondisabled children in the regular class;
5. A statement of any individual modifications in the administration of state or district-wide assessments of student achievement or description of justification for use of alternative testing;
6. Projected date for beginning of the services and modifications and the anticipated frequency, location, and duration of those services and modifications;
7. Beginning at age 14, and updated annually, a statement of transition service needs;
8. A statement of how the child's progress toward meeting annual goals will be measured and how the child's parents will be informed of the child's progress.

The IEP Team is composed of (1) parents; (2) at least one regular education teacher (if the child participates in a regular education environment); (3) at least one special education teacher; (4) a representative of the LEA; (5) at the discretion of the parent or agency, other individuals who have knowledge or special experience; and (6) the child (if possible). Physical therapists are not required to attend IEP meetings, but it is in the best interests of the therapist and the child to participate if physical therapy is an integral part of the educational plan.

INDIVIDUALIZED FAMILY SERVICE PLAN

Federal legislation is very specific about the contents of the written IFSP. It must include:

1. A statement of the infant's or toddler's present levels of physical development (vision, hearing, motor, and health), cognitive development (thinking, reasoning, learning), communication development (responding, understanding, using language), social or emotional development (feelings, playing, interacting), and adaptive development (bathing, feeding, dressing, etc.) based on objective criteria.
2. A statement of the family's resources, priorities, and concerns related to enhancing the development of the family's infant or toddler with a disability.
3. A statement of the major outcomes expected to be achieved for the infant and the family (criteria, procedures, and timelines).
4. A statement of specific early intervention services necessary to meet the unique needs of the infant, toddler, and family, including frequency, intensity, and method of delivering services.

5. A statement of the natural environments in which early intervention services shall appropriately be provided.
6. Projected dates for initiation of services and anticipated duration of services.
7. Identification of the service coordinator from the profession most immediately relevant to the infant's or toddler's or family's needs.
8. Steps to be taken to support the transition of the toddler with a disability to preschool or other appropriate services.

Both the IEP and the IFSP require measurable goals and objectives, stated in functional behavioral terms which can be difficult for physical therapists unaccustomed to the educational environment. Indicators of high-quality goals and objectives include the following[36]:

1. Functionality—the identified skill will:
   a. Increase a child's ability to interact with people and objects within the daily environment.
   b. Have to be performed by someone else if the child cannot do it.
2. Generality—the identified skill:
   a. Represents a general concept as opposed to a particular task.
   b. Allows for individual adaptations and modifications for a variety of disabling conditions.
   c. Can be generalized across settings, materials, and people.
3. Ease of integration—work on skill can be incorporated into daily routines
4. Measurability—a skill is measurable if it can be seen and/or heard, can be directly counted (frequency, duration, or distance measures), and lends itself to determination of performance criteria.
5. Hierarchial relationship exists between long-range goals and short-term objectives (i.e., the skill complements the long-term goal).

Campbell urges physical therapists to consider the long-term needs of the children they serve.[37] Research indicates that the concerns of adults with cerebral palsy or myelodysplasia are related to secondary disabling conditions, including musculoskeletal impairments, low self-esteem, and poor educational and vocational attainment. In planning for children, physical therapists must help empower individuals and their families, promote the functional use of movement in age-appropriate activities, allow conservation of energy for the things that really matter in life, and promote gradual assumption of personal responsibility for health and fitness[37] (Tables 15–2 and 15–3).

Administration/Management

Management functions are important in the educational environment to ensure that decisions affecting job descriptions, delivery of care, supervision, and so on, are compatible with best practice models. It is not possible, as it was in the 1930s, for physical therapists to have the same job description and qualifications as teachers. Shortages are common, and therapists must understand and communicate to school administrators recruitment and retention strategies for physical therapists that are often very different than those for educational personnel. In the survey of physical therapists practicing in educational settings, the areas of job dissatisfaction most frequently mentioned were lack of continuing education opportunities, insufficient peer contact, lack of an identified place to work, lack of time allotted for administrative tasks and meetings, and too much travel.[19]

A variety of other management tasks are essential as a framework for best practice, and time should be negotiated to ensure that they can be given adequate attention. Efficient systems should be in place for documentation, recordkeeping, and billing, and these components should be reviewed on a regular schedule. Job

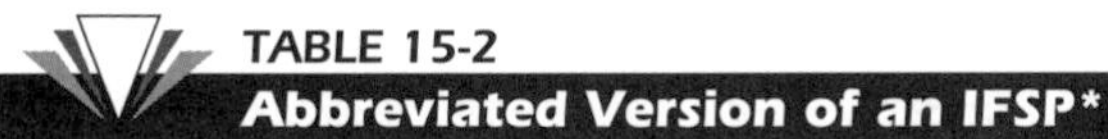

TABLE 15-2
Abbreviated Version of an IFSP*

WESTERN EARLY INTERVENTION PROGRAM
Individualized Family Service Plan

1. **Cover Page:** Families are encouraged to personalize the cover page in any way that they want. Suggestions include photographs, poems, list of important dates and events, or a drawing by the child.
2. **IFSP Information:** Includes usual identifying information about the child and family (name, address, phone, date of birth, date of referral, language spoken in the home, etc.) and a list of the members of the IFSP Team.

IFSP Team

Name	Relationship/Role	Phone Number	Address	Date
Amanda Jones	Mother	704 586-5922	108 Hill Street, Mountain	1/2/98
Mike Jones	Father	704 586-5922	108 Hill Street, Mountain	1/2/98
Bob and Mary Jones	Grandparents	704 586-5216	42 Blue Bird Road, Mountain	1/2/98
Amy Smith	Child Service Coord	704 227-7456	Mountain DEC, Cullowhee	1/2/98
Tom Bryson	Physical Therapist	704 227-7456	Mountain DEC, Cullowhee	1/2/98

3. **Family's Concerns, Priorities, and Resources.** Optional for the family to complete. A list of suggested topics on *"What you want the IFSP team to know about your child"* is helpful to include (e.g., pregnancy and birth history, medical information, child's likes/dislikes, effect of child's needs on the family, etc.).
4. **Summary of Child's Present Abilities and Strengths:** Summary of functional assessments, evaluations and observations of the child in his day-to-day environment; evaluators, procedures, and child's strengths for each of the five domains:
   a. Adaptive/self-help skills (bathing, feeding, dressing, toileting, etc.)
   b. Cognitive skills (thinking, reasoning, learning)
   c. Communication skills (responding, understanding, and using language)
   d. Physical development (vision, hearing, motor, and health)
   e. Social-emotional skills (feelings, playing, and interacting)

Date	Description
12/16/97	*Tom Bryson, Physical Therapist* conducted a physical therapy assessment using *the Motor Scale (of the Bayley Scales of Infant Development II) observation,* and *parent report.* Brian has some gross and fine motor delays. His strengths are head control and sitting. Brian is able to sit with slight support for an extended time and sits alone for several seconds. He supports himself on partially extended arms when positioned on his stomach but cannot shift his weight for functional reach and play with one hand. He has no means of independent mobility at this time.

5. **IFSP Outcomes:** The changes the family wants for themselves or for their infant or toddler. Outcomes should be discussed at the IFSP meeting by all team members as related to the family's concerns, priorities and resources, the child's abilities and needs, or both.
   a. Family's concerns (needs, issues, or problems they want addressed), priorities (things and accomplishments important to the family), and resources (formal and informal means that can help the family)
   b. Child's abilities and needs
   c. Specific outcome number, target date, start date, specific activities, person responsible, date and outcome status

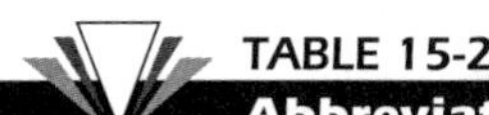

TABLE 15-2
Abbreviated Version of an IFSP* (Continued)

Family's Concerns, Priorities, and Resources:
"We want Brian to be able to get around on his own."

Child's Abilities/Needs:
Brian is ready to start crawling.

Outcome #3
Brian will develop a means of mobility on the floor.

Target Date:
5/1/98

Start Date	Activities	Person(s) Responsible	Date/Outcome Status
1/2/98	Provide family with activities that fit into their daily routine to encourage Brian to pull himself forward on his stomach.	Tom Bryson, Physical Therapist	3/1/98—Ongoing
	Evaluate progress and modify suggestions as needed.		3/1/98—Ongoing
	Monitor receipt of physical therapy, Brian's progress, family satisfaction.	Amy Smith, Child Service Coordinator	
	Do activities suggested by Tom with Brian. Give him frequent opportunities on the floor. Give feedback to Tom.	Amanda and Mike Jones, Parents	

6. IFSP Service Delivery Plan

Service	Provider	Start Date	Location/ Most Natural Environ- ment	Frequency/ Intensity	Cost of Family/ Payment Arrange- ment	Antici- pated Duration	Date Ended	Parent/ Coord. Agency Initials
Child Service Coordination	Valley River PACT	1/2/98	Home and community	Monthly and as needed	None	2/4/99		
Physical Therapy	Mountain DEC	1/2/98	Home	Once a week for 1 hour	None	2/4/99		

7. **Parent/Coordinative Agency Agreement:** Formalized agreement with signatures of parents and agency representative and child service coordinator and dates
8. **IFSP Review:** Summary of progress towards meeting each outcome, including feedback from parents; the review cycle (e.g., semiannual, annual) and the target date for next review.

*Adapted from unpublished training materials developed by Becca Moon, Western Regional Infant/Toddler Coordinator, NC.

descriptions should be comprehensive, state essential functions, and form the basis for annual performance evaluations of individual physical therapists. Both the job descriptions and performance evaluations should be reviewed annually. A plan for program evaluation, quality assurance, and peer review should be in place and reviewed regularly (at least annually). Agreement should be reached on reasonable caseloads and guidelines for determining eligibility for physical therapy as a related service. Lines of communication and authority should also be clearly established.

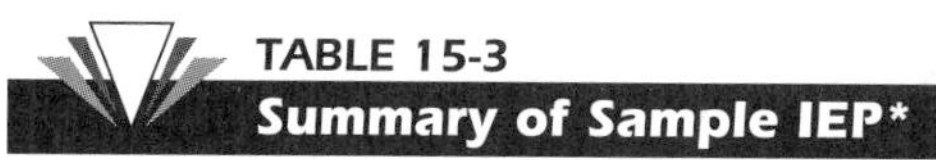

TABLE 15-3

Summary of Sample IEP*

Mountain School District
Individualized Education Program (IEP)

Student: Suzanne Wilson **Grade:** 3 **School: Mountain Elementary**

1. **Present Level(s) of Performance:** *(Describe, using objective and measurable terms, specific strengths, and needs that apply to academic performance as determined by evaluation and classroom observation. This may include behavior, social/emotional development, learning styles, physical limitations, and other relevant information.)*
   Strengths: Suzanne is able to walk with bilateral ankle-knee-hip orthoses and a posterior wheeled walker in the classroom and to propel her wheelchair on level surfaces within the school environment.
   Needs: Suzanne requires assistance to don her orthotics, to transition from sitting to standing, and to navigate ramps and nonpaved areas of the school grounds in her wheelchair.
2. **Annual Goal:** *(One goal per page. Functional outcome stated in objective, measurable terms that is reasonable for the student to accomplish in 1 year as a result of receiving special education. Must state who will do what and how accomplishment will be determined.)*
   Suzanne will be able to independently push to stand from her wheelchair and lock her orthotics in preparation for classroom ambulation. The physical therapist will design a program of fading physical and verbal prompts (based on MOVE curriculum) and instruct classroom personnel to help Suzanne gradually increase her level of independence with this functional classroom activity. Classroom personnel will implement program each time Suzanne needs to transition to standing and will keep a weekly log of her progress. The physical therapist will assess Suzanne's progress in meeting this goal on a monthly basis and consult with classroom personnel as needed (at least monthly). Suzanne's parents will be informed of the program and her progress so that they can reinforce her independent function at home. The goal will be accomplished when Suzanne can transition consistently from her wheelchair to standing without having to request assistance.
3. **Date of Beginning/Duration of Special Education and Related Services: From 8/19/98 To 6/1/99**
4. **Short-Term Instructional Objectives**

Short-Term Instructional Objectives (in measurable terms)	**Evaluation Procedures (How progress will be measured)**	**Evaluation Schedule (When progress will be measured)**	**Date Reviewed/ Progress Noted**
Suzanne will be able to independently: Push herself to the edge of her W/C seat	Fading system of physical and verbal prompts. (See separate program.)	Weekly progress notations by classroom personnel and at least monthly reassessment/consultation by PT	11/5/98 Consistently gets herself to edge of W/C seat
Push herself to a standing position using the arms of her W/C, then grasp her walker, first with one hand and then the other.	As above	As above	11/5/98— Requires verbal prompts and support at her waist/hips
Fully extend her knees when standing so that locks on orthotics engage and her knees are locked in an extended position.	As above	As above	11/5/98— Locks left leg without physical assist in three of five trials and right leg in two of five trials.
Turn 180 degrees so that she is properly positioned in her walker for ambulation.	As above	As above	11/5/98— Independent!

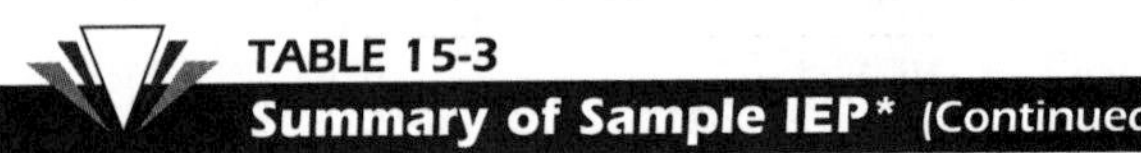

TABLE 15-3
Summary of Sample IEP* (Continued)

Individualized Education Program/Service Delivery Plan
(To be completed after the IEP is developed)

I. Area of Eligibility		**II. Related Service(s)**
Orthopedically impaired		Physical Therapy
III. Least Restrictive Environment (Placement) **A. Regular Program Participation**	**B. Appropriate Modification in Regular Classroom**	
All except reading, math, and physical education	Assistive Devices—wheelchair, walker, standing frame with raised desk	
B. Amount of Time in Exceptional Education **Type of Service**	**Amount of Time Per Session**	**Sessions Per Week**
Consultation		
Direct Special Education	90 Minutes	5 Sessions per week
Related Services		
Physical Therapy Consultation	30 Minutes	Once a month
Continuum of Services	**Where Services Received**	**Transition Component**
Resource–21% to 60% of day with nondisabled peers	LEA/School in Attendance Area	Not applicable
State Testing Program—Needed Modifications	**Adaptive Physical Education Required?**	**Extended School Year Status**
None	Yes	Not Eligible
IEP Committee/Placement Committee. The following were present and participated in the development and writing of the IEP: **Signature**	**Position**	**Date**
Mark Swanson	LEA Representative	8/19/98
Bruce Henson	Teacher	8/19/98
Martha Jones	Mother	8/19/98
Paul Jones	Father	8/19/98
Jeannette Willow	Physical Therapist	8/19/98

*Based on NC guidelines.

Many references are now available to guide the physical theapist in the educational environment. Many states have published guidelines for physical therapy in the schools. Other resources include the Pediatric Section of the American Physical Therapy Association and the Council for Exceptional Children.

Summary

The educational environment is a challenging and rewarding environment for the physical therapist. To be effective in the public school setting in the United States, a physical therapist must have an understanding of the federal legislation that has shaped the delivery of special education for children from infancy to young adulthood. Most significant was PL 94-142, passed in 1975, which mandated physical therapy as a related service and created a variety of conceptually new ways of thinking about the educational needs of children with disabilities.

Local, state, and federal rules and regulations must be understood and adhered to. Physical therapists must be willing and able to participate actively as part of a multidisciplinary team and to consider parents an integral part of that team. They must acknowledge that their intervention is limited to the educational needs of the child. They must appreciate and utilize models of service delivery that most effectively address the individualized needs of the child. Practice in the educational environment requires the knowledge, skills, and abilities of a specialist in pediatric physical therapy, but with the grounding to always be able and willing to interpret physical therapy intervention so that it is understood and appreciated by nonmedical personnel. The rewards include the benefits of functioning as part of a team, following a child long-term, and having the opportunity to observe the child in his or her daily functions within the school environment.

Acknowledgment

Grateful appreciation is extended to Diane Lindsey, State Physical Therapy Consultant with the NC Department of Public Instruction, who has been mentor and guide to many physical therapists since the enactment of PL 94-142, myself included. After listening patiently to our struggles to define our role in the educational environment and offering sound advice, Diane would often summarize a lengthy conversation with, “You need to do the right thing.” She has had a second sense about what constitutes the “right thing” in the educational environment for a long time. Her guidance has made a significant difference, not just for professionals but for countless children and families who have benefited from appropriate service.

REFERENCES

1. Sweeney JK, Heriza CB, Markowitz R. The changing profile of pediatric physical therapy: A 10-year analysis of clinical practice. *Pediatr Phys Ther*. 1994; 6:113–118.
2. Pratt RE. Physical therapy in schools for crippled children. *Phys Rev*. 1950.
3. DeYoung R. Child cripples get full course at Morton High. *Phys Rev*. 1932;24.
4. Hutchinson E. The physical therapist looks at the school child. *Phys Rev*. 1944;24:6–9.
5. Section 504 of the Rehabilitation Act. U.S. Congress. Senate. 1973.
6. Education for All Handicapped Children Act. Public Law 94-142. U.S. Congress. Senate, 94th Congress; 1975.
7. Simunds EE. Physical therapy in educational environments. Judicial interpretation of related service guidelines: A commentary. *Physical Therapy Practice in Educational Environments: Policies and Guidelines*. American Physical Therapy Association; 1990.
8. Education of the Handicapped Act Amendments of 1986, Public Law 99-457. U.S. Congress Senate, 99th Congress; 1986.
9. Individuals with Disabilities Education Act of 1990, Public Law 102-119. U.S. Congress Senate, 102nd Congress; 1990.

10. Technology-Related Assistance for Individuals with Disabilities Act, Public Law 100–40, 1991.
11. Medicare Catastrophic Coverage Act, Public Law 100-360.
12. Americans with Disabilities Act, Public Law 101-336, 1990.
13. Amendments to Individuals with Disabilities Act, Public Law 105-17, 1997.
14. DeHaven GE. Is selective hearing an occupational hazard in physical therapy? *Phys Ther.* 1974;54: 1301–1305.
15. Martin KD, ed. *Physical Therapy Practice in Educational Environments: Policies and Guidelines.* American Physical Therapy Association; 1990: 214–216.
16. Effgen SK, Bjornson K, Chiarello L, et al. Competencies for physical therapists in early intervention. *Ped Phys Ther.* 1991;3:77–80.
17. Connolly BH, Anderson RM. Severely handicapped children in the public schools: A new frontier for the physical therapist. *Phys Ther.* 1978;58: 433–438.
18. Long TM. Administrative issues. In Long TM, Cintas HL, eds. *Handbook of Pediatric Physical Therapy.* Baltimore: Williams & Wilkins; 1995.
19. Effgen SK, Keppler S. Survey of physical therapy practice in educational settings. *Pediatr Phys Ther.* 1994;6:15–21.
20. Rainforth B. Analysis of physical therapy practice acts: Implications for role release in educational environments. *Pediatr Phys Ther.* 1997;9:54–61.
21. Bundy AC. Assessment and intervention in school-based practice: Answering questions and minimizing discrepancies. *Phys Occup Ther Pediatr.* 1995; 15(2):69–87.
22. McEwen IR, Shelden JL. Pediatric therapy in the 1990s: The demise of the educational versus medical dichotomy. *Phys Occup Ther Pediatr.* 1995; 15(2):33–45.
23. Lindsey D, O'Neal J, Haas K, et al. Physical therapy services in North Carolina's schools. *Clin Man Phys Ther.* 1984;4:40–43.
24. Hardy DD, Roberts PL. The educational needs assessment on physical therapy for special educators: Enhancing in-service programming and physical therapy services in public schools. *Ped Phys Ther.* 1989;1:109–114.
25. Borkowski MA, Wessman HC. Determination of eligibility for physical therapy in the public school setting. *Pediatr Phys Ther.* 1994;61–67.
26. *Waukesha Delivery Model: Providing OT/PT Services to Special Education Students.* Milwaukee: Wisconsin Department of Public Instruction; 1987.
27. Carr SH. Louisiana's criteria of eligibility for occupational therapy services in the public school system. *Am J Occup Ther.* 1989;43(8):503–506.
28. Giangreco MF. Related service decision-making: A foundational component of effective education for students with disabilities. *Phys Occup Ther Pediatr.* 1995;15(2):47–68.
29. Rapport MJ. Laws that shape therapy services in educational environments. *Phys Occup Ther Pediatr.* 1995;15(2):5–32.
30. King-Thomas L, Hacker BJ, eds. *A Therapist's Guide to Pediatric Assessment.* Boston: Little, Brown, 1987.
31. Long TM. Measurement. In Long TM, Cintas HL, eds. *Handbook of Pediatric Physical Therapy.* Baltimore: Williams & Wilkins; 1995.
32. Bruininks RH. *Bruininks-Oseretsky Test of Motor Proficiency.* Circle Pines, MN: American Guidance Service; 1978.
33. Russell DJ, Rosenbaum PL, Gowland C, et al. *Gross Motor Function Measure.* Hamilton, Ontario: Gross Motor Measures Group; 1990.
34. Bidabe L, Lallar JM. *MOVE/Mobility Opportunities Via Education.* Bakersfield, CA: MOVE International; 1990.
35. Linehan SA, Brady MP, Hwang C. Ecological versus developmental assessment: Influences on instructional expectations. *JASH.* 1991;16(3): 146–153.
36. Notari-Syverson AR, Shuster SL. Putting real-life skills into IEP/IFSPs for infants and young children. *Teaching Exceptional Children* (a publication of the Council for Exceptional Children). 1995; Winter:29–32.
37. Campbell SK. Therapy programs that last a lifetime. *Phys Occup Ther Pediatr.* 1997;17(1):1–15.

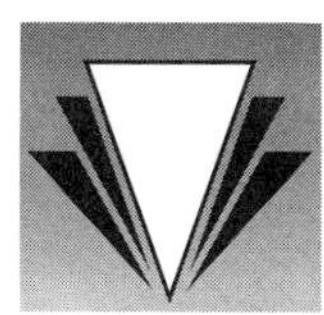

Index

Page numbers followed by *t, f,* and *d* denote tables, figures, and displays, respectively.

C

D

I

M

N

O

P

Q

R

T